S0-ADE-766

FROM THE EDITORS OF BOTTOM LINE HEALTH

BOTTOM LINE'S BIG BOOK OF PAIN-RELIEVING SECRETS

1,253 Unique Remedies to Keep You PAIN-FREE for Life

BottomLineBooks
BottomLineInc.com

Bottom Line's Big Book of Pain-Relieving Secrets

Copyright © 2018 by Bottom Line Inc.

10 9 8 7 6 5 4 3 2 1

All rights reserved. No part of this book may be reproduced, scanned, distributed or transmitted in any form, by any means, electronic or mechanical, without written permission from the publisher.

ISBN 0-88723-811-4

Bottom Line Books® publishes the advice of expert authorities in many fields. These opinions may at times conflict as there are often different approaches to solving problems. The use of a book is not a substitute for legal, accounting, investment, health or any other professional services. Consult competent professionals for answers to your specific questions.

Offers, prices, rates, addresses, telephone numbers and websites listed in this book are accurate at the time of publication, but they are subject to frequent change.

Bottom Line Books® is a registered trademark of Bottom Line Inc.
3 Landmark Square, Suite 201, Stamford, CT 06901

BottomLineInc.com

Bottom Line Books® is an imprint of Bottom Line Inc., publisher of print periodicals, e-letters and books. We are dedicated to bringing you the best information from the most knowledgeable sources in the world. Our goal is to help you gain greater wealth, better health, more wisdom, extra time and increased happiness.

Printed in the United States of America

Contents

2 • ARTHRITIS AND JOINT PAIN

3 • AUTOIMMUNE AND RELATED DISEASES

15 • MUSCLE CRAMPS AND WEAKNESS

16 • MYSTERY ILLNESS: WHAT'S THAT PAIN MEAN?

17 • NECK AND SHOULDER PAIN

18 • NEUROPATHY AND OTHER NERVE PAIN

19 • TEETH, FACE AND MOUTH PAIN

20 • VERY PERSONAL PAIN

PART II—MODALITIES FOR A PAIN-FREE LIFE

21 • PAINKILLER DOs AND DON'Ts

PART 1

Conditions

CHAPTER 1

Abdominal Pain

What's Really Causing Your Gas and Bloating?

Ugh! Here comes another gas attack. Or maybe it's bloating that's got you feeling so out of sorts. If you're lucky, you can avoid gas and/or bloating by forgoing the usual triggers—carbonated drinks…some high-fiber foods such as beans…chewing gum…and artificial sweeteners and the fruit sugar fructose.

But sometimes the source of this all-too-common gastrointestinal (GI) discomfort isn't so obvious. If your symptoms don't ease within a few weeks…or they have no apparent reason and tend to come and go, you and your doctor may need to do some investigating. The following health problems can cause gas and/or bloating but often go undetected—especially in the early stages…

- **Aerophagia (air swallowing).** Swallowing too much air can stretch the stomach and cause bloating. This often occurs when people are experiencing anxiety or can even become an unconscious habit. It can also happen when chewing gum, using a straw or drinking carbonated beverages.

What to do: Consider stress-reducing activities like deep breathing, meditation or yoga. If symptoms are severe, see a counselor for stress-management techniques.

- **Irritable bowel syndrome (IBS).** As many as one in five adults experiences the chronic symptoms of IBS—abdominal pain, bloating, gas, diarrhea and/or constipation—to some degree. IBS can have many causes, but typically nerves in the GI tract are extremely sensitive to food and gas passing through the bowel, triggering discomfort.

What to do: An IBS diagnosis includes regular abdominal pain that is relieved by a bowel

Douglas A. Drossman, MD, codirector emeritus at the University of North Carolina Center for Functional GI and Motility Disorders and professor emeritus of medicine and psychiatry at the University of North Carolina School of Medicine in Chapel Hill.

movement, along with symptoms of bloating, diarrhea and/or constipation.

If you have IBS, your doctor may prescribe antispasmodics, such as *dicyclomine* (Bentyl) and *hyoscyamine* (Levsin), that may help relieve your symptoms. Since stress can trigger IBS symptoms, try to manage it with yoga, massage, meditation and counseling, if needed.

• **Functional dyspepsia.** After eating, the stomach in a healthy adult can expand in volume up to four times its normal size. But with functional dyspepsia, the muscles don't relax properly and the stomach remains small, leaving you feeling full and bloated after just a few bites.

What to do: If symptoms are stress-related, relaxation techniques, such as deep breathing or biofeedback, may be effective. An antianxiety drug, such as *buspirone* (BuSpar), can also help because it helps to relax the stomach.

• **Celiac disease.** People with celiac disease are sensitive to gluten, a protein in wheat, barley and rye that can produce inflammation in the bowel, resulting in bloating, gas, abdominal cramps and diarrhea.

What to do: If you suffer from the digestive symptoms described above—especially if you also have any nutritional deficiencies and/or experience frequent fatigue—see your doctor. Celiac disease is diagnosed with a blood test followed by an endoscopic biopsy. By avoiding foods and products that contain gluten, most sufferers can eliminate symptoms. For a list of hidden sources of gluten, go to Celiac.org.

More serious but less common causes of gas and/or bloating...

• **Diverticulitis.** This condition occurs when small pouches in the walls of the colon become inflamed and/or infected—often due to small tears caused by stool trapped in the pouches. It not only causes gas and bloating but also pain in the lower left side of the pelvis, where pouches get infected.

What to do: If you're having severe abdominal pain with fever and vomiting, see your doctor right away—you could have a serious infection that requires antibiotics and possibly emergency surgery. Sometimes, however, diverticulitis is mild, and symptoms may improve if you apply heat to the painful area...go on a liquid diet—including clear broth, clear fruit juice (such as apple), gelatin and plain tea—for a few days to "rest" your digestive system...and/or take antibiotics if needed to treat an infection.

• **Gallstones.** They often cause no symptoms, but if gallstones block the duct where the gallbladder empties, the gallbladder stretches, resulting in distension and pain, as well as bloating and gas.

What to do: If you suffer bloating and gas, pain in the upper-right abdomen (where the gallbladder is located), nausea and fever, see your doctor. He/she will perform an ultrasound to check for gallstones. Gallstone removal, which is routinely performed via laparoscopic surgery or, in some cases, endoscopy, is often recommended.

• **Certain cancers.** With advanced colorectal cancer, the bowel can become blocked, which leads to gas, bloating and blood in the stool. Ovarian cancer often causes subtle symptoms that may include bloating and feeling full quickly.

What to do: With colorectal cancer, regular colonoscopies after age 50 (or after age 40 if a close family member has had the disease) will catch suspicious polyps before a malignancy develops. Women who experience the symptoms described above for more than two or three weeks—especially if they are accompanied by pelvic pain and/or an urgent or frequent need to urinate—should see a gynecologist.

QUICK RELIEF

If your gas and/or bloating is only occasional, consider trying...

• **Probiotics,** which promote the growth of "good" bacteria in the bowel. One study found that *Lactobacillus acidophilus* and *Bifidobacterium lactis* helped bloating by replacing the bad (gas-causing) bacteria with good (gas-relieving) bacteria in people with bowel disorders, such as IBS or functional dyspepsia. In another study, probiotics were found to relieve intestinal gas.

What to do: Try a daily probiotic in supplement form or via probiotic-rich fermented foods and beverages such as kefir, miso or kimchi.

Could You Have Celiac Disease and Not Even Know It?

Peter H.R. Green, MD, director of the Celiac Disease Center at Columbia University and professor of clinical medicine at Columbia University College of Physicians and Surgeons, both in New York City. Dr. Green is coauthor of *Celiac Disease: A Hidden Epidemic*. CeliacDiseaseCenter.columbia.edu

Celiac disease is the most underdiagnosed autoimmune condition in the US. This gastrointestinal disorder affects one in every 100 Americans—yet only about 3% of those afflicted get properly diagnosed and treated. It takes 11 years, on average, from the time symptoms appear until the diagnosis is made. In the interim, as the disease progresses, patients are increasingly at risk for complications that can harm their bones, blood and nervous system…or even lead to cancer.

Women are twice as likely as men to have celiac disease. Contrary to what many doctors believe, it can develop at any time, even among seniors.

New finding: Celiac disease is now four times as common as it was 50 years ago, tests of old blood samples show.

CONFOUNDING SYMPTOMS

When a person who has celiac disease consumes gluten—a protein in wheat, rye, barley and triticale (a wheat-rye hybrid)—her immune system attacks the protein. This inflames and damages the intestinal lining and interferes with absorption of nutrients. *The person may develop…*

- **Classic, overt symptoms.** Typically, celiac disease causes severe chronic or recurrent diarrhea. Poor nutrient absorption leads to weight loss, smelly stools, gassiness and/or weakness. Many doctors, mistaking these symptoms for irritable bowel syndrome or inflammatory bowel disease, advise eating more high-fiber grains—which only makes patients sicker.

- **Silent symptoms.** When there is no diarrhea, it's called silent celiac disease. In some silent cases, there are no symptoms at all. In others, atypical symptoms—abdominal pain, migraines, numbness or pain in hands and feet—lead to various wrong diagnoses. Silent celiac disease nonetheless continues to cause intestinal damage.

- **Skin symptoms.** Dermatitis herpetiformis (DH) is a chronic itchy, blistery rash. Only people with celiac disease get DH—but the vast majority of DH patients do not develop intestinal symptoms. Consequently, they often are misdiagnosed with eczema, psoriasis or "nerves."

Untreated, celiac disease creates an ever-increasing risk of developing very serious complications, such as osteoporosis, anemia, infertility, neurological problems (poor balance, seizures, dementia) and/or various cancers (melanoma, lymphoma). A missed diagnosis also represents a missed opportunity to watch for other autoimmune disorders that often go hand-in-hand with celiac disease, including thyroid disease, rheumatoid arthritis and alopecia areata (patchy hair loss).

GETTING DIAGNOSED AT LAST

Celiac disease is genetic—you cannot get it by eating too much gluten. The genes can "express" themselves at any point in life, and the disease is never outgrown.

Vital: Get tested if you have any of the following…

- **Possible celiac symptoms.**

- **A family history of the disease.** Almost 10% of family members of celiac patients also have it, even if they have no symptoms.

- **Type 1 diabetes.** Genetic factors link this autoimmune disorder to an increased risk for celiac disease.

- **Down syndrome.** Again, there appears to be a genetic link.

Celiac disease usually can be diagnosed with blood tests for certain antibodies. A biopsy of tissue from the small intestine then is needed to confirm the diagnosis. If a patient has skin symptoms, a skin biopsy that confirms the DH rash also confirms the celiac diagnosis.

Sometimes nutritionists or naturopaths will recommend that patients adopt the gluten-free diet used to control celiac disease—but without first confirming the diagnosis with a blood test or biopsy.

Problem: Starting a gluten-free diet before you complete the diagnostic tests will yield a false-negative result. If you do not actually have celiac disease, you subject yourself to needless limitations...you incur the extra cost of buying gluten-free foods...and your diet may lack adequate fiber.

THE DIET SOLUTION

Currently there are no drugs or supplements available to treat celiac disease. However, following a strict gluten-free diet can work wonders at alleviating celiac symptoms.

Important: If tests confirm celiac disease, the diet is essential even if you have no symptoms—otherwise, intestinal damage continues.

The diet can be tricky because gluten is in all foods that contain wheat, rye, barley and triticale. What's more, gluten grains have many aliases.

Example: Bulgur, couscous, dinkle, durum, einkorn, emmer, fu, graham, kamut, matzah, mir, seitan, semolina and spelt all are wheat products. Avoid oats, too—these often get tainted from being processed in proximity to gluten grains—unless labeled "gluten-free."

Unexpected: Gluten may be found in processed luncheon meat, imitation seafood, canned soup, frozen entrées, soy sauce, beer, medications, supplements and lipsticks.

Adhering to a gluten-free diet is easier than it used to be because all products with wheat now must be labeled as such. Though products containing gluten-grain-derived ingredients are not all necessarily labeled that way, requirements for allowing a food to be labeled gluten-free have become stricter. Now gluten-free breads, cereals, pastas and other foods are sold in supermarkets and health-food stores. Do be sure to get enough fiber from gluten-free grains and other sources.

After adopting a gluten-free diet, some patients see radical improvement within weeks... for others, it takes months or longer. If improvement is slow, your gastroenterologist should investigate possible underlying conditions (such as infection or hormonal problems) that can exacerbate celiac symptoms.

Information: Celiac Disease Foundation (818-716-1513, Celiac.org)...Celiac Sprue Association/USA (877-272-4272, CSAceliacs.org).

Natural Remedies for Celiac Disease

Jamison Starbuck, ND, naturopathic physician in family practice and a lecturer at the University of Montana, both in Missoula. She is past president of the American Association of Naturopathic Physicians and a contributing editor to *The Alternative Advisor: The Complete Guide to Natural Therapies and Alternative Treatments.* DrJamisonStarbuck.com

The next time a waiter puts a basket of fresh bread on your restaurant table, think twice before you eat it. Experts believe that at least one out of every 100 American adults has celiac disease, a condition that can make sufferers ill after eating even a single slice of bread. The culprit is gluten—a type of protein found in wheat, barley, rye and, in some cases, oats that creates an autoimmune, inflammatory reaction in the small intestine. The usual symptoms are bloating and diarrhea, but some people also experience abdominal pain and/or constipation. In some cases, celiac disease causes only a blistery, itchy skin condition (dermatitis herpetiformis) or fatigue.

If you think you might have celiac disease, discuss it with your doctor. A diagnosis requires specific blood tests and, in some cases, an intestinal biopsy. If you do have celiac disease, your medical doctor will tell you to completely avoid gluten. This may sound like hard work, since gluten is in all sorts of things you might not suspect, such as many kinds of soy sauce, creamed soups and salad dressings. But it is definitely doable and gets easier as you learn where gluten-free products (even bread and pasta) are available—for example, in many health-food stores and a growing number of restaurants.

Payoff: Once you start avoiding gluten, your celiac symptoms will disappear over a period of weeks and months. *Other steps to consider...**

• **Take supplements.** Inflammation in the small intestine interferes with the absorption of key nutrients. I advise my celiac patients to take a daily regimen that includes 5 mg of folic acid...800 international units (IU) each of vitamins E and D...25,000 IU of vitamin A...and 2 mg of vitamin K.

Note: Vitamin K supplements should be avoided by patients taking *warfarin* (Coumadin) or another blood thinner. I also recommend taking a botanical formula that contains one or more of these herbs (in powdered form)—deglycyrrhizinated licorice root, slippery elm and marshmallow root. Follow label instructions and take until inflammatory bowel symptoms abate.

• **Eat healthful fats daily and fish twice a week.** Olive oil, avocado, soy milk and small portions of unsalted nuts (eight to 12) are good sources of healthful fat. (However, celiac patients should avoid peanuts, which can be hard for them to digest.) Fatty fish, such as salmon or halibut, is an easily digested protein source.

Warning: In people with celiac disease, high-fat dairy products, as well as fried foods, tend to worsen diarrhea.

• **Use plant-based enzymes.** Enzyme supplementation helps break down food and reduces post-meal bloating. Plant-based enzymes (available at natural-food stores) are usually derived from pineapple or papaya, and they are safe for just about everyone unless you have ulcers or are allergic to pineapple or papaya.

Typical dose: One or two capsules per meal.

• **Get support.** Avoiding gluten isn't easy, but you'll feel much better if you do. For more advice, consult the Celiac Sprue Association/USA, 877-272-4272, CSAceliacs.org.

*To minimize inflammation, follow the dietary advice indefinitely—and also continue to take the vitamin supplements to guard against a nutritional deficiency.

Don't Let Them Tell You Gluten Intolerance Isn't Real

Study titled "Small Amounts of Gluten in Subjects with Suspected Nonceliac Gluten Sensitivity—a Randomized, Double-Blind, Placebo-Controlled, Cross-Over Trial," by researchers in the department of internal medicine at University of Pavia, and the department of medical and surgical sciences at University of Bologna, both in Italy, published in *Clinical Gastroenterology and Hepatology.*

You may have been told that unless you have the autoimmune disorder celiac disease, you're not gluten intolerant, and the symptoms of pain and bloating you blame on sensitivity to gluten are all in your head. Meanwhile, the gluten-free food industry is booming as never before, and many people are singing the benefits of a gluten-free life. So...is gluten sensitivity real? Or is it just the latest craze?

GLUTEN SENSITIVITY IS REAL—BUT NOT ALWAYS

According to a new study, it is entirely possible to be sensitive to gluten without having a wheat allergy or celiac disease. But it's also possible that gluten exerts a nocebo effect on some folks. A nocebo effect is an ill effect caused by the suggestion or belief that something—in this case gluten/wheat—is harmful.

The study, conducted by researchers from the Universities of Pavia and Bologna in Italy, involved 59 participants who had self-described gluten intolerance. They reported symptoms such as bloating, gassiness, diarrhea, headache and brain fog. Before starting the study, all of the participants had blood work and biopsies of the small intestine to rule out wheat allergies and celiac disease.

To identify whether gluten was actually causing symptoms, the researchers put participants on a strict gluten-free diet for five weeks, and during part of that time had them take one of two daily pills—either wheat gluten or a placebo. Participants switched off during the study so that everyone had a chance to take gluten pills and placebos during different weeks (but without knowing which was which, of course). Each gluten pill contained about the amount of gluten found in two slices of white bread.

Participants completed daily questionnaires that measured the severity of a wide range of symptoms on a scale of zero (not affected) to three (severely affected). In addition to intestinal symptoms, such as pain, bloating and gas, nonintestinal symptoms frequently associated with gluten intolerance, such as headache, tiredness, malaise, brain fog and anxiety, were also asked about.

The results: The participants' total average symptom severity score was 30% higher during the week they were given gluten compared with the week they received placebo pills, showing that gluten did make a difference for some. However, when the researchers plotted each participant's weekly scores on grids to view correlations between how each person felt during gluten and gluten-free weeks, they found that about half of the participants complained about symptoms to the same degree whether they were receiving gluten or not. The remaining participants logged in more symptoms when they were receiving either gluten or placebo. Of the nine patients who recorded more symptoms while on gluten than placebo, three (amounting to 5% of the study group) had scores that consistently showed symptom flares when exposed to gluten but not placebo. Symptoms of bloating, abdominal pain, brain fog, depression and canker sores—the most common intestinal and nonintestinal symptoms experienced across the board—were consistently and significantly worse during the week of gluten exposure in these patients compared with the rest of the study group. The researchers commented that these participants likely had true gluten intolerance despite lack of wheat allergy or celiac disease and that the other six participants may have had a lesser level of gluten sensitivity. They also point out that the dose of gluten given was low, and so higher amounts might have shown greater sensitivity in more of the participants.

DO YOU REALLY NEED TO BE GLUTEN-FREE?

These study findings add weight to both sides of the argument...yes, gluten intolerance does seem to occur in a small percentage of people. On the other hand, gluten may not actually be behind symptoms that many people experience and attribute to gluten intolerance.

If you notice that you have abdominal pain or bloating, fogginess or low mood after eating foods with gluten, you can test whether you are truly sensitive to it by going gluten-free for one or two weeks, evaluating whether symptoms improve and then reintroducing bread or pasta back into your diet and again evaluating symptoms. A better strategy, though, would be to consult a dietitian or naturopathic doctor who can expertly evaluate your symptoms and guide you through a diet regimen to correct the problem without compromising nutrition—whether that means avoiding gluten or following some other strategy.

Beware: Signs of an Abdominal Aortic Aneurysm

Christopher J. Abularrage, MD, assistant professor of surgery, division of vascular surgery and endovascular therapy, The Johns Hopkins Hospital, Baltimore.

A pulsating sensation in the abdomen can be a sign of many health problems, such as a hernia or an enlarged spleen. However, the most serious cause is an abdominal aortic aneurysm.

This type of aneurysm is an enlargement of the abdominal aorta, the large blood vessel that extends from the heart to the legs. As the aneurysm enlarges, there is a greater risk for rupture, which is often fatal.

Aneurysms usually develop slowly over many years and often have no symptoms. Signs that an aneurysm may be starting to rupture include severe, sudden, persistent pain in the abdomen or back...dizziness...nausea...and a rapid heart rate. If you have any of these symptoms, get to a hospital emergency department. If your only symptom is a pulsating sensation in the abdomen, your doctor can screen for an aneurysm with an ultrasound (this procedure should be covered by insurance).

Depending on the size of the aneurysm and your overall health, the aneurysm may need to be repaired with traditional open surgery or with a minimally invasive procedure that uses a stent.

Finally...a Way to Prevent IBD

Jenifer Fenton, PhD, MPH, assistant professor, department of food science and human nutrition, College of Osteopathic Medicine, Michigan State University, East Lansing. Her study was published in *The Journal of Nutrition*.

Life can be a waiting game—an anxious and decidedly unfun game—for people whose family history puts them at high risk for inflammatory bowel disease (IBD).

An umbrella term for a group of digestive disorders, IBD includes ulcerative colitis, which usually is confined to the colon and rectum... and Crohn's disease, which can appear anywhere along the lining of the digestive tract.

Symptoms can be really terrible, including diarrhea, constipation, abdominal pain, gas, bloating, bloody stools, malnutrition and more.

Do you know if IBD has affected anyone in your family?

You should—because you no longer have to just wait for it to hit you. *You can lower your risk of getting it...*

FEEDING THE GOOD

A recent study examined the effects of something called a prebiotic—but first, here's a reminder about the workings of the bacteria in your gut.

In your intestines are trillions of bacteria, with the specific types varying from person to person based on factors such as diet and environment. One theory about IBD suggests that it is caused by an overactive immune response to some "bad" bacteria in the intestines.

The "good versus bad bacteria" idea is nothing new—in fact, it's one reason why you want that "live, active cultures" label on your yogurt. Those live, active cultures are probiotics, beneficial bacteria that you can ingest directly. A prebiotic is different—it is food for bacteria, so you can use it to support certain types of beneficial bacteria that are already in your gut.

TESTING, TESTING

For this study, the researchers wanted to use a prebiotic supplement (basically a type of fiber) to feed and thus increase a specific population of beneficial bacteria before IBD developed. The goal was to see whether the prebiotic might help prevent the development of the disease or make it less severe if it did develop.

Researchers performed the study on mice that did not have symptoms of the disease but were genetically predisposed to develop colitis after infection with "bad" bacteria. One group of mice received a prebiotic supplement of galacto-oligosaccharides (GOS) daily for six weeks...a second group did not get GOS. After the first two weeks, the researchers purposely infected all the mice with a pathogen to trigger the onset of colitis.

Results: Compared with mice that did not get GOS, those that were fed the prebiotic developed significantly less severe colitis...and their lab tests showed much less inflammation and dysplasia (abnormal tissue development) in their digestive tracts.

Researchers hypothesize that the prebiotic helps by increasing the number of protective bacteria in the gut, which in turn enhances immune function, reduces intestinal inflammation and/or reduces colonizing of harmful pathogens.

IS IT RIGHT FOR YOU?

Lead researcher Jenifer Fenton, PhD, MPH, emphasized that because this study was conducted in mice, the results—though encouraging—cannot be directly translated to people. So human studies definitely are needed. *In the meantime, however...*

Patients who already have IBD should consult the physician treating their IBD before deciding whether to take GOS. The problem with having a chronic disease such as IBD for years is that it leads to a dramatic change in the intestinal tissue. A supplement could theoretically make it worse. What's more, because GOS is a type of fiber, it may not be well-tolerated by IBD patients, who often cannot eat a high-fiber diet.

So who is most likely to benefit from GOS? People with a family history of IBD (meaning that a parent, sibling or child has or had the disease)...and perhaps those who are at risk for exposure to pathogenic gut bacteria (for instance, because they are traveling to a new country).

To determine whether GOS is appropriate for you, consult a doctor with expertise in nutrition. You may be given a test called a comprehensive digestive stool analysis. As for dosage, follow your doctor's guidelines. (By way of comparison, in one human study published in *American Journal of Clinical Nutrition,* participants took daily doses of up to five grams of GOS.) GOS generally is safe, though it may cause an increase in flatulence and/or mild gastrointestinal discomfort, particularly in people who are not accustomed to consuming much fiber.

Crohn's/Colitis Drug

The FDA recently approved the intravenous drug *vedolizumab* (Entyvio) for ulcerative colitis and Crohn's disease patients who have not responded to standard medications. In clinical trials of 2,700 patients with either of these inflammatory bowel conditions, about 50% of symptoms eased for at least a year. When given at least every eight weeks, Entyvio blocks certain inflammatory cells from entering areas in the gastrointestinal tract. Side effects may include headache, joint pain and liver damage.

Stephen Hanauer, MD, medical director, Digestive Health Center, Northwestern University Feinberg School of Medicine, Chicago.

7 Steps to Controlling Crohn's Disease Naturally

Andrew L. Rubman, ND, director, Southbury Clinic for Traditional Medicines, Southbury, Connecticut.
American Society for Microbiology, ASM.org

For people with digestive issues, life tends to revolve around what you can and can't eat and how far away from the nearest bathroom you dare to venture. That's certainly the case with Crohn's disease, which along with ulcerative colitis is one of the two most common forms of inflammatory bowel disease. Symptoms include wrenching stomach pain soon after eating (typically in the lower right side) and relentless diarrhea. It's relatively rare, but a new research finding suggests that people with Crohn's are seven times more apt to carry bacteria that cause a related gastrointestinal disease in cattle. The bacteria—*Mycobacterium avium* subspecies paratuberculosis or MAP—has been found in milk in American supermarkets, and some studies have found it in meat and cheese, raising the possibility that it may be passed up the food chain to people.

IT'S GUT WRENCHING

Whether or not bacteria such as MAP cause disease in the intestinal tract is largely a matter of threshold. A person with a healthy, intact digestive tract will likely be able to resist infectious bacteria. But the large intestine is the body's center of immunity, and when the digestive tissue becomes damaged and inflamed, it becomes more susceptible to invasive microorganisms, be it MAP or the increasingly infectious species of *E. coli, Salmonella,* and other causes of food poisoning. If the balance of healthy versus harmful bacteria is disrupted and/or tissue is damaged, people become less able to resist disease and it becomes more difficult to treat.

Little is known about the causes of Crohn's disease, although family history, an overactive immune system and inflammation response, and environmental triggers are all believed to play a role. It differs from ulcerative colitis (which causes similar symptoms) because inflammation is deeper in the intestinal wall and also potentially affects the entire gastrointestinal tract from mouth to anus. Ulcerative colitis primarily affects the colon. There's no known cure for Crohn's and remedies offered by conventional medicine are riddled with problems.

In September 2008, the FDA ordered stronger warnings for common Crohn's drugs—*infliximab* (Remicade), *adalimumab* (Humira) and *certolizumab pegol* (Cimzia)—after an association with the risk of developing fungal and yeast infections such as *Candidiasis* was found. Because conventional treatments have significant side effects—even when they work, and they don't always—more than half of people with Crohn's disease turn to natural therapies.

NATURAL SOLUTIONS

Since Crohn's disease affects different people in different ways, Dr. Rubman individualizes treatment for each patient, working in collaboration with his/her gastroenterologist—a strategy he suggests for all Crohn's patients since a combination of natural and mainstream treatments seems to be most effective.

Natural solutions include...

• **Probiotics.** Health requires maintaining a balance between good and bad bacteria in the digestive tract. Poor diet, stress or a digestive disorder such as Crohn's can result in a takeover of the system by "bad" bacteria, resulting in symptoms such as diarrhea and gas. To restore a proper floral balance, Dr. Rubman frequently prescribes a seven- to 10-day course of a probiotic supplement composed of *Lactobacillus acidophilus* and *Bifidobacterium bifidus*. However, it is important to have a stool test before treatment, in order to ensure the proper probiotic formula is administered.

• **Fish oil.** A small British study found that fish oil taken with antioxidants may help reduce the inflammation associated with Crohn's disease. Eat fatty fish such as salmon, mackerel or sardines two or three times a week. In addition, Dr. Rubman often prescribes one or more grams of an EPA-DHA fish oil capsule or liquid daily.

• **Vitamin B-12.** When the bowel has been damaged by Crohn's disease, it may no longer effectively absorb B-12. If you are tired and run-down, ask your doctor to test you. Dr. Rubman prefers to prescribe sublingual B-12 rather than B-12 shots. It's as effective, less expensive and certainly more comfortable.

• **Acupuncture.** Acupuncture has traditionally been used to treat inflammatory bowel disease in China and is meeting with increasing mainstream acceptance in the US. A small German study suggests that acupuncture may help improve quality of life and general well-being in people with Crohn's disease by modulating symptoms and may even result in a small decrease in inflammatory markers in the blood. Find an acupuncturist in your area at the website of the American Association of Acupuncture and Oriental Medicine at AAAOMonline.org/45000.asp.

• **Focus on whole foods, fresh fruits and vegetables.** A diet that contains lots of processed and fast foods—like white bread, sugary desserts, etc.—stresses the bowel and may trigger inflammation and worsen symptoms of Crohn's disease. Disease-causing microorganisms thrive on foods like these. Many people with Crohn's report that they feel better when they eliminate or significantly cut back on processed foods and place a greater emphasis on whole foods, fresh fruits and vegetables and moderate amounts of protein. Avoid milk and dairy products as well as trans fats, as they can also irritate the intestinal track.

• **Decompress.** Many people with Crohn's find that their symptoms worsen during stressful periods. If you find this to be the case, take steps to effectively manage stress. Do whatever works best for you—whether that is yoga or meditation or dancing or tennis.

• **Stay away from colonics.** Many people are tempted to turn to this "quick fix," but colonics can backfire and worsen symptoms. The large intestine requires a healthy balance of microorganisms to function properly, and colonics indiscriminately wipe out the good with the bad under the thinly supported premise of detoxification.

To feel more in control of your disease and your life, learn more about Crohn's and connect with others who are going through the same things you are. Join message boards, chats, blogs and support groups (online or offline) at websites such as CrohnsColitisFoundation.org, or those listed at Crohns-disease-and-stress.com and IBDcrohns.about.com/od/onlinesupport/a/supportgroups.htm.

Acknowledging that a diagnosis of Crohn's disease is never good news, those who have the problem should stay optimistic—it can often be controlled without drastic drugs or a draconian diet, and quality of life need not suffer.

The Baffling Bladder Condition Antibiotics Can't Cure

Kristene E. Whitmore, MD, professor and chair of urology and female pelvic medicine and reconstructive surgery at Drexel University College of Medicine, and medical director of the Pelvic and Sexual Health Institute, both in Philadelphia. She is coauthor of *Overcoming Bladder Disorders.* PelvicAndSexualHealth Institute.org.

Perplexing, painful and inconvenient, the chronic condition interstitial cystitis/painful bladder syndrome (IC/PBS) affects women more than nine times as often as men. Its symptoms, including bladder pain and frequent urination, often are mistaken for those of a bladder infection—yet tests reveal no bacteria, and antibiotics bring no relief.

Though IC/PBS affects up to 6% of American women, its cause is a mystery.

What is known: The bladder wall becomes inflamed and super-sensitive...pinpoints of bleeding and ulcers often appear...stiffness and scarring may develop.

Many women suffer for years without a proper diagnosis, taking antibiotics for infections that they do not actually have. This delay causes needless pain...raises the odds of becoming resistant to antibiotics...and increases the risk that an IC/PBS–triggered inflammatory reaction will spread to other organs. In severe cases, surgery may be needed to remove part or all of the bladder. IC/PBS cannot be cured—but treatment can relieve symptoms and reduce complications.

GETTING DIAGNOSED

If you have symptoms that suggest IC/PBS, visit your doctor. If no infection is found or symptoms persist despite treatment, consult a urologist or urogynecologist.

IC/PBS symptoms...

- **Bladder pain or pressure**
- **Frequent urination** (more than eight times in 24 hours)
- **Urgent need to urinate**
- **Discomfort, pain or pressure in the lower pelvis or vulva**
- **Pain during or after sex**
- **Flare-ups during menstruation**

There is no definitive test for IC/PBS. Diagnosis involves excluding other conditions, such as a bladder infection, overactive bladder or bladder cancer. Testing may include blood and urine tests, bladder biopsy and cystoscopy (exam of the bladder using a viewing instrument).

Good news: For about 70% of patients, natural remedies ease symptoms with few or no side effects.

SOOTHING DIETARY STRATEGIES

Your diet affects how your bladder feels. *Helpful...*

- **Identify foods that spark symptoms.** A chief culprit is cranberry juice. Yes, this juice combats bladder infections—but with IC/PBS, you aren't fighting an infection. And cranberry juice is acidic, so it irritates a sensitive bladder.

Other top troublemakers: Alcohol...artificial sweeteners...caffeine (coffee, soda, tea)... carbonated drinks...citrus fruits, citrus juic-

Breakthrough: Antibiotic Relieves IBS

The antibiotic rifaximin can relieve irritable bowel syndrome (IBS) symptoms, such as bloating, abdominal pain and diarrhea, for up to 10 weeks after patients take it for two weeks. It is equally effective in men and women. Rifaximin was not tested in people whose IBS causes constipation.

Mark Pimentel, MD, director of the GI Motility Program at Cedars-Sinai Medical Center, Los Angeles, and principal investigator in a study of rifaximin use, published in *The New England Journal of Medicine.*

es...spicy foods...and tomato products. For a comprehensive list of problematic foods, visit the website of the Interstitial Cystitis Association (IChelp.org, click on "Living with IC" and then "Interstial Cystitis and Diet"). To identify your personal triggers, for one month do not eat anything on the ICA list. Then, reintroduce one food from the list every three to five days. If symptoms flare up, swear off that food.

• **Drink more, not less.** You may think that limiting fluids reduces your need to urinate—but skimping on water makes urine more concentrated and thus more irritating. Drink six to eight cups of water daily—and sip, don't gulp.

• **Take supplements.** With your doctor's okay, try the following...

• **Prelief (sold at drugstores) contains calcium glycerophosphate,** which makes food less acidic.

• **CystoProtek** (sold at Cysto-Protek.com) has antioxidants and anti-inflammatories (glucosamine, quercetin, rutin) that help repair the bladder lining.

Note: If you take a multivitamin or other supplement that contains vitamin C, choose one with ascorbate, not ascorbic acid.

MIND OVER BLADDER

Try any or all of the following mind-body therapies...

• **Bladder retraining.** Urinating temporarily relieves pain, so patients use the toilet often—in some cases, up to 60 times a day—but this habit further reduces the bladder's capacity to comfortably hold urine.

Best: Try to increase your typical time between bathroom trips by 15 minutes. After two weeks, increase by another 15 minutes. Continue until you can wait at least two hours.

• **Stress reduction.** Practice relaxation techniques daily, such as deep breathing, meditation and yoga. Also consider craniosacral therapy (gentle head and spine massage).

Practitioner referrals: Upledger Institute, 800-233-5880, Upledger.com.

• **Acupuncture.** This reduces IC/PBS pain for some patients.

Referrals: American Association of Acupuncture and Oriental Medicine, 866-455-7999, AAAOMonline.org.

MEDICAL TREATMENT OPTIONS

Persistent bladder pain eventually can cause pelvic muscles to spasm, worsening IC/PBS. *Helpful...*

• **Intravaginal Thiele massage.** To relieve spasms, a physical therapist massages muscles inside the vagina and/or rectum...and patients learn to do the procedure themselves at home. In one study, this reduced symptoms for 90% of patients.

• **Electrical nerve stimulation.** Stimulating the sacral nerves in the back with a mild current helps pelvic floor muscles function normally. If symptoms are severe, a urologist or urogynecologist can implant a nerve stimulator under the skin near the tailbone for continuous stimulation.

• **Medication.** About 5% to 10% of IC/PBS patients must resort to narcotic prescription painkillers—but these can have adverse effects, including a risk for dependence.

Better: First consider one or more of the following non-narcotic prescription drugs, discussing the pros and cons with your doctor...

• ***Dimethyl sulfoxide* (DMSO).** This pain-relieving anti-inflammatory and antispasmodic is infused into the bladder through a catheter and kept in place for about 20 minutes. The procedure typically is done once a week for six weeks. Relief lasts three to 12 months... treatment is repeated as needed. Side effects may include garlic taste in the mouth, headache and dry nasal passages. DMSO is the only drug approved for this treatment, but for some patients, other anesthetics (such as lidocaine) work as well with fewer side effects.

• ***Pentosan* (Elmiron).** This oral drug helps heal the bladder lining. It can thin the blood, however, so it may be inappropriate if you use a blood thinner, such as *warfarin* (Coumadin).

• ***Potassium citrate* (Urocit-K).** Taken orally, this makes urine more alkaline. Possible side effects include nausea, muscle weakness and irregular heartbeat.

• **Urelle.** This brand-name oral medication is a five-drug formulation that reduces pain and spasms. Side effects may include nausea, dizziness and blurred vision.

LIFESTYLE CHANGES

To make day-to-day life with IC/PBS more comfortable, try...

• **Modified exercise routines.** When symptoms flare up, reduce the intensity and duration of workouts—for instance, by walking instead of running. Rinse off after swimming to remove irritating chlorine.

• **Bathing.** Soak in bathwater mixed with colloidal oatmeal (sold at drugstores). Avoid bubble baths and bath oils—these can be irritating.

• **A personal lubricant for sex.** This makes intercourse more comfortable.

Try: The organic Good Clean Love line (541-344-4483, GoodCleanLove.com).

Is It Just a Bladder Infection...or Are Your Kidneys in Danger?

Mildred Lam, MD, associate professor at Case Western Reserve University School of Medicine and an attending physician in the division of nephrology at MetroHealth Medical Center, both in Cleveland. She specializes in the care of patients with acute and chronic kidney disease.

In most cases of urinary tract infection (UTI), bacteria get into the urethra (the tube that carries urine out of the body), travel into the bladder and multiply. Called a bladder infection or cystitis, this generally is easily treated with antibiotics.

But sometimes the bacteria travel farther and invade the kidney itself, causing a kidney infection. Possible consequences of this type of UTI include temporary or permanent kidney failure...chronic kidney disease...and potentially life-threatening septicemia if bacteria enter the bloodstream.

Women are more vulnerable to UTIs than men because in women, the urethra and bacteria-laden anus are closer together...and the urethra is shorter, so bacteria don't have to travel as far to reach the bladder and kidneys. *Other risk factors...*

• **Being postmenopausal**—accompanying hormonal changes can diminish muscle tone in the urinary tract, making it easier for bacteria to invade.

• **Sexual activity, especially with a new partner**—perhaps because, over time, a woman develops antibodies to her partner's bacteria.

• **Diabetes**—sugar in the urine promotes bacterial growth.

• **Kidney stones**—these provide a place for bacteria to grow and also impede the flow of urine (and therefore bacteria) out of the body.

• **Congenital defects that let urine travel upward from the bladder to the kidney**—normally urine only travels downward from kidney to bladder.

Because a kidney infection can quickly become serious, Dr. Lam urges women to be on the lookout for symptoms. *Call your doctor today if you notice...*

• **Discomfort or burning pain when urinating.**

• **Frequent urge to urinate** (even if little comes out).

• **Cloudy or blood-tinged urine.**

• **Low-grade fever.**

• **Mild to moderate pain in the middle of the lower back.**

These symptoms suggest a bladder infection. A urine test can confirm the diagnosis.

Remember: Prompt treatment—typically a three-to-five-day course of oral antibiotics—helps keep a bladder infection from moving to the kidneys. If you need a pain reliever, your doctor may recommend *acetaminophen* (Tylenol). High-dose aspirin, ibuprofen and naproxen carry a small risk for kidney failure.

• **Severe pain in the "flank" area of the back,** at the lower edge of the ribs on the left or right side.

• **Chills and/or fever above 102°.**

• **Nausea and vomiting.**

These symptoms suggest a kidney infection. To minimize the risk for permanent kidney damage, high-dose IV antibiotics are needed to quickly achieve high antibiotic levels in both the blood and the urine. You may be given IV fluids if dehydrated or very nauseated. Once fever subsides and you can take fluids and medication by mouth, you'll switch to oral antibiotics, taking these for 10 to 14 days to eradicate the bacteria.

Bladder and kidney infection prevention strategies...

- **Don't hold your urine too long**—going when you need to go helps flush bacteria out of the bladder.
- **Always wipe from front to back after using the toilet.**
- **Drinking cranberry juice or taking cranberry supplements may help**—cranberries contain a compound that makes it difficult for bacteria to cling to the bladder walls.
- **Stay hydrated.**
- **Urinate before and after intercourse.**

If you are especially prone to UTIs (getting more than two in a six-month period), ask your doctor about taking a single dose of an antibiotic immediately after intercourse.

Kidney Stones...Never Again! How to Avoid This Painful Condition

Fredric L. Coe, MD, nephrologist and professor of medicine at The University of Chicago Pritzker School of Medicine. Dr. Coe has published more than 250 peer-reviewed medical journal research articles and an additional 200 reviews, chapters and books.

If you've ever endured the searing pain of a kidney stone—it's often described as worse than childbirth—then you probably felt like celebrating once the pain was gone and now consider yourself home free. But that's a mistake.

What most people don't realize: Once you've suffered a kidney stone, which can be as small as a grain of sand or as large as a golf ball, you have a chronic condition that must be managed over a lifetime to prevent a repeat performance.

Here's what you need to know to control this condition over the long haul—and prevent it in the first place if kidney stones run in your family...

A GROWING PROBLEM

Even if you've never had a kidney stone, that doesn't mean you're in the clear. About one in every 10 Americans will have a kidney stone during his/her lifetime.

Eye-opening new finding: For unknown reasons, the prevalence of kidney stone disease has doubled in the past 15 years—more than three million Americans receive medical care for the condition each year.

BEST TREATMENT OPTIONS

Treatment for a kidney stone mainly depends on its size. If you develop a small stone (less than 4 mm—or about one-sixth of an inch), count yourself lucky. You may be able to simply drink lots of water (about three liters per day)...take an over-the-counter nonsteroidal anti-inflammatory drug, such as *ibuprofen* (Motrin)...and wait for it to pass on its own within a few days, though it sometimes takes a week or longer. A prescription medication, such as *tamsulosin* (Flomax), may also be used to help pass the stone.

Important: It's crucial that a urologist monitor the patient (for example, with an abdominal X-ray or ultrasound), since the stone may cause an obstruction that damages the kidney—even if the pain has subsided.

A larger stone (4 mm or more) usually needs more extensive medical intervention. While doctors once relied on external sound waves (shock wave lithotripsy), which was only moderately successful at breaking apart a kidney stone in the body, there's now a more effective method. An ultra-thin lighted tube (ureteroscope) can be threaded into the urethra, into the bladder, then up to the ureter. A laser at the tip of the scope pulverizes the stone, turning it into dust that is urinated out.

When a kidney stone exceeds 2 cm (or about three-quarters of an inch), surgery is usually required. With percutaneous nephrolithotomy, the surgeon creates a small incision in your back to remove the stone.

KNOW YOUR STONE

To avoid a recurrence, the key is to know the composition of your kidney stone. *Main types of stones...*

- **Calcium oxalate.** These small, black or dark brown stones account for about 80% of all kidney stones.
- **Calcium phosphate.** These stones, which are usually tan to beige, form when urine is more alkaline.
- **Uric acid.** These red or orange stones form when urine is too acidic due to heredity, obesity or kidney disease.
- **Cystine.** These lemon-yellow stones are associated with the hereditary disorder cystinuria, which causes high urine concentrations of the amino acid cystine.
- **Struvite.** These brownish-white stones are produced when bacteria get introduced into the urinary tract—due, for example, to the use of a urinary catheter.

PREVENTION SECRETS

To prevent a kidney stone recurrence, your goal is to stop the stone-forming process by changing the composition of your urine. *Here's how to do that...*

STEP 1: **Get your kidney stone analyzed.** If you pass a stone at home, save it so that your doctor can have its composition analyzed. Urine analysis shows what stone-causing compounds are in your urine so that you can take appropriate preventive steps.

What to do: Strain your urine through gauze in a funnel and then put the stone into a small plastic bag.

Important: It's best to have all stones analyzed, since your kidneys can produce stones of varying crystals at different times in your life, which may require a change in treatment. Anyone who has ever suffered a kidney stone should also see a doctor at least once a year for urine analysis.

STEP 2: **Provide two 24-hour urine samples after the stone has passed.** This requires catching and saving all your urine for 24 hours after you've resumed your normal diet and lifestyle habits. Getting two samples provides a more accurate view than a single sample.

STEP 3: Raise your urine volume. The more dilute your urine becomes, the less likely that stones will form. The goal is to produce about 2.5 liters daily in urine volume. This will require drinking three liters or more of fluid daily (spaced out during waking hours). People who sweat a lot due to heat or physical activity may need to drink four to six liters of water per day.

Note: High water intake can sometimes be harmful for people with heart, kidney or liver disease...the elderly...and people taking certain medications (such as diuretics). Consult your physician for advice on how much water you should drink.

STEP 4: Change your diet. This should start immediately when you have a kidney stone and continue for a lifetime. *A kidney stone prevention diet is...**

- **Low sodium and high calcium.** If your daily sodium intake is below 1,500 mg, you can eat 1,000 mg to 1,200 mg of calcium daily (mainly from dairy foods and leafy green vegetables, except for spinach), and urine calcium losses will be as low as possible. Why do you need calcium? High calcium intake will reduce oxalate absorption—oxalate is a component of most kidney stones.

Helpful: After following a low-sodium/high-calcium diet for about a month, repeat the 24-hour urine test to see if additional dietary restrictions are required.

Important: If urine oxalate remains high (over 30 mg per day) despite a high calcium intake, then you need to go low oxalate. To reduce your risk for calcium oxalate stones, avoid high-oxalate foods (such as spinach, rhubarb, beets, cocoa, raspberries and soy products).

Note: Even though many of these foods are healthful, there are safer substitutes—for example, instead of spinach, you can try arugula

*If you have chronic kidney disease, your dietary and treatment needs may differ—consult your doctor.

or kale. For a full list of high-oxalate foods and good substitutes, go to KidneyStones.UChicago.edu/how-to-eat-a-low-oxalate-diet.

• **High potassium.** When food sources of potassium—all fruits and most vegetables—are consumed, they are converted to bicarbonate. This process reduces the risk for calcium and uric acid stones.

Recommended daily potassium intake: 4,700 mg.

• **Low protein and high refined sugar intake.** These foods can promote uric acid stones. Ideally, intake of refined sugar should be less than 10% of total caloric intake, and protein intake should be about 0.8 g to 1 g of protein per 2.2 pounds of body weight.

STEP 5: **Ask your physician about medication.** A variety of medications can help prevent a kidney stone recurrence. These include potassium citrate tablets for people who have had uric acid stones or calcium stones...thiazide diuretics, which help prevent calcium stones...and antibiotics for struvite stones that are triggered by, say, a urinary tract infection.

For more on kidney stones, go to the website KidneyStones.UChicago.edu.

KIDNEY STONE BASICS

When a stone forms in the kidney, it typically moves through the urinary tract to exit the body in urine. At various points along that journey, the stone may become lodged, leading to extreme pain (usually in one's side or back near the bottom of the rib cage, though it may spread to the lower abdomen and groin).

Important: Kidney stones may also cause blood in the urine, an inability to pass urine, nausea and vomiting and/or fever and chills. Get to an emergency room if you suffer from any of these symptoms—they may signal an infection that requires immediate medical care.

Help for Large Kidney Stones

More than 83% of patients whose stones measured 5 mm to 10 mm passed them within 28 days after being given tamsulosin (sold as Flomax and used to improve urination in men)—compared with 61% who passed stones of that size when given a placebo. Tamsulosin does not help patients pass smaller stones, which usually pass on their own.

Jeremy Furyk, MBBS, senior staff specialist and director of emergency research at The Townsville Hospital, Queensland, Australia, and leader of a study published in *Annals of Emergency Medicine.*

Best and Worst Drinks for Preventing Kidney Stones

Pietro Manuel Ferraro, MD, physician, department of internal medicine and medical specialties, Catholic University of the Sacred Heart, Rome, Italy. His study was published in *Clinical Journal of the American Society of Nephrology.*

Mention kidney stones and everyone within earshot winces—because we've all heard how painful these stones can be. So if you want to be stone-free, you're probably following the common advice to drink lots of liquids. But instead of focusing on how much you drink, the crucial question is what you drink, a new study reveals. Certain beverages—including some very surprising ones, such as beer!—are particularly helpful in protecting against stones, while other drinks do more harm than good.

Unfortunately, kidney stones are common, plaguing 19% of men and 9% of women in the US at least once in their lifetimes—and recurrences are quite common. Drinking plenty of water helps prevent stones from forming...but actually, there are other fluids that can be even more effective.

DRINK THIS, NOT THAT

Using data from three large studies, researchers followed 194,095 people, none of whom had a history of kidney stones, for more than eight years. Participants periodically completed questionnaires about their diet and overall health. During the course of the study, there were 4,462 cases of kidney stones.

Researchers adjusted for health factors (age, body mass index, diabetes, medications, blood pressure) as well as various dietary factors (including intake of meat, calcium and potassium) known to affect kidney stone risk. Then they calculated the stone risk associated with various types of beverages.

How the comparison was done: For each analysis, the effects of drinking an average of one or more servings per day were compared with drinking less than one serving per week. Because data from three different studies were used, serving sizes were not necessarily alike across the board. But in general, a serving was considered to be 12 ounces of soda or beer…eight ounces of coffee, tea, milk or fruit punch…five ounces of wine…and four to six ounces of juice. The researchers' findings were eye-opening.

Kidney stone risk boosters…

- **Sugar-sweetened noncola sodas increased kidney stone risk by 33%.**
- **Sugar-sweetened colas increased risk by 23%.**
- **Fruit punch increased risk by 18%.**
- **Diet noncola sodas (but, surprisingly, not diet colas) increased risk by 17%.**

Kidney stone risk reducers…

- **Beer reduced kidney stone risk by 41%.**
- **White wine reduced risk by 33%.**
- **Red wine reduced risk by 31%.**
- **Caffeinated coffee reduced kidney stone risk by 26%.**
- **Decaf coffee reduced risk by 16%.**
- **Orange juice reduced risk by 12%.**
- **Tea reduced risk by 11%.**

Consumption of milk and juices other than orange juice did not significantly affect the likelihood of developing kidney stones.

Theories behind the findings: Because sugar-sweetened sodas and fruit punch are associated with higher risk, researchers suspect that their high fructose concentration may increase the amount of calcium, oxalate and uric acid in the urine—and those substances contribute to kidney stone formation. So how to explain the beneficial effects of orange juice, which is also high in fructose? Perhaps orange juice's high concentration of potassium citrate offsets the fructose and favorably changes the composition of urine.

Regarding the beneficial effects of coffee and tea, it could be that their caffeine acts as a diuretic that promotes urine production and thus helps prevent stones. Tea and coffee, including decaf, also contain antioxidants that may help combat stone formation. Alcohol, too, is a diuretic, and wine and beer contain antioxidants as well—though of course, with any type of alcoholic beverage, moderation is important.

Get Rid of a Gallstone—Naturally

Andrew L. Rubman, ND, founder and medical director Southbury Clinic for Traditional Medicines, Southbury, Connecticut. SouthburyClinic.com

People who develop painful gallstones are generally given one of three treatments—a drug to dissolve the stone slowly over several months or even years…a tube down the throat through which a doctor removes the stone…or surgery to remove the entire gallbladder. None of these options sounds particularly appealing. Is there a natural way to treat gallstones? It turns out, for a certain subset of people who have a gallstone, there is.

If a gallstone is causing pain, it's important to treat it—not only to relieve your pain. If you let a painful gallstone linger, it could lead to serious problems, such as inflammation and degeneration of the gallbladder or blockage or infection of the bile duct. This is a life-threatening condition that needs emergency medical treatment. (If a gallstone isn't causing pain, it's probably very tiny and may pass through your body without treatment, but check with your doctor to see whether treatment is a good idea.)

A NATURAL ALTERNATIVE

The following botanical remedy has cured many of my patients. It won't work on every patient with a gallstone—only those with a gallstone that's no more than about eight millimeters in diameter (about the size of half a dime) and causes only mild to moderate pain. The patient also needs to have a healthy gallbladder and no signs of total bile duct obstruction or infection (fever, chills, vomiting or jaundice). If you meet the criteria, ask a naturopathic doctor about trying the following two-pronged, week-long approach—but only under the ND's careful supervision. In other words, make sure that an ND gives you these supplements…tells you how much and when and how to take them…and checks in with you regularly to see how much they're helping. Sometimes I give my patients both of the following supplements at once and sometimes I give them one first and the other second—it depends on a variety of factors, and your doctor can make the call.

1. Release the grip on the gallstone. The first daily supplement is an extract from the *Hyoscyamus niger* plant that is known for its antispasmodic effects. It allows the bile duct to relax its grasp on the stone, so it helps push the gallstone through the colon and out of the body. This particular extract can be harmful, even lethal, if misused, and it is sold exclusively to physicians (not to general consumers). Your ND can prescribe it safely based on your age, weight, medical history and whatever medications and/or supplements you may already be taking.

2. Shrink the gallstone. In addition to prescribing the above supplement, I prescribe an additional supplement that improves the flow of bile and degrades the gallstone, allowing it to pass through the digestive system more easily. The dose is usually two or three daily tablets of Priority Lipo. It's a blend of about 16 different botanicals and nutrients such as vitamin B-6, magnesium and choline. It's made by a company called Priority One—a bottle of 120 capsules (a 30-day supply, according to the dosing instructions on the bottle) costs about $50 at Accutrition.com. Side effects may include temporary indigestion, upset stomach or loose stools. It does contain an extract of a plant called barberry, which should not be consumed by pregnant or lactating women. Anyone who has chronic liver disease may need extra supervision while taking the supplement, since it stimulates liver function.

This program usually works within a week, and you'll know that it has worked when you stop feeling pain. (Even if the gallstone shifts in position but doesn't actually pass, you'll still feel pain.) Whenever you have a bowel movement that week, you can look for your gallstone in the bowel movement if you feel like digging for it, but since it was relatively small to begin with and since this natural treatment can degrade it and make it even smaller, you might not feel it pass. If you want to know for sure that it's gone, ask an MD or ND to give you a scan (either an ultrasound, MRI or CT).

If you and your doctor decide that you should try this gallstone treatment and the regimen is unsuccessful, you and your ND may decide to consult a gastroenterologist to discuss other treatment options.

Hidden Hernia

J. Scott Roth, MD, assistant professor of surgery at the University of Maryland School of Medicine, director of the University of Maryland Hernia Center and head of surgical endoscopy at the University of Maryland Medical Center, all in Baltimore.

Most people are familiar with the type of hernia that appears as a bulge in the groin. Much more common in men than in women, this type of hernia (known as an inguinal hernia) occurs when part of the intestine protrudes into the groin, possibly as a result of pressure caused by lifting heavy objects and/or straining during a bowel movement.

What you may not know: There is another type of hernia, called a hiatal hernia, that far fewer people are aware of, even though estimates show that it occurs in up to six out of 10 people over age 60. A hiatal hernia, in which a portion of the stomach protrudes into the chest cavity, usually causes no symptoms. When symptoms do occur, however, they are often misdiagnosed as ordinary heartburn and/or nausea.

WHEN THE STOMACH MOVES

The diaphragm (a dome-shaped muscle that helps with breathing) separates the abdominal and chest cavities. The esophagus passes from the throat through an opening in the diaphragm (hiatus) to the stomach. The diaphragm opening is normally less than one inch across.

In patients with hiatal hernias, the opening is larger—sometimes up to 4.7 inches. Result: The upper portion of the stomach can poke through the enlarged hole into the chest cavity. As the hernia enlarges, an increasing amount of the stomach may enter the chest. Large hiatal hernias may cause swallowing difficulties, nausea and vomiting.

Very large hiatal hernias, in which a significant portion of the stomach has entered the chest, can sometimes be detected during a physical exam. A doctor may be able to detect bowel sounds inside the chest cavity. In most cases, hiatal hernias can be diagnosed only with a barium X-ray (the patient drinks a chalky liquid that coats—and illuminates—the upper digestive tract) or an endoscopic procedure, in which a doctor uses a lighted tube to view the esophagus and stomach.

RISK FACTORS FOR HERNIAS

Some people have a genetic susceptibility to hernias—they're born with an unusually large hiatus or the opening enlarges due to weakness in the surrounding muscles.

As with inguinal hernias, repeated abdominal pressure—from lifting heavy objects, straining to have bowel movements, being overweight, and/or severe coughing, sneezing or vomiting—may increase risk for hiatal hernias.

Two types of hiatal hernias...

- **Sliding hernias are the most common.** They occur when a small portion of the stomach (typically about an inch) "slides" into the chest cavity, then returns to its normal position. This movement reduces pressure on the lower esophageal sphincter (LES), a circular band of muscle at the base of the esophagus, allowing reflux (backing up) of stomach acid.
- **Paraesophageal hernias, though quite rare, are potentially more serious.** The upper part of the stomach rises until it's next to the LES. This can restrict (strangulate) blood flow in the stomach, which if untreated can result in necrosis (death) of the stomach. If the necrosis is not treated, it can be fatal.

If a paraesophageal hernia causes symptoms, such as chest pain, it should be surgically repaired.

CONTROLLING HEARTBURN

Without treatment, the chronic surge of stomach acid that occurs in patients with symptomatic hiatal hernias can cause inflammation of the esophagus...iron-deficiency anemia from esophageal bleeding...or premalignant changes (Barrett's esophagus) that can lead to esophageal cancer. Some patients experience difficulty breathing or even severe chest pain that resembles a heart attack.

Most people with hiatal hernias don't require surgical repair as long as they can minimize discomfort and damage caused by the reflux of stomach acid. *My advice...*

Make lifestyle changes. Most patients with hernia-related heartburn require medication, but some improve significantly with lifestyle adjustments...

- **Avoid eating within four to five hours of bedtime.** Eating stimulates the production of stomach acid, which is more likely to cause heartburn when patients lie down soon afterward.
- **Avoid peppermint and caffeine.** Both reduce muscle tension in the LES, the muscular band that helps prevent reflux.
- **Raise the head of the bed about six inches.** Gravity can prevent stomach acid from moving into your esophagus while you sleep. Use bricks, wood or plastic risers designed to elevate the head of the bed.
- **Consider taking medication.** For most medical conditions, doctors usually prefer to start treatment with the mildest drugs first. In my experience, the opposite approach—starting strong, then tapering off, if possible—seems to work better for hernia-related heartburn...
- **Proton-pump inhibitors (PPIs)** are considered the strongest heartburn medication, so your doctor may advise you to start with one of these drugs. PPIs, such as *omeprazole*

(Prilosec) and *esomeprazole* (Nexium), inhibit acid production in the stomach and allow damaged tissues to heal. If a PPI taken twice daily improves symptoms within about six weeks, your doctor may suggest that you cut back to one dose a day.

- **Antacids and H2-blockers.** If heartburn symptoms continue to improve over roughly a six-week period, you can probably switch to a milder (and less expensive) drug, such as an over-the-counter antacid or H2-blocker, including *famotidine* (Pepcid) or *cimetidine* (Tagamet), for occasional relief.

WHEN TO CONSIDER SURGERY

Most people with hiatal hernias can control heartburn with drugs alone. Therefore, surgery is recommended only if you have a twisted stomach that endangers your stomach's blood supply...complications, such as scarring or bleeding due to reflux...or severe discomfort or reflux of stomach contents (such as bile or digestive enzymes) that isn't relieved by medications. Surgery also is recommended for patients who no longer wish to take reflux medications.

Most hernias, including hiatal hernias, are repaired with laparoscopic "keyhole" surgery, in which the surgeon inserts a camera and instruments through four or five small (less than half an inch) incisions in the abdomen.

About 95% of patients who receive surgery for hiatal hernias will no longer need medication to control symptoms.

Is Surgery a Must When You Have a Hernia?

Hien Tan Nguyen, MD, assistant professor of surgery, Johns Hopkins University School of Medicine, director, Johns Hopkins Comprehensive Hernia Center and assistant professor of biomedical engineering and associate medical director, Johns Hopkins Center for Bioengineering Innovation and Design, all in Baltimore.

A hernia can be a serious problem—or not. For example, the average hernia causes little or no discomfort...and may not get any worse. Nevertheless, doctors often recommend surgery due to the risks that hernias can pose.

When is a hernia about to change from "harmless" to "extremely dangerous?" Are you getting the latest and most effective therapies?

WHAT IS A HERNIA?

A hernia is a protrusion of tissue, such as intestine, through a weak spot in the abdominal muscles. *Types of hernias...*

Both inguinal and umbilical hernias are easy to diagnose and rarely require an imaging test because your doctor can see and feel them. The bulge can cause discomfort or even severe pain.

Where to look: Inguinal hernias appear on either side of the groin or, in men, within the scrotum. Umbilical hernias appear near the belly button. Both types tend to get larger and more tender during activities that increase abdominal pressure, such as while straining with a bowel movement, during a sneezing or coughing fit or just from standing up.

A special warning for women: Women are more prone than men to occult (hidden) hernias—too small to be seen or felt by touch—that can press on nerves and cause pain. Often, these hernias get misdiagnosed as endometriosis or another gynecological problem. A woman with pelvic pain should start by consulting with her gynecologist and make sure to ask whether a hernia could be the cause.

What you can do: The size and discomfort of inguinal or umbilical hernias can vary over time. *What helps...*

- **A cold compress.** Encourage protruding tissue to retreat back into the abdomen or groin, thus "reducing" a hernia, by lying down and applying a cold compress for about 10 minutes. Use gentle pressure to slowly press downward on the bulge.

- **Wear a truss.** Some people wear a truss (hernia belt). While this may help, it isn't a cure, and wearing a truss can cause the wearer to forget about the hernia and overexert, making a small hernia larger.

- **Try yoga.** A study found that men with reducible inguinal hernias (they readily retract) who practiced a daily one-hour program of yoga followed by relaxation for three months rated their pain up to five points lower on a 10-point scale compared with before starting yoga. Yoga and other gentle workouts won't cure a hernia but can help to minimize symptoms, such as pain and cramps.

Hernias tend to get bigger over time, so to avoid possible future complications, many doctors recommend surgery to minimize the risk for complications. But painless inguinal or umbilical hernias are unlikely to need emergency surgery.

My advice: Consult your doctor if you are concerned that you have a hernia. Don't delay too long—you'll have fewer surgical complications when a hernia is repaired before the symptoms are severe.

Latest treatment options: Most surgeries for inguinal or umbilical hernias can be performed on an outpatient basis with minimally invasive surgery, using small incisions that allow for faster recovery and less pain following surgery. You'll be sore for about two weeks, and able to resume normal activities in about a month.

Caution: Hernias can come back. Reduce risk by maintaining a healthy weight, not smoking and exercising to strengthen abdominal muscles.

Best exercise: Cardio helps manage weight, especially abdominal weight.

With a hiatal hernia, the upper part of the stomach pushes through an opening in the diaphragm. You can't see or feel a bulge, but you might notice heartburn—or have no discomfort at all.

Most people only discover their hiatal hernia from an imaging test done for another condition. In severe cases, the hernia protrudes into the chest and interferes with normal function of the lungs or heart, causing symptoms that include shortness of breath.

If your doctor suspects a hiatal hernia, he/she will order an upper endoscopy to check your stomach and esophagus for inflammation and/or ulcers. A manometry test to measure pressure inside the esophagus...an esophogram to look for abnormalities...a pH test to measure the amount of acid flowing into your esophagus...or a CT scan to see how much of the stomach protrudes into the chest cavity also may be done.

What you can do: If you have heartburn that is mild/occasional and your hiatal hernia is small, your doctor is likely to prescribe medication rather than recommend surgery. Acid-blocking drugs such as *omeprazole* (Prilosec) or *cimetidine* (Tagamet) can reduce discomfort. Lifestyle changes, such as eating smaller, more frequent meals, not lying down immediately after eating and avoiding foods that trigger heartburn, won't heal the hernia but can alleviate symptoms.

Caution: Acid-suppressing drugs can have side effects such as increased risk for pneumonia and nutritional deficiencies, including vitamin B-12. Your doctor should supervise your use of these drugs.

Hiatal hernias that require surgery usually can be repaired with a minimally invasive procedure, but larger incisions may be needed in some cases. Surgery commonly involves pulling the stomach down through the diaphragm and narrowing the esophageal opening...and wrapping the stomach around the lower end of the esophagus, a procedure called Nissen fundoplication. The tighter fit keeps the stomach where it belongs and increases pressure on the esophagus—important for relieving heartburn. Most patients spend a night in the hospital and resume their regular activities within a few weeks.

WHEN ANY HERNIA "GOES BAD"

Whether it's an inguinal, umbilical or hiatal hernia, if your doctor believes that there is a risk for strangulation (twisting), in which the protruding tissue gets trapped between the muscle layers, you'll need surgery. With strangulation, the blood supply to the twisted tissue is cut off, causing it to become damaged or to die, leading to sepsis or gangrene—both life-threatening complications.

Critical symptoms: With an inguinal or umbilical hernia, sudden, worsening pain, nausea, vomiting, fever, inability to move bowels or pass gas...with a hiatal hernia, hoarseness or difficulty breathing.

Protect Your Pancreas!

Jerry R. Balentine, DO, vice president for medical affairs and global health at New York Institute of Technology (NYIT) and professor of emergency medicine at NYIT College of Osteopathic Medicine.

This crucial gland can be damaged by certain drugs, infections and more.

Pancreatitis is a condition that most people associate with heavy drinking.

Facts not widely known: Nearly two-thirds of the pancreatitis cases in the US may be caused by using certain prescription medications, including antibiotics, blood pressure drugs and antidepressants...or by having other conditions, especially gallstones...high triglycerides (a type of blood fat)...infection (such as mumps, herpes or food poisoning)...or autoimmune disease (such as lupus or Sjögren's syndrome). Trauma that damages the pancreas also can lead to pancreatitis.

Why this is important: Pancreatitis is not only painful but also associated with an increased risk for pancreatic cancer. Even if you don't have pancreatitis now, you still want to do everything you can to avoid the condition. Fortunately, if you do develop pancreatitis, the simple steps described in this article will help prevent attacks...

THE DANGER OF INFLAMMATION

When the pancreas gets inflamed, digestive enzymes that normally travel from the pancreas to the small intestine get trapped. These enzymes, which are potent enough to digest food in the stomach, start "digesting" the pancreas itself.

Result: Tissue damage and intense pain. With treatment, attacks due to acute pancreatitis usually subside within about one week. However, about 20% of patients who suffer acute pancreatitis go on to develop *chronic pancreatitis*, in which lingering inflammation may cause extensive damage and scarring.

RED FLAGS

Most patients with acute pancreatitis experience sharp pains in the upper-left part of the abdomen, and the pain may extend all the way to the back. The pain, which usually is accompanied by nausea and/or vomiting, may be mild initially but almost always gets more severe over a period of hours.

With chronic pancreatitis, flare-ups can be mild. But you'll probably lose weight, get occasional indigestion and have pale or clay-colored stools—all due to impaired digestion from a reduced supply of pancreatic enzymes.

GETTING THE RIGHT CARE

The pain of acute pancreatitis is very intense, so you will probably need to be hospitalized during an attack. Your doctor will give you medications for pain and probably administer IV fluids to keep you hydrated. Because the pain worsens after eating, people often stop eating and drinking during a pancreatitis attack.

Your doctor will then focus on what's causing the pancreatitis. For example, you may need surgery to remove gallstones or the gallbladder. Gallstones can cause reflux of bile into the pancreas, producing inflammation. Other treatments might include antibiotics that don't damage the pancreas to treat infection...or treating an alcohol addiction.

The conditions that cause pancreatitis are easily diagnosed with blood tests, stool tests to check for proper digestion/absorption of nutrients and/or imaging tests, such as ultrasound or a CT or MRI scan, to detect pancreatic inflammation, gallstones and blockages.

THE NEXT STEP

Doctors routinely review medications in people who have been diagnosed with acute pancreatitis. In some cases, discontinuing a "problem" medication (see box on next page) will eliminate the risk for future flare-ups. Lifestyle changes and other self-care measures can help you reduce discomfort and prevent future attacks. *Steps to follow...*

- **Use the right painkiller.** *Ibuprofen* (Motrin) and aspirin are among the best choices. Do not take *acetaminophen* (Tylenol). People with pancreatitis are at greater risk for liver damage, which can occur in anyone who takes acetaminophen.
- **Don't drink.** You'll want to avoid alcohol if you've been diagnosed with pancreatitis. It can trigger flare-ups even if the initial inflammation wasn't caused by alcohol.

• **Limit dietary fat.** It's harder for the body to digest fat than the carbohydrates and protein in foods such as legumes, fresh vegetables and whole grains. In addition to fast food and most desserts, foods that are relatively high in fat include meats, eggs and whole-fat dairy products.

• **Eat frequent, small meals.** Large meals stress the pancreas. I advise patients with pancreatitis to eat six or eight times a day instead of the traditional three daily meals.

• **Try supplemental enzymes.** They seem to ease symptoms in some patients with acute or chronic pancreatitis. Products such as Nature's Life Pancreatin or Pancreatic Enzyme Formula haven't been proven to help, but they're worth a try if you're having trouble with digestion and/or abdominal pain.

• **Get a lipid test.** For reasons that aren't clear, some pancreatitis cases are caused by very high triglycerides (above 1,000 mg/dL in a blood test). If you test high, you can lower triglycerides with exercise, weight loss, fish-oil supplements and a diet that's low in saturated fat. Medications, including niacin or a fibrate drug, such as *gemfibrozil* (Lopid), also may be needed if your triglycerides are this high.

DRUGS THAT CAN HARM YOUR PANCREAS

The following are among the frequently prescribed drugs that may trigger pancreatitis...*

• **Antibiotics** such as *ciprofloxacin* (Cipro), *azithromycin* (Zmax) and *demeclocycline* (Declomycin).

• **Antidepressants** such as *escitalopram* (Lexapro) and *bupropion* (Wellbutrin).

• **Blood pressure drugs** such as *enalapril* (Vasotec), *amlodipine* (Norvasc) and *metolazone* (Zaroxolyn).

• **Cholesterol drugs** such as *atorvastatin* (Lipitor) and *gemfibrozil* (Lopid).

• **Heartburn drugs** such as *omeprazole* (Prilosec) and *cimetidine* (Tagamet).

To check other drugs, go to the FDA website, FDA.gov/drugs.

*Do not discontinue any drug without consulting your doctor.

What to Do About Pancreatic Attacks

Mark A. Stengler, NMD, naturopathic doctor and founder of the Stengler Center for Integrative Medicine in Encinitas, California. He is author or coauthor of numerous books, including *The Natural Physician's Healing Therapies* and *Bottom Line's Prescription for Natural Cures*, and author of the newsletter *Health Revelations*. MarkStengler.com

The pancreas is a gland located behind your stomach and close to your small intestine. It secretes digestive enzymes and hormones involved in blood sugar regulation. If your attacks are caused by the disease called pancreatitis, your pancreas is probably inflamed, and the digestive enzymes are becoming activated prematurely and damaging your pancreas. Pancreatitis produces abdominal pain that may radiate to the back and/or cause nausea, vomiting and fever. The most common causes include alcohol abuse or gallstones, but in roughly 15% of cases, the cause remains unknown.

My recommendations: Avoid alcohol and, to reduce inflammation, cut out caffeine and simple sugars, such as soda, cookies and crackers. Have your holistic doctor test you for food allergies, which can aggravate this condition. Take a full-spectrum digestive-enzyme complex (available at health-food stores) at mealtimes for improved digestion. Finally, consider seeing an acupuncturist (find one at the website of the American Association of Acupunc-

Diverticulitis Linked to Red Meat Consumption

Men who ate the most red meat—more than six servings per week—were up to 58% more likely to develop diverticulitis (infected "pouches" in the lining of the colon that lead to abdominal pain, nausea and constipation) than those who ate the least.

Theory: Eating a lot of red meat may promote chronic, low-level inflammation, which may increase risk for diverticulitis.

Andrew T. Chan, MD, MPH, program director, gastroenterology training program, Massachusetts General Hospital, Boston.

ture and Oriental Medicine, AAAOMonline.org) or a homeopathic practitioner (get a referral from the National Center for Homeopathy at 856-437-4752, Homeopathycenter.org). I have seen good results from both in my patients who have pancreatitis.

Diverticulitis? Don't Be Too Quick to Get Surgery

Arden M. Morris, MD, MPH, division chief and associate professor of surgery, division of colorectal surgery, University of Michigan Health System, Ann Arbor, and coauthor of a recent study on diverticular disease published in *JAMA*.

Imagine having abdominal pain so severe that you're curled up in the emergency room, screaming. Your diagnosis is diverticulitis, an inflamed or infected "pouch" in the intestinal wall. A surgeon recommends that you have an operation to remove the inflamed portion of your intestine. If you don't, you're warned, the diverticulitis will come back…and the next time, it might rupture, requiring emergency surgery and perhaps even a colostomy (when the colon is diverted to an opening in your abdomen and you have to collect your feces in a plastic bag). So, of course, you have the surgery, right?

Not necessarily—because the operation could be a complete waste. Doctors are now realizing that, in many cases, diverticulitis is treated too aggressively, as a large-scale new study shows.

Diverticulitis is a fairly common ailment, so if you haven't experienced it yet, your day may come. And in recent years, hospital admissions for elective diverticulitis surgery have increased by about 25% to 30%. *Here's what you need to know to avoid unnecessary surgery…*

PAINFUL POUCHES

Diverticula are small, bulging pouches that can form anywhere along the digestive tract but most commonly develop in the large intestine. About half of Americans over age 60 have these pouches, which are typically the size of a marble. Most pouches cause no problems, so people don't even know that they have them. But if a pouch gets infected or inflamed, the likely symptoms include sudden and severe abdominal pain, fever, nausea, vomiting, constipation or diarrhea and/or rectal bleeding.

The majority of diverticulitis cases are uncomplicated, albeit painful. However, in some cases, serious complications do develop. These include a perforation (a hole in the intestinal wall)…fistula (a hole that creates a passageway between the intestine and the abdominal wall, bladder, uterus or vagina)…abscess (a collection of pus in the swollen pouch)…or obstruction (intestinal blockage). Fear of such complications—or fear of a recurrence that might lead to complications—has been a driving force behind the common practice of doing surgery even in uncomplicated diverticulitis cases.

Recently, researchers from the University of Michigan conducted a review of 80 scientific studies on diverticulitis to evaluate the effectiveness of current treatments. *Here are some main factors behind the study's conclusion that surgery often is not warranted…*

- **Recurrence is not as common as was thought.** Some patients are told that, once diverticulitis develops, a recurrence or multiple recurrences are practically guaranteed unless surgery is done. However, in one study of 2,366 diverticulitis patients who did not have surgery only 13% had experienced a recurrence and less than 4% had more than one recurrence after nearly nine years of follow-up.

- **Recurrence is not as dangerous as had been believed.** Even for people who do have a recurrence or who develop chronic diverticulitis, fewer than 5% developed one of the dreaded complications. In fact, it now appears that subsequent episodes of diverticulitis typically are less severe, not worse, than initial episodes. No one knows exactly why that's the case, but one theory is that the inflammation in the first episode triggers nearby structures to reinforce themselves and bolster the area to help guard against perforation in the event that the inflammation recurs.

- **Surgery provides no guarantee against future problems.** Diverticulitis surgery itself has a fairly high complication rate...and up to 25% of patients who did have the operation still experienced unresolved symptoms afterward. Also, in more than one in three cases of recurrences, the inflammation or infection developed in a different area of the intestine than the original attack—so surgery that removed the initial pouch would not have prevented the second pouch from becoming symptomatic.

• **Complications are even more common in a first episode than in a recurrent episode.** In one study of patients who did have complicated diverticulitis (with an abscess or perforation), nearly three-quarters had had no previous "warning" episode—contradicting the idea that the surgery prevents most complications.

THE RIGHT TREATMENT

None of this is to say that surgery is never appropriate for diverticulitis—because sometimes it is absolutely essential. *Urgent surgery is needed if any of the following occurs...*

• **A patient develops sepsis,** an overwhelming immune response to a bacterial infection in which chemicals released into the blood trigger widespread inflammation, leading to blood clots and leaky blood vessels.

• **There is an obstruction blocking the intestine.**

• **An infected pouch perforates,** spilling intestinal contents into the abdominal cavity.

Elective surgery should be scheduled if...

• **A patient has a fistula.**

• **A patient has a compromised immune system** (for instance, from HIV or an organ transplant), because this creates a greater infection risk overall.

When surgery is not warranted, what treatment is appropriate? It depends on the individual case, so patients need to work closely with a doctor who is knowledgeable about the latest research. *Generally, though, the options include...*

• **Antibiotics—maybe.** In the past, patients often were kept in the hospital for several days of intravenous antibiotics. However, recent studies have found no advantage in using intravenous rather than oral antibiotics...and even oral antibiotics don't help much in cases of uncomplicated diverticulitis, having no effect on the rate of complications or recurrence and doing little to relieve symptoms. This means that some patients are getting antibiotics that aren't doing them any good—and that may do harm, considering that the drugs can disrupt the normal beneficial bacteria in the gut and worsen diarrhea.

Exceptions: For complicated diverticulitis, antibiotics are likely to reduce symptoms by helping limit infection and inflammation. And the drugs are absolutely warranted when a CT scan (typically done during diagnosis) shows either an abscess or a phlegmon, an area of inflammation that has not yet developed into an abscess. An abscess also requires drainage, which can be done through a small puncture in the skin.

• **Probiotics—maybe.** Some experts believe that an imbalance of the normal gut bacteria contributes to chronic inflammation and diverticulitis. This study's review included one small study of people who were randomly assigned to take either a placebo or a supplement containing probiotics (beneficial digestive bacteria) after their diverticulitis was treated with antibiotics. There was no difference in the rate of diverticulitis recurrence between the two groups. However, those who used probiotics reported less abdominal pain and bloating.

• **Anti-inflammatory medication.** Diverticulitis appears to share some traits with inflammatory bowel disease (IBD), a broad term that describes several conditions characterized by chronic or recurring inflammation of the gastrointestinal tract. An anti-inflammatory drug called *mesalamine* (Pentasa), which is used to treat IBD, shows some promise for also reducing the underlying inflammation of the colon wall that may contribute to diverticulitis.

• **Clear liquid diet at first...followed by an increase in fiber.** Consuming only water, tea, broth and juice for three or four days reduces abdominal pain and gives the digestive tract a chance to recover. Generally, after several days, solid food can be gradually reintroduced. Going forward, it's a good idea to increase your intake of fiber. Some studies show that people who eat a high-fiber diet have lower risk of ever developing diverticulitis, so even though there's no evidence that fiber helps prevent a recurrence, it can't hurt. As for the old admonishment that people with a history of diverticulitis should avoid nuts, seeds and popcorn like the plague—for fear that these small, hard foods would get trapped in the pouches and trigger another flare-up—that notion has been debunked. These foods are nutritious and high in fiber, so it's fine to go ahead and enjoy them.

The Worst Drugs for Gut Health

Anita Gupta, DO, PharmD, MPP, board-certified anesthesiologist, pharmacist and former FDA adviser. She currently is a physician with Penn Medicine Princeton Health in Princeton, New Jersey.

Antibiotics are known to upset the harmonious balance of the microbiome—the trillions of bacteria in your gastrointestinal (GI) tract that are critically important to maintaining your overall health. As antibiotics eradicate harmful bacteria, they may inadvertently target the good-for-you ones, too, that keep this balance in check.

Shocking new finding: One out of four non-antibiotic drugs also inhibits the growth of at least one strain of healthy gut bacteria, according to a new study in *Nature*.

Among the medications known to disrupt your friendly microbiome flora...

- **Acid-reducing medications.** Proton pump inhibitors (PPIs) such as *omeprazole* (Prilosec OTC) and *esomeprazole* (Nexium) treat heartburn, ulcers and reflux by reducing acid production in the stomach. That ultimately lessens the amount of acid that reaches your gut.

But your gut microbiome wants an acidic environment, which helps healthy bacteria, such as *Lactobacillus* and *Bifidobacterium,* thrive and keeps harmful ones at bay. So while changing the gut's pH to a more basic, less acidic level may improve symptoms, it allows dangerous bacteria to proliferate.

Recent finding: A review of studies that included about 300,000 patients found a 65% increase in the incidence of *Clostridium difficile* (*C. difficile*)–associated diarrhea among PPI patients. C. difficile releases toxins that damage the intestinal wall, causing pain, diarrhea and fever. Unwanted *Streptococcus* and *Staphylococcus* bacteria and *Escherichia coli* (*E. coli*) also tend to be more prevalent in the gut microbiome of PPI users.

Note: H2 receptor antagonists, known as H2 blockers, such as *ranitidine* (Zantac) or *cimetidine* (Tagamet), exert similar effects on the microbiome, though their impact is less potent than that of PPIs.

Try instead: As many as 70% of PPI patients may be taking them unnecessarily. Ideally, you want to take the smallest dose of these drugs for the shortest duration possible. Talk to your doctor about possibly tapering off by switching to a 20-mg dose of a mild PPI, such as omeprazole...then to an H2 blocker for a week or two...then slowly stopping altogether. Lifestyle modifications, including weight loss, smoking cessation and dietary tweaks to curb acid reflux, often are a first line of defense for indigestion.

Algae-based heartburn medicines such as Gaviscon may ease stomach upset by coating the stomach lining and, in turn, have less impact on the microbiome. Most people take two to four tablets after meals and at bedtime, up to four times daily.

Bifidobacterium has been shown to inhibit or prevent C. difficile infections, so consider a Bifidobacterium-containing probiotic, such as MegaFlora for Over 50 ($41.90 for 60 capsules, MegaFood.com) when taking a PPI.

If you use both a PPI and a probiotic, take them separately to avoid canceling out the effects of each one. Most people take the PPI first and wait several hours before taking the probiotic. Talk to your physician to determine the best timing based on the PPI you're taking.

• **Nonsteroidal anti-inflammatory drugs (NSAIDs).** NSAIDs, such as over-the-counter *ibuprofen* (Advil, Motrin) and *naproxen* (Aleve) and prescription *celecoxib* (Celebrex) and *meloxicam* (Mobic), relieve pain by blocking the formation of inflammatory compounds called prostaglandins. But there actually are several types of prostaglandins in the body, including one that protects the lining of the GI tract. Chronic NSAID use can erode this lining, causing leaky gut syndrome. That's when dangerous bacteria "leak" into the bloodstream where they don't belong and can wreak havoc by triggering inflammation, allergies, autoimmune disease and more damage to the microbiome.

Even worse: As the lining erodes, stomach bleeding and ulcers can occur. Patients end up using an acid-blocking medication to get relief, further compromising the microbiome.

Recent findings: NSAIDs also change the composition and diversity of gut microbes. In a study published in *Clinical Microbiology and Infection*, taking celecoxib or ibuprofen was linked with a surplus of *Enterobacteriaceae* bacteria, which can lead to serious infections in older adults.

Other research shows that when NSAIDs alter the microbiome, how the drug itself is broken down is impacted and its effectiveness is diminished. So when you must use an NSAID, take the lowest dose for the shortest duration possible.

Try instead: Yoga and physical therapy may ease pain and help you avoid NSAIDs altogether. Acupuncture stimulates the production of endogenous opioids, your body's own natural pain relievers, and may ease back, neck and shoulder osteoarthritis and headache pain.

A combination of feverfew, an anti-inflammatory plant in the daisy family, and ginger was shown to eliminate or significantly reduce migraine pain in 63% of participants within two hours, according to a study in *Headache*. Run-of-the-mill headaches should respond, too. (*Try*: GelStat Migraine.) Drinking 10.5 ounces of anti-inflammatory tart cherry juice can ease muscle soreness after a workout.

According to a study in *Phytotherapy Research*, rheumatoid arthritis patients who took 500-mg supplements of curcumin, a natural anti-inflammatory compound found in turmeric, experienced more pain relief after eight weeks than those taking an NSAID.

Note: Avoid curcumin if you have ulcers or gallstones or take an anticoagulant.

• **Iron supplements.** Do you take an iron supplement or a multivitamin with iron? Many older adults begin taking these on their own to avoid anemia. If you have colon cancer or a GI disorder such as ulcerative colitis or Crohn's, you may have been prescribed iron pills to counter the iron deficiency that often accompanies these conditions.

The problem: Less than 20% of the iron in most supplements is absorbed, mostly in the small intestine. The rest makes its way to the colon where nasty bacteria, including *Salmonella*, *Shigella* and E. coli, depend on it to survive and proliferate. So once that unabsorbed iron reaches the colon, it fuels bad bugs.

Try instead: Most healthy people can get enough iron through diet. In fact, women typically experience an increase in iron stores postmenopause, as they're no longer losing iron through menstruation. A simple blood test can determine whether you need supplements.

If so, try a brand containing ferrous sulfate, which is better absorbed than other forms. (*Try*: Nature Made Iron.) That said, ferrous sulfate is notoriously constipating, so up your daily fiber intake to 30 g, drink plenty of water and get regular exercise to keep things moving.

After a few months, you may be able to switch to less constipating ferrous gluconate (it has less elemental iron by weight than ferrous sulfate, making it a step-down choice).

Tip: Look for the words "Slow Fe" on the bottle. This means the iron is released at a slower rate, which can be less constipating.

What's Really Causing That "Stomach Bug"

Deborah A. Fisher, MD, associate professor of medicine in the division of gastroenterology at Duke University School of Medicine, associate director of gastroenterology research at Duke Clinical Research Institute and director of social and digital media accounts for Duke's GI division, all in Durham, North Carolina.

When stomach upset hits, if you're like most people you blame that awful cramping, diarrhea, nausea and other gastrointestinal (GI) distress on something you ate. It's true that one in six US adults do experience a bout of food poisoning every year (see box on next page). *But there are other culprits that are less recognized...*

- **Medications.** Certain prescription and over-the-counter medications can cause GI distress...

- **Nonsteroidal anti-inflammatory drugs (NSAIDs).** *Ibuprofen* (Advil, Motrin), *naproxen* (Aleve) and other NSAIDs are known to cause dyspepsia. Dyspepsia, better known as indigestion, is marked by pain and burning in the upper abdomen, below the breastbone, and queasiness without vomiting. Dyspepsia can also occur with other drugs such as some antibiotics (see below).

In one Canadian study, up to 30% of patients with dyspepsia were found to be taking an NSAID.

What helps: Try lowering your NSAID dose, but realize that some people cannot tolerate even a low dose. If this approach doesn't help, try switching to *acetaminophen* (Tylenol), which may be equally effective in treating pain but without stomach discomfort.

Note: Long-term use of an NSAID or acetaminophen can have side effects. Both types of pain relievers are for occasional use only.

- **Proton pump inhibitors (PPIs).** These stomach acid medications have been linked to higher rates of diarrhea caused by the dangerous *Clostridium difficile* bacterium. Chronic PPI use (generally, more than six months) reduces the diversity of bacteria in your GI tract, possibly allowing unhealthy bugs to thrive.

Commonly used PPIs include *esomeprazole* (Nexium), *lansoprazole* (Prevacid) and *omeprazole* (Prilosec). If you experience persistent, watery diarrhea, stomach pain and fever, and are taking a PPI, talk to your doctor. He/she may test you for *Clostridium difficile*–associated diarrhea, which can be treated with antibiotics. If PPI use causes GI distress, ask your doctor about taking *ranitidine* (Zantac) on an as-needed basis—it's less likely to cause stomach problems than PPIs.

- **Antibiotics.** *Azithromycin* (Zithromax, Zithromax Z-Pak) and *erythromycin* (Eryc, Ery-Tab) are among the antibiotics most likely to cause diarrhea by speeding up food's transit time through the intestine. Typically, you just have to ride it out, being sure to stay hydrated.

Helpful: Water with a splash of orange juice and a pinch of salt is an effective, inexpensive substitute for store-bought, electrolyte-infused water.

Also: Ask your doctor whether your antibiotic can be taken with food—such as crackers—to help prevent GI symptoms. Some data suggest that taking probiotics may help counteract the GI effects of antibiotics. Get them via fermented foods such as kefir, sauerkraut, yogurt, kimchi and miso soup. Never stop an antibiotic without first consulting your doctor.

- **Selective serotonin reuptake inhibitors (SSRIs).** This class of antidepressants, including *fluoxetine* (Prozac), *sertraline* (Zoloft) and *paroxetine* (Paxil), can cause nausea and diarrhea in some patients. This usually subsides in a few weeks.

FODMAPs, or fermentable oligosaccharides disaccharides monosaccharides and polyols. These are difficult-to-digest sugars such as lactose, found in dairy products...fructose, in fruit...fructan, in wheat and good-for-you veggies including asparagus, onions, garlic and artichokes...and galactans, in complex carbohydrates such as beans, including kidney beans, chickpeas and soybean products.

For unknown reasons, in some people, the carbohydrates in high-FODMAP foods don't get digested in the small intestine. The undigested carbohydrates advance to the large intestine, where bacteria feast on them, causing cramping and gas, and draw excess water into the colon, triggering diarrhea. If your GI discomfort flares up when eating one of the foods above, see a gastroenterologist to find out if FODMAPs are to blame.

Helpful: The American Gastroenterological Association offers a downloadable guide for following a low-FODMAP diet.

- **Stomach flu.** At least 20 million Americans are hit with acute gastroenteritis (commonly known as "stomach flu") every year. It's usually caused by the norovirus, which spreads rampantly through crowded areas such as hospitals, airplanes, cruise ships and nursing homes. The virus makes its way from an infected person's feces or vomit into your mouth, usually when you touch a contaminated surface (a toilet handle or an ATM machine, for example) or eat food prepared by a person who is infected.

Symptoms such as diarrhea, vomiting, stomach pain, fever, headache and body aches usually begin within 12 to 48 hours of exposure, and most individuals recover in one to three days. There is no effective treatment. Protect yourself with thorough handwashing using soap and water. An alcohol-based hand sanitizer should not be used as a substitute for soap and water. Good handwashing is essential to avoid transmission. If you become sick, avoid preparing food for others.

Note: Stomach flu is not the same as the flu, which is a respiratory illness caused by the influenza virus. For this reason, getting a flu shot won't protect you from stomach flu. Also, stomach flu is easily confused with food poisoning, which causes similar symptoms. For more on food poisoning, see the end of this article.

- **Too much fiber.** Following a high-fiber diet is a healthy move. But consuming too much fiber too quickly can cause cramping, bloating and gas.

Better: Gradually increase your consumption of produce (such as broccoli, carrots, avocado, apples, pears and figs) and beans by one to two servings a day—or a fiber supplement by one tablespoon a day. As long as you experience no adverse GI symptoms, continue increasing your intake slowly for a total of 30 g of fiber per day for men...and 21 g for women. If you are taking a laxative for constipation, synthetic fibers such as *methylcellulose* (Citrucel) may be less gas-forming than natural fibers such as *psyllium* (Metamucil).

- **Stress.** If you've ever been stuck on the toilet due to nerves, you know that the brain and belly are linked. Numerous studies have suggested that some GI problems may have a neurological component.

Why: More than 100 million neurons (cells that carry messages from the brain to other parts of the body) line the human GI tract—creating "the second brain." Not only can stress lead to upset stomach, new research suggests that the effect may also work in reverse, possibly explaining why many people with irritable bowel syndrome and other GI disorders develop depression and/or anxiety. Cognitive behavioral therapy or hypnotherapy tailored for GI issues may help. Ask your doctor for a referral.

WHAT IF IT IS FOOD POISONING?

Food poisoning is no fun! If you consume food that has been contaminated with bacteria, such as *E. coli* or *Staphylococcus aureus,* the telltale symptoms, including abdominal cramps, diarrhea and vomiting, often come on suddenly and typically last for 72 hours or so.

Due to the "transit time" it takes food to make its way through your body's digestive system, it's likely that something you ate a few hours before symptoms began—or even a few days earlier—is to blame.

Foods that most often cause food poisoning: Undercooked meat or poultry, ground meat, unpasteurized dairy, improperly washed fresh produce and food contaminated by a sick food handler.

Note: Many fast-food chains source their meat and eggs from multiple farms, increasing your risk for exposure to bacteria.

If you get food poisoning, be sure to stay hydrated (drink enough fluids so that your urine is light colored). Dizziness when standing can be caused by dehydration. Uncontrolled vomiting requires prompt medical attention.

Important: If you experience vomiting and diarrhea for more than 72 hours—or bloody diarrhea at any time—call your doctor. You may have a particularly virulent strain of E. coli that can cause kidney failure and may require IV fluids and perhaps even short-term dialysis. (For natural relief, see the following article.)

How to Bounce Back from Food Poisoning

Jamison Starbuck, ND, naturopathic physician in family practice and a guest lecturer at the University of Montana, both in Missoula.

So you had a great time at an outdoor cookout. The barbecued chicken was delicious, and you even had seconds of the potato salad. But now you're struck with a queasy, sick feeling. As you rush off to the bathroom, a sinking realization takes hold—you have food poisoning.

If you've ever had this extremely uncomfortable condition, the symptoms are unmistakable: nausea, stomach pain and loose bowel movements that come fast and furious every half hour or so. As the infecting organisms invade your intestines, it gets even worse. You're likely to start vomiting...have a mild fever and ongoing abdominal cramps—and just feel lousy.

The good news is that natural medicine can shorten an episode of food poisoning from three to four days to a day or two and dramatically reduce the severity of symptoms. *Here are my favorite methods...**

- **Take activated charcoal.** At the first sign of food poisoning, take two capsules of activated charcoal and repeat every four waking hours until your symptoms are gone. Activated charcoal can be purchased from a natural-food store. Inside your system, toxins attach to the surface of the activated charcoal and are drawn out of the stomach and intestines.

- **Use antiseptic herbs.** Oregon grape root, uva ursi and gingerroot will help kill the organism causing your food poisoning. You can use any of these herbs individually or buy a tincture that contains all three of them for the greatest benefit.

Typical adult dose: Sixty drops (about one-quarter teaspoon) in one ounce of water every four waking hours for up to three days.

- **Try carob powder.** Unsweetened carob powder, available in bulk at most natural-food grocers, has a "binding" effect and will ease diarrhea. I usually prescribe it along with slippery elm powder, an herb that soothes the digestive tract and helps reduce abdominal pain. Add two teaspoons of carob powder and two teaspoons of slippery elm powder to one-quarter cup of unsweetened applesauce. Eat the mixture slowly throughout the day. Repeat daily until symptoms are gone.

- **Drink clear liquids.** If you limit your diet to mostly clear liquids, you can reduce diarrhea by slowing down the activity of your gut.

Good choices: Vegetable broth...peppermint, chamomile and/or raspberry leaf herbal teas...and plain water.

Also helpful: Try rice water—cook one cup of brown or white rice in four cups of water, strain off the liquid and drink six ounces several times a day. This gives you starch, which slows diarrhea, without taxing your gut to digest the rice. Avoid dairy products, meat, eggs and beans—these foods are hard to digest when the body is fighting a bug and will worsen your symptoms.

Caution: Seek prompt medical attention if you experience diarrhea for more than three days. Also see a doctor if you have a fever above 101.5°F...blood in the stool or in vomit...severe abdominal pain...lack of urination...or more than one episode of difficulty swallowing, vision changes, fainting or dizziness. These can be signs that infection has spread throughout your body.

*Check with your doctor before using herbal therapies.

Get Rid of That Tummy Ache Naturally

Lori DiBacco, ND, naturopathic doctor in private practice at Northeast Integrative Medicine in Bedford, New Hampshire, and Winchester Natural Health Associates in Winchester, Massachusetts.

If you are like a lot of healthy-minded people, you try not to overdo it, especially over the holidays or during vacations. But with all the temptations, it's sometimes difficult not to eat or drink those special foods that you normally avoid—let alone eat too much of them. To make sure that you know about easy-to-take natural remedies if you do hit a brief period of indigestion, we turned to Lori DiBacco, ND, a naturopathic doctor in private practice in New Hampshire and Massachusetts, who specializes in detoxification and endocrinology. *Here is what she recommends to her patients with bouts of indigestion...*

For occasional periods of indigestion, there are several safe natural remedies to choose from that have very few or no adverse side effects when taken as directed on the label.

WHAT CAN HELP

While many people may turn to conventional over-the-counter treatments for indigestion, such as antacids, these may actually hinder the stomach's natural production of acid. We need this acid to help break down our food and make nutrients more easily absorbed by the body.

What many naturopathic doctors find: The root of many people's digestive problems, especially as they get older, is lack of stomach acid or insufficient digestive enzyme production. Several natural remedies can help—some by stimulating the body's production of enzymes...others by soothing irritated tissues. Patients are encouraged to experiment to find the remedy that works best for them.

- **Digestive enzymes.** Digestive enzymes, which are readily available in supplement form at drugstores and health-food stores, help to increase the supply of enzymes produced by the body.

Best choice: "Full-spectrum" enzymes, a type of supplement that may contain as many as a dozen or more enzymes that help with the breakdown of all types of foods.

When to take them: Right before or in the early part of every meal.

- **Herbal teas.** Ginger tea can help stimulate digestion—and your body's production of digestive enzymes.

When to drink: Drink a cup right before or in the early part of a meal. Slippery elm or licorice tea can help soothe irritated tissues and reduce inflammation.

When to drink: When symptoms occur. These teas are available either in tea bags or loose at health-food stores.

- **Apple cider vinegar.** This type of vinegar is known to help stimulate your body's production of digestive enzymes.

When to take: Start with one teaspoon of apple cider vinegar mixed in any amount of warm water. If that doesn't help, gradually increase the amount of apple cider vinegar up to three teaspoons.

When to drink: Right before eating meals.

PREVENTING STOMACH UPSET

One way to prevent future bouts of indigestion is simply this: Slow down. Eat slowly and chew your food completely. This gives the enzymes in your saliva time to begin digesting food...and signals the stomach to start making and secreting your digestive enzymes.

WHEN TO SEEK HELP

If your indigestion continues, your symptoms might be a sign of an underlying digestive problem, such as gastroesophageal reflux disease (GERD), gastritis, ulcers, gallbladder disease or irritable bowel syndrome. If that's the case, speak to a holistic doctor who can help you figure out exactly what is causing the indigestion and can treat it accordingly.

Is Your Sugarless Gum Giving You a Stomachache?

Andrew L. Rubman, ND, director, Southbury Clinic for Traditional Medicines, Southbury, Connecticut.

Sugarless gum seems practically virtuous—a sweet treat with few, if any, calories and no sugar. Yet a report in the *British Medical Journal* told of two patients who experienced serious and inexplicable pain or gas and diarrhea, along with extreme weight loss...which doctors finally tracked down to their heavy gum-chewing habits—around 20 sorbitol-sweetened sticks a day.

THE SORBITOL STORY

Commercially produced sugar alcohols such as sorbitol—and indeed, all its cousins with the "ol" suffix, including xylitol, erythritol and mannitol—are widely used as substitute sweeteners. Sorbitol, in particular, is used in cough drops and a wide variety of diet and diabetic food products, including candies, cookies, cakes and sugar-free maple syrup. Labels proudly proclaim the sugar-free, low-calorie status of these foods—what they don't say, however, is that ingested in large quantities, the sweetener they are formulated with is known to cause abdominal pain, bloating, gas and diarrhea. Interestingly, few people have such troubles with natural sorbitol, found in some fruits such as apples, cherries, peaches, pears, plums and prunes. According to naturopath Andrew L. Rubman, ND, excessive sorbitol disrupts the large intestine's natural function of recapturing water from the mass that passes through it. This potentially creates wider imbalances in the microfloral community in the gut and the underlying tissues, which—as regular readers have heard before—creates a difficult set of problems.

In fact, the FDA regulates sorbitol, requiring information about gastrointestinal side effects on the label if the sorbitol-containing foods might result in a total daily consumption of 50 grams. A stick of gum or a candy contains only a gram or two of sorbitol, so it carries no cautionary information.

This is unfortunate, to say the least, since much lower levels have been known to cause harm. The patients described in the study lost 20% of their body weight, consuming 20 to 30 grams of sorbitol daily for months. Study authors warned that as little as 5 to 20 grams a day could result in bloating and cramps. The severity of symptoms is a question of sensitivity and degree of exposure. Some people—especially children, people who are chronically ill and individuals with digestive issues—are naturally more sensitive than others, and cumulative exposure to even small amounts of sorbitol can quickly add up in the short run. If you are indeed sensitive, you have probably noticed this effect already.

Your best bet: Eat real foods. Time and again, we see new evidence that the empty calories and additives in processed foods are just not worth it.

Natural Therapies for Ulcers

James N. Dillard, MD, DC, former assistant clinical professor at Columbia University College of Physicians and Surgeons and past clinical director of Columbia's Rosenthal Center for Complementary and Alternative Medicine, both in New York City.

If you've got an ulcer, chances are you're taking an over-the-counter (OTC) antacid and/or prescription medication to neutralize gastric acid or inhibit its production. These medications include proton pump inhibitors (PPIs), such as *esomeprazole* (Nexium) and *lansoprazole* (Prevacid), and H2-blocking drugs, such as *cimetidine* (Tagamet) and *ranitidine* (Zantac).

What most people don't realize: There are several natural, complementary remedies that help reduce ulcer symptoms and promote healing while conventional treatment is under way. Some of these treatments also can help prevent ulcers in some patients.

WHAT CAUSES ULCERS

It's been more than 20 years since doctors learned that an infectious disease—rather than emotional stress—was the primary cause of most ulcers.

A screw-shaped bacterium, *Helicobacter pylori*, or *H. pylori*, burrows through the protective mucous lining in the small intestine and/or stomach, allowing harsh digestive fluids to accumulate and ulcerate the lining. About 50% of Americans over age 60 are infected with H. pylori. The bacterium doesn't always cause ulcers—but about 60% of patients with ulcers harbor H. pylori.

The remainder of ulcers are caused by regular use of stomach-damaging nonsteroidal anti-inflammatory drugs (NSAIDs), such as aspirin, *ibuprofen* (Advil) and *naproxen* (Aleve)...alcohol...and/or smoking. Excessive alcohol wears down the lining of the stomach and intestines. Nicotine causes the stomach to produce more acid.

Best complementary treatments...*

NONDRUG THERAPIES

• **Probiotics.** The intestine contains up to four pounds of "friendly" bacteria, which aid digestion. There's some evidence that maintaining adequate levels of beneficial bacteria helps create an inhospitable environment for H. pylori and makes it harder for this ulcer-causing bacterium to thrive.

Self-defense: Take a probiotic supplement that contains *Lactobacillus acidophilus* and *Bifidobacterium bifidus*. These organisms create a healthful mix of bacteria and can inhibit the growth of harmful organisms. Probiotics are helpful if you've taken antibiotics, which can kill off some beneficial bacteria.

The optimal dose for probiotics hasn't been determined. Preliminary research cites a daily dose of up to 10 billion organisms—the amount usually included in one to two capsules. Probiotics are available at health-food stores.

• **Cabbage juice.** This folk remedy has some evidence to support it. Cabbage is high in vitamin C, which seems to inhibit growth of H. pylori. It also contains glutamine, an amino acid that may strengthen the protective lining in the stomach.

A small Stanford University School of Medicine study found that ulcer patients who drank about a quart of cabbage juice daily healed significantly faster than those who didn't drink it.

Self-defense: If you have an active ulcer, consider drinking a quart of cabbage juice (about the amount in half a head of cabbage) once daily for up to two weeks.

• **Deglycyrrhizinated licorice (DGL).** Herbalists often recommend fresh licorice root to heal ulcers. Licorice contains mucin, a substance that protects the stomach lining, and antioxidants that may inhibit H. pylori growth.

However, natural licorice can increase the effects of aldosterone, a hormone that promotes water retention and can increase blood pressure in some people. DGL supplements (available at health-food stores) are a better option, because the substances that increase blood pressure have been removed.

Self-defense: Take one DGL tablet before meals, and another before bed. DGL may be effective for people with ulcers whose H. pylori has been successfully treated with antibiotics but who still have some stomach irritation.

• **Vitamin A.** Vitamin A helps repair damaged mucous membranes. A report in the British medical journal *The Lancet* suggests that ulcers heal more quickly in patients given supplemental vitamin A.

Caution: High-dose vitamin A therapy can be toxic, so get your vitamin A from dietary sources along with a daily multivitamin—not from a separate vitamin A supplement.

Self-defense: Get 10,000 international units (IU) of vitamin A daily if you're undergoing ulcer treatment. (A multivitamin typically contains 3,500 IU to 5,000 IU of vitamin A.)

Good food sources: Beef liver (1½ ounces contains 13,593 IU)...carrots (one raw carrot contains 8,666 IU)...and spinach (one cup of raw spinach contains 2,813 IU).

• **Zinc.** Like vitamin A, zinc is involved in tissue healing. In Europe, a drug compound made with zinc plus an anti-inflammatory is often used for treating ulcers. Early studies indicate that zinc alone can speed ulcer healing and possibly even help prevent some ulcers.

Self-defense: Don't exceed the recommended daily intake (15 mg) of zinc. Take a daily multivitamin that includes zinc...and get ad-

*Check with your doctor before taking supplements. They can interact with prescription medications.

equate intake from dietary sources (five medium fried oysters, 13 mg...3⁄4 cup fortified breakfast cereal, 15 mg...three ounces lean beef tenderloin, 5 mg).

ANOTHER WAY TO FIGHT ULCERS

NSAIDs alleviate pain by inhibiting the production of pain-causing chemicals called prostaglandins. However, the body produces several kinds of prostaglandins, including some that protect the stomach lining. That's why NSAIDs, which block the production of pain-causing and stomach-protecting prostaglandins, make people who regularly use the drugs more susceptible to ulcers.

Self-defense: If you require regular pain relief, start with *acetaminophen* (Tylenol). It relieves pain without depleting stomach-protecting prostaglandins.

Caution: Taking more than the recommended dosage or drinking alcohol with acetaminophen can cause liver damage.

Also helpful: Ask your doctor about taking Arthrotec, a prescription drug combination that includes the NSAID diclofenac along with misoprostol, which protects the stomach and intestinal lining. One study found that patients taking Arthrotec experienced up to 80% fewer ulcers than those taking an NSAID alone.

Quick and Easy First Aid for Indigestion, Constipation And Diarrhea

Andrew L. Rubman, ND, founder and medical director, Southbury Clinic for Traditional Medicines, Southbury, Connecticut. He writes the "Nature Doc's Patient Diary" blog at BottomLineInc.com/blogs.

Even if you eat a healthy diet and get plenty of exercise, digestive problems still happen. If they happen a lot, you should check with your doctor to rule out underlying serious health issues. But for once-in-a-while indigestion, constipation and/or diarrhea, there are easy, natural remedies that will soon have your gut feeling better.

FOR OCCASIONAL INDIGESTION

If you ate too much...or too fast...or if something you ate "didn't agree with you," you can try...

- **Baking soda.** Sodium bicarbonate, commonly known as baking soda, neutralizes the acidity in your stomach. Mix about one-half teaspoon of baking soda with four ounces of water, and slowly sip the mixture. Relief should come quickly (and maybe a belch or two).

Important: Wait for at least two hours after eating to drink this remedy—you do not want to partially neutralize the acid that is needed to digest food and absorb nutrients.

FOR OCCASIONAL CONSTIPATION OR DIARRHEA

Both of these conditions can be the result of a poor diet...the wrong mix of organisms in the gut microbiome...and/or certain medications. Not drinking enough water also can cause constipation. *What can help...*

- **Probiotics.** There are many different kinds of beneficial probiotic bacteria that we need to have in our guts for good digestive health. Some of the most well-studied strains with evidence of gut benefit are Lactobacillus casei, Lactobacillus acidophilus and Lactobacillus rhamnosus GG—all particularly good for treating diarrhea but also helpful for treating constipation. Lactobacillus supplements are available over-the-counter in grocery and drugstores.

Align is a good product with a patented strain of another probiotic (*Bifidobacterium infantis*) that works well with Lactobacillus and that has shown gut benefits in industry-sponsored studies.

Follow the label directions for the correct dose. You should get relief within 12 to 18 hours, although complete healing can take three to five days.

Bonus: Probiotic products containing Lactobacillus have been found to significantly reduce flatulence.

- **Glucomannan.** This water-soluble fiber supplement is made from the root of the konjac plant. It is an effective "bulk-forming" laxative, so it helps with constipation but not diarrhea. As a bonus, glucomannan also helps relieve nausea.

This type of laxative swells in the intestine, softening the stool and making it easier to pass. When using to relieve constipation, take one 575-mg capsule of glucomannan with at least a full eight ounces of water up to three times a day, away from meals.

HOW TO KEEP YOUR DIGESTION WORKING GREAT

While the remedies above are good to have on hand, it's best if you don't have to use them often. *Here are some strategies to keep your digestion functioning smoothly...*

• **Chew thoroughly.** You'll eat more slowly, enjoy your food more—and give your stomach a break. Chewing sufficiently allows enzymes in saliva to start digestion in your mouth, as they're meant to do—and breaking the food into smaller particles lets your intestines better absorb nutrients.

• **Drink water, but not with your meal.** Drinking water or other liquids at mealtime dilutes the hydrochloric acid your stomach needs to digest food, slowing digestion and inhibiting absorption of nutrients.

It's OK to slowly sip just enough liquid at a meal to help you wash down mouthfuls of food if you want—but keep it to no more than four ounces. It's best not to drink close to meals—aim for a half hour before to an hour after. On the other hand, do be sure to drink enough liquids during the rest of the day.

Burning Abdominal Pain

Mark A. Stengler, NMD, naturopathic doctor and founder of the Stengler Center for Integrative Medicine in Encinitas, California. MarkStengler.com

By the time he consulted me, 57-year-old Shawn was fed up. For four decades, he had suffered from unpredictable bouts of burning abdominal pain that occurred about once a month and lasted for days. Each attack was accompanied by excessive burping and a bitter taste.

Over the years, Shawn had consulted half a dozen gastroenterologists and had numerous tests—including ultrasound and endoscopy—but no abnormalities had been found. Antibiotics provided only temporary relief. Shawn also took *pantoprazole* (Protonix), a prescription heartburn drug that reduces stomach acid. It did ease his heartburn but did not alleviate his sporadic abdominal pain.

A stool test showed undigested meat fibers, indicating poor protein digestion. This made sense, since Shawn was still taking the acid-suppressing medication. It also showed an overgrowth of the fungus *Candida albicans*—a common side effect of antibiotics, which destroy beneficial bacteria in the digestive tract that keep fungi in check.

Blood tests showed no signs of a food allergy but did show a deficiency of vitamin B-12, which is common in people with low levels of the stomach acids that promote absorption of certain nutrients. A B-12 deficiency also can result from excessive alcohol use—clearly the case for Shawn, who had several alcoholic drinks per day.

Since Shawn's abdominal pain was not the result of any single cause, we took an integrated approach. He agreed to cut back to three alcoholic drinks weekly and limit foods that contain simple sugars, such as soda and white bread. He began taking a daily B-12 supplement and, to reduce inflammation, an ingestible blend of aloe vera juice plus deglycyrrhizinated licorice root (DGL). (These shouldn't be used while pregnant or nursing.) I prescribed the homeopathic remedy *Chelidonium majus* (from the juice of a plant with the same name), to take at the first sign of abdominal pain (from Remedy Source, 301-908-7203, RemedySource.com).

A month later, Shawn reported that the Chelidonium majus brought quick relief during bouts of pain. I prescribed a supplement of antifungal herbs, including oregano oil and pau d'arco (from the taheebo tree), to halt the Candida overgrowth. After several months, Shawn was able to stop using his heartburn medication—and his abdominal pain became a thing of the past.

Peppermint Oil for Irritable Bowel Syndrome

Alexander Ford, MD, senior lecturer, section of molecular gastroenterology, Leeds Institute of Molecular Medicine, Leeds University, UK.

Peppermint oil can alleviate the gastrointestinal symptoms associated with IBS, including flatulence and abdominal pain and distension, by blocking the flow of calcium into muscle cells in the intestines, which in turn reduces muscle contractions.

Best: When symptoms are present, take two coated capsules of peppermint oil three times daily.

Herbs and More for Leaky Gut

Jamison Starbuck, ND, a naturopathic physician in family practice and writer/producer of Dr. Starbuck's Health Tips for Kids, a weekly program on Montana Public Radio, MTPR.org, both in Missoula. DrJamisonStarbuck.com

If you've got celiac disease, food allergies or an autoimmune bowel disease, such as Crohn's disease or inflammatory bowel disease, you probably have leaky gut syndrome. Also known as gastrointestinal permeability, leaky gut syndrome is a condition in which microscopic "holes" develop in the lining of the digestive tract as a result of medications, allergies to foods, genetics and other causes. Your digestive tract, or gut, is designed to keep food particles in your intestines and out of your bloodstream. When food is properly digested and broken down, food nutrients pass through the filter of the intestinal wall and into the bloodstream. This is how your body gets the nutrition it needs to survive.

With leaky gut syndrome, your gut wall is like a torn window screen. Insects that are meant to stay outside enter your home. When leaky gut occurs, overly large food molecules pass through these microscopic holes into your bloodstream. To the body, these large molecules are an enemy. The immune system responds protectively and makes defenders known as antibodies. If you have a lot of food-related antibodies, you have food allergies (or a food sensitivity). You'll also have an inflamed bowel and leaky gut syndrome.

One way to heal the symptoms of leaky gut syndrome, which include indigestion, irregular stools, generalized fatigue and inflammation, skin rashes and migraines, is to avoid the foods to which you are allergic. That can help. However, if you don't repair the intestinal wall, you'll continue to suffer with many of the above symptoms and may even become allergic to other foods.

How, then, do you treat the gut wall? *What I recommend...*

- **Eat the right foods.** Sauerkraut is rich in probiotics, which help crowd out pathogens that damage the gut wall. Do not use canned sauerkraut—the probiotics are killed in the heating process that is required for canning. Plant-based oils, such as olive, sunflower and borage, are nourishing to the intestine. Fish, baked or cooked on a grill, can also help heal a leaky gut. It is easy to digest, anti-inflammatory and contains helpful proteins and oils. Just be sure to avoid fried fish and fried foods generally. You may also want to try a probiotic supplement. Follow label instructions.

Caution: People with weakened immune systems (such as those using chemotherapy) should consult their doctors before eating probiotic-rich food or taking a probiotic supplement.

- **Consider these herbs.** My favorite herbs for leaky gut are slippery elm...marshmallow root...and plantain (a medicinal plant not to be confused with the banana-like food). You can use one of these herbs or combine two or more.

To treat leaky gut: You need to take herbal medicine between meals—60 minutes or more after a meal or 30 minutes or more before a meal—to ensure that the herb comes into direct contact with the gut wall.* You can take these herbs in capsules, tea or bulk powders.

*If you use any prescription medication, have a chronic medical condition (such as diabetes) or are pregnant or nursing, consult your doctor before taking any herbs.

Typical daily dose: Three standard-sized capsules two times a day...three cups of tea...or two teaspoons of the bulk-powdered herb. For convenience and taste, put the powdered herb in a small amount (one-eighth cup or less) of applesauce or oatmeal.

With my patients, treatment usually takes about three months to heal leaky gut. Assuming that one's diet stays healthy, the regimen above can often be discontinued when symptoms subside.

Use Your Mind to Heal Your Stomach

Miranda van Tilburg, PhD, assistant professor of medicine, University of North Carolina School of Medicine, Chapel Hill, commenting on research that was published in the *American Journal of Gastroenterology*.

Stomachaches—ugh! Whether you have chronic abdominal pain due to irritable bowel syndrome (IBS) or another health problem, such as Crohn's disease or functional abdominal pain (FAP), ongoing belly discomfort can rob the joy from your life. According to a recent study, "gut-directed" hypnotherapy can alleviate the pain.

ADJUSTING YOUR STATE OF MIND

The study, done by researchers from the Netherlands, tracked the impact of "gut-directed" hypnotherapy in girls and boys between the ages of 12 and 17 and young adults up to age 23 who had chronic abdominal pain.

All patients had participated in an earlier hypnotherapy study done by the same researchers five years before. In the earlier study, the patients had been split into two groups. Half underwent six sessions of hypnotherapy—including at-home "self-hypnosis"—while the rest were offered standard abdominal pain treatment consisting of pain medications, dietary changes and stress-reduction techniques.

About 68% of the participants who had been taught hypnosis were free or mostly free of abdominal pain five years later, compared with only 20% of those who had received standard therapy alone. Scores for headache, chronic fatigue and joint pain were markedly lower among the hypnosis group as well.

TRANCES AREN'T TRICKY

What is hypnotherapy? It's not as theatrical as television might lead you to believe. In general, it's done in a quiet room, where the patient sits, eyes closed, and imagines something fun—if the patient is a child, this could be going down a waterslide or riding a roller coaster. In this state of focused attention, while patients' eyes are still closed, they're given suggestions relating to how their bellies feel—for example, they might be told that there's a "protective layer" inside that prevents anything from bothering them. Hypnotherapy may help by reprogramming how signals from the gut are processed by the brain. In other words, hypnotherapy can help you trick yourself into feeling less pain.

If you suffer from abdominal pain, whether you're a child or an adult, ask your doctor about trying hypnotherapy, since there are no side effects. To find licensed health professionals who practice hypnosis, visit the website of the American Society of Clinical Hypnosis (Asch.net).

Digestive Enzymes May Be The Answer to Your Gut Pain

Leo Galland, MD, director of the Foundation for Integrated Medicine in New York City. He is coauthor of *The Allergy Solution: Unlock the Surprising, Hidden Truth About Why You Are Sick and How to Get Well.* DrGalland.com

If you watch the TV ads, you might think that a good probiotic is the answer for all your digestive problems. Don't believe it.

While it is true that probiotic supplements can help relieve gas and diarrhea—and boost your immunity—when your intestinal bacteria are out of whack, that's not always the issue.

Perhaps your gut has plenty of "friendly" bacteria, but you are still plagued by gut-related problems such as flatulence, heartburn, lactose intolerance, diarrhea or abdominal pain. What then?

It is time to think about taking digestive enzymes.* These supplements not only help relieve the digestive problems described above, they can also have powerful healing effects for other ailments, such as arthritis and sinusitis, that have nothing to do with the digestive system.

WHAT ARE DIGESTIVE ENZYMES?

Digestive enzymes are present in saliva, the stomach and the small intestine. Their job is to break down the food you eat into smaller components.

After about age 50, the pancreas produces only about half the amount of digestive enzymes that it did when you were younger. Some individuals find that they have less gas, bloating or fullness when they take an enzyme supplement during or after meals.

When to consider taking a digestive enzyme—most are available at drugstores or health-food stores…

• **Flatulence.** Most people have heard of the over-the-counter flatulence preventive known as Beano, but they do not necessarily know how it works. This product is actually a digestive enzyme called alpha-galactosidase. Taken just before consuming gassy foods, such as cabbage, beans, cauliflower and broccoli, it breaks down some of the complex carbohydrates into easily digestible sugars, thus preventing intestinal gas.

• **Heartburn.** I have seen some great responses in patients with frequent heartburn who take digestive enzymes along with—or instead of—over-the-counter remedies such as Tums with calcium, which tightens the valve between the stomach and esophagus. It is not clear how these enzymes help. It is possible that they deactivate some of the body's pepsin, a stomach enzyme that plays a crucial role in digestion but that surges upward from the stomach in some patients, damaging tissue in the esophagus. This is what causes the "burn" in heartburn.

What to try: A blend that includes different enzymes, such as lipase, protease and amylase. Some good products include AbsorbAid Digestive Support powder, Botanic Choice Digestive Enzyme Complex and Twinlab Super Enzyme Caps.

How to use it: Take the supplement with or just after meals.

• **Dairy Sensitivity.** It's estimated that up to 50 million Americans have symptoms of lactose intolerance, a sensitivity to dairy foods that can cause bloating, gas, cramps and other digestive problems. Humans are born with high levels of lactase, the enzyme that is required to digest a sugar (lactose) in dairy foods. But the levels drop in the first years after birth, so by adulthood, many people don't have enough lactase to comfortably digest dairy.

What to try: Supplemental lactase will replace the enzyme that's missing from the intestine. People who take lactase supplements can usually enjoy dairy foods without discomfort.

How to take it: Chew or swallow a tablet just before eating dairy…for milk and other liquidlike dairy, you can use lactase drops if you prefer.

Yet another option: Lactaid Milk, which comes with added lactase.

• **Gluten Intolerance.** If you are one of the millions of Americans who is sensitive to gluten, a protein that is contained in wheat, barley and rye, you already know that a simple slice of bread or a bowl of wheat cereal can lead to hours of digestive problems, such as diarrhea, stomach cramps and flatulence.

Important: Many people who think that they're gluten-intolerant actually have fructose malabsorption, which occurs when the small intestine can't absorb fructose, a plant sugar. Get checked by a doctor before assuming that gluten is the problem. Fructose malabsorption is typically diagnosed with a hydrogen breath test—after ingesting a fructose solution, the amount of hydrogen in your breath is measured. An increase in hydrogen means that the fructose has not been properly digested.

What to try: If you are sensitive to gluten, you can try taking a supplement such as GlutenEase, which contains a blend of protease enzymes. You might be able to eat small

*Digestive enzymes are generally safe, but check first with your doctor if you have a chronic condition or regularly take any medication or supplement.

amounts of wheat and other gluten-containing foods without discomfort.

How to use it: Take one capsule with meals. Double the dose if one capsule isn't effective.

If your gluten sensitivity is caused by celiac disease: Don't depend on any supplement. Patients with celiac disease must avoid even trace amounts of gluten, and supplements are unlikely to help.

IT'S NOT WHAT YOU EAT—IT'S HOW YOU EAT

If your gut acts up during or after a meal, you may want to change how you eat before trying a digestive enzyme. *What to do...*

- **Eat slowly and chew your food well.** This gives the enzymes in your saliva a better chance to start breaking down your food before it reaches your stomach.
- **Enjoy your food and relax.** People who are stressed have an increase in dopamine and adrenaline, hormones that inhibit normal digestion.
- **Be aware of any tension you feel in your body...**relax your shoulders and jaw... and breathe slowly (your abdomen should expand and your chest should not rise when you breathe in).
- **Take a walk after eating.** It increases metabolism and helps you digest more efficiently. It also stimulates motility, the intestinal movements that move food (and wastes) through your system. Walk for at least five minutes—a leisurely pace is fine to promote digestion.

Before You Give Up Gluten, Try a Low-FODMAP Diet

Peter Gibson, MD, professor and director of gastroenterology, Alfred and Monash University, Melbourne Australia. He is a recipient of the Gastroenterological Society of Australia's Distinguished Research Prize. For more information on FODMAP diets, check his department's website, Monashfodmap.com

These days just about everyone has a friend who has gone on a gluten-free diet and raves about it. Perhaps you've tried it yourself. Perhaps digestion improves, and so does well-being. Does that mean that you or your friend is sensitive to gluten?

Maybe not. Surprisingly, you may actually be reacting to a different ingredient in wheat... and in many other foods. Avoiding this particular class of hard-to-digest carbohydrates, called FODMAPs, may improve digestive symptoms in people who believe that they are sensitive to gluten.

That's not to say that gluten is suddenly fine for everyone. It's pure poison for the two million Americans with celiac disease, a digestive disease in which the body can't digest gluten, a protein found in wheat, rye and barley. Nor does it mean that non-celiac gluten sensitivity (NCGS) isn't real. It's just that the population with NCGS may be smaller than once believed—and certainly fewer than the 30% of Americans who currently try to avoid gluten in their diets.

The good news is that a careful plan to remove just the FODMAPs that are causing your particular reaction may lead to a less restrictive diet than a gluten-free one—and be more effective in fixing your digestion.

IS FODMAP THE NEW GLUTEN?

To understand the FODMAP/gluten story, step back to 2011. Australian researchers studied people who didn't have celiac disease but did have irritable bowel syndrome (IBS), with its symptoms of bloating, stomach pain, and diarrhea and constipation. (As many as 20% of Americans experience these symptoms in this often-undiagnosed and poorly understood condition.) In a randomized placebo-controlled study, the Australians reported that gluten made the 34 study participants' IBS symptoms worse and that a gluten-free diet reduced symptoms.

That very influential study helped establish the concept of non-celiac gluten sensitivity and boosted the popularity of gluten-free diets.

But then a couple of years later, the same researchers revisited the topic. They examined whether gluten was indeed the cause of symptoms in a group of people who had NCGS. These 37 patients "felt that gluten was the cause of their gut symptoms" explained the study's lead author, Peter Gibson, MD, professor and director of gastroenterology at The Alfred and Monash University in Melbourne, Australia. The study also looked at the effects of FODMAPs, which stands for fermentable oligosaccharides, disaccharides, monosaccharides and polyols. They're found in many foods, and some studies were starting to find that they could trigger IBS symptoms.

What the study found was surprising...

- **A low-FODMAP diet significantly reduced gastrointestinal symptoms.**
- **Participants who had reported improvements in GI symptoms on a gluten-free diet** before the study had even fewer symptoms on a low-FODMAP diet.
- **When the researchers "challenged" 37 of the participants by giving them food that contained either no gluten,** a small amount of gluten (2 grams), or a large amount of gluten (16 grams, about the amount in 10 slices of wheat bread), there was no difference in symptoms. In other words, gluten had no effect on symptoms.

While the study had a small number of subjects (as did the 2011 one), it was carefully designed to provide reliable clinical results. Not only was it double-blind, so that neither researcher nor subject expectations could affect the results, and placebo controlled, but it was a "cross-over re-challenge" study—each participant got each one of the different diets. "This kind of study is the gold standard way of determining whether a food is causing symptoms," said Dr. Gibson. "If gluten was the cause of the symptoms, then it would cause greater symptoms than the placebo. It did not. That is why gluten is unlikely to be the culprit in those subjects studied."

THE LOW-FODMAP DIET TAKES OFF

Since that study was published, the benefits of a low-FODMAP diet for people with digestive symptoms has become even clearer. Researchers who've been looking for ways to help people with IBS, for example, are almost giddy with excitement—well, as giddy as scientists get in print—with editorials such as "Diet as a Therapy for Irritable Bowel Syndrome: Progress at Last." One 2014 study of the low-FODMAP diet for IBS concluded: "This high-quality evidence supports its use as a first-line therapy." A recent study of dieticians found that in their experience, a low-FODMAP diet helps patients with GI symptoms better than the old advice to "eat a healthy diet" while restricting lactose-containing foods and cutting back on caffeine.

To be sure, the debate over whether NCGS is a distinct clinical diagnosis, unrelated to FODMAP sensitivity, at least for some people, continues. One 2015 scientific review concluded that it is not clear whether what is thought to be NCGS is caused by gluten or FODMAPs, for example. However, Alessio Fasano, MD, director of the Center for Celiac Research and Treatment at the Mass General Hospital for Children in Boston, pointed out in a 2015 scientific review that people with NCGS often have immunological reactions to wheat and other grains—not just stomach problems. NCGS may contribute to other conditions including chronic fatigue syndrome and autoimmune diseases, he argues. To make matters even more complicated, there are other ingredients in wheat, rye, and barley, such as amylase-trypsin inhibitors (ATIs), that may trigger immune response–related symptoms. Dr. Fasano said that a better name for NCGS is non-celiac wheat sensitivity. Going on a low-FODMAP diet wouldn't address these concerns.

For now, though, if you have unresolved digestive symptoms, it's clearly time to give a low-FODMAP diet a close look. "Our advice is to try reducing FODMAPs first, since this is an easier diet than a gluten-free diet," explained Dr. Gibson. Based on research, he estimates that about 70% of people with IBS symptoms will benefit.

HOW TO GO ON A LOW-FODMAP DIET

"The major argument against the low-FODMAP approach is that it is too difficult, but that is the opinion of people who do not know much about how easy the low-FODMAP diet is to implement," said Dr. Gibson.

It is true that FODMAPs are very common in a typical Western diet. FODMAPs include fructans, found in wheat as well as onions and garlic...fructose, high-fructose corn syrup, and some fruits such as apples and pears...lactose, the sugar in milk and other dairy products... polyols, found in the sweetener sorbitol and in stone fruits such as plums and cherries...and galacto-oligosaccharides, found in beans, lentils and soybeans. However, many individuals are more sensitive to some FODMAPs than others. It's also the dose of FODMAPs that counts—a little bit is OK but a lot will cause symptoms. So you may need to reduce FODMAPs a small amount to feel better. (That's why it's a "low-FODMAP" diet, not a "FODMAP-free diet.")

That's good, because many of these foods are very nutritious. It's best, by far, to get help from a dietician if you want to see whether you would feel better on a low-FODMAP diet—a dietician will guide you through a FODMAP-elimination process in which you will get rid of most or all FODMAPS and then carefully add each type back, in turn, to see which ones cause your symptoms. A dietician can also help make sure you eat a nutritious diet even if you need to eliminate certain classes of foods. To learn more, Stanford University has a good list of FODMAPs at StanfordHealthcare.org/medical-treatments/l/low-fodmap-diet.html and Monash University has created Monashfodmap.com with information on low- and high-FODMAP foods as well as meal plans.

If you continue to have problems and suspect gluten, on the other hand, do get it checked out. The first action is to find out if you have celiac disease, and there are well-established tests for this. Don't give up gluten until you know, because having eaten gluten is key to the diagnosis. You may also want to check for a wheat allergy, which is a different beast entirely. If the FODMAP diet doesn't help and other conditions such as Crohn's have been ruled out, you may want to consider gluten. Unfortunately, there aren't lab tests that can establish gluten sensitivity, but you can work with your doctor to go on a gluten-free diet to see if it helps your symptoms. But that should be your last step in this process—not your first!

Surprising Foods That Can Upset Your Stomach

Christine L. Frissora, MD, assistant attending physician at New York-Presbyterian Hospital and an associate professor of medicine at Weill Medical College of Cornell University, both in New York City.

If you have a sensitive stomach, you probably experience frequent bouts of digestive distress. While in some cases it's obvious what has caused the discomfort—for example, eating spicy foods or taking seconds, or even thirds—other times it seems to be a mystery.

What you may not know is that it could have been something seemingly harmless, or even healthful—like green tea or yogurt—that caused you to feel nauseated or bloated.

FOODS TO AVOID

Surprising triggers of digestive discomfort...

- **Energy bars.** Because these bars, such as Zone Perfect bars and PowerBars, contain added nutrients and vitamins, they typically are eaten as a healthful snack, a meal replacement or for a preworkout energy boost. Some bars, especially low-sugar or low-carb varieties, contain sugar alcohols, such as glycerin and maltitol syrup, which can cause bloating, gas and diarrhea. Other bars are simply too high in complex carbohydrates and calories for someone with a sensitive stomach to digest easily.

What to do: If you want to have an energy bar, be sure to eat only a small portion of it at a time.

- **Green tea.** Although green tea is widely recognized for its disease-fighting properties—it's full of antioxidants and other compounds that help fight cancer and heart disease and stave off diabetes, stroke and dementia—it contains irritants that can make you feel nauseated.

For example, green tea contains caffeine—anywhere from 24 mg to 40 mg per eight-ounce cup—which can irritate the gastrointestinal (GI) tract. Even decaffeinated green tea has some caffeine. But it's not the caffeine by itself that makes green tea a cause of digestive distress in some people. Green tea is also very high in tannins (polyphenols responsible for its astringent taste), which are associated with nausea and stomach upset in some individuals.

What to do: If green tea makes you nauseated, avoid it altogether or have a very weak cup. Chamomile tea is soothing to the GI tract and is a good alternative.

• **Vegetable skins.** Eggplant, bell pepper and potato skins can be difficult to digest, especially if you have diverticulitis (inflamed or infected pouches in the intestinal wall) or colitis (inflammation of the large intestine)... or have had complicated abdominal surgery (involving infection or perforation).

What to do: Peel thick-skinned vegetables, then purée, mash or stew the insides before eating to aid digestion.

• **Grapes.** Red and black grapes contain the phytochemical resveratrol, a powerful antioxidant thought to help protect against coronary disease, some cancers and viral infections. But eating too many grapes—or even just a few if you are sensitive to them—can cause nausea and diarrhea.

Reason: Grapes are high in fructose, a natural sugar that often causes gas. Green grapes contain a lot of tannins, like green tea, which can lead to stomach upset.

What to do: Eat only a small amount of grapes, or avoid them altogether if you are sensitive to them. Instead, try eating other fruits rich in resveratrol, such as cranberries, blueberries and bilberries.

• **Nuts.** The high fiber and fat content of nuts slow their movement through the digestive tract, which increases the risk for gas and bloating. Nuts also contain stomach-irritating tannins.

What to do: Avoid eating nuts if you experience digestive discomfort when consuming them...have had a complicated abdominal surgery...have peritonitis (inflammation of the inner abdominal wall)...or have diverticulosis (small pouches that bulge through the large intestine) or diverticulitis. Some alternatives to whole nuts include nut butters or oatmeal with berries.

• **Probiotics.** The balance of healthful and potentially unhealthful bacteria in your digestive system can be thrown off due to illness, medications and diet, causing diarrhea and constipation. Probiotic supplements and foods contain live, healthful bacteria that can help restore balance to the digestive system. Examples of the bacteria contained in probiotics include *Lactobacillus* and *Bifidobacterium.*

Certain probiotic supplements and foods are helpful for specific situations. For example, Activia yogurt can help alleviate constipation... the supplement Align can ease bloating...and Florastor (*Saccharomyces boulardii lyo*) helps diarrhea caused by antibiotics.

What to do: Many probiotic supplements and foods can produce bloating (due to the ingestion of billions of bacteria). Avoid probiotics if this is a problem for you.

Caution: If you are severely ill or your immune system is compromised, avoid probiotics (and check with your doctor before having yogurt). Probiotics can enter the bloodstream and cause sepsis, a potentially life-threatening condition caused by the body's inflammatory response to bacteria or other germs.

Important: A sensitive stomach, marked by gas and bloating, may be caused by celiac disease, an immune reaction to gluten in wheat, barley and rye. If you have these symptoms, get tested for celiac disease.

BETTER-KNOWN TROUBLEMAKERS

You may already know that the following foods can cause stomach upset, but they're worth a reminder...

• **Artificial sweeteners.** Some artificial sweeteners, such as Splenda (sucralose), Equal

Try Yogurt!

Lactose-intolerant people may be able to eat yogurt. Yogurt has less than half the lactose of milk.

Reason: The live cultures in yogurt secrete lactase in the intestine and stomach, which reduces the lactose content and prevents gastrointestinal symptoms, such as abdominal pain, diarrhea and flatulence.

Vicki Koenig, RD, registered dietitian and nutritionist, New Paltz, New York.

(aspartame) and Sweet'N Low (saccharin), are difficult for the body to break down, which can lead to bloating, nausea, headache and other symptoms.

What to do: Be on the lookout for artificial sweeteners, which are found not only in diet sodas and sugarless gum, but also in many other processed foods, including some yogurts, cereals, snacks and juices.

• **Carbonated beverages.** These drinks contain carbon dioxide gas, which distends the stomach.

What to do: Avoid beer, soda, seltzer and other "fizzy" drinks if you have bloating. Plain water is best.

• **Monosodium glutamate (MSG).** This flavor enhancer often is added to Chinese food, canned vegetables, soups and processed meats. It can cause nausea, headache, cramping, fatigue and other symptoms.

What to do: Avoid Chinese food, unless it is free of MSG, and avoid canned or processed foods with MSG on the label.

WHAT HELPS

How you eat and drink also can help prevent discomfort. For example, it's widely known that having six small meals per day, rather than three larger meals, makes it easier for the stomach to empty properly. *Other helpful approaches...*

• **Drink liquids between meals.** While the digestive system needs to be well-hydrated to function optimally, too much water or other liquids during meals can overdistend the stomach, especially in patients with gastroesophageal reflux disease (GERD), in which stomach contents backwash into the esophagus...hiatal hernia, in which part of the stomach sticks upward into the chest through an opening in the diaphragm...and gastroparesis, delayed emptying of the stomach.

• **Small sips of liquid during a meal are fine.**

Helpful: Avoid having a lot of liquids about 15 minutes before you eat and at least an hour after you eat.

• **Don't talk while eating.** This can lead to aerophagia, a condition caused by swallowing too much air, which can result in abdominal bloating, frequent belching and gas.

• **Eat slowly and chew well.** Make sure to thoroughly chew foods—especially hard foods, such as nuts—before swallowing.

• **Stew meats.** They are digested more easily than those that are broiled, grilled or fried.

• **Take chewable supplements.** Many supplements can cause bloating or nausea. If possible, use chewable forms, which are less likely to cause discomfort.

WHAT CAUSES A SENSITIVE STOMACH?

Your stomach mixes food with digestive juices, then empties its contents into the small intestine. If you have a sensitive stomach, the muscles of the stomach may function more slowly, which can lead to indigestion. Or the nerves of the stomach may be overly sensitive to distension (enlargement of the stomach after eating), resulting in uncomfortable bloating. Eating certain foods, including onions, garlic, apples and pears, can make these symptoms worse.

Coca-Cola Cures Bezoars

Dimitrios Kamberoglou, MD, consultant gastroenterologist, gastroenterology division, First Department of Medicine–Propaedeutic, Medical School, Athens University, Laikon Hospital, Greece.

You probably assume that the food you eat starts getting digested in your stomach, finishes the digestion process in your intestines and then leaves your body via the "back door." And usually that is what happens. But not always!

Sometimes foods don't get fully digested—and the undigested bits clump together to form a hard chunk that gets stuck in your intestines. This chunk is called a bezoar.

Bezoars can cause nasty symptoms, such as feeling full after eating only a small amount of food, abdominal pain and vomiting. The chunks also can lead to gastric ulcers, intestinal bleeding, intestinal obstruction and even gangrene of the digestive tract. So treatment is definitely warranted—yet treatments can be invasive and costly and they have side effects and risks, as well.

BEZOAR BASICS

People at highest risk for bezoars are those with diabetes or end-stage kidney disease or those who have had gastric surgery. Seniors also are at increased risk because aging decreases stomach acid and diminishes chewing efficiency. Use of certain drugs that interfere with digestion can contribute to risk, too. But the fact is that anyone can develop a bezoar.

Of the several different types of bezoars, the most common is a phytobezoar, which is composed of indigestible food fibers, such as cellulose from fruits and vegetables. Not all high-fiber foods are problematic—but particular culprits do include prunes, raisins, persimmons and pineapples...beets, celery, pumpkins and leeks...and sunflower seed husks.

FIZZY SOLUTION

Scientists in Greece combed through 10 years of research done in various countries—24 studies covering 46 patients in total—showing that using Coca-Cola was an effective treatment for phytobezoars.

Most patients either drank the Coke or got it via a nasogastric tube. Different amounts of Coke were used in different studies, and the frequency of the dosages also varied. But typically, patients drank the soda over the course of as little as 24 hours or as long as six weeks. When the Coke was given through a nasogastric tube, it was usually administered over a 12-hour period.

Results: Using Coke alone completely dissolved half the bezoars. For another 40%, Coke was used first to make the bezoar smaller and softer, and then the remaining chunk was either broken up or removed using an endoscopic tool inserted into the stomach.

This is very encouraging news, when you consider the other treatment options for bezoars. Sometimes doctors have patients ingest an enzyme such as papain or cellulase, for example. But papain may increase the risk for gastric ulcer, and cases of small bowel obstruction have occurred after treatment with cellulase. There's also endoscopy and, as a last resort, surgery—both of which are expensive, invasive and carry risks (such as infection).

In comparison, the Coke treatment holds appeal even for people who normally avoid soda like the plague. In fact, 50% of all bezoar patients in the studies who got the Coke therapy were able to avoid all of the other treatments mentioned above—and 90% of them were able to avoid surgery.

COKE MIMICS STOMACH ACID

Only regular (full-sugar) Coke was used in the studies, but past research has shown that Diet Coke and Coca-Cola Zero are equally effective at breaking down bezoars. That's because all versions are highly acidic and resemble the natural stomach acid that's necessary to properly digest fiber. Also, the fizzy drinks' carbonation may enhance this dissolving effect. Researchers did not think that the caffeine in cola was a factor in combating bezoars.

Could other brands of cola be as effective as Coke? They probably would be, but researchers have no experience with using other brands for this purpose. And there is no data to suggest whether noncola soft drinks (such as Sprite) would be effective against bezoars.

Are you at high risk of developing a bezoar, or have you had one in the past? *Here are prevention strategies...*

- **Chew your food thoroughly.**
- **Drink plenty of water throughout the day to avoid dehydration.**
- **Don't stop eating fruits and veggies (you need their nutrients!),** but avoid persimmons and pineapples because those fruits can cause especially hard bezoars that are difficult to treat.
- **Consider drinking a daily glass or two of cola.** Although this hasn't been studied explicitly, the drink may help prevent bezoars from forming in the first place.

Caveat: Drinking regular Coke, of course, increases your risk for obesity, high blood sugar and other health problems...and though Diet Coke and Coca-Cola Zero have no calories, there are concerns about their artificial sweeteners—so first discuss the benefits and risks with your doctor.

And if you ever do experience possible symptoms of a bezoar? Visit your doctor, who can diagnose the problem with either an imaging test or endoscopic test. Then show this article to your physician—in case he or she isn't aware of this "Coke therapy."

The Right Way to Chew (It's Not as Simple as You Think)

Karyn Kahn, DDS, staff member of the Head and Neck Institute in the dentistry department and consultant for craniofacial pain and jaw dysfunction at Cleveland Clinic, and associate professor at Case Western Reserve University School of Dentistry, both in Cleveland.

Mastication, or chewing, begins the digestive process and prepares food for swallowing. Front teeth cut and tear the food...back teeth crush and grind it, increasing its surface area so that digestion of carbohydrates can begin. *Be careful about chewing...*

- **Too little.** Often the result of eating too fast, this can cause choking or pain upon swallowing. Additionally, heartburn or stomach pain can occur because saliva's digestive enzymes don't have time to work. And because gobbling food inhibits the release of hormones that tell you when you're full, you may overeat.

Solution: Start with smaller bites, and use your molars more; you should barely feel food going down when you swallow.

To slow down: Put your fork down between bites, and take a deep breath after each swallow.

- **Too long.** Once a bite is ready to be swallowed, teeth should separate and not touch. Chewing past the point when the normal swallowing reflex occurs can overload jaw muscles, resulting in muscle pain and/or dysfunction. This is one reason why gum chewing in which teeth touch during chewing can lead to disorders of the temporomandibular joint (TMJ), or jaw joint.

- **On just one side of your mouth.** If you have a full set of teeth and a normal diet, having a favorite side on which to chew, as many people do, is not a problem.

But: If you wear full dentures, food must be distributed during the chewing process from one side of the mouth to the other to maintain the dentures' stability.

Important: If you avoid chewing on one side because it is painful, see your dentist.

Stomach Comfort in a Cup: Healing Herbal Teas

Brigitte Mars, adjunct professor of herbal medicine at Naropa University in Boulder, Colorado. She is a professional member of the American Herbalists Guild and author of *Healing Herbal Teas*. BrigitteMars.com

Herbal teas help soothe pain, ease stress and treat disease—more economically and with fewer side effects than drugs.

For convenience: Use tea bags.

For potency: Use loose organic herbs (sold in health-food stores).

Instructions: Boil eight ounces of water. Remove from heat. Stir in one heaping tablespoon of dried herbs or three level tablespoons of fresh herbs. Steep 10 minutes. Remove tea bag or strain off loose herbs. Drink hot or iced. Have two to three cups daily until symptoms subside...then one cup every few days to maintain health.*

Chamomile tea eases...

- **Insomnia**
- **Gastrointestinal upset**
- **Inflammation**

How it works: It has mild sedative properties to calm nerves...stimulates production of digestive fluids...and may inhibit metabolism of arachidonic acid, an inflammatory omega-6 fatty acid.

*Some herbs can interact with drugs or cause allergic reactions. Always consult your doctor before using herbal tea, especially if you have heart disease, diabetes, ulcers, gallbladder problems, a bleeding or seizure disorder, or a kidney or liver disorder, or if you are anticipating surgery.

Keep in mind: Steep no longer than three to five minutes to prevent bitterness. Discontinue two weeks before any surgery. Do not use if you are allergic to ragweed, celery or onion or take blood-thinning drugs.**

Ginger tea eases...

- **Nausea, motion sickness, morning sickness**
- **Colds and flu**
- **Pain (sore throat, arthritis, migraine)**

How it works: It stimulates secretion of digestive fluids...reduces congestion and inflammation...and bolsters the immune system. It also reduces risk for blood clots.

Keep in mind: Steep it in hot (but not boiling) water. Discontinue two weeks before any surgery. Do not use if you have heartburn, ulcers or gallbladder problems or take blood-thinning or diabetes drugs.

Nettle tea eases...

- **Arthritis pain**
- **Bloating**
- **Allergies, asthma**

How it works: It reduces inflammation... acts as a diuretic...and may deactivate mast cells (which release histamine, a chemical that provokes mucous membrane hyperactivity).

Keep in mind: It is best to use dried nettle —the fresh plant can cause a stinging rash. Discontinue if it causes gastrointestinal upset. Do not use if you have any problems with blood sugar.**

Peppermint tea eases...

- **Stomach upset**
- **Bad breath**

How it works: It increases circulation to the digestive tract...improves flow of digestive fluids...calms intestinal spasms...suppresses mouth chemicals that contribute to bad breath.

Keep in mind: It is safe to use when pregnant or breast-feeding. Do not use if you have a hiatal hernia or gallbladder problems.

**Do not use if you are pregnant or breast-feeding.

Acupressure Cure for Stomach Pain

This remedy came to us from an Asian massage therapist. If you are having stomach discomfort, massage the acupressure points at the sides of your knees, just below the kneecaps. This will relieve your stomachache.

Joan Wilen and Lydia Wilen, folk-remedy experts based in New York City who have spent decades collecting "cures from the cupboard." They are authors of *Bottom Line's Treasury of Home Remedies & Natural Cures* (Bottom Line Books).

Easy Yoga Exercises for Stomach Pain

Susan Winter Ward, a Pagosa Springs, Colorado–based yoga instructor and the author of *Yoga for the Young at Heart: Accessible Yoga for Every Body.* She has taught yoga worldwide and is the creator of the Yoga for the Young at Heart video series, which can be ordered on her website, Yogaheart.com.

Spinal twist. This stretches the rib cage and spine and eases back strain. It also aids digestion by massaging the stomach and intestines.

What to do: Sitting up straight, cross your right leg over your left and place your left hand on the inside of your left knee. Inhale deeply as you twist to the right, pulling your right elbow and shoulder around toward the back of the chair. Keeping your back straight, take three to five deep breaths as you hold the pose. Lengthen your spine by lifting through the top of your head with each inhalation, and twist a bit farther to the right with each exhalation. Return to center, then repeat on the opposite side.

- **Gas.** Try this yoga pose called the wind-relieving pose. Lie on your back with your legs and arms extended. As you exhale, draw both knees to your chest. Clasp your hands around them. While holding only your right knee with both hands, release your left leg and extend it along the floor. Hold this pose for one minute. Draw your left knee back in toward your chest, and clasp your hands around both knees again. Then while holding only your left knee, release your right leg and extend it along the floor. Hold this pose for up to a minute. Finally, draw both knees to your chest. Then with an exhalation, release and extend both legs.

Exercise Eases IBS Symptoms

E. Johannesson, et al., "Physical Activity Improves Symptoms in Irritable Bowel Syndrome: A Randomized Controlled Trial," *American Journal of Gastroenterology* (2011).

Researchers from the University of Gothenburg in Sweden have found that patients with irritable bowel syndrome (IBS) who participated in moderate-to-vigorous exercise for 20 to 30 minutes three to five times weekly had a decrease in abdominal pain and stool problems. Patients reported a reduction in these symptoms by about 50 points (on a scale of one to 500), whereas the group that did not increase their physical activity had only a five-point decrease in symptoms. Even a slight increase in physical activity was found to reduce IBS symptoms.

Foot Reflexology to Relieve Intestinal Pain

Jamison Starbuck, ND, a naturopathic physician in family practice Montana, Missoula. She is past president of the American Association of Naturopathic Physicians and a contributing editor to *The Alternative Advisor: The Complete Guide to Natural Therapies and Alternative Treatments.* Dr.JamisonStarbuck.com

Massaging reflexology points on the feet is thought to help increase blood flow to and improve the function of corresponding organs or body parts.

What to do: Whenever you have GI discomfort, firmly massage (for five to seven minutes) with your thumb and forefinger the outside portion of the middle one-third of the soles of the feet. According to reflexologists, this area corresponds to the colon. Your strokes should move toward the heel.

CHAPTER 2

Arthritis and Joint Pain

Best Ways to Make Arthritis Pain Disappear

Arthritis is a major cause of disability in the US, and the numbers are rising fast. About 21 million Americans suffer from osteoarthritis (the most common form of the disease), and the total number of arthritis patients is expected to double in the next few decades as baby boomers reach the highest-risk years.

In late 2004 and early 2005, patients lost access to two of the most popular arthritis drugs—Bextra and Vioxx, both COX-2 selective inhibitors ("coxibs"). They were withdrawn because of concerns about heart disease risk... but patients still have many effective options.

BAD TO THE BONE

In osteoarthritis, the cartilage that cushions the ends of bones gradually roughens and breaks down after decades of pressure and friction. Bone ends start to "grab" instead of glide, causing pain and inflammation.

Weight-bearing joints in the hips and knees are most susceptible because they're subjected to daily pressure—especially for people who are obese or have joint injuries.

There isn't a cure for osteoarthritis, but most patients can significantly reduce pain and maintain full mobility with a combination of medical and lifestyle approaches. *Best strategies...*

ANTI-INFLAMMATORY DRUGS

Nonsteroidal anti-inflammatory drugs (NSAIDs), including *ibuprofen* (Advil, Motrin), *naproxen* (Aleve) and coxibs such as *celecoxib* (Celebrex), reduce pain and inflammation. They're an effective treatment for most people with osteoarthritis—though new studies indicate that these drugs may slightly increase heart disease risk. For patients without serious cardiac risk factors such as a history of

Roland W. Moskowitz, MD, rheumatologist and professor of medicine, Case Western Reserve University School of Medicine, Cleveland. He is codirector of the Arthritis Translational Research Program at University Hospitals of Cleveland.

heart disease, NSAIDs remain an important therapeutic option.

The main risk of NSAIDs is gastrointestinal (GI) upset and bleeding, though coxibs are less likely to cause GI distress than traditional NSAIDs, such as ibuprofen and naproxen. For any of these agents, take the lowest possible dose that provides adequate pain relief. This is particularly important in the case of aspirin. The risk of bleeding from aspirin can double or quadruple at higher doses.

People with a history of ulcers and/or GI bleeding can try *acetaminophen* (Tylenol), which is somewhat less effective than an NSAID but less likely to cause stomach damage. Or you can combine an NSAID with a proton pump inhibitor such as Nexium, Prevacid, Prilosec, which reduces the risk of GI bleeding.

JOINT INJECTIONS

Injecting a corticosteroid such as cortisone into a joint stops inflammation usually within a few days and can reduce or eliminate pain for six months or more. Injected steroids don't cause the systemic side effects that may occur with oral drugs. Injections can be repeated several times a year.

Injections of hyaluronic acid also can relieve pain and reduce inflammation. Many patients with chronic arthritis pain get very good results with these injections, which usually are given weekly for three to five weeks. Most experience much less pain—or are pain-free in some cases—for at least six months after getting the injections. Side effects are minimal and may include mild joint pain for a day or so afterward.

Steroids usually are used for flare-ups and hyaluronic acid for persistent pain.

QUELL SLEEVE

The Food and Drug Administration recently approved the first nondrug noninvasive treatment for knee osteoarthritis (along with other forms of chronic pain). The product, Quell, comes in a sleeve that fits over the calf and stimulates nerves with pain-free electrical impulses. It is used for six to eight hours a day and can be worn while sleeping. More study is needed, but it seems to be effective for some patients. Ask your doctor. (For more information, see page 450 in chapter 22, "Drug-Free Protocols for Pain Relief.")

DAILY EXERCISE

Exercise is one of the best arthritis treatments. I recommend two types—targeted, which builds up muscles surrounding painful joints...and aerobic. Most patients should engage in both types several times a week.

Targeted exercise, which can be done with weights or isometric (muscle contraction) movements, strengthens muscles and improves joint stability. It also provides almost as much pain relief as simple analgesics, such as acetaminophen or low-dose NSAIDs.

Example: A patient with knee osteoarthritis might be advised to strengthen the quadriceps (thigh) muscles with leg lifts or isometric exercises in which the thigh muscle is tightened for 30 seconds, then relaxed. Strengthening thigh muscles helps support the knee joint.

Work with a physical therapist or trainer. Doing exercises incorrectly or too vigorously can exacerbate joint damage and pain.

Aerobic exercise elevates levels of endorphins, pain-killing chemicals that are produced in the brain. It also increases the flow of nutrients to the joint. Good choices include biking, swimming, fast walking, etc. Ask your doctor which is best for you.

WEIGHT LOSS

Obesity increases the pressure on—and subsequent damage to—the hips, knees and ankles. The National Health and Nutrition Examination Survey found that obese men are about five times more likely to develop knee osteoarthritis than men of normal weight. For obese women, the risk is four times higher.

Every extra pound can increase joint pressure by a factor of three or four.

Example: A woman who weighs 160 pounds experiences 80 pounds of pressure on each leg when standing still. When she's walking, all of her weight is intermittently transferred from one leg to the other—and the actual pressure can quadruple. If she is 10 pounds overweight, the stress on each knee increases by an additional 30 to 40 pounds.

Most patients who exercise regularly, watch calories and eat nutritious foods can lose at least 10 pounds. Often, that's enough to significantly decrease the pain as well as the frequency of arthritis flare-ups.

SUPPLEMENTS

Daily use of a combination supplement containing 1,500 milligrams (mg) of glucosamine and 1,200 mg of chondroitin can reduce pain in many patients. Glucosamine, extracted from the shells of shellfish, and chondroitin, made from animal cartilage, may inhibit cartilage breakdown.

Caution: Avoid glucosamine if you are allergic to shellfish. Avoid chondroitin if you are on a blood thinner—it has a mild blood-thinning effect.

TOPICAL TREATMENTS

Applications of heat, cold and/or medicated ointments can be helpful.

Cold packs (or ice wrapped in a washcloth or towel) cause blood vessels to constrict and help minimize inflammation during flare-ups.

Heat is better than cold for improving range of motion. Heat increases blood flow and is helpful when the joint is a little achy—but it can increase inflammation during acute flare-ups. In general, patients do better with heat than with cold.

Moist heat works well for many people. Try a hot 15-minute shower or bath. Or ask your doctor or pharmacist about moist heat appliances, such as heating pads.

Medicated ointments that contain capsaicin (made from the seeds of chili peppers) or methyl salicylate (found in products such as Bengay) may relieve pain in joints close to the skin surface, such as fingers, knees and elbows. Ointments may be used two to four times a day—follow package directions.

JOINT REPLACEMENT

Between 300,000 and 400,000 Americans undergo joint-replacement surgery annually to relieve pain and stiffness from osteoarthritis and other causes. Usually it is a knee or hip that is replaced, but artificial joints also are available for the shoulder, elbow and ankle.

Doctors used to advise adults younger than age 65 to refrain from surgery because it was thought that artificial joints would last only 10 years—so someone with decades of life ahead of him would require additional surgery.

Not true. Studies suggest that prosthetic joints last at least 15 to 20 years. Most people who undergo joint replacement are very happy with the results and have few complications.

Joint replacement typically requires a two- to three-day hospital stay and physical therapy for weeks or months afterward.

Arthritis? No...Bursitis—Here's Why It Matters

James V. Luck, Jr., MD, orthopedic surgeon, professor and residency program director of the UCLA/Orthopaedic Hospital Department of Orthopaedic Surgery. He is chairman of the national Medical Advisory Board for the Shriners Hospital for Children.

Don't assume that an aching joint means that you have arthritis. If the pain came on suddenly, hurts more at night and gets better when you're active, you might have bursitis.

Many of the body's joints have one or more bursae (bur-SEE), fluid-filled sacs that rest between bones and tendons. Irritation of a bursa (the singular form) can cause intense pain that makes it difficult to move.

Bursitis usually occurs in the shoulder, hip, elbow or knee, but it also can occur in the heel and base of your big toe. Depending on the location and the degree of irritation, the pain can range from merely irritating to excruciating.

WHAT GOES WRONG

Bursae provide a lubricating surface between joint bones and the tendons and muscles that lie above. When you move, the tendons/muscles glide, with almost no friction, across the bursae.

Bursitis is caused when pressure and/or repetitive movements irritate a bursa and cause inflammation. Inflammation not only is painful, but it also increases the friction of moving tendons/muscles, which exacerbates the problem.

Bursitis can be triggered by trauma, such as a hard knock to the elbow or knee. However, most cases are due to repetitive movements (such as frequently lifting your arms over your head) or pressure (from kneeling or leaning on your elbows). People with hobbies or professions—electrician, carpet installer, musician, factory worker—that involve repetitive movements and/or pressure have the highest risk.

If the discomfort from the bursitis severely inhibits your range of motion and you quit moving normally, you can develop scar tissue that can lead to chronic inflammation and stiffness.

Example: One common disorder, adhesive capsulitis, often occurs in patients who first had shoulder bursitis and then put up with limited joint motion. This condition, also known as "frozen shoulder," can cause severe pain and take many months to resolve.

Another risk: An infected bursa, known as septic bursitis.

BURSITIS OR SOMETHING ELSE?

Your doctor will press on different points around your painful joint to see if there's tenderness above one or more bursae. It's difficult to distinguish bursitis from tendonitis, inflammation of a tendon. Patients with bursitis often have tendonitis as well, because the increased friction from an inflamed bursa can irritate the tendon. Also, tendonitis can spread to the adjacent bursa. The distinction usually isn't important because the treatments for each condition typically are the same.

Your doctor usually can distinguish bursitis from arthritis by your symptoms. In general, the pain caused by osteoarthritis (the most common form of arthritis) is more persistent...gets worse rather than better with continued movements...and usually is worse during the day, when patients are most active.

If your doctor isn't sure what's causing your pain, you probably will need an X-ray. It's the only way to definitively distinguish arthritis from bursitis.

If your doctor suspects that a bursa might be infected, he/she will remove fluid with a needle and test it for infection.

Bonus: Although the procedure is mildly uncomfortable, it usually will reduce bursitis pain almost immediately.

SELF-HELP FOR BURSITIS

Apply ice or a cold pack as soon as you feel pain. Chill the area for 10 to 15 minutes at a time, and repeat it once or twice an hour—or as often as you can—for at least 48 hours. Applying cold will help reduce swelling as well as pain. After 48 hours, intermittent heat is appropriate to increase circulation and promote healing.

You also can take an over-the-counter anti-inflammatory, such as *ibuprofen* (i.e., Advil, Motrin), following the directions on the label.

MEDICAL HELP

If you have severe pain, your doctor can inject the bursa with a mixture of cortisone and an anesthetic. The anesthetic will stop the pain instantly. The cortisone gradually will reduce swelling as well as pain. Most patients with bursitis who get an injection need only one treatment.

If you have septic bursitis, you'll need antibiotics—the type will depend on the bacterium that's causing the infection. Most patients will take antibiotics orally. Severe infections might need to be treated with intravenous antibiotic therapy.

When bursitis is severe and doesn't improve after treatment, surgery may be needed to remove the bursa—but this is rarely necessary.

PREVENTION

To avoid bursitis...

Protect your joints as much as possible. For example, someone who spends a lot of time kneeling can wear knee pads. Or rest your weight on your forearms rather than on your elbows.

Take frequent breaks. If you're laying tile, for example, stand up and walk around every 15 or 20 minutes.

Routinely move your joints through their full range of motion.

Examples: Periodically move your arm in a complete circle—from front to back and from side to side. You can work the knee joint by lying on your back, with your knees bent, and slowly bringing the heel of your foot close to the buttocks.

Walking also is helpful, and using a bicycle is an excellent exercise for knees and hips. Doing shoulder exercises in a warm shower often is beneficial.

Could Your Arthritis Be an Infection?

David Lans, DO, FACP, clinical assistant professor of medicine at New York Medical College in Valhalla, New York, chief of rheumatology at NewYork-Presbyterian/Lawrence Hospital in Bronxville, New York.

When you think of arthritis, what probably comes to mind is osteoarthritis, the wear-and-tear disease that affects more than 30 million Americans.

What you may not realize: Other types of arthritis can ravage joints, including arthritis caused by infection. For example, a recent study published in *Arthritis Care & Research* found that more than 16,000 people go to the emergency room every year with septic arthritis, an infection that can cause irreversible damage and deformity to joints.

Infections play a role in many cases of arthritis, both acute and chronic. Because these types of arthritis are less common than osteoarthritis, they are often misdiagnosed or overlooked. *What you need to know about...*

- **Septic arthritis.** Triggered by bacteria in the bloodstream that settle in a joint, this is the most serious form of infectious arthritis. Without prompt treatment, deep bone infections may occur and take months to resolve. One-third of people with septic arthritis suffer joint damage—and 10% die.

About half the time, the infection is in the knee, and pain and swelling are so severe that walking is difficult. The joint will also be red and hot. And you'll have a fever and chills and feel very sick. The knee is a common site for septic arthritis because of its large size and location.

People who have weakened immune systems, including adults over age 65 and children, are the most common victims of septic arthritis. You're also at higher risk if you already have a joint problem, such as osteoarthritis, gout or rheumatoid arthritis, which is an autoimmune disease...if you're taking medications for rheumatoid arthritis, which suppress the immune system...if you have an immune-weakening disease, such as diabetes or cancer...or if you have fragile skin that is easily injured and heals poorly (a fairly common problem among older adults and those with diabetes), allowing bacteria ready access into your bloodstream.

Many types of bacteria can cause septic arthritis. The most common bacterial culprits are Staph and Streptococcal species. If the infection isn't stopped, bacteria can destroy cartilage, causing permanent damage.

What to watch out for: Sudden, severe pain in a knee or other joint, and flulike symptoms, including fever and chills.

Treatment: Go to the emergency room or see a doctor—immediately. The joint will be drained with a needle or tube (arthroscopy), and the fluid will be cultured to identify the bacteria. It's likely you'll also get blood tests to help pinpoint the infection and X-rays to see if the joint has been damaged.

If you're diagnosed with septic arthritis, you'll receive IV antibiotics, followed by oral antibiotics. The usual antibiotic treatment duration is about six weeks. If antibiotics aren't effective, you may need surgery to drain the infection.

- **Reactive arthritis.** This type of arthritis can plague joints for weeks to years. Doctors aren't certain if reactive arthritis is an infection of the joint...or a joint-centered inflammation triggered by an infection elsewhere in the body. Either way, the arthritis is typically caused by either a sexually transmitted bacterial infection, such as chlamydia or gonorrhea, or a gastrointestinal infection, such as *C. difficile* or *Salmonella*. Food poisoning is a common trigger.

What to watch out for: Joint pain that develops a few weeks or months after a sexually transmitted or gastrointestinal infection.

Treatment: A blood test will be given to detect the bacteria. If it's positive, you'll take antibiotics that target the organism. Nonsteroidal anti-inflammatory drugs (NSAIDs), such as *ibuprofen* (Motrin)...corticosteroids...or antirheumatic drugs, such as *methotrexate* (Trexall), may also be prescribed.

• **Lyme arthritis.** Lyme disease, a bacterial infection from a tick bite, is found throughout the US, but mainly in the Northeast, from Maine to Virginia, and in Minnesota, Wisconsin, Michigan and northern California. Some people never overcome the infection and develop chronic Lyme disease. Among those, more than half develop Lyme arthritis—one or more swollen joints (usually a knee), with pain (typically mild) that is intermittent or constant.

What to watch out for: Lyme arthritis usually develops several months after the tick bite. As with all types of arthritis, joint swelling and pain can occur.

Treatment: Lyme arthritis often resembles reactive arthritis. To make a definitive diagnosis, your doctor will order a blood test to detect antibodies to *B. burgdorferi*, the bacterium transmitted from the tick bite. The doctor may also remove fluid from your joint for a polymerase chain reaction (PCR) test, which detects the presence of DNA from B. burgdorferi.

If one or both of these tests are positive, your doctor will probably prescribe oral or intravenous antibiotics for one to three months. In most cases, this treatment cures Lyme arthritis, especially if it's initiated early on.

However, in some patients, the treatment fails, and chronic arthritis, as well as other symptoms (such as fatigue, headache and difficulty concentrating), may persist. If the disease isn't controlled, a drug used for rheumatoid arthritis—a disease modifying antirheumatic drug, or DMARD—often helps control the Lyme arthritis. Some patients require long-term treatment, while others improve over a period of months.

• **Viral joint infections.** Many viruses can trigger acute arthritis, but the joint pain that results is usually mild and goes away on its own after a few weeks. *Viral infections that can cause arthritis include...*

• **Zika virus,** from mosquitoes that carry it.

• **Epstein-Barr,** the virus that causes mononucleosis.

• **Hepatitis A and B,** the liver-infecting viruses that cause about one-third of virus-triggered arthritis.

• **Parvovirus,** a respiratory infection common in adults who are routinely exposed to children, the primary carriers of this infection, which causes a distinctive face rash.

What to watch out for: Sudden, mild joint pain (viral arthritis can affect almost any joint).

Treatment: Your physician will order a blood test for antibodies to specific viruses that can cause acute arthritis. Pain control is the goal, typically with an over-the-counter NSAID, such as ibuprofen or *naproxen* (Aleve).

Best Treatments for Ankle Arthritis

Judith F. Baumhauer, MD, MPH, professor and associate chair of the department of orthopedics at University of Rochester School of Medicine, New York. She is the recipient of the American Orthopaedic Foot & Ankle Society's Roger A. Mann Award for outstanding clinical study in 2017.

Remember that sprained ankle you suffered years ago? Or maybe it was an ankle fracture that left you hobbling around for weeks. Whatever the specific problem, be forewarned that ankle injuries can come back to haunt you—years or even decades later. *Here's how...*

SELF-CARE FOR ANKLE ARTHRITIS

The ankle is vulnerable to the same types of arthritis that affect other joints. Post-traumatic arthritis is the most common form in the ankle, followed by age-related osteoarthritis and rheumatoid arthritis. For these forms of ankle arthritis, you might be able to manage discomfort with simple remedies.

But self-care is tricky. You can't "go easy" on the ankles in the same way that you would with certain other joints. People use their ankles all day, every day. *My advice for people with ankle arthritis...*

- **Choose activities that minimize ankle wear and tear.** To stay active and keep the muscles supporting the ankle strong, try biking, swimming, walking, rowing, elliptical workouts or other low-impact, weight-bearing exercises that don't cause relentless pounding.

- **Keep your weight down.** People with ankle arthritis tend to gain weight because they find it too painful to walk or exercise much... and the extra pounds accelerate joint damage by increasing the weight load on the ankles.

Helpful: Losing even five pounds can reduce the ankle load by 20 pounds, which may be enough to minimize symptoms.

- **Exercise the ankles.** Ankle-specific exercises will build up the muscles surrounding the joint, keep the joint from getting stiff and reduce the bone-on-bone friction that occurs with arthritis.

Example: Several times a day, flex your foot upward (dorsiflexion) as far as it will go... hold for a few seconds...then flex it downward (plantarflexion). You can find dozens of ankle exercises on the Internet.

- **Wear shock-absorbing shoes.** Also known as "stability sneakers," they have a densely cushioned heel/sole that absorbs shocks when you walk, exercise, etc.

NOT READY FOR SURGERY

In addition to the steps above, some simple therapies can help slow the progression of arthritis. For example, it may help to wear an over-the-counter ankle brace that gives support and stability...apply cold packs when the ankle is hurting...and/or take as-needed doses of a nonsteroidal anti-inflammatory drug (NSAID), such as *ibuprofen* (Motrin) or *naproxen* (Aleve).* If you're lucky, these and other self-care therapies—including physical therapy—may be the only treatments you'll ever need.

Very helpful: A cortisone injection. Cortisone (sometimes combined with lidocaine) is a strong anti-inflammatory that can reduce or eliminate pain within a day. The shot is good for patients who are having moderate daily pain—and might be helpful for an upcoming vacation, for example, or when the pain is unusually severe. This shot won't stop the arthritis but can get you through a rough patch. In some cases, hyaluronic acid injections may be used but may not be covered by insurance.

WHEN SURGERY IS NEEDED

Even with the approaches described earlier, many people will eventually develop "end-stage" arthritis that does not improve and interferes with their daily activities. Once ankle arthritis progresses to that extent, it's serious business.

Until about 10 years ago, most patients with end-stage ankle arthritis were advised to have a procedure called ankle arthrodesis, commonly known as ankle fusion because affected bones are fused together to reduce pain and inflammation. Now patients (based on their age and other factors) have a second option—a total ankle replacement.

Because long-term comprehensive studies haven't yet been done, there's still debate about which approach is better. Both procedures are effective...and both have downsides that patients need to know about. *Specifically...*

- **With ankle fusion, the affected bones are locked together** (with screws alone or plates and screws) and eventually fuse into a solid mass of bone. This eliminates the rubbing/friction that causes the pain and disability of ankle arthritis. Most patients will walk in a shoe (without a cast) in eight to 12 weeks. And unlike ankle replacement (discussed below), the procedure is permanent. You're unlikely to require an additional procedure unless it doesn't fuse.

Downside: Bone fusion eliminates ankle mobility. You might walk haltingly when you go up hills or down a flight of stairs. And because the ankle is locked in place, other structures in the foot assume more of the burden of daily movements—and could become more susceptible to arthritis.

*Discuss the use of NSAIDs with your physician—they can cause side effects such as stomach upset, ulcers and high blood pressure.

Ankle fusion might not be the best choice if you have a highly active lifestyle that involves, for example, strenuous hiking, tennis, etc., and want your ankle to move "naturally"...or if you have other arthritic areas of your foot that couldn't take on more responsibility when the ankle is locked up.

• **With a total ankle replacement,** the arthritic surfaces are replaced—as also occurs with a knee or hip replacement—with an artificial joint. Surgeons advise patients that the implants might last for eight to 12 years. A recent study found that 73% were still working after 15 years.

The advantage of total ankle replacement is that the ankle will flex. Patients retain a greater degree of motion and experience less stress on surrounding joints.

Downside: The risk for additional procedures to repair/replace a damaged implant.

My take: I might recommend joint replacement for someone who's over age 60 and in good health but has other arthritis in the foot...or a person who is active with sports, such as tennis, that involve jumping and cutting. However, the choice between fusion and replacement is highly individualized.

Important: See a surgeon who's experienced in both procedures to get an unbiased opinion about the pros and cons of each. To find such a surgeon near you, consult the American Orthopaedic Foot & Ankle Society, AOFAS.org.

Insurance typically covers these procedures, but be sure to ask.

Better Joint-Replacement Recovery

Stavros G. Memtsoudis, MD, PhD, attending anesthesiologist and senior scientist, Hospital for Special Surgery, New York City.

Peripheral nerve blocks (PNBs)—the injection of an anesthetic near nerves to block pain in a specific area during surgery—improve pain control after joint replacement.

Now: An analysis of more than one million knee- and hip-replacement surgeries found that PNBs also improve complication rates, resulting in fewer infections and shorter hospital stays than reported in patients who did not receive a PNB.

Possible reason: Patients with PNBs have less need for opioids to control pain and fewer side effects than when general anesthesia is used and are able to participate in rehabilitation sooner after surgery.

The Real Reason Your Joints Won't Stop Hurting

Harris McIlwain, MD, board-certified specialist in rheumatology and geriatric medicine who practices with the Tampa Medical Group in Florida, TampaMedicalGroup.com. He is coauthor of *Pain-Free Arthritis—A 7-Step Program for Feeling Better Again.*

That stabbing, aching pain in your joints may mean that you just have a touch of garden-variety osteoarthritis. Or so you tell yourself.

What most people don't realize: When osteoarthritis wears down the cartilage covering the ends of your bones, it can lead to bony growths known as osteophytes, an often undetected source of severe joint pain.

Commonly known as bone spurs, these smooth or pointed growths on normal bone tissue also can form in response to stress on a joint—as may occur from repetitive motion activities, such as running or typing. Regardless of the trigger, bone spurs can rub against other bones, ligaments, tendons or nerves and are marked by painful inflammation.

Why this matters: It's important to distinguish bone spurs from run-of-the-mill arthritis so that you can take the necessary steps to stay ahead of potentially debilitating joint inflammation. If not dealt with in the right way (and at the right time), bone spurs often require powerful additional treatment to control the pain, and this treatment can have bad side effects. You want to deal with bone spurs early.

What you need to know to determine whether you have bone spurs—and the therapies that help most...

MORE THAN ARTHRITIS

How do you tell whether your joint pain is partly or completely due to bone spurs?

Clues to watch for: Osteoarthritis pain tends to come and go gradually—like the general stiffness that affects a large area of your body, such as your lower back, in the morning but eases by afternoon.

A bone spur, on the other hand, may cause chronic localized pain that's bad enough to make you not want to move your back, neck, hip, finger or some other joint that may be affected. You may have bone spurs in more than one place, but one spur could cause more pain, depending on its location and the amount of physical activity in that area.

The more sudden and severe the pain, the more likely that a bone spur is the culprit. Numbness, tenderness and weakness may also occur. If a parent or sibling has suffered from bone spurs, you're at increased risk, too—research suggests there is a genetic component.

HOT SPOTS FOR BONE SPURS

Any joint can develop a bone spur, but here are the most common locations and how the pain and other symptoms may vary in each part of your body...

- **Knees.** Bone spurs in the knee—a common location for those that occur with osteoarthritis—often resemble a pointy bird's beak on X-rays. The resulting discomfort is typically a blend of arthritis and bone spur pain—both sore and sharp.

- **Feet and/or heels.** Acute pain that occurs with every step—the kind that makes you want to avoid walking—can signal bone spurs in the feet and/or heels (often called "heel spurs"). Corns and calluses may also build up over heels or toes as the body tries to protect the area by providing added padding. Therefore, if you have pain along with corns and/or calluses, ask your doctor to check for a bone spur.

- **Hips.** Arthritis in the hips generally produces a deep aching and stiffness that occurs when you stand or walk. Bone spurs at the side of the hip—where the bony prominence can sometimes be felt—trigger pain when the hip is flexed, such as when riding a bike.

- **Hands and/or shoulders.** Jabbing pain (rather than a dull throb) is the telltale sign.

- **Neck and/or spine.** Bone spurs at these locations usually do not cause pain unless accompanied by arthritis, but they can pinch the spinal cord and irritate surrounding nerves.

GETTING DIAGNOSED

If you have one or more bone spurs, the usual arthritis treatments—including nonsteroidal anti-inflammatory drugs (NSAIDs), such as *ibuprofen* (Motrin) and *naproxen* (Aleve)... stretching...and warm heat—often don't make a dent in your joint pain.

Because bone spurs usually are not large enough to feel externally, an X-ray is the easiest way to diagnose them. In certain areas, such as the neck, more advanced imaging tests, such as MRI or CT scans, may be needed to diagnose them.

My advice: If your joint pain doesn't respond to the therapies described earlier and you suspect that you may have bone spurs, you don't need a definitive diagnosis provided by an X-ray. Ask your physician whether you may have bone spurs, and get his/her OK to promptly try the approaches below. If you don't start treatment quickly, the serious pain that bone spurs typically cause may limit your use of the joint, progressively weakening muscles surrounding it and creating an even worse problem.

Joint Surgery Reduces Heart Disease Risk

People with osteoarthritis who received knee- or hip-replacement surgery had a 40% lower risk for a heart attack, stroke or other cardiovascular event, compared with those who did not have surgery.

Theory: Debilitating arthritis limits patients' ability to do heart-healthy exercise...and joint replacement reduces pain, inflammation and depression—risk factors for cardiac events.

Seven-year study of 306 people by researchers at University of Toronto, Canada, published in *BMJ.*

FINDING THE BEST TREATMENT

Among the best therapies for joint pain due to bone spurs...

- **Alternate heating pads and ice packs in 20-minute intervals.** Use ice first to ease acute pain, then moist heat to penetrate inflamed areas. Do this twice a day.
- **Get acupuncture.** Acupuncture has been shown to reduce pain and improve functional mobility. Your acupuncturist will tailor a treatment plan for your bone spur.
- **Eat inflammation-fighting foods.** Processed foods promote inflammation, while certain whole foods, such as salmon, nuts, beets, leafy greens, olive oil and berries, fight it. Include as many of these foods in your daily diet as possible.
- **Use targeted supplements.** These include fish oil, turmeric and ginger. There is strong research showing that these supplements help fight painful inflammation.

My advice: You can take one or all of these supplements, depending on the intensity of your pain. Daily dosages are up to 3 grams (g) of fish oil...three 400-milligram (mg) to 600-mg tablets or capsules of turmeric...and two 500-mg to 1,000-mg capsules of ginger, taken with food. It usually takes about two months for turmeric to work.

Caution: Talk to your doctor before using any of these supplements if you take any type of medication (especially a blood thinner) or have a chronic medical condition.

- **Try ultrasound therapy.** Ultrasound uses sound waves that can penetrate more than two inches into the body to reach the painful area. Often used for shoulder or heel pain caused by bone spurs, it can be administered by a medical doctor or physical therapist.

Caveat: The pain relief provided by ultrasound may be long-lasting but sometimes lasts only a few weeks.

WHEN TO CONSIDER SURGERY

One of the biggest misconceptions about bone spurs is that they need to be removed surgically. The truth is, when strategies such as those described in this article are used, the inflammation may lessen after a period of weeks or months even though the spur does not go away.

In determining the need for surgery, location of the bone spurs is the key factor. For example, bone spurs located in the neck can press on nerves or even the esophagus, which can interfere with swallowing.

Generally, however, the risks associated with surgery, such as infection, outweigh the benefits for most bone spurs. If you have tried the regimen described above for bone spurs for about a year but still have not gotten adequate pain relief, then ask your primary care doctor for a referral to an orthopedic surgeon.

Women...Reasons Why Your Joints Hurt

Beth E. Shubin Stein, MD, orthopaedic surgeon and sports medicine specialist at the Women's Sports Medicine Center at the Hospital for Special Surgery and an assistant professor at Weill Medical College of Cornell University, both in New York City.

We women have lots of joint pain. A study by the Centers for Disease Control and Prevention found that nearly one-third of adult women in the US have some type of chronic joint pain or have been diagnosed with arthritis.

Despite what's commonly believed, it's not that women have more trouble with their joints than men, but that they tend to have different types of problems.

Example: In general, women's joints tend to be looser than men's joints, particularly the knees and shoulders, which can reduce stability and lead to damaging wear patterns and pain. *What you need to know to protect and soothe your joints...*

TROUBLE SPOT #1: KNEES

Women have inherent difficulties with their patellofemoral joints—or kneecaps—and how they join with the thigh bone. Because women have wider pelvises than men, the hip-to-knee line is less vertical than it is in men, which places more stress across women's knees.

Another reason for knee pain in women is that their soft tissue, including ligaments, is often more lax than that in men.

A third cause of female-specific problems is muscular imbalance. The muscles that support and control the knees include the quadriceps (front of the thighs), the hamstrings (back of the thighs) and the gluteal (buttocks) muscles. Many women do not have the proper balance of strength among these muscles to support and protect knees.

Weakness in the hamstrings may increase risk for traumatic injuries, such as tears to a ligament when jumping or turning quickly. Weakness in the quadriceps or gluteals may predispose a woman to "overuse" problems, such as pain in the kneecap area due to pressure from body weight on the knee.

What to do: Knee pain often can be treated with physical therapy to strengthen the proper muscles, including the quadriceps, hamstrings and gluteals—and followed up with a long-term exercise program incorporating the fundamentals learned in physical therapy. You can't change the alignment of your hips and knees or the laxity of your ligaments, but how strong you are is something you can control with exercise.

Also helpful: Don't wear high heels more often than necessary. They worsen knee pain by increasing pressure behind the kneecap.

For mild-to-moderate arthritis in the knee that doesn't respond well to physical therapy and home exercise, your doctor may want to try viscosupplementation, in which a lubricant based on hyaluronic acid, a substance that occurs naturally in the body, is injected into the knee. This procedure doesn't build back cartilage or bone damaged by injury or arthritis, but it can reduce pain for six months or more and it is safe.

TROUBLE SPOT #2: SHOULDERS

The rotator cuff, a group of muscles and tendons that attaches the arm to the shoulder joint and lets the arm rotate up and around, can become irritated and/or inflamed. Continued irritation can cause tendonitis and bursitis.

What to do: A physical therapist can help you strengthen muscles, often using a stretchy exercise band. It's a good idea to fortify the scapulothoracic muscles of the back (they come into play when you squeeze your shoulder blades together).

Smart: Don't carry a heavy purse or other bag on one side of your body—it will promote shoulder and back pain. Instead, distribute weight evenly across your body, such as with a backpack-style purse.

Best of all: A small bag on wheels with an extendable handle. That's what I use to take my patients' charts between my office and the hospital.

TROUBLE SPOT #3: THUMBS

The base of the thumb, called the carpometacarpal (CMC) joint, is prone to pain from arthritis in women. We aren't sure why, but it may have something to do with the fact that this joint is smaller in women than in men, yet women must bear the same loads while pinching and grasping as men do. With CMC arthritis, a simple activity like holding a fork can be painful.

What to do: A special splint fitted by an occupational therapist can support your thumb joint and limit the movement of your thumb and wrist. If a splint is going to help, you should start to feel relief within a few days to a week.

If a splint isn't effective, you may need an injection of a steroid into the thumb, which can reduce pain and inflammation. Although most such injections help for only six to eight weeks, that sometimes lets the joint heal enough to stay pain free.

If a steroid injection doesn't solve the problem and arthritis progresses to an advanced stage, you may require one of two kinds of surgery...

- **Replacement of damaged portions of the joint with tendon from the wrist.** This preserves mobility but usually results in a loss of strength.
- **Fusing together of bones in your thumb.** This maximizes strength but limits mobility.

AEROBICS–PLUS

It's important to get aerobic exercise at least several days a week. Besides improving your cardiovascular health, it will help keep your weight down—and excess weight is an enemy of your joints, especially your weight-bearing joints, such as the knees and ankles.

Best: Aerobic activities that also put joints through ranges of motion, such as using an elliptical training machine, swimming and cycling.

However, to slow age-related bone loss, it's vital to do weight-bearing exercise, which stimulates growth of new bone. The easiest way for most people is to walk a lot. To involve the upper body, use a variety of weight-lifting machines or handheld weights.

Natural Cures for Arthritis: Research Shows They Really Work!

Steven Ehrlich, NMD, naturopathic physician and founder of Solutions Acupuncture & Naturopathic Medicine in Phoenix. He has spent the last decade using natural medicine to treat chronic pain and illness. Dr. Ehrlich has also taught naturopathic techniques to both conventional and alternative medicine practitioners.

If you have arthritis, you may have shied away from natural medicine in the past because you didn't think that it would relieve your pain.

After all, there is no rigorous scientific evidence to back up these remedies, right?

Wrong.

Now: While it's true that many nondrug approaches for pain relief have been based primarily on their thousands of years of use by Asian, Indian and other traditional cultures, there is now an impressive body of scientific evidence that makes natural medicine a smarter choice than ever before for many arthritis sufferers. (These therapies have been studied most often for osteoarthritis but may also relieve pain due to rheumatoid arthritis. Check with your doctor.)

PAIN RELIEF WITH LESS RISK

Millions of Americans depend on high-dose pain relievers that cause side effects, including gastrointestinal upset or bleeding, in up to 60% of patients.

What you may not realize is that some natural therapies, which are far less likely to cause side effects, work just as well as the powerful pain-relieving drugs that are so commonly used for arthritis.

Many Americans take glucosamine (a dietary supplement that stimulates production of key components in cartilage) to help fight arthritis. However, arthritis pain symptoms improve only slightly or moderately in some patients—even when they take glucosamine sulfate, the most widely studied form of this supplement. (Research currently indicates that adding chondroitin, a supplement derived from shark or bovine cartilage or produced synthetically, isn't necessarily helpful for arthritis).

In my practice, I often recommend the following regimen (with or without glucosamine) to relieve arthritis pain—the typical arthritis patient might start with curcumin and fish oil (pain relief should begin within one week to a month). *Ginger can be added if more pain relief is needed...**

- **Curcumin.** A chemical compound in the spice turmeric, it helps inhibit inflammatory enzymes and reduces joint pain without the gastrointestinal side effects that often occur with aspirin and related drugs.

Scientific evidence: A study published in *The Journal of Alternative and Complementary Medicine* found that curcumin reduced arthritis pain and improved knee function about as well as *ibuprofen* (Motrin).

How to use curcumin: To obtain a concentrated dose of the active ingredient, try curcumin supplement capsules with a standardized curcuminoid complex (rather than kitchen turmeric, which would be difficult to consume in therapeutic amounts). Follow the label instructions—typically taking it three times daily during flare-ups. Between arthritis episodes, you can take half this amount to prevent inflammation.

*Consult a doctor before trying these supplements—especially if you have a chronic condition or take medication. To find a physician near you with experience prescribing botanical medicines, consult the American Association of Naturopathic Physicians at Naturopathic.org.

Caution: Curcumin can inhibit the ability of blood to clot. Use this supplement only under a doctor's supervision, particularly if you're also taking a blood-thinning medication such as *warfarin* (Coumadin) or aspirin.

• **Fish oil.** The omega-3 fatty acids in fish oil supplements increase the body's production of inhibitory prostaglandins, substances that prevent inflammation.

Scientific evidence: A study published in *Arthritis & Rheumatism* discovered that some arthritis patients who took fish oil improved so much that they were able to discontinue their use of conventional painkillers.

How to use fish oil: The amount of omega-3s found in dietary sources is insufficient for pain relief. Use a fish oil supplement—doses range from about 2,000 mg to 6,000 mg daily. Start with the lower dose, then gradually increase it until you notice improvement in pain and stiffness (the rate at which the dose is increased depends on the patient). If you take more than 2,000 mg of fish oil daily, you should be monitored by a physician—this supplement has a blood-thinning effect.

• **Ginger.** This spice has compounds that inhibit the effects of cyclooxygenase, an inflammatory enzyme.

Scientific evidence: A study that looked at 261 patients with knee arthritis discovered that those who took ginger supplements had less pain—and required fewer painkillers—than those taking placebos.

How to use ginger: Ginger spice will not provide enough of the active ingredient, so use a ginger supplement. The standard dose is 250 mg taken four times daily. Talk to your doctor before trying ginger—especially if it's used with a blood-thinning drug, curcumin and/or fish oil. Ginger can increase the risk for bleeding in some patients.

OTHER THERAPIES THAT HELP

The following approaches can accelerate and increase the pain-relieving effects offered by the supplements described earlier...

• **Balance Method acupuncture.** Acupuncture can be extremely effective because it increases the flow of blood and oxygen into painful areas while accelerating the removal of inflammatory chemicals.

Scientific evidence: A study involving more than 3,500 patients with chronic hip and/or knee arthritis found that those given acupuncture (in addition to conventional care, including doctor visits and use of painkillers) had fewer symptoms and a better quality of life than those given only conventional treatments.

My advice: Consider trying Balance Method acupuncture. Rather than inserting needles above or near the painful areas (as occurs with standard acupuncture), the practitioner will use points on your arms or legs that "remotely" affect the joints. It seems to be more effective than standard acupuncture.

How acupuncture is used: Virtually all arthritis patients improve by the end of the third session—some after the first session. Most practitioners advise an initial series of 12 to 15 sessions, given once or twice a week, followed by monthly "tune-ups."

• **Meditation.** Meditation works in part by lowering levels of stress hormones. This decreases inflammation as well as the perception of pain. Patients who do meditation may still have pain, but it won't bother them as much as it did before.

Scientific evidence: In a study reported at an American College of Rheumatology meeting, arthritis patients who did meditation for 45 minutes a day, six days a week for six months had an 11% decrease in symptoms, a 46% decrease in erythrocyte sedimentation rate (a measure of inflammation) and a 33% reduction in psychological stress.

How meditation is used: Practice meditation for five to 10 minutes, once or twice a day—even during symptom-free periods.

Helpful: "Tapping meditation," which incorporates elements of acupressure as the patient taps different areas of his/her body. It has been especially helpful for arthritis patients in my practice. Most health practitioners who recommend meditation can teach you how to perform tapping meditation.

• **Yoga.** Any form of exercise is helpful for arthritis as long as it doesn't put excessive pressure on the joints. Yoga is particularly beneficial because it gently stretches and strengthens the muscles. It also increases the movement of synovial (lubricating) fluid across bone surfaces.

Scientific evidence: Researchers recently found that patients with knee osteoarthritis who took a weekly yoga class had improvements in pain and mobility after just eight weeks.

How yoga is used: The yoga that's practiced in many health clubs and yoga studios may be too aggressive for patients who have arthritis. Start with a beginner's class, preferably one that's taught by an instructor who specializes in therapeutic yoga, which is designed to treat specific medical conditions. To find a yoga instructor who specializes in therapeutic yoga, consult the International Association of Yoga Therapists at IAYT.org.

Turmeric Relieves Arthritis Pain

In India, turmeric is a popular remedy for indigestion. It contains curcumin, an oily, yellow pigment that appears to prevent gut muscles from contracting and cramping.

What else turmeric can do: Relieve arthritis, morning stiffness and minor sprains. Turmeric reduces levels of an inflammatory, hormone-like substance known as PGE2.

Holly Phaneuf, PhD, expert in medicinal chemistry and author of *Herbs Demystified.*

Ice Is Nice for Arthritis

Bill Gottlieb, CHC, health coach certified by the American Association of Drugless Practitioners. Based in Middletown, California, he is author of 16 health books that have sold more than three million copies and been translated into 10 languages, including *Speed Healing: More Than 2,000 Quick Cures and Fast Fixes to Ease Everything from Arthritis to Wrinkles.*

Nearly half of Americans age 60 and older suffer with the pain of knee arthritis. Ice is the fastest way to relieve that pain—faster than taking a pain pill, says Jason Theodosakis, MD, coauthor of *The Arthritis Cure* and associate clinical professor at University of Arizona College of Medicine in Tucson. But ice often is used incorrectly, undercutting its pain-relieving power. Many people find the feeling of cold uncomfortable, so they either don't ice often enough or at all.

Rapid Remedy: Buy a freezable soft gel ice pack and a compression (ACE-type) bandage. Store the gel pack in the freezer. When your knee hurts, place the pack on your knee over a pant leg or a towel, securing it to your knee with the compression bandage. (Never put the ice pack directly on your skin.) Keep the ice pack on for about 15 minutes—just the right amount of time to provide an hour or two of pain relief. Ice packs can bring relief to other parts of the body, too, including the ankle, shoulder and neck.

If You Have Arthritis: Strive for a Healthy Mind...and Gut

Jamison Starbuck, ND, naturopathic physician in family practice and writer and producer of Dr. Starbuck's Health Tips for Kids, a weekly program on Montana Public Radio, MTPR.org, both in Missoula. She is a past president of the American Association of Naturopathic Physicians and a contributing editor to *The Alternative Advisor: The Complete Guide to Natural Therapies and Alternative Treatments.* DrJamisonStarbuck.com

People with arthritis often suffer from indigestion, constipation or irritable bowel syndrome—all of which inflame and irritate the gastrointestinal tract.

Good natural remedy: The amino acid glutamine, which helps strengthen the lining of the gastrointestinal tract. Glutamine is abundant in cabbage and okra and can be taken as a supplement—typical dose is 1,000 mg in powdered form added to four ounces of water and taken three times a day, between meals.

- **Get positive.** You may be surprised to learn that in arthritis patients, 85% or more of their 50,000 or so daily thoughts are negative, critical and self-defeating. To curb thoughts that increase pain perception and worsen joint stiffness, try to become more self-supportive through therapy, meditation, biofeedback or stress-management counseling.

An increasing body of evidence now shows that stress reduction really does reduce pain. You may have noticed this through your own experiences—for example, your pain lessens while you're on vacation or during a relaxed weekend. Three stress-reducing methods that I highly recommend are yoga, meditation and massage. I advise patients to engage in one or more of these practices on a regular basis. An ideal stress-reducing regimen might include daily meditation, yoga three times a week (or as much as you're physically able) and/or massage once a week.

- **Watch out for "trigger" foods.** Coffee, sugar, alcohol, red meat, dairy products and processed foods promote inflammation, increasing risk for joint pain. To prevent arthritis, cut back or eliminate these foods and increase your intake of anti-inflammatory foods—for example, vegetables, fruits, plain water and healthful oils (such as those from fish and olives).

- **Move your body.** Physical activity improves circulation and sends nourishing nutrients to joints and surrounding tissue. It also helps keep body weight under control—an important factor in fighting joint pain. Regular movement will not worsen arthritis. Start slowly with simple stretches or walking. Consult a physical therapist if you need help setting up an exercise program that's right for you.

The Anti-Arthritis Diet

Harris McIlwain, MD, board-certified specialist in rheumatology and geriatric medicine who practices with the Tampa Medical Group in Florida, TampaMedicalGroup.com. He is coauthor of *Pain-Free Arthritis—A 7-Step Program for Feeling Better Again.*

In my rheumatology practice I often treat patients suffering from painfully arthritic joints who have been unable to get relief, despite seeing many doctors. I tell them that one of the most important things they can do for their arthritis is to change their diets. After just a few weeks on my pain-free diet plan, I've had many patients cut back on their anti-inflammatory medications and even put off joint-replacement surgery. The diet helps alleviate pain and stiffness in most types of arthritis, including rheumatoid arthritis and osteoarthritis.

How it works: The pain-free diet guides you toward healing foods that are known to reduce inflammation and boost the immune system. It helps you eliminate those foods that promote inflammation and might trigger symptoms. The diet also includes recommendations on nutritional supplements.

Bonus: This nutritional approach makes it easier to maintain a healthy body weight, which is essential for patients who need to take pressure off their joints. Maintaining a healthy body weight also produces metabolic changes that lessen the body's inflammatory response.

Helpful: It's easier to maintain a healthy weight when you eat frequent, smaller meals. Instead of three large meals, eat about six mini-meals throughout the day. In addition to a breakfast, lunch and dinner of about 300 calories each, eat three snacks between meals of about 150 to 200 calories each.

FOODS THAT HEAL

Foods that are high in antioxidants and other inflammation-fighting nutrients can noticeably reduce arthritis pain and stiffness when consumed daily. *The following are especially effective...*

- **High-antioxidant fruits and vegetables.** Antioxidants help reduce inflammation.

Several years ago, the US Department of Agriculture ranked the following foods according to their antioxidant activity. Among the top 10 fruits and vegetables from highest to lowest were blueberries, kale, strawberries, spinach, Brussels sprouts, plums, broccoli, beets, oranges and red grapes. Eat a variety of these foods, raw and cooked, to get the greatest benefit.

Also beneficial: Asparagus, cabbage, cauliflower, tomatoes, sweet potatoes, avocados, grapefruit, peaches and watermelon.

• **Oil-rich fish.** Research has shown that the omega-3 fatty acids contained in anchovies, mackerel, salmon, sardines, shad, tuna, whitefish and herring help reduce inflammation—particularly levels of leukotriene B4, a chemical that contributes to many types of arthritis. Researchers have found that women who ate at least three servings of baked or broiled fish weekly had about half the risk of getting rheumatoid arthritis as those who ate only one serving.

• **Soy.** Studies have found that a diet rich in soy may help reduce inflammation-related pain and swelling. Try tofu, soy milk, soy yogurt, soybeans or miso, a traditional Japanese food consisting of fermented soybeans and made into a thick paste.

• **Green and black tea.** Green tea contains a polyphenol (a chemical found in plants that acts as an antioxidant) called EGCG, which can inhibit a key gene involved in the arthritis inflammation response. Research suggests that the more you drink, the more benefit you'll get. Black tea, while processed differently than green, also provides benefits. It contains anti-inflammatory chemicals of its own called theaflavins. The Iowa Women's Health Study found that women who drank three or more cups of tea (not including herbal tea) reduced their risk of rheumatoid arthritis by 60%.

• **Pineapple.** This tasty fruit contains bromelain, an enzyme that reduces inflammation associated with arthritis. Fresh pineapple is the most beneficial, but canned is also good.

• **Onions and apples.** Both of these foods are especially high in flavonoids, which are also inflammation-fighting compounds. Eat a variety of these foods, both raw and cooked.

FOODS TO AVOID

The only way to know which of the foods below affect your joint pain is to eliminate each one for at least two weeks and assess your symptoms. That way, you'll know which type of food increases your inflammation and pain.

• **Avoid foods that increase inflammation.** There are a variety of foods that trigger the body to produce cytokines—naturally occurring proteins that can promote inflammation, leading to pain and deterioration of cartilage in the joints. These include beef and other red meat...foods cooked at high temperatures, particularly fried foods...and any foods containing man-made trans fats (often called partially hydrogenated fats or oils on food labels), including junk food and commercial baked goods. Eat these types of foods sparingly.

• **Reduce intake of foods from animal products.** I tell my patients to eat turkey and chicken in moderation. But the fact is that all animal products—including poultry, some farm-raised fish, egg yolks and other dairy products—contain arachidonic acid, a fatty acid that is converted by the body into prostaglandins and leukotrienes, two other types of inflammation-causing chemicals. I've had many patients tell me that they reduced arthritis symptoms by adopting a "modified vegetarian" diet.

Key: Decrease your intake of animal protein and increase the amount of protein you get from fish and plant sources, such as beans, nuts, soy, portobello mushrooms (a common meat substitute) and whole grains. Start by substituting one-fourth of the animal protein you normally eat with plant-based foods, cold-water fish and low-fat dairy. After two or three months, increase the substitution to half—adding more vegetables, fruits, lentils, beans, fish, whole grains and low-fat dairy. After a while, many of my patients choose to give up all animal protein because they enjoy the benefit of reduced pain and inflammation.

Note: A small percentage of people find that certain vegetables—including tomatoes, white potatoes, peppers and eggplant—make their arthritis worse. These nightshade family plants contain solanine, a substance that can be toxic if not sufficiently digested in the intestines. Eliminate all of these foods, then add them back one at a time—as long as you do not have pain or inflammation.

• **Stay away from foods with a high glycemic index.** While high-glycemic foods (foods that quickly raise your blood sugar) should be avoided by people with diabetes or prediabetes, they pose problems for people with arthritis as well.

Reason: They increase insulin production, which promotes accumulation of body fat and causes a rebound sensation of hunger a few hours after eating—making it harder to maintain a healthy weight, which is important for reducing arthritis symptoms. High-glycemic foods include table sugar, baked white potatoes, French fries, pretzels, white bread and rolls, white and brown rice, potato and corn chips, waffles, doughnuts and corn flakes.

SUPPLEMENTS THAT CAN EASE ARTHRITIS

The following supplements may also help reduce arthritis inflammation. Always check with your doctor before taking any dietary supplement—even a "natural" one.

- **Glucosamine (1,500 mg/daily).** While the data on this nutritional supplement are mixed, it's perfectly safe. Some studies suggest that it may slow arthritis progression. It's often combined with chondroitin (1,200 mg), another nutritional supplement that may help relieve arthritis symptoms for some people.
- **Vitamin C (500 mg to 1,000 mg/daily)** plays a key role in building and protecting collagen, an important component of cartilage. Among other things, it contains antioxidants that fight inflammation and help regenerate damaged joint tissue.
- **Bromelain.** This anti-inflammatory enzyme is found in pineapple, but it's also available in pill or capsule form. Include fresh pineapple (two servings daily) in your diet or take capsules (follow directions on label for amounts)—or do both.
- **Fish oil capsules.** For people who aren't eating two or more servings of fish per week, this is a good option. Your dose should provide 600 mg of combined DHA and EPA in a 2:1 ratio—the ratio that occurs naturally in wild salmon. Read your product's label for its DHA/EPA content.
- **Ginger.** Clinical studies have found that this herb reduces arthritis symptoms and inflammation. It can be taken in the form of tincture, capsules, as a spice added to foods or as a tea made from boiling gingerroot. You may benefit by drinking ginger juice or extract. Since ginger inhibits blood clotting, don't consume more than four grams a day.

Arthritis Supplements Do Help

Mark A. Stengler, NMD, naturopathic doctor and founder of the Stengler Center for Integrative Medicine in Encinitas, California. He is author or coauthor of numerous books, including *The Natural Physician's Healing Therapies* and *Bottom Line's Prescription for Natural Cures*, and author of the newsletter *Health Revelations*. MarkStengler.com

Almost a decade ago, researchers in a well-publicized study (the Glucosamine/Chondroitin Arthritis Intervention Trial) concluded that "glucosamine and chondroitin sulfate alone or in combination did not reduce pain effectively in the overall group of patients with osteoarthritis of the knee." As a result, many media outlets reported that glucosamine and chondroitin were ineffective for the treatment of osteoarthritis. While the combination wasn't effective for mild sufferers in the study, it was more effective than Celebrex for participants with moderate to severe osteoarthritis pain of the knees. Yet most of the mainstream media did not report this finding. Interestingly, for the group of patients with moderate to severe pain, Celebrex was only mildly more effective than the placebo.

My view: If you are being helped by these supplements, keep taking them. It's also worthwhile to try them before taking Celebrex or a similar drug, since glucosamine and chondroitin have a much lower risk of side effects, such as digestive upset. Even if you have only mild pain, these supplements can help prevent cartilage breakdown so that the problem does not worsen. For high-quality formulas, use brands sold at health-food stores.

Caution: Glucosamine and chondroitin may increase insulin resistance, so people with diabetes should monitor blood sugar levels carefully. The combination supplement should not be used by people with shellfish allergies.

Supplement Combinations That Work for Arthritis

Peter Bales, MD, board-certified orthopedic surgeon and member of the clinical staff, department of orthopedic surgery, University of California at Davis Health System. He is author of *Osteoarthritis: Preventing and Healing Without Drugs.*

The most widely used supplements for osteoarthritis are glucosamine and chondroitin, taken singly or in combination. Several studies show that they work.

Better: A triple combination that contains methylsulfonylmethane (MSM) as well as glucosamine and chondroitin. MSM is a sulfur-containing compound that provides the raw material for cartilage regrowth. Glucosamine and chondroitin reduce osteoarthritis pain and have anti-inflammatory properties.

What to do: Take daily supplements of glucosamine (1,500mg)...chondroitin (1,200 mg) ...and MSM (1,500 mg).

Instead of—or in addition to—fish oil and the triple combination, you may want to take...

- **SAMe.** Like MSM, S-adenosylmethionine (SAMe) is a sulfur-containing compound. It reduces the body's production of TNF-alpha, a substance that's involved in cartilage destruction. It also seems to increase cartilage production.

In one study, researchers compared SAMe to the prescriptionanti-inflammatory drug *celecoxib* (Celebrex). The study was double-blind (neither the patients nor the doctors knew who was getting which drug or supplement), and it continued for four months. Initially, patients taking the celecoxib reported fewer symptoms—but by the second month, there was no difference between the two groups.

Other studies have found similar results. SAMe seems to work as well as over-the-counter and/or prescription drugs for osteoarthritis, but it works more slowly. I advise patients to take it for at least three months to see effects.

What to do: Start with 200 mg of SAMe daily and increase to 400mg daily if necessary after a few weeks.

Oregano for Arthritis

The late James A. Duke, PhD, an economic botanist with the USDA, where he developed a database on the health benefits of various plants. He is the author of numerous books including *The Green Pharmacy Guide to Healing Foods: Proven Natural Remedies to Treat and Prevent More Than 80 Common Health Concerns.*

Oregano helps alleviate osteoarthritis and other inflammatory conditions, such as rheumatoid arthritis. You might be surprised to learn that this favorite spice of Italian cooking contains natural compounds that have many of the same effects as the powerful anti-inflammatory COX-2 inhibitor drug *celecoxib* (Celebrex).

In addition, oregano contains dozens of other anti-inflammatory compounds that act as muscle relaxants and pain relievers. Unlike celecoxib, which may increase heart attack risk in some people, oregano actually protects the heart by helping to prevent blood clots and irregular heart rhythms.

Best uses: Use oregano liberally on salads or on pizzas. Oregano also can be mixed with peppermint and/or spearmint for a hot or iced mixed-herb tea. If you prefer to take an anti-inflammatory supplement, oregano is one of the half dozen spices in a product called Zyflamend (its ingredients also include rosemary and turmeric). The herbs in Zyflamend act synergistically to provide a more powerful effect than each would when used individually. Zyflamend can be purchased in health-food stores and online. Follow label instructions.

Milk's Good for Pain

Study of 1,260 women and 888 men with knee arthritis by researchers at Brigham and Women's Hospital, Boston, published in *Arthritis Care & Research.*

Milk may slow the progression of knee osteoarthritis in women.

Recent finding: The more low-fat or fat-free milk women drank, the more slowly the disease progressed. The same benefit was not found in men.

But: Increased intake of cheese made knee osteoarthritis progress more quickly. Yogurt was not found to have any effect.

Black Pepper for Pain... And More

Bill Gottlieb, CHC, editor of *Healing Spices: How to Use 50 Everyday and Exotic Spices to Boost Health and Beat Disease*, founder and president of Good For You Health Coaching, former editor in chief of Rodale Books and Prevention Magazine Health Books and author of 14 health books that have sold more than two million copies.

Black pepper is rich in piperine, the pungent compound that triggers a sneeze when it hits the nerve endings inside your nose. Hundreds of studies show that piperine also triggers healing—energizing and protecting nearly every organ and system in your body. Black pepper can help relieve the pain of arthritis and gout.

Piperine is anti-inflammatory—and studies show that it can stop destructive inflammation in cartilage cells (loss of cartilage is the cause of osteoarthritis) and reduce inflammation associated with gout. It also reverses the symptoms of arthritis in lab animals.

How to use: For the highest level of piperine, buy whole black peppercorns and grind as needed. (Green and white peppercorns are not as rich in piperine, and once the peppercorn is ground, piperine begins to decrease.) Add freshly ground black pepper liberally and often—in cooking and at the table. Try to add freshly ground pepper at the end of cooking because the benefits break down the longer the spice is heated.

Also helpful: Studies show that just smelling black pepper (in the form of black pepper oil) can cut nicotine cravings in smokers and strengthen "postural stability" in older people (thereby helping to prevent falls). Put a drop of oil on a tissue, and inhale for two minutes, two to three times a day. Black pepper oil is available at Amazon.com and other online retailers.

Healing Vegetable For Joint Pain

Joan Wilen and Lydia Wilen are folk-remedy experts based in New York City who have spent decades collecting "cures from the cupboard." They are authors of *Bottom Line's Treasury of Home Remedies & Natural Cures* and *Bottom Line's Household Magic.*

If your joints ache with gout, rheumatism or minor arthritis pain, you might want to take a bite out of celery. *Here's why...*

Celery contains many nourishing properties, such as potassium, magnesium and luteolin, an anti-inflammatory. Some modern herbalists believe that celery has the power to help neutralize uric acid and other excess acids in the body that can cause painful inflammation. Eat fresh celery daily (be sure to wash it thoroughly). The leaves on top of celery stalks are also good to eat.

If so much roughage is rough on your digestive system, place five or six clean celery stalks (including the tops and the tough parts) in a nonaluminum pan. Cover with at least three-and-a-half cups of water, and slowly bring to a boil. Then simmer for 10 to 15 minutes. Strain and pour into a jar.

Dose: Drink eight ounces three times a day, a half hour before each meal. You can vary your celery intake by drinking celery seed tea and/or juiced celery stalks, or do as the Romanians do and cook celery in milk. (Eat the celery, and drink the milk!) Celery is a diuretic, so plan your day accordingly.

Caution: Celery can interact with some medications, such as levothyroxine and lithium. Be sure to talk to your doctor before increasing your intake.

Super-Broth for Super-Healing

Sally Fallon Morell, founding president of The Weston A. Price Foundation, which champions nourishing, traditional foods from grass-fed animals. She is author of *Nourishing Traditions* and coauthor of *Nourishing Broth: An Old-Fashioned Remedy for the Modern World.* NourishingTraditions.com

Before the 20th century, almost all soups and stews were made with a stock of bone broth—bones and other animal parts slowly simmered in a cauldron or stockpot, producing a nutrient-rich concoction. Today's processed "broth" often is nothing more than a powder or cube dissolved in water and spiked with additives such as MSG that mimic the taste of broth.

What most people don't realize: Traditional bone broth delivers unique, health-giving components that can be hard to find anywhere else in the diet. And a brothless diet may be hurting your health—contributing to painful arthritis and other nagging injuries.

Good news: Bone broth is simple to make or buy (see next page). The optimal "dose" is one cup daily. If you are trying to heal, increase this to two cups.

SUPER-HEALTHY INGREDIENTS

Bone broth, whether it's made from the bones of a chicken, cow, lamb, pig or the like, is extraordinarily rich in the following...

• **Collagen.** The number-one health-giving component of bone broth is melted collagen, or gelatin. Collagen is the most abundant protein in the body, providing strength and structure to tissue. In fact, microscopic cables of collagen literally hold your body together—in joints, tendons, ligaments, muscles, skin and membranes around internal organs.

It becomes harder for your body to make collagen as you age, leading to arthritis, wrinkled skin and other degenerative conditions.

• **Glucosamine and chondroitin sulfate.** These two nutrients are well-known for helping to ease arthritis pain—and bone broth supplies ample amounts of both.

Glucosamine is created from glucose (sugar) and glutamine (an amino acid, a building block of protein). It's found in cartilage, the part of the joint that provides cushioning and lubrication between bones.

Chondroitin sulfate is a proteoglycan, a type of molecule that helps hydrate cells. It also supplies sulfur, a mineral that nourishes cartilage and balances blood sugar.

• **Glycine.** This amino acid supports the health of blood cells, generates cellular energy, aids in the digestion of fats, speeds wound healing and helps the body rid itself of toxins, such as mercury, lead, cadmium and pesticides. Glycine also regulates dopamine levels, thereby easing anxiety, depression and irritability and improving sleep and memory.

• **Glutamine.** This amino acid nourishes the lining of the gut, aiding the absorption of nutrients. It boosts the strength of the immune system. It helps the body recover from injuries such as burns, wounds and surgery. It also strengthens the liver, helping the body process and expel toxins. And glutamine boosts metabolism and cuts cravings for sugar and carbohydrates, aiding weight loss.

FEEL-BETTER BROTH

Bone broth delivers extra-high levels of all those health-giving compounds, so it's not surprising that it can help prevent and heal many health problems, including...

• **Arthritis and joint pain.** By supplying collagen, glucosamine, chondroitin and other cartilage-nourishing factors, bone broth can repair and rebuild cartilage, preventing osteoarthritis or easing arthritis pain. In fact, bone broth might be the best food for osteoarthritis, which affects more than 30 million Americans.

Compelling research: In a review of seven studies on osteoarthritis and melted collagen (collagen hydrolysate), researchers at University of Illinois College of Medicine in Chicago found that ingesting the compound helped create new cartilage, thus lessening pain and improving everyday functioning.

• **Digestive problems.** In the 19th century, broth and gelatin were widely prescribed—by Florence Nightingale and many others—for convalescents who lacked the strength to digest and assimilate food properly.

Sadly, nutritional therapy for digestive problems went out of fashion after World War II, replaced by pharmaceuticals.

Example: A form of gelatin (gelatin tannate, or Tasectan) is being used as a digestive drug, with studies showing that it can help heal gastroenteritis (stomach and intestinal irritation). The new drug is being hailed as a "gut barrier protector"—but wouldn't it be better to prevent digestive diseases by strengthening your gut with bone broth?

- **Injuries and wounds.** The components in bone broth are crucial for healing broken bones, muscle injuries, burns and wounds—a key benefit for seniors, whose injuries can take longer to heal.

The use of cartilage (a main component of bone broth) for wound healing was championed by John F. Prudden, MD, whose published papers include "The Clinical Acceleration of Healing with a Cartilage Preparation," in the May 3, 1965 issue of *JAMA*. In his research, Dr. Prudden showed that cow cartilage could speed wound healing, produce stronger healing that was less likely to be reinjured and produce smoother, flatter and more natural-looking scars.

More recently, studies have shown that bone broth ingredients—particularly glycine and other amino acids—are uniquely effective at healing wounds, including hard-to-heal diabetic foot ulcers.

- **Infections.** Chicken soup—"Jewish penicillin"—is a classic home remedy for a cold, flu, pneumonia and other infectious diseases. Over the years, researchers studying broth and its components have noted their ability to strengthen immune cells, fight off viruses and calm down the overactive immune system caused by autoimmune diseases such as rheumatoid arthritis, Crohn's disease and psoriasis.

HOW TO MAKE BONE BROTH (OR BUY IT)

Making a very healthful and delicious bone broth may seem daunting—but it's not. Here's a simple way to make a chicken bone broth. You can use the same method for any kind of animal bones. Beef bones (such as rib bones, short ribs and beef shanks) should be browned first in the oven for the best flavor.

How to prepare bone broth: Whenever you eat chicken, save the bones. You can save skin and meat, too—the skin is rich in collagen, and there is some collagen in the meat. Just put all these leftovers in a zipper freezer bag, and store in the freezer until you have enough to fill a standard six-to-seven-quart slow cooker, about six to eight cups. Add a splash of vinegar and one sliced onion. Fill up the slow cooker with filtered water.

Slow-cook on low overnight. (If you don't have a slow cooker, you can make the broth by simmering it all day in a stockpot.)

In the morning, ladle the broth through a strainer and put the broth in the refrigerator. Fill up the slow cooker with water, and cook the bones again overnight, producing a second batch. As with the first batch, ladle the broth through a strainer. You now have about one gallon of chicken broth, which you can refrigerate or freeze.

What to look for: A sign that your broth is rich in collagen is that it gels when chilled. To get a good gel, it is helpful to add chicken feet or a pig's foot to the bone mix.

You can use your broth as a basic ingredient in soups, stews, sauces and gravies. Or just add a little salt, heat it and drink it in a mug.

Try this simple Thai soup: Two cups of chicken broth with one can of coconut milk, the juice of one lime and a pinch of red pepper flakes.

If you want to purchase healthful bone broth, good sources include Bare Bones Broth Company (BareBonesBroth.com), OssoGood (OssoGoodBones.com), Stock Options (StockOptionsOnline.com) and the Brothery (BoneBroth.com). These broths are available by mail order, but you may be able to find them in some gourmet and specialty shops.

The Amazing Gin-Soaked Raisin Remedy for Arthritis

Joan Wilen and Lydia Wilen are folk-remedy experts based in New York City who have spent decades collecting "cures from the cupboard." They are authors of *Bottom Line's Treasury of Home Remedies & Natural Cures* and *Bottom Line's Household Magic.*

We demonstrated this remedy on national television, and the feedback has been incredible. One woman wrote to tell us that she had constant pain and no mobility in her neck.

Her doctor finally told her, "You'll just have to learn to live with the pain." Although that was unacceptable, she didn't know what else to do. And then she saw us on television, talking about a remarkable raisin remedy. We got her letter two weeks after she started "The Amazing Gin-Soaked Raisin Remedy." The woman had no pain and total mobility. She also had all of her friends waiting for their gin to be absorbed by their raisins.

This is one of dozens and dozens of success stories we've received. Some people have dramatic results after eating the raisins for less than a week, while it takes others a month or two to get results. There are some people for whom this remedy does nothing. But it's inexpensive, easy to do, delicious to eat and worth a try. Be consistent—eat the raisins every day. Expect a miracle...but have patience!

Recipe:

1 lb golden raisins
Gin (approximately 1 pint)
Glass bowl (Pyrex is good—crystal is bad)
Glass jar with lid

Spread the golden raisins evenly on the bottom of the glass bowl, and pour enough gin over the raisins to completely cover them. Let them stay that way until all the gin is absorbed by the raisins. It takes about five to seven days, depending on the humidity in your area. (You may want to lightly cover the bowl with a paper towel so that dust or insects don't drop in.) To make sure that all of the raisins get their fair share of the gin, occasionally take a spoon and stir the mixture, bringing the bottom layer of raisins to the top of the bowl.

As soon as all the gin has been absorbed, transfer the raisins to the jar, put the lid on and keep it closed. Do not refrigerate. Each day, eat nine raisins—exactly and only nine raisins a day. Most people eat them in the morning with breakfast.

The Research Triangle Institute (RTI.org) tested "The Amazing Gin-Soaked Raisin Remedy" for alcohol content.

The result: Less than one drop of alcohol was left in nine raisins. So when people who take the raisins are feeling no pain, it's not because they're drunk—it's because the remedy works.

Even so, be sure to check with your health professional to make sure that gin-soaked raisins will not conflict with any medication you may be taking or present a problem for any health challenge you may have, particularly an iron-overload condition. Also, do not give the gin-soaked raisins to children or women who are pregnant or nursing.

Special Tea for Arthritis Pain

Joan Wilen and Lydia Wilen are folk-remedy experts based in New York City who have spent decades collecting "cures from the cupboard." They are authors of *Bottom Line's Treasury of Home Remedies & Natural Cures* and *Bottom Line's Household Magic.*

Do your joints ache with arthritis pain? *Here's a remedy to soothe the soreness without dangerous side effects:* Bring one-half cup of water to a boil. Lower the heat to a slight boil. Peel and slice thinly a two-inch piece of fresh ginger, add to the water, and let it simmer for five minutes. Remove and discard the ginger. Turn off the heat, and add one-quarter teaspoon of turmeric powder, one tablespoon of unflavored gelatin and one tablespoon of coconut oil. Stir until the gelatin is dissolved, then add one-half to one cup of calcium-enriched orange juice. Drink this beverage twice a day, and you may begin feeling relief within days.

Fight Osteoarthritis Pain With the Mighty Grape

Shanil Juma, PhD, associate professor, department of nutrition and food sciences, Texas Woman's University, Denton, Texas. His research was presented at the Experimental Biology Conference in San Diego.

When osteoarthritis sets in, people often turn to nonsteroidal anti-inflammatory drugs for pain relief even though long-term use of these drugs can cause serious side effects—including gastrointestinal bleeding, stroke and heart attack. But certain foods contain compounds known to be powerful, natural anti-inflammatories. One fruit, loved from earliest history—the grape—is just such a food, and a recent study has found that grapes actually can help with arthritis. There's even some evidence that grapes can help prevent damage to cartilage.

WHAT CAUSES OSTEOARTHRITIS PAIN?

First, to understand why grapes, among all foods, might be so good for arthritis relief, it helps to know a little more about osteoarthritis. In osteoarthritis, pain is caused by joint inflammation which, in turn, is caused by the destruction of articular cartilage. Articular cartilage is the cushiony stuff between the joint and bones. When it wears away, bone rubs directly against bone, causing thickening and spurs that aggravate the tissue around the joint. This is the process that makes activities such as kneeling, walking, standing up, holding a pen or unscrewing a bottle top so painful—sometimes nearly impossible. Strategies that keep the inflammation to a minimum and promote cartilage formation are the key to pain relief in conditions such as osteoarthritis, which is the most common form of arthritis in the United States.

GRAPE EXPECTATIONS

Research from the Texas Woman's University in Denton uncovered the power of the grape for osteoarthritis pain in a small study of 56 adults, mostly women (42 women versus 14 men) with osteoarthritis of the knee. The study participants were randomly assigned to either a treatment or control group. Each member of the treatment group consumed 47 grams of freeze-dried grape powder, dissolved in a glass of water, each day for four months. (This dosage is roughly the equivalent of two cups of fresh whole grapes per day.) Meanwhile, the control group consumed a powder that resembled the grape powder but was really a placebo.

The grape powder was not an extract but made from whole freeze-dried California grapes and included all colors and seeded and seedless varieties. This sort of grape powder isn't on the market for regular people—it is made available by the California Table Grape Commission only to scientists who want to study how humans might benefit from grapes. The powder is, however, essentially equivalent to real, whole California grapes.

Before the study began and at its completion, all of the participants had blood tests to examine signs of inflammation and cartilage health. Participants also reported their levels of activity and pain using a questionnaire that rates pain, stiffness and ability to perform various activities, such as sitting or lying down, standing up, bending, walking, climbing stairs, getting in and out of a car or bathtub, putting on or taking off socks, shopping, and doing light and heavy household chores. Participants also received physical exams. *The results...*

- **Pain.** Pain improved significantly in the group consuming the grape powder, com-

Delicious Juice Cure for Osteoarthritis

Fight osteoarthritis with pomegranate juice. It has antioxidants and an anti-inflammatory effect that can block enzymes involved in cartilage deterioration by up to 68%. It also may protect against cancer and heart disease. Pomegranate juices are available at health-food stores.

Best: Mix at least two tablespoons of 100% pomegranate juice with another juice or seltzer daily.

Tariq Haqqi, PhD, professor of medicine and director of rheumatology research at Case Western Reserve University in Cleveland. His study was published in *Journal of Nutrition.*

pared to the placebo group, which reported very minor improvement.

• **Activity.** Improvement in activity level was strongly seen in the grape-powder group—but only in participants who were younger than age 65. These folks were able to increase activities that they had originally rated as "very hard" by 70%, on average. Meanwhile, participants of every age in the placebo group participated less in such activities, and older folks in the grape group participated less in moderate-to-difficult activities as the four-month study progressed. This slowing down is common in osteoarthritis because activities become more difficult as time passes. But in light of the overall benefits seen in the grape group, researchers theorized that the older people perhaps needed to continue the grape-powder regimen for a longer time to see improvement in physical activity.

• **Cartilage health.** Markers in blood revealed that the grape-powder treatment improved cartilage health, but only in men. (Interestingly, although this same cartilage-boosting effect was not seen in women, women reported greater pain relief than men from the grape powder.) And again, it's possible that improvements in cartilage might have been seen in the women if they had consumed the grape powder for a longer period of time. More research is needed to investigate this and why grape powder seems to have different effects in men and women.

THE WHOLE GRAPE IS BETTER THAN EXTRACTS

Of course, the grape is not a stand-alone magic bullet. Also, know that the grape-powder study was funded through a research grant from the California Table Grape Commission, which, of course, wants to promote grape consumption—but also wants to know exactly how the health benefits of grapes really work and whether the many nonscientific claims out there are really true. Research is increasingly showing that whole grapes—that is, all of the good things in grapes taken together—have superior health benefits compared with single grape extracts, such as resveratrol. Grapes are high in sugar, though. So, rather than eating large portions of them daily, you may want to include them in moderate proportions in a broader anti-osteoarthritis strategy that combines a variety of nutritional anti-inflammatory foods.

Supplements for Stiff Joints

Michael T. Murray, ND, naturopathic physician in Paradise Valley, Arizona, and coauthor of *The Encyclopedia of Natural Medicine.*

Stiff joints? Staying well hydrated (with water, herbal tea and fresh, raw vegetable juice) helps keep joints lubricated. Also, exercise for a half hour five days a week to help pump nutrition in and waste products out of joint tissues.

For supplements, I recommend glucosamine sulfate (1,500 mg daily), natural eggshell membrane (500 mg daily) and Celadrin (1,000 mg daily). Glucosamine and eggshell membrane promote the manufacture of cartilage components, while Celadrin, a mix of fatty acids, reduces inflammation. Check with your doctor first if you have a chronic condition, such as diabetes, or take medication.

Cherry Pills Ease Arthritis Pain

John J. Cush, MD, rheumatologist, Baylor Research Institute, Dallas.

In a new study of 20 patients with osteoarthritis of the knee, more than half the patients experienced significant improvement in knee pain after taking tart-cherry supplements daily for eight weeks.

Theory: Cherry extracts contain flavonoids and anthocyanins, which have been shown to have anti-inflammatory effects.

If you have osteoarthritis: Ask your doctor about trying tart-cherry supplements.

Unusual Herbs That Help Treat Arthritis

Andrew Heyman, MD, adjunct clinical instructor in family medicine, University of Michigan Medical School, Ann Arbor.

Devil's claw has an anti-inflammatory component that may relieve pain.

Suggested dose: 750 mg of standardized 3% iridoid glycosides three times a day.

- **Extract of avocado and soybean oil can reduce pain and stiffness**—300 mg a day.
- **Phytodolor,** a mixture of ash, aspen and goldenrod, may also reduce symptoms—30 drops three times a day.
- **Niacinamide can ease pain and swelling**—100 mg three to four times a day.
- **Tart cherry juice.** A daily cup can ease mild arthritis.

Note: Check with your doctor before taking any dietary supplements.

Relieve Arthritis Pain With Ayurvedic Herbs

Nancy Lonsdorf, MD, adjunct clinical faculty in Vedic medicine, Maharishi University of Management, Fairfield, Iowa. She maintains private practices in Fairfield, Iowa and Los Angeles. Dr. Lonsdorf also is the author of *The Ageless Woman: Natural Health and Beauty After Forty with Maharishi Ayurveda*.DrNancyLonsdorf.com

Your poor joints are stiff, inflamed and achy from osteoarthritis—but the medications that reduce your pain also can have serious side effects, such as gastrointestinal bleeding, liver and kidney damage, and increased risk for heart attack and stroke.

Safer solution: Consider the Ayurvedic approach to osteoarthritis treatment, which relies on natural herbs and spices to bring relief.

The following four Ayurvedic arthritis remedies have been used in ancient Indian medicines and in cooking for more than 5,000 years. And they really work—a study presented at a meeting of the American College of Rheumatology showed a combination herbal Ayurvedic therapy to be as effective in treating knee osteoarthritis as the commonly prescribed medication *celecoxib* (Celebrex). *Recommended...*

- **Boswellia (Indian frankincense).** This comes from the resin of the *Boswellia serrata* plant. It works by blocking an enzyme involved in the formation of leukotrienes, chemicals that trigger inflammation.

Note: Boswellia may cause a reaction in people who are allergic to ragweed, and it can irritate the gastrointestinal tract (especially if taken alone rather than in a balanced combination formula as traditionally used) .

- **Turmeric.** The active ingredient in this spice, curcumin, interferes with three important inflammation-producing enzymes—so it disrupts the inflammatory process at three different stages. Turmeric also may provide some protection against the damage that pain-relieving medications can do to the gastrointestinal tract.
- **Ginger.** Various studies have demonstrated ginger's ability to reduce pain and inflammation by interfering with inflammatory enzymes.

Bonus: Ginger also aids digestion. Why should that matter? Because according to Ayurvedic principals, poor digestion is a primary trigger for arthritis. When we eat improper foods or our digestion is weak, food is not broken down into small molecules, so larger-than-normal molecules get absorbed into the bloodstream. These biochemical impurities circulate, eventually getting localized in a tissue and initiating swelling. When the affected tissue is a joint, the result is arthritis.

- **Ashwagandha.** This herb is also known as winter cherry or Indian ginseng. Lab studies suggest that it has anti-inflammatory properties that protect against cartilage damage. In addition, animal studies provide evidence that the herb combats stress. When we are stressed, the hormones cortisol and epinephrine cause a breakdown of various body tissues. Ashwagandha helps alleviate the damaging effects of stress by restoring the proper hormonal balance to the nervous system, which in turn strengthens the immune system and further reduces inflammation.

Caution: Since Ashwagandha makes your immune system more active, it is not appropriate for people who have an autoimmune disorder, including rheumatoid arthritis. Rarely, Ashwagandha can irritate the gastrointestinal tract.

USING AYURVEDIC HERBS

Ayurvedic herbal products are available in health-food stores and online. For maximum convenience and effect, I recommend that osteoarthritis patients take an herbal supplement that combines several of the herbs and spices listed above, such as Maharishi Ayurveda's Flexcel, which contains boswellia, ashwagandha and ginger as well as other natural ingredients that further support joint and bone health. This product does not contain turmeric, so try using the spice liberally in the kitchen. Turmeric added to food can be more effective than in a formula because you can get much a greater quantity that way. I recommend adding turmeric to every meal and cooking it into each dish, even if only in small amounts, for its cumulative anti-inflammatory and antioxidant protection.

Important: According to a Boston University study, some commercial Ayurvedic herbal remedies contain lead, mercury and/or arsenic in amounts exceeding regulatory standards. One reputable manufacturer is Maharishi Ayurveda (MAPI.com), a company that has been in business for nearly 30 years. If you are interested in a different brand, to guard against contamination, contact the seller to make sure the company tests every batch in the US for heavy metals, as well as for parasites and fungus.

To make sure that the specific ingredients are safe and appropriate for you and to get dosage recommendations, consult a physician who is knowledgeable about Ayurvedic medicine. To find such a practitioner, visit the website of the Light on Ayurveda Education Foundation.

Try this Ayurvedic approach for eight weeks to see whether these remedies relieve your osteoarthritis symptoms. If they do, you can continue to take them indefinitely, reducing to the lowest dose that maintains your improvement.

Rhus Toxicodendron—A Soother for Arthritis

Mark A. Stengler, NMD, naturopathic doctor and founder of the Stengler Center for Integrative Medicine in Encinitas, California. He is author or coauthor of numerous books, including *The Natural Physician's Healing Therapies* and *Bottom Line's Prescription for Natural Cures*, and author of the newsletter *Health Revelations*. MarkStengler.com

Rhus toxicodendron (pronounced roos tox-ih-ko-den-dron) is the homeopathic dilution of poison oak.

Rhus tox is commonly used for osteoarthritis and rheumatoid arthritis. This is probably the right remedy for you if you notice certain characteristics about your symptoms—they are worse in the morning, improve with motion and activity during the day and then get worse again at night while in bed.

Rhus tox is also a good remedy if these arthritic symptoms flare up before a storm or in damp weather. It's probably the right remedy for you if hot baths and showers also provide joint pain relief.

Dosage: The typical dosage for rhus tox is 30C potency taken two to three times daily for a day or two for conditions such as stiffness from overexertion. For long-term use for eczema or arthritis, I generally start with a lower dose such as 6C taken two to three times daily.

What are the side effects?: While rhus tox has few side effects, some people may experience skin irritation. People with chronic eczema or arthritis may experience a flare-up of their condition at the beginning of treatment. This is usually a sign that the remedy is working (known as a healing aggravation).

Rose Hip Powder Is Flower Power for Osteoarthritis Pain Relief

Study titled, "Low-dose Seed and Shell Powder from Rose-hip (*Rosa Canina*) Can Alleviate Symptoms of Osteoarthritis and Reduce C-reactive Protein in Patients Suffering from Osteoarthritis," presented at the 2014 World Congress of The Osteoarthritis Research Society International in Paris.

Although nonsteroidal anti-inflammatory drugs aspirin, *ibuprofen* (Motrin), the COX-2 inhibitor *celecoxib* (Celebrex) and *acetaminophen* (Tylenol) are the standard fare for osteoarthritis (OA) pain relief, you know that they can cause an array of side effects, from stomach upset to liver damage and even cardiovascular risks. But what Europeans have known for years is that a common, poetic and romantically beautiful flower—the rose—holds the secret to safer relief of OA pain. A new study has even confirmed that a low dose of a powder made from rose hip (the fruit that grows once the blossom fades) provides true OA pain relief.

Yes, the rose—my favorite flower, scent and tea. Scandinavians and other Northern Europeans have known about it and have been studying its pain-relieving properties—specifically, from rose hip powder—for years. New Zealand and Australia have gotten into the act, too. But American medical news on this breakthrough is virtually nil. So—just for you—here is the latest from this year's meeting of the Osteoarthritis Research Society International and more on the value of rose hip powder for OA.

EFFECTIVE AND SAFE

Rose hip powder is made from the ground shell and seeds of the fruit of a common species of rose—*Rosa canina*. Rose hip powder, of course, is widely available, but a standardized formulation of it, marketed as Litozin, is used in Scandinavia and other countries for OA pain relief. Is it any different from other rose hip powder supplements? It's vitamin-C (80 mg per dose) and flavonoid fortified, and the manufacturer says that only wild Chilean rose hips, which are particularly nutrient-rich, are used. But wild Chilean rose hip powder is easily found, even through Amazon.com, and it can certainly be taken with a bioflavonoid-fortified vitamin C supplement—which you might already be taking.

The standard dosage of rose hip powder is one-half to one teaspoon twice a day, equaling 5,000 mg to 10,000 mg per day. This dosage is based on studies such as those from the University of Copenhagen. Effects aren't immediate, though…give it up to three weeks.

Rose hip powder can help you completely drop use of standard painkillers…or at least allow you to lighten up on how much and how often you use them, according to the research. Also, there are no known side effects associated with the standard dosages or even slightly higher dosages, but very high dosages beyond the standard dose have been shown to cause either diarrhea or persistent constipation in some people.

LESS IS MORE

One of the most recent scientific studies on rose hip powder and OA found that taking one teaspoon a day for three weeks and then reducing the dosage to one-half teaspoon effectively relieves pain and reduces inflammation—so, although "more" won't hurt you, it is not necessarily "better." (But be aware that the study used Litozin, so results may vary with another brand of rose hip powder.)

HOW WELL DOES IT WORK?

The value of rose hip powder for OA is widely recognized. In one study of hip and knee OA pain published in the *Scandinavian Journal of Rheumatology*, 82% of patients receiving rose hip powder reported improvement compared with 49% of patients receiving placebo. Plus, patients receiving rose hip powder supplements cut their use of acetaminophen and mild opioid-based pain killers nearly in half, while use of standard painkillers increased among the folks receiving placebo. In another study that looked at wrist OA pain, which was published in the *Open Journal of Rheumatology and Autoimmune Diseases*, 90% of patients receiving rose hip powder reported improvement compared with 36% of patients receiving placebo.

If you are dealing with OA pain and are concerned about the damaging effects that long-term use of standard pain relievers can have on your heart, stomach and liver, talk to your doctor about trying this European standard—"flower power" rose hip powder—for a safe way to ease or completely give up your reliance on pharmaceutical pain relievers.

Sex Can Relieve Arthritis Pain

Warren Katz, MD, chairman of medicine, Penn-Presbyterian Medical Center, Philadelphia.

Seventy percent of people in one study said their arthritis pain was relieved for up to six hours after intercourse.

Possible explanation: Sex triggers the release of natural cortisone and betaendorphins—two chemicals that relieve pain naturally.

Helpful: A warm bath or shower before sexual activity to relieve any initial stiffness.

Sweet Therapy for Knee Osteoarthritis

David Rabago, MD, assistant professor and associate research director of department of family medicine, University of Wisconsin, Madison, and leader of a study in *Annals of Family Medicine*.

Sugar injections may help knee osteoarthritis that has not responded to physical therapy or nonsteroidal anti-inflammatory drugs (NSAIDs). The reason dextrose prolotherapy—an injection of a sugar solution into and around the knee joint to relieve pain and stiffness—helps is not known. The shots may trigger a healing response.

To find an experienced prolotherapist: Visit the website of the American Association of Orthopaedic Medicine (AAOMed.org under "Find Experienced Orthopaedic Doctors" click on "Prolotherapy Injections").

Sugar injections typically are not covered by insurance.

Arthritic Knees? Surprising Shoe Recommendation...

Najia Shakoor, MD, associate professor of internal medicine at Rush Medical College, Chicago.

If you have painful arthritic knees, you probably think that you should be wearing shoes that look and feel supportive—thick-soled, sturdy ones like super-structured sneakers. Not so! A recent study from Rush University Medical Center in Chicago discovered that such footwear doesn't help the problem. In fact, the research concluded that shoes offering the least amount of foot support are better for folks who suffer from osteoarthritis in their knee or knees.

Rheumatologist and study author Najia Shakoor, MD, associate professor of internal medicine at Rush, explained that when people who have knee arthritis walk around, it increases the load (or force) exerted on the inner knee, which is where arthritis most commonly occurs. This additional pressure erodes cartilage even further, eventually resulting in the hideously painful bone-on-bone contact that characterizes arthritis at its worst.

Dr. Shakoor's team evaluated the differences in load created by walking in a variety of types of shoes—heavy-soled clogs (Dansko)...walking shoes with sturdy foot support (Brooks Addiction)...lightweight, flexible sneakers with thin soles (Puma H Street)...ordinary rubber flip-flops...as well as going barefoot.

LESS IS BEST

To the surprise of many, researchers found that the biomechanics of the foot and knee working together created the least load when patients walked barefoot. Next best were the most minimal of shoes, such as thin-soled sneakers and even rubber flip-flops! Far better for the knees than the rigid structure of clogs and heavy-duty athletic shoes, these flexible types of shoes reduced knee load by as much as 15%.

Now, before anyone runs out to Walmart to buy flip-flops, take note. While they may have their place (the beach, for instance), Dr. Shakoor and many other experts caution against flip-flops for many folks—most particularly those with balance issues, because they may cause you to trip. Instead, look for something that has flat, flexible soles but doesn't "flip or flop" while you walk—for example, it's not hard to find sandals that strap the foot securely to the sole. Ballet flats or slip-on boat shoes (such as Docksides) are also good choices. And, when you get home, this is a great excuse to kick them off—which is what feels best of all!

Walking: A Drug-Free Rx for Arthritis

Susan Besser, MD, primary care physician, Mercy Personal Physicians in Baltimore, Maryland.

Study titled "Effectiveness of a Scaled-Up Arthritis Self-Management Program in Oregon: Walk With Ease," led by researchers at Oregon State University, published in *American Journal of Public Health*.

Getting on a smart walking program can help with inflammatory conditions such as rheumatoid arthritis and psoriatic arthritis and "wear and tear" osteoarthritis.

Walking is so beneficial that it's considered a natural medication for arthritis. It makes your muscles stronger, which takes pressure off your joints...and boosts the health of your cartilage, your joints' shock absorbers, by increasing circulation and bringing nutrients and oxygen to the area. And while walking specifically targets the joints in your lower body, the feel-good endorphins released during exercise should make you feel better from head to toe.

As a calorie-burning exercise, walking can also help with weight loss—and every pound of overweight puts added pressure on your joints. Weigh less, and you have less pain. *Here's what to do...*

How long to walk: Your goal is to walk for 30 to 60 minutes at a time, but if you can handle only five minutes to start, that's OK—start there and go a little longer every day.

How often to walk: Remember, walking is medicine for arthritis—so aim to take this medicine every day! If you're new to walking, begin with two or three days a week and build up from there.

How fast to walk: Walk fast enough to increase your heart rate while still being able to have a conversation. The key is to push yourself but not to the point that you're tiring too quickly or adding to your joint pain.

Of course, if you have any additional mobility issues or other chronic conditions, ask your doctor whether you should refine these guidelines.

You can follow a plan on your own, no gym membership needed. But you might find needed motivation through a walking group with friends or with a formal program such as Walk with Ease from the Arthritis Foundation. This six-week course, held in cities across the country, shows you how to manage arthritis as well as begin a walking routine. Researchers at Oregon State University surveyed 598 sedentary people with arthritis who participated in the program and found that those who completed it reported significantly less pain and fatigue. Not near a group? You purchase a self-guide book ($12) with all the information from their website and start reaping the benefits.

To make your walks more comfortable, warm up for a few minutes with easy walking in place, then stretch. Stretch again after walking—you should be able to increase your range of motion as these muscles will be quite warm.

Whenever your joints feel sore, use a shorter stride. This puts less pressure on them.

Maintain good posture, with your core engaged and your upper body relaxed.

Don't let pride or even forgetfulness keep you from wearing a brace if your doctor has recommended one. The support it offers will help stabilize the joint, make walking easier, and potentially prevent a fall.

Note: If starting out walking on land is simply too painful for you, get in a pool, said Susan Besser, MD, a primary care physician with Mercy Personal Physicians in Baltimore, Maryland. Walking in water is gentler on your joints yet adds some resistance, giving you an even better workout.

Even if You Have Arthritis, High-Impact Exercise Can Help Your Knees

Study titled "Effect of Exercise on Patellar Cartilage in Women with Mild Knee Osteoarthritis" by researchers at Central Finland Central Hospital, Oulu University Hospital, University of Oulu, University of Helsinki and Helsinki University Hospital, Finland, published in *Medicine & Science in Sports & Exercise.*

When your knees hurt climbing the stairs, you don't exactly feel like jumping for joy. But that may be exactly what you need to do to strengthen the cartilage in your knees and slow the progression of osteoarthritis. While you shouldn't run outside and starting playing hopscotch right away, a carefully structured jumping program may benefit your knees without hurting them.

STEP JUMPING BUILDS CARTILAGE

Until now, high-impact exercise has been thought to be harmful to people with knee arthritis. The surprising finding that it may not only be safe but actually beneficial comes from a Finnish study. It helps build knee cartilage, which no- or low-impact aerobic exercise has not been shown to do.

The researchers looked at the effect of a high-impact exercise program on knee cartilage, osteoarthritis symptoms and physical function in 76 women, ages 50 to 65, who had knee pain on most days. The women had patellofemoral joint osteoarthritis, a common form of the disease that causes pain under the kneecap (aka the patella) and often makes climbing stairs painful. Sound familiar? Men often get this kind of knee arthritis, too, so let's all pay attention.

The women were randomly assigned to either an exercise group or a control group. The control group went about their normal daily routines. The exercise group went to supervised classes of about an hour three times a week.

Their jumping exercises started out very gentle and gradually increased in intensity. The women did aerobics while jumping over foam blocks that were two inches from the ground and jumped up and down steps that were four inches high. Every three months, the heights were raised until eventually they were about eight inches for both the aerobics and the steps. There were no deep squats. (Squats can be very tough on knees.) On average, each exerciser did 44 high-impact jumps per exercise session, which is less pounding than you'd get from, say, running for the same amount of time. A few women (six, to be exact) had some joint problems at one time or another, but they just took a week or more off and then returned to the classes.

The results were modest but significant. At the end of the 12-month period, the investigators found that when measured via magnetic resonance imaging (MRI), the thickness of the kneecap cartilage among women assigned to the jumping group had a 7% increase. For the control-group there was no improvement. They also found the knee extension force of those in the jumping group increased by 11% compared with controls. Self-reported pain was about the same in the jumping and the control group. The women got a little fitter, too.

Added bonus: Although this study did not look at bone strength, high-impact exercise is exactly what's been shown to help strengthen bones against osteoporosis.

SHOULD YOU JUMP TO IT?

The current study suggests that adding a little jumping—carefully—to your routine might be reasonable. But don't neglect low-impact exercises such as cycling or aquatic classes either. In the end, any exercise that doesn't hurt you is good for your knees. You might call it the arthritis paradox—it may hurt to be active, but being active reduces the hurt. When it comes to the knees in particular, there is growing evidence that exercise reduces pain and improves function.

Ease Arthritis in Just Eight Weeks with Tai Chi

Leigh Callahan, PhD, professor in the departments of medicine and social medicine at the Thurston Arthritis Research Center of the University of North Carolina at Chapel Hill. She has more than 20 years of experience in arthritis and health outcomes research.

Paul Lam, MD, family physician, tai chi master, and director and cofounder of the Tai Chi for Health Institute in Sydney, Australia. He is the author or coauthor of numerous books, including *Overcoming Arthritis: How to Relieve Pain and Restore Mobility Through a Unique Tai Chi Program* and *Teaching Tai Chi Effectively*. TaiChiForHealthInstitute.org

When arthritic joints ache, the last thing you may want to do is work out. But a new study shows that a certain kind of exercise actually can relieve arthritis symptoms fairly quickly—no drugs involved.

The secret weapon: Tai chi, a gentle form of martial arts.

The study participants included 247 patients (mostly women) who had osteoarthritis, rheumatoid arthritis or another type of arthritis. Lead researcher Leigh Callahan, PhD, a professor at the University of North Carolina at Chapel Hill's Thurston Arthritis Research Center, told me that after only eight weeks of twice-weekly sessions of tai chi, participants experienced significantly reduced joint pain, stiffness and fatigue...improved ability to extend their reach while maintaining balance (which can be challenging for arthritis patients)...better sleep...and an increased sense of well-being.

For some specific moves that can give readers a taste of tai chi, we contacted Paul Lam, MD, a family physician, tai chi master and coauthor of *Overcoming Arthritis: How to Relieve Pain and Restore Mobility Through a Unique Tai Chi Program*. Dr. Lam suggested that as you practice the two techniques that follow, you try to move slowly, continuously and gracefully (as you become more familiar with the movements, they will start to flow)... breathe slowly, naturally and easily...and never lock your joints. (Of course, as with any new exercise activity, get your doctor's OK before you begin.) *Tai chi moves to try...*

- **Spine stretch.** *To start:* Stand with feet shoulder-width apart and knees slightly bent... or sit in a sturdy chair. Hold your hands out in front of you, about eight inches from your torso, elbows somewhat bent, left hand at collarbone height (palm facing down) and right hand at belly-button height (palm facing up). Palms should be approximately 12 inches apart, as if holding the top and bottom of a beach ball.

Move: Slowly raise your right arm, bringing it overhead and turning your right palm up toward the ceiling...at the same time, lower your left arm until your left hand is near your left hip, left palm still facing toward the floor. (Both elbows should stay slightly bent throughout.) Pause, visualizing the gentle stretch that your spine is getting. Then slowly return to the initial position, but with the right hand on top and the left hand on the bottom of the imaginary beach ball. Repeat the move on the other side, raising your left arm and lowering your right arm.

Video demo: Visit Arthritis.org/living-with-arthritis/exercise/videos/tai-chi/.

- **Arm circles.** *To start:* Stand with feet shoulder-width apart, knees slightly bent...or sit in a sturdy chair. Arms are at your sides, elbows slightly bent.

Move: Slowly lift your arms, opening them out to your sides and turning the palms upward. Keeping elbows somewhat bent, continue raising your arms until they create a large circle overhead. Then slowly lower your arms, bringing your palms together as your hands move down past your face to heart level...then return to starting position and repeat.

To learn more: Check for tai chi classes at your local community center, health clubs or martial arts schools (be sure to ask if the instructor has experience in working with arthritis patients)...and/or contact your local Arthritis Foundation chapter (Arthritis.org) for referrals to approved tai chi instructors, Dr. Lam suggested.

Yoga Cure for Arthritis

Tara Stiles, founder and owner of Strala Yoga in New York City. She is the author of two books, *Yoga Cures* and *Slim Calm Sexy Yoga*. Stiles has also created several yoga DVDs with Jane Fonda, Deepak Chopra and others. TaraStiles.com

Yoga aficionados know that this ancient practice can tone muscles and calm the mind. But few people are aware of yoga's ability to cure everyday ailments that can cause pain.

As a low-impact exercise that focuses on physical postures (asanas) and breathing techniques, yoga helps relieve a number of chronic conditions—by increasing blood flow, for example, and improving range of motion.

And even though regular yoga practice offers the broadest range of health benefits, doing targeted yoga moves, as needed, can often help you feel better within minutes. Do not worry about doing the move perfectly—simply breathe deeply while gently moving your body into position.

If you suffer from arthritis, consider trying the single, carefully chosen yoga pose described here. This can help other treatments, such as medication, work more effectively—(stay in the pose for five to 10 deep, long breaths)...*

Pose to try: "Hands and knees fist release." For many people, this pose helps the swelling, joint pain, stiffness and limited range of motion that accompany rheumatoid arthritis and osteoarthritis—especially in the hands.

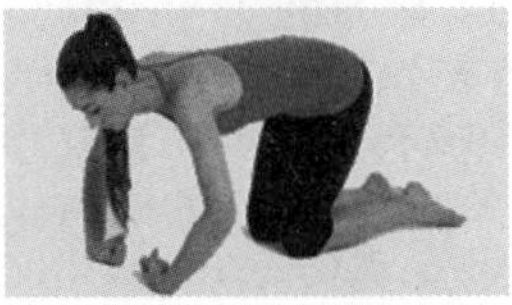

What to do: Gently, get on your hands and knees. Make tight fists with both hands. Bend your elbows out to your sides, and place the tops of your hands on the ground, with your knuckles facing each other. Begin to straighten your elbows, but keep your fists tight and only do as much as you can without causing pain. You should feel a stretch on the tops of your wrists.

How it works: Whether you have arthritis or just sit at a desk all day, which dramatically limits your range of motion, this move increases flexibility in the wrists, hands, arms and back—important in easing arthritis pain.

*If your joint pain is severe, or you have a chronic medical condition in addition to arthritis, check with your doctor before doing this pose, which should be done on a mat or carpeted floor.

Photo Credit: Thomas Hoeffgen

Exercises for Pain-Free Joints

Harris H. McIlwain, MD, rheumatologist and pain specialist with Tampa Medical Group and adjunct professor at University of South Florida College of Public Health, both in Tampa. He is coauthor, with Debra Fulghum Bruce, PhD, of *Diet for a Pain-Free Life* and *Pain-Free Arthritis*.

Stretching makes joints more limber, prevents muscles from becoming short and tight, and protects against injury. Stretch gently, moving each joint to the maximum range of motion possible without causing unusual discomfort. Do these moves daily, working up to 15 repetitions of each.

- **Shoulder stretch.** Sit with back straight and clasp hands behind your head. Move elbows forward as if trying to get them to touch in front of your face. Hold five seconds. Next, move elbows back until they point out to the side...hold five seconds. This increases shoulders' range of motion—making it easier, for instance, to style your hair.
- **Bathtub stretch.** Moist heat eases movement by increasing flow of blood, oxygen and nutrients to joints. During a warm bath or while seated on a shower stool, "circle" wrists by rotating hands, envisioning fingertips tracing the face of a clock. Next, circle ankles by rotating feet.
- **Finger flexion.** Bring the tips of your right thumb and forefinger together, making as round an "O" as possible...hold five seconds... repeat with other fingers. Switch hands.

- **Resistance training strengthens muscles that surround joints, easing pain by providing muscular support.** Try these exercises three times weekly, building up to 15 repetitions of each.

- **Hand helper.** Hold a tennis-ball–sized foam (Nerf) ball in one hand...squeeze, hold five seconds, release. Switch hands.

- **Hip extension.** Lie facedown on a mat or bed, legs extended. Bend arms and turn head to one side, resting your cheek on the backs of your hands. Knees straight, raise your right leg until your ankle is eight to 12 inches above the mat...hold five seconds...lower. Switch legs.

- **Knee extension.** Sit in a chair, feet flat on floor. Raise your left foot, straightening knee completely so the leg is parallel to the floor... tighten knee and thigh muscles...hold five seconds...lower foot to floor and relax. Switch sides.

- **Foot and ankle strengthener.** Sit in a chair. Place your bare foot on top of a tennis ball on the floor. Bearing down slightly, roll the ball underfoot, using the muscles of the toes, arch and ankle to move the ball back and forth and side to side. Continue for 30 seconds. Switch feet.

- **Aerobic activity,** such as walking, rowing and stair-climbing, burns calories and helps you lose excess weight that stresses joints.

For sore shoulders: Swim in a heated pool.

For problem knees and hips: Try biking or stationary cycling. Build up to five 30-minute sessions weekly.

Pain-Free Gardening

Jim Miller, an advocate for older Americans, who writes "Savvy Senior," a weekly information column syndicated in more than 400 newspapers nationwide. Based in Norman, Oklahoma, he also offers a free senior news service at SavvySenior.org.

Gardening is a favorite outdoor activity for millions of Americans, but it can be tough on the body and difficult for individuals with physical limitations, such as arthritis or back pain. Garden work often requires a lot of repetitive stooping, squatting, kneeling, gripping and lifting, which can lead to numerous strains and injury.

To help make your gardening chores a little easier, a wide variety of gardening gear is available now that is lightweight, comfortable to use and ergonomically designed to help protect your body from the physical strains of gardening. *Here are the best of these...*

GLOVES

Specially designed gloves can improve your grip and protect your hands.

- **Atlas Nitrile Touch 370 Garden Club Gloves** are form-fitting and made of a breathable nylon knit with palms and fingers that are coated with nitrile. This thin and flexible synthetic rubber provides excellent grip with less effort and can withstand punctures from small thorns. Available in four sizes and six colors. $5.90. (Amazon.com)

- **ReliefGrip Gardening** leather gloves have durable silicone fingertips and extra padding in the palm and finger joints that can improve gripping power and reduce calluses and blisters. $39.99. (877-524-6642, BionicGloves.com)

DIGGING AND WEEDING TOOLS

Ergonomically designed tools can help take stress off your wrists by reducing the bending and twisting wrist movement that often comes with digging and weeding.

- **CobraHead Weeder and Cultivator** is a steel hook-shaped blade that flares at the tip, resembling the head of a cobra. It requires you to primarily use your arm muscles (rather than your wrists) to dig and chop into the soil.

Available in various versions: A short-handled version (13 inches) for close-up work, $24.95...or a long-handled version (48-, 54- and 60-inch options) for standing work, $59.95. (866-962-6272, CobraHead.com)

- **Miracle-Gro Five-Piece Ergonomic Garden Tool Set** has hand tools with curved handles that keep your wrist in a natural, straight position. The set includes a scooper, weeder, transplanter, cultivator and trowel. $54.99. These tools also are sold separately for $9.99 each ($14.99 for the scooper). (734-222-8044, RadiusGarden.com)

• **Radius Pro Stainless Transplanter** is a multipurpose shovel that has a large O-shaped handle that allows you to comfortably grip it with both hands for better leverage. It also has a narrow blade and oversized areas for foot placement on the blade to provide better balance and ease of use. $46.99. (734-222-8044, RadiusGarden.com)

PRUNING TOOLS

Fiskars makes three types of pruning tools that have earned the Arthritis Foundation's Ease-of-Use Commendation, which recognizes products that make life easier for people who have arthritis and other limitations. *These tools all have "PowerGear" mechanisms that increase leverage to make cutting easier than with traditional pruners...*

• **Fiskars PowerGear Hand Pruner** is for cutting stems and branches up to three-quarters-of-an-inch thick. It has a contoured handle that rotates toward you when you squeeze it to reduce hand and wrist strain. $24.99. Fiskars also offers the same pruner in a large size for people with big hands for $29.99 and a soft-grip version for extra comfort, $13.99. (866-348-5661, Fiskars.com)

• **Fiskars PowerGear Loppers** cut tree and shrub branches up to two inches thick. Loppers come in five different lengths, ranging from 15 to 32 inches, and cost between $26.99 and $47.99. (866-348-5661, Fiskars.com)

• **Fiskars PowerGear Hedge Shears** are for shaping and trimming hedges and shrubs. These shears give you up to three times more power on every cut. $41.99. (866-348-5661, Fiskars.com)

• **Corona Razor Tooth Folding Saw,** used for pruning branches, offers a seven-, eight- or 10-inch razor-toothed curved blade that folds into the handle for safe, easy storage. It has an ergonomic grip for comfort. $26.70 to $30.34. (800-847-7863, CoronaToolsUSA.com)

KNEE AND BACK AIDS

Knee pads and garden seats can protect your knees and save your back when you are working close to the ground. The Gardener's Supply Company (888-833-1412, Gardeners.com) offers a number of well-designed products...

• **Jolly Kneeler** is a lightweight polyurethane knee rest that is molded to support your knees and has a built-in handle. $29.95.

• **Garden Kneeler** is a multipurpose knee pad with steel support handles to help you raise and lower yourself. Or flip it over, and it becomes a padded bench to sit on for weeding or planting. $34.95. There also is the Deep-Seat Garden Kneeler with a 30% larger knee pad/seat. $44.95.

And there is the GardenEase Kneeler, with easy-to-grip round handles and a removable foam pad that you can use separately for indoor chores. $69.95.

• **Deluxe Tractor Scoot with Bucket Basket** is a height-adjustable, swivel garden seat on four wheels. It has a pull handle that doubles as a support to help you get up and sit down, a built-in accessory tray under the seat and a rear basket mount that lets you carry tools, plants or other gardening paraphernalia. $89.95.

CHAPTER 3

Autoimmune and Related Diseases

When Your Immune System Fights Itself

How many autoimmune diseases can you name?

If you're like most Americans, the answer is "none"...and that's a bigger problem than you might guess. Why? Because autoimmune diseases affect as many as one in 20 Americans, and if anyone in your family has one, you are at risk, too. Autoimmune diseases can be painful and debilitating, even fatal—and with this type of illness, patient awareness is particularly important.

Scientists have identified more than 100 autoimmune illnesses, and the list includes some names that you surely will recognize—such as multiple sclerosis, diabetes and celiac disease, not to mention rheumatoid arthritis and psoriasis. The American Autoimmune Related Diseases Association (AARDA) is trying to educate people about the fact that all autoimmune diseases are genetically linked to one another...your mother's psoriasis is related to your brother's arthritis and your cousin's Crohn's disease.

CONNECTING THE DOTS

It's not always clear what the trigger is (more about that in a minute), but all autoimmune diseases occur when your immune system attacks your body's own proteins, mistakenly identifying them as invaders and producing antibodies or T cells to overcome them. The result is any one of a number of serious and chronic illnesses that can develop in any bodily system, but most commonly in the nervous, gastrointestinal and endocrine systems, blood, kidneys, lymph nodes, heart and liver.

Noel R. Rose, MD, PhD, director, Autoimmune Disease Research Center, The Johns Hopkins University, Baltimore, and chairman emeritus, National Scientific Advisory Board, American Autoimmune Related Diseases Association, Inc. (AARDA), Eastpointe, Michigan.

Virginia T. Ladd, president and executive director, American Autoimmune Related Diseases Association, Inc. (AARDA), Eastpointe, Michigan.

While their symptoms vary widely, autoimmune diseases share several common threads…

• **They can run in families,** although they may take different forms in different family members. The shared trait is an increased susceptibility to autoimmune disease in general.

• **Women are more susceptible than men as a result of their enhanced immune system.** Three out of four people with an autoimmune disease are women. Ethnicity is a factor, too, with African American, Hispanic and Asian women more prone than Caucasians to certain autoimmune disorders.

• **Environmental factors also can trigger autoimmune disease.** Research has found links with viral and bacterial infections, toxins, drugs, chemicals and even sunlight.

DO THESE SOUND FAMILIAR?

Here are some of the most common autoimmune diseases (you can view a more comprehensive list at AARDA.org)…

• **Celiac disease.** An intolerance for gluten in wheat and other grains.

• **Crohn's disease.** A form of inflammatory bowel disease. (See more on celiac, Crohn's and gluten disorders in chapter 1, "Abdominal Pain.")

• **Diabetes type 1.** A lifelong endocrine condition resulting from the autoimmune destruction of the cells in the pancreas that manufacture insulin.

• **Hashimoto's disease.** An autoimmune disease in which the thyroid is gradually destroyed.

• **Lupus.** A chronic, inflammatory disorder that damages the joints, skin, kidneys and other parts of the body.

• **Multiple sclerosis.** A crippling autoimmune disease that affects the brain and spinal cord.

• **Psoriasis.** An inflammatory skin disorder characterized by redness and silvery scales.

• **Rheumatoid arthritis.** A painful autoimmune joint disease that involves other organs.

• **Scleroderma.** A disorder in which inflammation infiltrates the skin, esophagus, lungs and other organs. (See chapter 6, "Chest Pain," for more information on scleroderma.)

WATCH THE SYMPTOMS

Many autoimmune disorders have symptoms that are vague, transitory and hard to pin down, which is undoubtedly a factor in a common complaint among people with autoimmune diseases—that doctors don't take them seriously. It's not uncommon for people to see four or five different doctors over a period of five years or so before finding one who pays close attention, orders the appropriate tests and pins down a diagnosis. The process can be incredibly frustrating, especially given that patients often get sicker and sicker before getting any meaningful treatment.

Does any of this sound familiar to you? Are any members of your family struggling with similar stories of disconnected symptoms that are not part of an identifiable disease, or has anyone already been diagnosed with an autoimmune disease? If so, you need to take your symptoms very seriously. *Here are the steps you should take to find the true cause of your symptoms and get a proper diagnosis and treatment…*

• **Research your family's medical history, and share it with your doctor.** Collect information about not just your immediate family, but also grandparents, aunts, uncles and cousins.

• **Write down all your symptoms**—even if they appear unrelated—and tell your doctor about them.

Note: The single most widespread symptom caused by autoimmune diseases is extreme fatigue, which goes way beyond ordinary tiredness—it's a state of exhaustion that makes it impossible to do what you need to do.

• **If many of your symptoms fall into a particular category** (say, gastrointestinal distress or joint pain), ask your primary care provider to refer you to an appropriate specialist (such as a gastroenterologist or a rheumatologist). When you see the specialist, share your family history and ask to have autoimmune disease investigated.

• **Get a second opinion**—or a third or fourth one, if necessary, if symptoms continue but no cause is discovered. And…if your doctor doesn't take your concerns seriously, you need a new doctor!

Living Well with Multiple Sclerosis

Patricia K. Coyle, MD, professor and acting chair of the department of neurology at Stony Brook University Medical Center, and director of the Stony Brook Multiple Sclerosis Comprehensive Care Center, New York.

The term multiple sclerosis (MS) conjures up frightening images of life in a wheelchair—but thanks to recent advances, an MS diagnosis no longer means that disability is inevitable. This is especially good news for women, given that MS is two to three times more common in women than men.

It is now possible to detect MS earlier...begin effective treatment just about as soon as symptoms appear...and slow the disease's progression. Yet despite this encouraging news, MS often goes undiagnosed for months or years—narrowing the window of opportunity that early treatment provides.

What women must know to protect themselves...

MS EXPLAINED

With MS, the immune system's white blood cells mistakenly attack the myelin (nerve fibers' protective coating) and nerve fibers themselves in the brain, spinal cord and optic nerves. This impairs the nerves' ability to transmit messages.

Women's greater vulnerability to MS may be related to hormones. MS typically strikes young adults, but it can appear as late as in one's 70s. People of northern European descent are more genetically predisposed to MS. Parents, siblings and children of MS patients have a 2% to 5% chance of developing it, too. Genes alone don't bring on the disease, however. Something in the environment—such as exposure to the Epstein-Barr virus (which causes mononucleosis) or vitamin-D deficiency at a young age—seems to help trigger MS.

DIAGNOSIS DIFFICULTIES

MS diagnosis often is delayed because the first symptoms can be vague. Patients tend to attribute them to a minor problem, such as a pinched nerve...doctors may mistake MS for spinal disk disease, vitamin B-12 deficiency or anxiety.

Any of the symptoms below merit a call to the doctor. If MS is suspected, a neurologist or MS center can run tests.

Referrals to a specialist: National Multiple Sclerosis Society, 800-344-4867, NationalMSSociety.org...Consortium of MS Centers, 201-487-1050, MScare.org.

Initial symptoms...

- **Clumsiness, loss of balance**
- **Double vision, blurred vision**
- **Eye pain, facial pain**
- **Numb face, limbs or torso**
- **Shocklike sensations upon bending the neck**
- **Stiffness, muscle spasms**
- **Weakness, extreme fatigue.**

Later symptoms...

- **Bladder or bowel incontinence**
- **Difficulty becoming sexually aroused or climaxing**
- **Paralysis, typically in the legs**
- **Poor concentration and memory**
- **Speech or swallowing problems.**

Diagnosis is based on a patient's medical history, a neurological exam and magnetic resonance imaging (MRI) to check for damaged tissue in the brain and spinal cord. *There are four types of MS...*

- **Relapsing-remitting MS,** which affects about 85% of patients, is characterized by sudden flare-ups (relapses) of symptoms followed by periods of improvement, during which patients are stable.
- **Primary progressive MS accounts for about 10% of MS cases.** Symptoms worsen progressively from onset with no improvement.
- **Progressive-relapsing MS,** which affects about 5% of patients, involves steady worsening of symptoms from onset, plus later flare-ups.

• **Secondary progressive MS** refers to relapsing-remitting MS that transitions to slow worsening. Patients become increasingly disabled instead of stabilizing between flare-ups.

MS is rarely fatal. Except when vital brain stem functions (such as breathing and heart rate) are affected or the disease has led to severe disability, most patients have a near-normal life expectancy.

MS TREATMENT TODAY

New disease-modifying therapy (DMT) drugs are key to treatment. Starting a DMT soon after MS develops can lower the risk for long-term disability...cut the number of relapses...and lessen symptom severity during flare-ups. DMTs cannot reverse existing damage but can forestall future damage and significantly reduce the likelihood that relapsing MS will transition to progressive MS. For patients who have had MS for years, DMTs also are helpful so long as relapses are still occurring.

Each MS medication has its own pros and cons, so doctors work with each individual patient to determine the optimal treatment. *Options...*

• **Glatiramer (Copaxone) and interferon betas (Avonex, Betaseron, Rebif)** are DMTs that reduce nervous system inflammation and protect nerve cells. They are given by self-injection once or more weekly.

• **Natalizumab (Tysabri),** a monthly DMT given by intravenous infusion (IV drip) at an infusion center, targets errant white blood cells.

• **Mitoxantrone (Novantrone),** an intravenous chemotherapy drug, suppresses the immune system.

• **Prescription steroids** are used during flare-ups to calm symptoms.

Natural therapies also ease MS symptoms. *Examples...*

• **Dietary changes.** MS patients may benefit from eating less saturated fat and more vitamin B-12 (found in dairy foods, eggs, meat, poultry and shellfish)...vitamin D (found in dairy foods and fish)...omega-3 fatty acids (found in fatty fish, cod liver oil and flaxseed oil)...and omega-6 fatty acids (found in safflower seed oil and sunflower oil). If blood tests show a deficiency, supplements may be recommended.

• **Exercise.** Aerobics help reduce fatigue, stress and incontinence...stretching eases stiffness.

Recommended: Yoga, tai chi, aquatics.

• **Acupuncture.** For many patients, this eases pain, numbness, spasms and incontinence.

• **Massage.** This may reduce pain, stiffness and spasticity.

On the horizon: Though still a long way off, novel therapies—such as oral DMTs and a DNA vaccine to treat MS—hold some promise that, in the future, MS may become a thing of the past.

How to Fight MS Without Drugs

George Jelinek, MD, emergency physician with professorial appointments at University of Melbourne and Monash University, both in Melbourne, Australia. He was the founding editor of *Emergency Medicine Australasia* and is author of *Overcoming Multiple Sclerosis: An Evidence-Based Guide to Recovery.* OvercomingMultipleSclerosis.org

---

Multiple sclerosis (MS) is one of the most common nerve diseases. It's also among the most frightening because there isn't a cure. Patients imagine a future that includes extreme fatigue, muscle weakness, pain and, in some cases, premature death.

Many patients have a form of MS known as relapsing-remitting, in which the disease generally flares up every year or two. The relapses are followed by periods of remission.

However, there's a way to reduce symptoms and the frequency of relapses by up to 95%. All you need to do is make some lifestyle changes. And these lifestyle changes may be more effective than medications at slowing, and sometimes stopping, the disease's progression.

Numerous studies have shown that people who modify their diets and make other lifestyle changes often can remain symptom-free for decades. I'm a good example—I was diagnosed with MS in 1999, when I was 45. I've had no relapses.

WHAT MS DOES

MS, an autoimmune disease, damages the fatty myelin sheath that surrounds nerves in the brain and spinal cord. The immune system kicks in and produces inflammation that strips away the myelin and causes nerve scarring. This impairs the transmission of nerve impulses.

The central nervous system can sometimes regenerate damaged nerve tissue—but only if there's minimal demyelination. The key way to reduce MS relapses is to reduce demyelination. *Here are the strategies that work best...*

ELIMINATE SATURATED FAT

One long-term study of MS followed the same group of patients for 34 years. At the beginning, participants averaged one to 1.2 relapses a year. This is typical for most MS patients. The patients who switched to a diet that was very low in saturated fat averaged just 0.05 relapses within three years. This translates to about one relapse every 20 years.

MS patients tend to accumulate more saturated fat in their cell membranes than those without the disease. Saturated fat is thought to stimulate the Th1 response, the release of myelin-damaging inflammatory chemicals by immune cells.

Patients who switch to a vegetarian diet—and avoid processed foods, which often are high in saturated fat—can reduce their relapse rate by about 95%. In contrast, most medications achieve only about a 30% reduction.

I advise patients not to eat fatty red meat (but see information on organ meats, page 89), commercial baked goods or anything that is deep-fried. They also should avoid eggs (except for the whites) and dairy, including reduced-fat cheese and reduced-fat milk. There's some evidence that a protein in dairy may be just as likely as saturated fat to trigger relapses.

MORE FISH

Patients who consume the most omega-3 fatty acids from fish (or fish-oil supplements) have about 30% fewer relapses than those who get the least. These fatty acids can reduce relapses even in patients who continue to eat meat or other foods that are high in saturated fat. The omega-3s make cell membranes more fluid and flexible. This improves their responsiveness to chemical signals and helps them resist attacks on the immune system. Omega-3s also help the body suppress inflammation.

The optimal amount is thought to be about 20 grams (g)—a little less than three-quarters of an ounce—of fish oil daily. I eat fish three or four days a week. I usually choose oily fish, such as sardines or mackerel. I take fish-oil supplements only on the days when I don't eat fish.

OMEGA-3S FROM FLAX

Flaxseed oil is the best nonfish source of omega-3s. It has a slightly buttery taste that I enjoy. I put it on salads or pasta. It's good for patients who don't like fish or who want a less expensive alternative to fish-oil supplements.

There's been a lot of debate about the use of flaxseed oil as a source of omega-3s. This is because only a small percentage of the alpha-linolenic acid in flaxseed oil is converted in the body into the healthful oils found in fish—EPA (eicosapentaenoic acid) and DHA (docosahexaenoic acid). I recommend two tablespoons of flaxseed oil daily.

VITAMIN D

Patients with MS tend to feel better, and have fewer relapses, when they spend time in the sun. A study published in *Occupational and Environmental Medicine* found that people with MS who got the most sun were 76% less likely to die from MS than those without sun exposure.

The body synthesizes vitamin D from sunshine. Vitamin D interacts with the receptors on white blood cells involved in the MS immune response. One study found that MS patients had the lowest relapse rates in mid-to-late summer, when UV exposure from sunlight is highest.

People are understandably nervous about getting too much sun. But in moderation, skin cancer risk is low. I advise patients to get 10 to 15 minutes of all-over sun (by wearing a bathing suit) three to five times a week. If you don't live where you can do that year-round, take a vitamin D supplement.

The long-running Nurses Health Study found that women who took a daily multinutrient that contained 400 international units (IU) of vitamin D were 40% less likely to get MS than those who didn't. Patients who already have MS are less likely to have relapses—and will probably have milder symptoms when they do—if they supplement regularly.

I recommend that MS patients take 5,000 IU of vitamin D on overcast days or on days when they don't get outside. Use the D-3 form—it's similar to the vitamin D from sun exposure.

BOOST ENERGY

Regular exercise improves energy and muscle strength and may reduce MS relapses. It also improves the body's ability to cope with the physical challenges that occur during relapses.

I live in a climate that's warm year-round, so I swim outdoors five or six days a week. It's good exercise, and I get my "dose" of sunshine at the same time.

Bonus: Being in water prevents overheating from exercise, a common problem for people with MS.

MEDITATE

A review in *Journal of Alternative and Complementary Medicine* found that meditation helps relieve symptoms of autoimmune illnesses. It also improves mood, which helps patients to deal positively with MS.

I meditate every day for 30 minutes, usually when I get home from work. The evidence suggests that people who can find the time to do this twice a day probably get even more benefits.

Meditation doesn't have to be a complex spiritual practice. You can just sit in a comfortable chair, relax and focus on your breathing. If you have stressful thoughts, notice them. Then let them go.

This Brain-Boosting Diet Can Conquer Multiple Sclerosis

Terry L. Wahls, MD, internist and clinical professor of medicine at the University of Iowa Carver College of Medicine in Iowa City and president of the Wahls Foundation (TheWahlsFoundation.com). She is the author of *Minding My Mitochondria: How I Overcame Secondary Progressive Multiple Sclerosis and Got Out of My Wheelchair.*

At age 44, I was diagnosed with multiple sclerosis (MS). Three years later, when I became dependent on a wheelchair, my MS was classified as "secondary progressive," meaning that the disease was steadily progressing with no periods of improvement. I kept getting weaker, even though I was receiving widely used treatments for MS including chemotherapy and immune-suppressing medications.

Now: Thanks to the regimen I designed, I haven't needed a wheelchair or even a cane for more than three years. I ride to work on my bicycle, my energy is good and I've stopped taking medication to treat my MS. What happened?

Here's what I credit for my dramatic turnaround—and a description of how it might help you, as well. Because MS is a neurological disease, this program is designed to also help people who are concerned about dementia or Parkinson's disease, have depression or have suffered a traumatic brain injury or stroke.

FINDING A SOLUTION

With the help of my medical training, I began poring over the medical literature and designed my own treatment protocol in 2007 based on my theories of what allowed MS to develop and progress.

In people with MS, immune cells damage the myelin sheath, protein and fatty substances that surround nerve cells in the brain and spinal cord. This results in slower nerve signals, which lead to muscle weakness, a lack of balance and muscle coordination, bladder or bowel spasms, blurred vision and other symptoms.

Medications can reduce symptoms, but they don't accelerate nerve signals. As a result, MS patients battle physical and neurological disability—experienced either episodically or in a steady, unrelenting course. The disease often continues to worsen despite therapy. Within 10 years of initial diagnosis, half of MS patients are unable to work because of disabling levels of fatigue, and one-third need a cane, scooter or wheelchair.

After thoroughly reviewing the research, I decided to put myself on a diet that increases the efficiency of mitochondria, units within cells that supply the energy that's needed for nerve activity. Although the effect of diet on MS was unproven, I firmly believed that this was my best hope for fighting MS.

My eating plan was designed to improve the balance of neurotransmitters and supply the mitochondria with the building blocks needed for healthy nerve activity.

MY BRAIN-HEALTH DIET

People who follow this diet typically notice improvements in neurological symptoms within weeks.*

Because natural foods contain a variety of nutrients that can work synergistically, I recommend taking supplements only when you are unable to get the following nutrients in your diet. Be sure to discuss the supplements (and dosages) with your doctor if you take blood-thinning medication—some supplements may have a blood-thinning effect.

In addition to taking such general steps as avoiding sugary and/or processed foods that are low in key nutrients, make sure you get enough...

- **Sulfur vegetables.** Cabbage, kale, collard greens and asparagus are excellent sources of sulfur, which is used by the body to produce gamma-aminobutyric acid (GABA). This "inhibitory" neurotransmitter counteracts the early brain-cell death that can occur if the neurotransmitter glutamate reaches excessive levels.

My advice: Consume three cups of greens each day, including one to three cups of sulfur-rich vegetables daily.

*Consult your doctor before trying the diet and/or supplements described here—especially if you take any medication or have kidney or liver disease.

Also: To get other important nutrients, consume one to three cups of brightly colored vegetables or berries each day.

- **Coenzyme Q-10.** Exposure to environmental toxins, such as detergents, pesticide residues and mercury, has been linked to MS and other neurological conditions, such as dementia and Parkinson's disease. Coenzyme Q-10 is a fat-soluble compound that helps minimize the effects of these toxins while increasing the amount of energy produced by mitochondria.

Organ meats, such as calf liver and chicken liver, are among the best sources of coenzyme Q-10. I particularly recommend organ meats for older adults because coenzyme Q-10 production declines with age. It's also suppressed by cholesterol-lowering statin drugs.

My advice: Eat organ meats at least once a week. If you don't like organ meats, sardines, herring and rainbow trout are also high in coenzyme Q-10. Coenzyme Q-10 is available in supplement form, too.

- **Omega-3 fatty acids.** The omega-3 fatty acids in cold-water fish, such as salmon and sardines, are used by the body to produce the myelin that insulates brain and spinal cord cells. Myelin is also used to repair damage caused by MS. Omega-3s are concentrated in the brain and are necessary to help prevent depression and cognitive disorders.

My advice: To avoid concern about mercury and other toxins in cold-water fish, such as salmon, get your omega-3s from fish oil supplements that are purified.

Recommended dose: 1 g to 3 g daily.

Processed Foods Linked to Autoimmune Disease

Study by researchers at Technion-Israel Institute of Technology, Haifa, Israel, published in *Autoimmune Reviews.*

Long-term exposure to the additives in processed foods—including glucose, sodium and fat solvents—is associated with a weakening of the intestine's resistance to bacteria and toxins. This weakening can contribute to the development of autoimmune diseases, such as type 1 diabetes, celiac disease, lupus and multiple sclerosis. This does not prove cause and effect, but you should consider eliminating processed foods from your diet, especially if you have an autoimmune disease or a family history of one.

How a Doctor Beat Her Thyroid Disease Naturally

Susan Blum, MD, assistant clinical professor in the department of preventive medicine at the Icahn School of Medicine at Mount Sinai in New York City, and an integrative medicine specialist in the medicine department at Greenwich Hospital in Connecticut. The founder and director of the Blum Center for Health in Rye Brook, New York, Dr. Blum is also the author of *The Immune System Recovery Plan.* BlumCenterforHealth.com

More than a decade ago, I was diagnosed with Hashimoto's thyroiditis (HT), the most common cause of hypothyroidism, a condition in which the thyroid gland doesn't produce enough thyroid hormones.

Hypothyroidism is more widespread than many people realize, affecting about 14 million Americans. And because thyroid hormones regulate metabolism—key functions such as breathing, heart rate, digestion and body temperature—symptoms are wide ranging. They can include daylong fatigue, weight gain, constipation, low libido, weakness, muscle cramps and aches, cold intolerance, dry skin, poor memory and depression.

HT is typically diagnosed with the same blood tests used to diagnose other causes of hypothyroidism (including those that measure thyroid hormone levels and antithyroid antibodies). With HT, however, an imaging test, such as ultrasound, might also be used to identify the characteristic inflammation of the thyroid gland that occurs with this disease.

My story: When I was diagnosed with HT, my primary care physician said, "No big deal. You'll just take thyroid hormone replacement medication and be fine." I disagreed. As a doctor board-certified in preventive medicine, I wanted to discover the causes of HT, an autoimmune disease in which the immune system mistakes the thyroid for a foreign invader, attacking it and destroying thyroid cells.

For years, I've researched HT for myself and for my patients. With the help of an increasing body of scientific evidence, I have identified key factors that often trigger and worsen most cases of HT—and the natural therapies that can help...

MERCURY

When I began to investigate my disease, I discovered that my body had trouble excreting mercury—a toxic metal that can damage tissues and cause autoimmune disease. I've now found that many patients with autoimmune disease have a high mercury level, based on blood and urine tests. One main source of mercury toxicity—eating lots of fish.

My advice: Large fish at the top of the food chain, such as swordfish and tuna, contain the most mercury, but all fish deliver some levels of the toxic metal. That's why I recommend eating fish only twice a week. Opt for varieties that are low in mercury (such as anchovies, sardines, salmon, sole, trout and Arctic char). If you limit your intake of mercury, your body will start to eliminate the excess stored in tissues via urine and stool.

MISSING NUTRIENTS

Two nutrients are key for preventing or healing HT...*

- **Selenium.** This mineral helps create thyroid hormone...helps convert T4 (the less active form of thyroid hormone) to T3 (the active form)...and protects the thyroid gland from oxidative damage. Selenium is so important for thyroid health that several studies suggest that a deficiency of the mineral might trigger HT.

My advice: Each day, take 400 micrograms (mcg) of selenomethionine (the form found in food, which is easier to absorb) for three to six months, then switch to a maintenance dose of 200 mcg.

*Check with your doctor before taking these supplements—they can interact with some medications and affect certain medical conditions.

Important: Selenium is therapeutic when taken in the appropriate dose but toxic in high doses. Never take more than 400 mcg daily. Once selenium levels are restored, you may be able to maintain adequate levels by eating selenium-rich foods (such as Brazil nuts, shrimp and sardines) instead of taking a supplement.

- **Vitamin D.** Researchers have linked low levels of this immune-strengthening nutrient to many autoimmune diseases, including multiple sclerosis, rheumatoid arthritis, lupus, inflammatory bowel disease—and now HT.

New research: Greek scientists studied 218 people with HT and found that 85% of them had a vitamin D deficiency.

My advice: Start by getting your vitamin D level checked. If your level is low, take a vitamin D-3 supplement. Most people can safely take up to 4,000 international units (IU) daily, but get your vitamin D level checked every three months. Once you reach an optimal vitamin D level (about 50 ng/mL), cut back to 1,000 IU to 2,000 IU daily.

GLUTEN

This protein, found in wheat, barley and rye, can damage the intestinal lining, triggering increased intestinal permeability (also known as leaky gut), in which gluten and other undigested proteins enter the bloodstream.

Once these undigested proteins are in the bloodstream, the immune system attacks them as if they were foreign invaders. People with gluten sensitivity can end up with leaky gut syndrome...diarrhea, bloating and/or fatigue...an immune system in constant overdrive...and an autoimmune disease such as HT.

Recent research: A study published in the journal *Gastroenterology* showed that people who were sensitive to gluten were seven times more likely to develop HT and other types of autoimmune disease compared with people who did not have gluten sensitivity.

My advice: Eliminate gluten for three weeks—and then eat gluten-containing foods for two or three days. Nine out of 10 of my HT patients feel a lot better after the three-week elimination period, with more energy and mental clarity—and their symptoms return after they reintroduce gluten. This is how you will know whether you are gluten sensitive.

Rice, buckwheat, millet and quinoa are gluten free. Gluten-free breads are often in the frozen section because they are not made with the usual chemical preservatives. For more on gluten-free foods, go to MassGeneral.org/digestive/assets/pdf/gluten_free_diet.pdf.

Surgery Could Be Best For Hashimoto's

Ivar Guldvog, MD, researcher, Telemark Hospital Trust, Porsgrunn, Norway.

People suffering from the autoimmune disorder known as Hashimoto's thyroiditis sometimes become so overwhelmed with fatigue, joint and muscle pain, and stiffness that they are unable to function. But preliminary results from a seven-year study suggest that removing the thyroid could bring about vast improvements for patients.

Why: Thyroid removal appears to normalize production of antibodies that attack the thyroid.

If you have Hashimoto's: Ask your doctor if surgery (which may be covered by insurance) is an option. Thyroid-replacement medication must be taken indefinitely.

Sjögren's Syndrome: The Mysterious Disease Defined

Alan Baer, MD, associate professor of medicine and clinical director, The Johns Hopkins University Rheumatology Practice, Good Samaritan Hospital, founder and director of the Johns Hopkins Jerome L. Greene Sjögren's Syndrome Center, Baltimore

When tennis superstar Venus Williams announced that she had been diagnosed with Sjögren's syndrome, the tennis world issued a collective gasp. It was followed by the question: *What on Earth is Sjögren's syndrome?* Venus had been plagued by, as she put it, an "energy-sucking" disease for some time. She suffered from so much fatigue and joint pain that it was sometimes hard for her to even lift her racket. Fans were incredulous. Venus appeared to be in such good shape and, in fact, had won her first match at the 2011 US Open. But then she withdrew from the competition suddenly. Many were bitterly disappointed and suggested that this was just an excuse for her to drop out of the tournament.

Nothing could be further from the truth. The idea that Sjögren's patients were "faking it" or were hypochondriacs is nothing new. That is due to two major factors—the disease is difficult to diagnose, and patients, like Venus, often appear to be perfectly healthy. So let's put this nonsense to rest and finally understand what we can about this mysterious—and serious—autoimmune disease.

FOUR MILLION AMERICANS HAVE THIS DISEASE

Sjögren's syndrome is a chronic inflammatory disorder in which disease-fighting white blood cells mistakenly attack the body's own moisture-producing glands, causing symptoms such as dry eyes and dry mouth. The disease can strike children and older adults, but typically, patients develop it between the ages of 40 and the mid-50s. (Venus, who is only 31 years old, got it very young.) Up to four million Americans have Sjögren's (90% of them are female, though doctors aren't sure why), and unfortunately there is no cure. However, it can be managed. Alan Baer, MD, director of the Johns Hopkins Jerome L. Greene Sjögren's Syndrome Center, explains…

MYSTERY DISEASE

Sjögren's can present many challenges…

- **It's tough to diagnose.** On average, it takes six and a half years for doctors to put the puzzle pieces together.

- **Symptoms seem unrelated.** When the body's immune system attacks the moisture-producing glands, it causes complications all over the body. The eyes and mouth become dry—without the benefit of cleansing saliva, teeth develop cavities…and fatigue and joint pain may develop. In women, there may be a lack of vaginal lubrication, which leads to increased risk for infection and pain during intercourse.

- **It's dangerous.** The longer a person goes without getting a diagnosis, the higher the health risks. If the disease advances undetected, it can set off a widespread inflammatory reaction that can harm the lungs, kidney, liver, pancreas and blood vessels as well as the gastrointestinal and central nervous systems. Up to 30% of Sjögren's patients suffer organ damage, and about 5% develop lymphoma (lymph node cancer).

An accurate diagnosis of the syndrome takes into account multiple factors, including a blood test to check for inflammation, antibodies and elevations in immune-related blood proteins. A biopsy from the inside of the lower lip is taken to assess the inflammatory reaction within the small salivary glands. The production of saliva and tears is also tested.

TOP TREATMENTS

Patients can choose from a variety of over-the-counter preparations that are generally very helpful for symptom relief, says Dr. Baer. Lubricants help with vaginal dryness. For dry

Fibromyalgia Underdiagnosed—Especially in Men

In a study of nearly 4,000 people, 6.4% reported having fibromyalgia symptoms, such as widespread pain, fatigue and memory problems, but only 1.1% had been diagnosed with the condition. Three times more women appeared to have fibromyalgia than were diagnosed—20 times more men had symptoms than were diagnosed. Fibromyalgia can be difficult to diagnose—there is no definitive lab test, and similar symptoms can occur with conditions such as chronic fatigue syndrome and depression.

Daniel Clauw, MD, director, Chronic Pain & Fatigue Research Center, University of Michigan Health System, Ann Arbor.

eyes, there are drops and ointments...and for dry mouth there are sprays, gums, gels, lozenges, mouthwashes and toothpastes.

More powerful prescription drugs can also help dry eyes and mouth. The drug *hydroxychloroquine* (Plaquenil), originally developed to treat malaria, is useful in Sjögren's to relieve fatigue and joint pain. To quiet an overactive immune system, patients can take *methotrexate* (Rheumatrex, Trexall)—it is used in high doses as chemotherapy, and now it's also used in low doses to treat autoimmune disorders. Methotrexate can be well-tolerated but can also cause some nasty side effects, including mouth sores, stomach upset, skin rash, hair loss and liver toxicity.

One bright spot: Research on drugs for autoimmune diseases is extremely active, and as general awareness of Sjögren's increases, patients are not likely to be left behind.

STEPS FOR QUALITY OF LIFE

Sjögren's can be mild, moderate or severe. Severe cases can cause renal failure, disability due to peripheral neuropathy, impaired vision, hepatitis or pneumonitis. But Dr. Baer says that most cases are mild. To help maintain quality of life, exercise of any kind is important for physical and psychological reasons. An anti-inflammatory diet built on healthy foods is essential—eat plenty of vegetables, fruits, fish and other proteins, and limit processed foods and refined grains. Dr. Baer says that fish oil supplements and flaxseed oil may help the problem of dry eyes. To maintain a good level of energy, patients need plenty of sleep. They also need to avoid triggers such as extreme heat, fumes, cigarette smoke, dust and winds—all of which can aggravate symptoms.

Quality of life also has much to do with finding doctors who are well-versed in Sjögren's. Rheumatologists are the primary doctors who handle it, but the nature of the disease also requires the involvement of ophthalmologists, otolaryngologists, dentists, neurologists and for women, gynecologists. Ideally, a patient will be treated at a Sjögren syndrome center, such as the one at Johns Hopkins, but these centers are relatively rare. More typically, doctors treat Sjögren's within rheumatology centers, where expertise on autoimmune diseases is available. Once a patient has been diagnosed, his/her primary care doctor will locate an appropriate place for treatment. For an impressive amount of information about the disease and tips for living well with it, go to the Sjögren's Syndrome Foundation website, Sjogrens.org.

Europe's Enlightened Fibromyalgia Approach: More Exercise, Fewer Drugs

Study titled "EULAR Revised Recommendations for the Management of Fibromyalgia" by researchers at University of Aberdeen, Scotland, published in *Annals of the Rheumatic Diseases.*

If you go on the website of the American College of Rheumatology and search for the best treatments for fibromyalgia, you'll find a detailed discussion of prescription medications first, followed by nondrug approaches.

That's precisely backward.

So concludes a distinguished European expert consortium, which has now released its first major updated evidence-based treatment recommendations for fibromyalgia in nearly a decade.

Their conclusion: To relieve symptoms of this often debilitating condition, which can cause widespread pain throughout your body, pharmaceuticals should be the last thing you try.

The Europeans didn't endorse all nondrug therapies, to be sure. One nondrug approach is strongly supported by evidence, others have some evidence behind them, a few are unproven—and one may be dangerous. They did find a few medications that may be helpful in certain circumstances—but never as a first-line treatment.

THE BEST TREATMENTS FOR FIBROMYALGIA

To determine the most effective treatments, the European League Against Rheumatism (EULAR) pulled together 18 clinicians and researchers from 12 different countries—experts

Supplements Fight Fibromyalgia

Sugar D-ribose decreases muscle pain in some people—take 5 grams twice daily (about two teaspoons of the powdered form). The amino acid 5-hydroxytryptophan (5-HTP) can relieve musculoskeletal and other symptoms, such as insomnia—take 100 milligrams (mg) three times daily. Do not take 5-HTP if you use an antidepressant or an antianxiety drug.

Also helpful: 500 mg of calcium twice daily and 200 mg of magnesium twice daily. Consult your physician before starting any supplement.

Mark A. Stengler, NMD, licensed naturopathic medical doctor in private practice, Encinitas, California...adjunct associate clinical professor at the National College of Natural Medicine, Portland, Oregon...author of *The Natural Physician's Healing Therapies* and coauthor of *Prescription for Natural Cures* (both from Bottom Line Books).

in rheumatology, internal medicine, pain medicine, epidemiology, occupational health and nursing plus patient representatives. Together, they reviewed 2,979 studies and reviews. The good news is that there is much better research than the last time they convened—in 2007. *Their evidence-based findings...*

• **Exercise.** This was the only "strong" recommendation—and it was unanimous. Exercise reduces pain, improves physical function, enhances well-being—plus it's widely available, safe and low-cost.

Research gap: It's not known yet whether aerobic or strength training or a combo is best.

• **Meditative movement therapies** (qigong, tai chi, yoga) was a "weak" recommendation—some evidence supports them. In particular, they can improve sleep, fatigue and quality of life.

• **Mindfulness-based stress reduction (MBSR),** another "weak" recommendation, improves pain and quality of life.

• **Acupuncture,** another "weak" recommendation, improves pain and fatigue.

• **Hydrotherapy,** also "weak," reduces pain and improves quality of life.

Not recommended: There wasn't enough evidence to support these approaches—biofeedback, capsaicin, hypnotherapy, massage... or SAMe, a supplement. That doesn't mean these don't work—just that there are not good studies to establish whether they do or not.

Caution: EULAR recommended against chiropractic care for fibromyalgia based on lack of evidence and safety concerns.

A SMALLER, SUPPORTIVE ROLE FOR MEDICATIONS

EULAR makes it clear that drugs should never be the first treatment option. But if the above approaches aren't working well enough, medications can be a second-line approach—based on individual symptoms and issues. *Their findings...*

• **Patients with "severe" pain** may benefit from *duloxetine* (Cymbalta), *pregabalin* (Lyrica) or *tramadol* (Ultram). This was a "weak" recommendation.

• **For patients with sleep disturbances,** there was another "weak" recommendation for *pregabalin* (Lyrica), *amitriptyline* (Elavil) and *cyclobenzaprine* (Flexeril).

Not recommended: NSAID painkillers such as ibuprofen and naproxen...as well as SSRI antidepressants such as Prozac—there isn't enough evidence that they work.

A strong warning: EULAR concluded with a "strong against" for medications such as growth hormones, strong opioids and corticosteroids. There's no evidence that they work, and there is a high risk of side effects.

If you have fibromyalgia or think you might have it—it often takes years to be properly diagnosed—it's important to discuss your individual condition with your doctor. The journey back to health and feeling better can be challenging, and it's very individual. Nor is it easy to start an exercise program when you're fatigued, in pain and having trouble sleeping, but there are ways to make exercise safer and more comfortable.

Good News for Fibromyalgia Sufferers!

Jarred Younger, PhD, assistant professor, Stanford University School of Medicine, Palo Alto, California.

In a recent study, 27 women with fibromyalgia received a low daily dose (4.5 mg) of *naltrexone* (Depade)—a drug normally used to treat narcotic addiction—for 12 weeks. They then took a placebo for four weeks. The drug reduced pain by an average of 48.5%, compared with 27.4% for the placebo.

Theory: Naltrexone may suppress functioning of hypersensitive immune cells, which can trigger fibromyalgia pain.

If you have fibromyalgia pain: Ask your doctor about an "off-label" prescription for naltrexone from a compounding pharmacy—the low dose used in the study isn't available at a regular pharmacy.

Make the Pain of Fibromyalgia Go Away

Alan C. Logan, ND, lecturer at Harvard School of Continuing Medical Education in Boston and nutrition editor of the *International Journal of Naturopathic Medicine.* He is coauthor of *Hope and Help for Chronic Fatigue Syndrome and Fibromyalgia.* DrLogan.com.

Muscle aches targeting your tenderest spots...fatigue so severe that you can scarcely stand up...sleep disturbances that keep you from ever feeling rested. If these symptoms sound familiar, the problem may be fibromyalgia.

Some doctors claim that fibromyalgia is "all in the head." Yet this potentially debilitating condition is very real to the estimated five million Americans who have it—with women outnumbering men nine-to-one. As yet, it has no known cause or cure. Conventional medical care often fails to bring relief—but many alternative therapies may ease fibromyalgia symptoms. *What you need to know to feel better...*

FIGURING IT OUT

No lab test can detect fibromyalgia, and patients' blood work often appears normal. Diagnosis is based on symptoms—widespread pain that persists for at least three months plus abnormal tenderness at 11 or more of 18 specific spots on the neck, shoulders, chest, back, hips, thighs, knees and elbows. Many patients also experience headache...stiff joints...constipation or diarrhea...depression...sleep problems...and/or sensitivity to lights, sounds or smells.

Theories as to the cause of fibromyalgia include an excess of, or oversensitivity to, the neurotransmitters (brain chemicals) that signal pain...or changes in muscle metabolism and/or hormones that affect nerve activity.

Anti-inflammatory drugs, painkillers and antidepressants are only moderately effective for fibromyalgia symptoms. What's more, because fibromyalgia patients often are very sensitive to medication, they're more likely than other people to experience side effects.

Bottom line: If drugs help you and do not cause side effects, consider complementing your medication with the therapies below. If medication is not effective or appropriate, alternative therapies offer the best chance for relief.

SOOTHING SUPPLEMENTS

The supplements below are listed in the order in which I believe they are likely to be effective for fibromyalgia. All are available at health-food stores and on-line. Try the first one for six to eight weeks. If it helps, continue indefinitely. If it doesn't help, discontinue use. For greater relief, try the others one at a time for six to eight weeks, continuing with any or all that work for you. They generally are safe and, unless otherwise noted, can be taken indefinitely—but get your doctor's approval before using them. As a general precaution, do not use while pregnant or breast-feeding.

- **Omega-3 fatty acids,** such as eicosapentaenoic acid (EPA) and docosahexaenoic acid (DHA), may ease pain by reducing inflammation.

Source: Fish oil liquid or capsules.

Dosage: 3 grams (g) daily of combined EPA and DHA.

• **S-adenosylmethionine (SAM-e),** a naturally occurring compound in the body, may reduce fatigue and depression by increasing levels of the neurotransmitter serotonin.

Dosage: 800 mg to 1,200 mg daily. Do not use SAM-e if you take antidepressants or have diabetes.

• **Coenzyme Q10 (CoQ10) and ginkgo biloba,** taken together, may have a synergistic effect. CoQ10, a vitamin-like substance, boosts cellular energy. Ginkgo biloba, an herb, improves blood flow.

Dosage: 200 milligrams (mg) daily of each.

• **Chlorella,** a type of green algae, reduced fibromyalgia pain by 22% in one study.

Possible reasons: It may boost the immune system and/or increase absorption of essential nutrients.

Dosage: 5 g to 10 g daily.

• **Nicotinamide adenine dehydrogenase (NADH),** a vitamin-like substance, may increase energy within cells and facilitate production of the neurotransmitter dopamine, which affects mood.

Dosage: 10 mg daily.

• **Melatonin,** a hormone that regulates the "body clock," can improve sleep.

Dosage: 3 mg daily. Melatonin can affect other hormones, so using it for more than one month requires close medical supervision.

• **Probiotics,** beneficial intestinal bacteria, combat harmful bacteria that cause digestive distress…and may influence inflammatory chemicals that trigger pain and depression.

Dosage: One billion colony forming units (CFU) of lactobacillus and/or bifidobacterium daily.

MORE ALTERNATIVE THERAPIES

Ask your doctor about…

• **Acupuncture.** This involves inserting thin needles into points along the body's meridians (energy pathways) to enhance flow of qi (life force). This may release endorphins that relieve pain.

Referrals: American Association of Acupuncture and Oriental Medicine, 866-455-7999, AAAOMonline.org.

• **Aromatherapy.** This lifts mood, making pain less bothersome.

To use: Place two or three drops of jasmine or lavender essential oil in an aromatherapy diffuser.

• **Mind-body techniques.** These reduce stress.

Try: Meditation, deep breathing, biofeedback. For DVDs and CDs on techniques, contact the Benson-Henry Institute for Mind-Body Medicine (617-643-6090, BensonHenry Institute.org).

• **Mud packs.** In one study, mud packs were heated to between 104°F and 113°F and applied to patients' sore areas for 15 minutes during 12 separate sessions. Pain, fatigue and physical function all improved.

Theory: Mud draws heat to muscles, reducing pain and stiffness.

Best: Ask a holistic doctor for a referral to a medical spa.

• **Myofascial trigger-point therapy.** This focuses on tender muscle areas that are anatomically similar to acupuncture points. Practitioners inject these "trigger points" with an anesthetic, then stretch muscles to relieve pain.

Referrals: National Association of Myofascial Trigger Point Therapists, MyofascialThe rapy.org.

• **Pool therapy.** Exercises done in a heated swimming pool for one hour three times weekly for several months can reduce fibromyalgia pain and increase stamina.

Referrals: Ask a physical therapist.

For a referral to a doctor who specializes in fibromyalgia, contact the National Fibromyalgia Association (NFA@FMaware.org).

SHINE Helps Fibromyalgia

Jacob Teitelbaum, MD, board-certified internist and nationally known expert in the fields of chronic fatigue syndrome, fibromyalgia, sleep and pain. Based in Kailua-Kona, Hawaii, he is author of numerous books, including *The Fatigue and Fibromyalgia Solution, Pain-Free 1-2-3* and *Real Cause, Real Cure.* Vitality101.com

SHINE stands for Sleep, Hormones, Infections, Nutritional supplements and Exercise —and this approach has led to improvements in 91% of fibromyalgia patients. Patients should get eight to nine hours of sleep a night...be tested for hormone deficiency and treated if necessary...get treated for any symptoms of infections...have nutritional supplementation, such as B-12 and magnesium...and exercise as much as possible. (See page 94 for more supplements that can relieve fibromyalgia.)

Fibromyalgia Breakthrough: Unlearn Your Pain

Howard Schubiner, MD, director of the Mind-Body Medicine Center of the St. John Providence Health System in Warren, Minnesota, clinical professor at the Wayne State University School of Medicine and author of *Unlearn Your Pain.*

Fibromyalgia pain is real. It is processed through the central nervous system along "learned nerve pathways" that are created and then repeatedly triggered by emotional trauma and stress—in exactly the same way you create nerve pathways when you learn to ride a bicycle and then use those same pathways for the rest of your life whenever you ride a bike. Sometimes the origin of the trauma and stress—the "priming" event that sets you up for fibromyalgia—is in childhood (for example, physical or sexual abuse, the death of a parent). Sometimes the priming event is in adulthood (for example, marital difficulties, problems at work).

Fact: Over half of people with fibromyalgia have post-traumatic stress disorder (PTSD) or PTSD-like symptoms, such as depression and anxiety. Research shows that people victimized by workplace bullying had a four times higher risk of fibromyalgia.

Striking research finding: A study by Howard Schubiner, MD, and his colleagues in the *Journal of Internal Medicine* shows that a focus on the pain-triggering role of negative emotions and stress in fibromyalgia can dramatically reduce pain—and even clear up the condition!

THE STRESS–PAIN CONNECTION

The researchers studied 45 middle-aged women who had been suffering from fibromyalgia for an average of 13 years.

The women were divided into two groups. One group received four weeks of a therapy called Affective Self-Awareness (ASA)—learning about and accepting the connection between emotions, stress, and the pain of fibromyalgia and learning and practicing techniques for expressing and releasing emotions and reducing stress. The other group was put on a waiting list to receive ASA. Pain levels were measured at the start of the study and six months later.

After six months, pain had been eliminated or reduced to very low levels in 25% of the ASA group—in effect, their fibromyalgia had gone into remission. Overall, nearly half of the ASA group had pain reduction of 30% or more.

Dr. Schubiner calls pain triggered by stress and emotion the Mind-Body Syndrome (MBS). If you accept that your pain is triggered by learned nerve pathways formed during sustained negative emotional experiences and stress—by the MBS, and not by any physical illness or problem—you can then unlearn your pain.

Good news: The understanding of MBS and the techniques of ASA may help reduce pain in many of the 50 million Americans who suffer from chronic pain problems, including low back pain, sciatica, neck pain, whiplash, tendonitis, tension headache, migraine headaches and irritable bowel syndrome.

AFFIRM HEALTH, WRITE FREELY

Here are two techniques that can help you "unlearn" your pain, says Dr. Schubiner.

• **Affirm your essential health.** When pain or other symptoms occur, stop and take a deep breath. Then take a moment to remind yourself that there is nothing seriously wrong with your body. You are healthy, and the MBS symptoms will subside soon. Tell your mind that you realize that the symptoms are just a way of warning you about underlying feelings of fear, guilt, anger, anxiety, shame, inadequacy or other emotions. Tell your mind to stop producing the symptoms immediately. Do this with force and conviction, either out loud or silently. Take a few deep breaths, and move on with what you were doing.

For the greatest benefits: Repeat whatever positive phrases you choose every time you encounter any of your triggers, until your brain unlearns MBS pathways.

• **Write away your pain.** "Writing about stressful situations allows you to become healthier, develop perspective, and learn to let go of the emotional reactions that have imprisoned you," says Dr. Schubiner.

One such exercise is free-writing—writing faster than you normally would...writing whatever comes in your mind...allowing any thoughts and feelings to be expressed...not crossing out anything out...and not worrying about spelling, punctuation and grammar.

For ten minutes a day, free-write in response to the following sentences (use one sentence per day)...

My feelings about me and________ include:

My understandings about me and ________ include:

"The idea is to process your feelings," said Dr. Schubiner. "Expressing emotions is important, but it is also critical to understand them, gain perspective on them and begin to move past them.

"Therefore in this free-write, make sure to use phrases such as 'I see that...,' 'I realize...,' 'I hope that...,' 'I need to...,' 'I want to...,' 'I can...,' 'I will...,' 'I understand that...,' 'I appreciate...' 'I wonder if...,' 'I have learned...' and 'I have discovered...' "

Write whatever comes to your mind with a focus on understanding the topic/issue as best you can.

Once the ten minutes is up, complete the free-write by copying the following affirmation three times: *Understanding these issues helps me feel better.*

Resource: The same techniques used in the study are in the book *Unlearn Your Pain,* available at UnlearnYourPain.com, where you can also enroll in Dr. Schubiner's Mind Body Program, read his blog and find other resources for overcoming MBS.

Hope for Lupus

Jennifer H. Anolik, MD, PhD, rheumatologist and associate professor of medicine in the immunology and rheumatology unit at the University of Rochester Medical Center in Rochester, New York, where she practices in the Lupus Clinic.

For the first time in more than 50 years, the FDA has approved a new drug for treating lupus. It's an important breakthrough because the drug, *belimumab* (Benlysta), may help reduce lupus flare-ups and could lead to more effective treatments. New treatments are needed because lupus is a systemic autoimmune disease that can affect virtually every part of the body, making it tough to treat.

WHAT IS LUPUS?

Lupus is an autoimmune disease that can cause inflammation in organs and tissues in many parts of the body. For reasons that still aren't clear, the body produces antibodies that trigger inflammation. Common symptoms include an unexplained rash, fatigue, persistent fever and joint pains.

Good news: It used to be that most patients with systemic lupus erythematósus (SLE), the most common form of lupus, typically had symptoms for three to four years before getting an accurate diagnosis—but today, the delay has been reduced to about two to three years. This is a significant improvement, but it's not ideal because the disease is chronic. Patients can develop irreversible organ damage if they don't get treated.

Important: Patients often think that a lupus diagnosis is a death sentence. This is not true. Between 80% and 90% of lupus patients have a normal life expectancy. With better treatments—and earlier diagnosis—an even larger percentage will go on to have normal lives.

EARLY DIAGNOSIS

About one in every 1,000 Americans has been diagnosed with SLE. For unknown reasons, women are disproportionately affected. About half of SLE patients have a mild form of the disease that mainly affects the joints and skin. The other half have a more serious form that affects the organs, including the heart and kidneys.

The challenge: SLE presents itself in a number of ways. One patient might have a skin rash but no joint pain. Someone else might have joint pain and fatigue but no rash. Others might have signs of kidney or heart disease. The disease is also episodic. Most patients will experience intermittent flare-ups, during which the disease is active…then, they'll have periods of quiescence, during which the disease is quiet, with no or only mild symptoms. *Main tests…*

- **Antinuclear antibody (ANA).** This blood test detects antibodies that indicate an immune response against one's self (autoimmune). More than 95% of SLE patients will have a positive ANA test. However, a positive result can also be caused by other autoimmune diseases, such as autoimmune thyroid disease or rheumatoid arthritis…an infection…certain medications (including some anticonvulsant medications)…or having a family history of lupus, even in someone who doesn't have the disease.
- **Anti-dsDNA antibody.** This blood test is often used to confirm a diagnosis of SLE in someone who has a positive ANA test or who has symptoms that indicate lupus.

Other blood tests, including an erythrocyte sedimentation rate, can indicate abnormalities that are associated with lupus.

BEST TREATMENTS

There isn't a cure for SLE, but most patients can significantly reduce flare-ups, disease activity and subsequent complications with a combination of medications and preventive care…

- **Nonsteroidal anti-inflammatory drugs (NSAIDs)** such as *ibuprofen* (Advil) and *naproxen* (Aleve) reduce joint pain and inflammation throughout the body in people with milder forms of SLE.
- ***Hydroxychloroquine* (Plaquenil).** Originally used to treat malaria, it also reduces inflammation caused by SLE. Studies have shown that most lupus patients who take hydroxychloroquine have a reduction of symptoms. It also can help reduce the severity/frequency of flare-ups.

Some patients may experience side effects such as headache or an upset stomach. Regular eye exams are also recommended—in rare cases, long-term use of the drug can lead to retinal damage.

- **Immune-suppressing medications,** such as *methotrexate* (Rheumatrex, Trexall) and *azathioprine* (Imuran), may be used for more severe cases of SLE. Steroids are potent anti-inflammatories and are frequently used to treat SLE—in low doses for milder manifestations such as arthritis and in high doses for severe features such as kidney inflammation (lupus nephritis). Other immunosuppressors, including *mycophenolate* (CellCept) or *cyclophosphamide* (Cytoxan), also are mainstays of treatment for lupus nephritis.

Benlysta is the first biologic medication that was designed specifically to treat SLE. It blocks the activity of B-lymphocyte stimulator, a protein that increases the production of antibodies and SLE.

Important: This medication is an important advance, but it's effective in less than 50% of patients—and it has not yet been studied in such conditions as lupus nephritis.

Benlysta is given in a doctor's office/medical center by IV infusion. The first three doses are given two weeks apart…then, the infusions are given monthly, although the schedule may be different for some patients. Common side effects include nausea, diarrhea and fever.

TRIGGERS TO AVOID

Every patient with SLE has triggers that increase the risk for flare-ups or worsen symptoms. *Helpful...*

• **Avoid the sun.** Exposure to UV radiation from sunshine is among the most common triggers. Patients with SLE are advised to use aggressive sun protection that includes a UVA- and UVB-protective sunscreen with an SPF of 50 or higher.

• **Protect yourself from infection.** Wash your hands several times a day...avoid contact with people with viral/bacterial infections... and get all recommended vaccinations. Viral and bacterial infections activate the immune system and can trigger a flare-up.

If you get an infection: Ask your doctor if it's safe to take sulfa antibiotics (such as Bactrim or Septra). Some patients with SLE are more likely to get a flare-up when they take these medications.

• **Eat well and emphasize fish.** The same diet that's good for the heart (high in complex carbohydrates, low in saturated fat) is good for lupus. Including several fish meals a week or a daily fish oil supplement is also helpful—there's some evidence that the omega-3 fatty acids in fish can help lower inflammation and reduce disease activity.

Herbs and Supplements That Relieve Lupus Symptoms

Sara Korsunsky, ND, licensed doctor of naturopathic medicine with a family-oriented private practice at the Centre for Natural Medicine in Winnipeg, Manitoba, Canada. NaturalMedicine.mb.ca and SunSkyWellness.com

When a doctor not only treats systemic lupus erythematosus but also has that disease herself, she has a unique kind of expertise.

An autoimmune disorder, lupus affects women eight times more often than men. There is no known cure, so treatment focuses on minimizing the disease's symptoms, such as skin rashes, fatigue, fever, gastrointestinal upset, and muscle and joint pain. By managing her own illness with a combination of supplements, herbs and very low-dose prescription drugs, Sara Korsunsky, ND, a naturopathic physician in Winnipeg, Canada, has been able to reduce her list of lupus symptoms from 10 to just three and now experiences only occasional, very mild flares. "I've maintained my health this way for five years now—even through a pregnancy, a time when lupus symptoms typically worsen." Many of her patients with lupus also have seen huge improvements by following her treatment guidelines.

Dr. Korsunsky said that, although prescription lupus drugs (such as corticosteroids, nonsteroidal anti-inflammatories and immunosuppressants) may offer quicker symptom relief, natural approaches generally have fewer side effects and bring about better overall health in the long run. She noted that, for maximum effectiveness and safety, it is vital to work directly with a qualified naturopathic doctor who can customize your treatment and suggest appropriate dosages. That's because autoimmune diseases manifest differently in different patients, and there are significant individual variations in body chemistry, diet and lifestyle.

Important: Do not stop taking your lupus medication on your own...and do not start taking supplements before checking with your doctor, as some supplements may cause side effects or stimulate your already overactive immune system. *Instead, talk with your doctor about complementing your conventional care with natural supplements that help to...*

• **Quell inflammation.** Because lupus is a systemic inflammatory disease, it can affect just about any part of the body—skin, joints, muscles, organs. That's why Dr. Korsunsky's number-one recommendation is to supplement with omega-3 fatty acids (in the form of fish oil) to help keep inflammation under control. Also potentially beneficial are flaxseed oil...antioxidants such as vitamins C and E...and the anti-inflammatory spices turmeric and ginger, both of which are available in capsule form.

• **Support digestion.** Nausea, constipation and other gastrointestinal problems are common among lupus patients because digestive function is strongly linked to immune function...and because nonsteroidal anti-inflammatory drugs can damage the gut wall. Supplementing with digestive enzymes, such as bromelain (which comes from the stem of the pineapple plant), can improve digestion, Dr. Korsunsky said.

• **Increase energy and improve adrenal function.** Lupus patients often feel fatigued due to underfunctioning of the adrenal glands. Also, the steroid drug prednisone, which many patients take, can worsen fatigue by further suppressing adrenal function.

Helpful: A multivitamin (particularly important are vitamins A, D and E)...an additional vitamin B complex supplement (since a multivitamin may not provide optimal amounts of the B vitamins needed for lupus)...and the herbs licorice root and ashwagandha.

More natural healing: Supplements and herbs are not the only natural therapies that are helpful to lupus patients, Dr. Korsunsky noted. You'll also want to talk with your doctor about the importance of an anti-inflammatory diet, including elimination of food allergens that tax the immune system...regular exercise...and stress management to keep flares at a minimum.

Best Care for Rheumatoid Arthritis

Harris H. McIlwain, MD, board-certified rheumatologist, founder of the McIlwain Medical Group, Tampa Florida, and former chair of the Florida Osteoporosis Board. He is author, with Debra Fulghum Bruce, PhD, of *Diet for a Pain-Free Life.*

The majority of rheumatoid arthritis (RA) sufferers eventually require prescription drugs, but everyone with the condition can benefit from natural approaches that reduce inflammation, pain and stiffness.

This blending of natural and conventional treatments often allows patients to reduce the frequency and doses of medications, which is important for curbing side effects, such as dizziness and increased risk for infection and, in rare cases, cancer.

Best natural treatments for RA...

• **Get regular low-impact exercise.** Any form of low-impact exercise, particularly walking and swimming, will increase joint lubrication and reduce inflammation, which helps people with RA perform daily tasks, such as dressing, without pain. Exercise will also increase endorphins, the body's natural painkillers.

• **Give up meat.** Studies have shown that RA sufferers who don't eat meat have less pain and greater mobility.

Reason: Beef (even organic, grass-fed beef) and other meats, such as lamb and pork, increase levels of arachidonic acid, a fatty acid that's transformed into inflammatory, pain-signaling compounds.

What we recommend for our RA patients: Avoid all meat (beef, lamb and pork), and replace it with other sources of protein—for example, from plants (such as legumes, including beans, and whole grains), poultry and fish. Fish is particularly good because the omega-3 fatty acids reduce inflammation. A fish oil supplement, which contains omega-3 fatty acids, also is sometimes advised. Consult your doctor for dosage.

• **Identify and manage food sensitivities.** The evidence isn't conclusive, but it appears that many people with RA are sensitive to one or more foods. For example, one of my patients has an immediate RA flare-up when he eats foods that contain corn syrup.

Helpful: An elimination diet to identify which food(s) you might be sensitive to.

How it works: Your doctor will advise you to stop eating certain foods, such as corn syrup, dairy, citrus, tomatoes, wheat and corn, for one to two weeks. Then, you reintroduce the foods, one at a time, over a period of weeks to see whether symptoms reappear.

• **Use anti-inflammatory spices,** such as ginger, turmeric, cumin, cinnamon, cardamom and garlic. They contain potent antioxidants that can reduce inflammation even in the amounts typically used in cooking.

DON'T NEGLECT CONVENTIONAL CARE

Natural approaches can help control RA, but unless you have an unusually mild case, you'll want to combine them with medication for the best results. That's because natural treatments help reduce pain and swelling but don't stop joint damage, which can become permanent if not promptly treated with medications.

Joint damage can be detected earliest with imaging tests, such as an X-ray, MRI or ultrasound.

Important: Start medications right away if imaging tests show any degree of "destructive" arthritis. The natural approaches outlined earlier can be continued while you are undergoing drug therapy.

The American College of Rheumatology's guidelines call for the aggressive treatment of RA. In the past, doctors were more likely to use "mild" medications, such as *ibuprofen* (Motrin) and other nonsteroidal anti-inflammatory drugs (NSAIDs), before escalating to more potent drugs. The problem is, NSAIDs are usually good at relieving pain and stiffness, but they won't prevent joint damage. *Also needed...*

- **DMARDs.** Most people who experience severe and frequent RA symptoms should take one or more disease-modifying anti-rheumatic drugs (DMARDs), such as *methotrexate* (Rheumatrex), *hydroxychloroquine* (Plaquenil) or *sulfasalazine* (Azulfidine).

DMARDs, which suppress the immune system, reduce RA flare-ups and reduce risk for serious joint damage. If a DMARD is effective, it is usually continued indefinitely.

Important: DMARDs may make you more susceptible to infection. Other side effects may include nausea, abdominal pain or, rarely, liver damage. Be sure to get the appropriate vaccinations for flu, pneumonia, etc.

- **Biologics.** If you don't get adequate relief from one or more of the DMARDs, your doctor might switch you to a biologic drug. Medications in this class include *etanercept* (Enbrel), *adalimumab* (Humira) and others, and can actually delay or prevent joint damage.

These meds also increase the risk for infection, so ask your doctor about prevention strategies. In rare cases, these drugs can increase cancer risk as well.

Cancer Drug Can Curb Rheumatoid Arthritis

Thomas W. J. Huizinga, MD, PhD, professor and chairman, department of rheumatology, Leiden University Medical Center, The Netherlands.

In an 18-month study of 110 people with an undetermined form of arthritis characterized by painful and stiff joints, those who took weekly doses of *methotrexate* (Rheumatrex) for 12 months were less likely to develop rheumatoid arthritis, one of the most debilitating forms of the disease—and more likely to go into remission—than those who took a placebo.

Theory: Methotrexate, a drug used to treat some cancers and severe psoriasis, works, in part, by curbing activation of white blood cells, which may play a role in causing rheumatoid arthritis.

Caution: For treatment of rheumatoid arthritis, methotrexate is taken once a week, not once a day, as it is for the treatment of cancer.

Slow Rheumatoid Arthritis With Early Detection

Beth L. Jonas, MD, assistant professor of medicine and rheumatology and director of the Rheumatology Fellowship Program at the University of North Carolina Thurston Arthritis Research Center in Chapel Hill.

Women are two to three times more likely than men to get rheumatoid arthritis. The disease can arise at any time but usually appears in midlife. While genetics may play some role, most RA patients have no close relatives with the disease—so we all should be on the lookout for RA. *See your doctor without delay if you experience any of the following...*

Pain, tenderness and/or stiffness in any of the small joints—fingers, wrists, toes, ankles—usually occurring symmetrically on both sides of the body. (As RA progresses, the neck, shoulders, elbows, hips and/or knees also may be affected.)

- **Morning stiffness** that lasts for more than 30 minutes.
- **Redness,** swelling and/or sensations of heat at the joints.
- **Numbness,** tingling or burning sensations in the hands or feet.

Confirming an RA diagnosis can be tricky because the symptoms mimic those of lupus, Lyme disease and other forms of arthritis. Diagnosis is based on a physical exam... blood tests for antibodies (including rheumatoid factor and anticyclic citrullinated peptide) plus various markers of inflammation... and imaging tests (ultrasound, MRI, X-ray).

So if your doctor suspects RA, ask to be referred to a rheumatologist or get a referral through the American College of Rheumatology (visit Rheumatology.org and click on "Find a Rheumatologist").

Important Info for Psoriasis Patients

Bruce F. Bebo, Jr., PhD, director of research and medical programs, National Psoriasis Foundation, Portland, Oregon.

Psoriasis is miserable...there's no question about it. But beyond dealing with those outbreaks of crusty, red patches on the body, nearly one in four psoriasis sufferers also has another potentially dangerous condition to worry about—and it's one that isn't being diagnosed promptly. It's a form of arthritis that specifically affects psoriasis suffers that is called (logically) psoriatic arthritis (PsA).

Don't Ignore Joint Pain If You Have Psoriasis

Having psoriasis is the single greatest risk factor for developing psoriatic arthritis (PsA), an autoimmune form of arthritis.

Recent research: A delayed diagnosis of even six months—from symptom onset to the first doctor's visit—can significantly increase risk for deformed joints and disability, according to a review of nearly 300 PsA patients.

Oliver FitzGerald, MD, professor of rheumatology, St. Vincent's University Hospital, Dublin.

CONNECTING THE DOTS

Researchers contacted 477 men and women with an average age of 59. About 58% of them had been diagnosed with psoriasis only... 2% had been diagnosed with PsA only...and 40% had been diagnosed with both conditions. *The researchers discovered...*

Of the psoriasis-only respondents, 22% reported having significant symptoms of PsA (more on those later), even though they had not been diagnosed with PsA.

Of the respondents who knew that they had both psoriasis and PsA, 15% weren't diagnosed with PsA until one to two years after their symptoms had started, and for 29%, it took two or more years to get a diagnosis.

Of the PsA-only group, none of them had been diagnosed with psoriasis, but researchers theorize that all of them will develop psoriasis at some point later in life, since it's impossible to have PsA without psoriasis. (Sometimes joint problems appear first.)

What are the telltale signs of PsA? The symptoms aren't much different from those of rheumatoid arthritis. They include pain and stiffness in one or more joints throughout the body...joints that are red or warm... pain in the feet, ankles and lower back... depressions in the nail surface or nails that separate from the nail bed...and, most especially, sausagelike swelling in one or more fingers or toes. Symptoms can be so debilitating that they affect a patient's ability to work and do active things, like get in and out of a car. So why aren't these symptoms being promptly diagnosed?

One main problem is that even though the symptoms seem impossible to miss, patients may not realize that they have a form of arthritis. They may just chalk up the symptoms to "getting older," so they don't tell their primary care physicians or their dermatologists about them. Patients need to speak up, so one of their doctors can refer them to a rheumatologist, the type of doctor that can diagnose and treat PsA. On the other side of the equation, all dermatologists (and even primary care physicians) need to be more informed about complications of psoriasis, like PsA, and should be regularly asking psoriasis patients questions about joint pain.

WHAT PEOPLE WITH PSORIASIS NEED TO KNOW

PsA is a form of inflammatory arthritis, so, like psoriasis, it's considered an autoimmune disorder. It's not like osteoarthritis, the most common form of arthritis, which is caused by wear-and-tear on the body—PsA occurs when your immune system, for unknown reasons, attacks your body. PsA also runs in families. The symptoms of and treatments for PsA are similar to those for rheumatoid arthritis, but they're not identical, so it's critical for a rheumatologist to tell you exactly which kind you have. Researchers aren't sure why some people with psoriasis develop PsA and others don't. More research should and will be done on the topic.

But here's what we do know: PsA usually strikes between ages 30 and 50, usually about 10 years after psoriasis is diagnosed. Both conditions are episodic, meaning that they flare up and recede over the course of a lifetime. Flare-ups are commonly responses to such triggers as infection (bacterial or viral) or trauma, but, interestingly, they don't tend to flare up at the same times—in other words, the severity of your psoriasis at any given time is not usually related to the severity of your PsA.

Sorry if this has been a downer thus far, but there is hope for a happy ending for people who have or are worried that they might develop this unpleasant condition. There is no cure, but there are treatments that can help control symptoms, such as over-the-counter and prescription medications, and there are even more treatments in the pipeline. Natural treatments can help, too, such as maintaining a healthy weight (since that puts less stress on joints), exercising regularly (to keep joints flexible), using cold or hot packs for 15 minutes at a time to numb pain in affected joints and changing the way you perform everyday tasks (such as carrying heavy pots with both hands instead of one and pushing doors open with your full body instead of just one arm). Some PsA patients may find relief by taking a variety of natural supplements and/or by making dietary changes—ask your doctor if making a change like this would be right for you.

The bottom line: Have psoriasis? Look out for PsA symptoms. If you think you may have PsA, speak up and tell your primary care doctor or your dermatologist—since he/she may not bring it up—and then he/she can refer you to a rheumatologist, who can give you the appropriate diagnostic tests.

Newer, More Effective Drug for Psoriasis Recently Approved for Psoriatic Arthritis

Andrew Blauvelt, MD, clinical dermatologist, dermatology researcher and president of Oregon Medical Research Center in Portland. He is an elected member of the International Psoriasis Council. PsoriasisCouncil.org

In clinical trials, the prescription drug *ixekizumab* (Taltz) was more than twice as effective as Enbrel, an older medication, in people with moderate-to-severe plaque psoriasis. After the initial dose, the new medication is injected by the patient or a health-care provider every two weeks for the first three months and every four weeks thereafter. Taltz was first approved by the FDA in early 2016 for treatment of adult patients with moderate-to-severe plaque psoriasis and was approved in late 2017 for active psoriatic arthritis.

Most common side effect: Upper-respiratory infections.

Watsu Water Massage For Arthritis, Fibromyalgia And More

Joyce Reim, director of The Watsu Institute School of Shiatsu and Massage in Middletown, California. WatsuCenter.com

Watsu massage is an intriguing form of bodywork, which incorporates numerous types of therapy, including the gentle Japanese finger-pressure technique called shiatsu...muscle stretching...joint mobilization...and massage, performed by a trained practitioner (or therapist) while the client soaks in warm water. It provides not only pain relief, but also emotional release that people really rave about.

The concept of Watsu massage was developed about 30 years ago, when a shiatsu practitioner named Harold Dull first combined Zen shiatsu stretches and movements as he worked with his students in the naturally therapeutic pools at Harbin Hot Springs in Northern California. Today, trained Watsu practitioners and therapists around the country treat patients for a variety of complaints, including stress, chronic back pain, arthritis, fibromyalgia and orthopedic problems.

To find out more about it, we spoke with Joyce Reim, director of the Watsu Institute at the School of Shiatsu and Massage in Middletown, California. Reim told us that she was a patient suffering from crippling arthritis pain when she herself first experienced Watsu. "Painkillers were all that traditional medicine had to offer me," she said. "After my first Watsu session, I felt invigorated and free of pain." Typically the pain is relieved while the patient is floating in the warm water, but does come back later, says Reim, noting that after regular Watsu sessions arthritis flare-ups are farther apart and the pain is less severe.

WHAT IS IT?

Watsu massage is given in a warm-water therapeutic pool about four feet deep, heated to body temperature (about 98 degrees). The massage therapist is in the water with you. You float on your back while he/she gently holds you, stretches and massages your tight muscles. Flotation devices are often used. The experience has been described as feeling like you are melting effortlessly into the warm water, blurring the boundaries between your body and the environment.

Water Exercise Is the Way to Go

Fibromyalgia can be relieved by water exercise. In an eight-month study of 33 women with fibromyalgia (characterized by painful muscles, ligaments and tendons), those who participated in a supervised exercise program in a heated swimming pool for 60 minutes three times weekly had fewer symptoms than nonexercisers.

Theory: Warm water induces relaxation, which helps fight pain. Ask your doctor if water workouts are an option for you.

Narcís Gusi, PhD, professor, University of Extremadura, Cáceres, Spain.

Yoga or water exercise can dramatically reduce common multiple sclerosis (MS) symptoms, such as fatigue, depression and paresthesia (pins and needles tingling), a study of women with MS found. Those who did these forms of exercise for at least 30 minutes three times a week had a 35-fold lower risk of developing moderate-to-severe depression, as well as less fatigue and paresthesia, than those who did no exercise.

Serge Brand, PhD, professor of affective, stress and sleep disorders, University of Basel, Switzerland.

According to Reim, warm water is an ideal medium for this kind of passive stretching. It provides support while also taking weight off the vertebrae, allowing the spine to be moved in ways that aren't possible on a solid horizontal surface. "Recipients feel profound physical release and a release from pain and tension," Reim said. Some describe the experience as intense and almost spiritual, as the practitioner cradles the client in his/her arms in the water, delivering physical and often emotional support. Reim also said that practitioners have a specific term for the profound connection that many givers and receivers report experiencing—it's called "heart wrap," and it delivers "a sense of oneness and peace."

WHAT'S WATSU GOOD FOR?

Research shows that the physical benefits are meaningful as well…

- **According to one study,** in the *Journal of Bodywork and Movement Therapies*, Watsu massage patients suffering from fibromyalgia experienced significant improvements in physical and social function, vitality and reduced pain.

- **A study found that after 18 months of twice-monthly, 30-minute Watsu sessions,** residents of a retirement community suffering a range of maladies, including knee replacement, cancer, Parkinson's disease and mild anxiety, reported substantial improvements in self-assessments of emotional stress, along with a reduction of aches and pains and improvements in flexibility, as well as in their ability to relax.

Watsu is generally considered a viable treatment for most people when given by a well-trained practitioner. To find a trained Watsu practitioner, go to the website of the Worldwide Aquatic Bodywork Association, Watsu.com/waba.html. It maintains a worldwide registry of therapists who have met requirements to practice and teach Watsu.

Can This Patient Be Cured? Rheumatoid Arthritis

Mark A. Stengler, NMD, naturopathic doctor and founder of the Stengler Center for Integrative Medicine in Encinitas, California. He is author or coauthor of numerous books, including *The Natural Physician's Healing Therapies* and *Bottom Line's Prescription for Natural Cures*, and author of the newsletter *Health Revelations*. MarkStengler.com

Sandy had been suffering from rheumatoid arthritis for 16 years. This inflammatory disease is characterized by joint pain on both sides of the body, most often in the hands, wrists and knees. It is an autoimmune condition—that is, the body's immune system attacks its own tissue, causing the cartilage in the joints to degrade over time. Sandy, a 43-year-old homemaker, had constant pain and inflammation in her hands and wrists.

When I first saw her, she was taking two prescription anti-inflammatory medications—*methotrexate* (Rheumatrex), which also is used as a chemotherapy agent, and *hydrochloroquine* (Plaquenil). To make matters worse, she had been in a car accident a year before, which injured her hands and back, further aggravating her condition. In addition to her pain, Sandy's digestion was not good—she was prone to diarrhea, gas and bloating—and for the past five years, she had not slept well.

Understandably, Sandy was concerned about the potential toxicity of her medications. For example, methotrexate can cause liver damage and anemia.

Sandy and I discussed the potential triggers of rheumatoid arthritis—stress (which was high in her life), food sensitivities, hormone imbalances, poor digestion, environmental toxins and nutritional deficiencies.

I started Sandy on enzymes that aid digestion, fish oil, a proteolytic enzyme (to reduce inflammation) and a formula containing the hormone melatonin and the amino acid 5-hydroxytryptophan to help her sleep. I had her tested for hormone imbalances as well as food and environmental sensitivities. I also tested the absorption status of her small intestine.

The tests showed that she had a mild problem with malabsorption—the food she ate was not being broken down and absorbed properly. This validated my prescription for supplements that support digestion. Hormone testing showed that her thyroid was underactive, so I prescribed natural thyroid hormone. The allergist I work with found that Sandy had several food sensitivities—to wheat, tuna, onions, yams and other foods. I suggested that she rotate these foods, since it is difficult to avoid them indefinitely. To reduce the reactions triggered by her overactive immune system, I also recommended that she take desensitization drops, with a homeopathic dilution of the foods to which she was sensitive.

On her follow-up visit two months later, Sandy reported that she no longer had any symptoms of arthritis in her joints and had stopped her medications (with her rheumatologist's knowledge). She did experience a mild flare-up midway through her menstrual cycle, indicating a hormone connection. For this, I prescribed the homeopathic remedy pulsatilla, known for its hormone-balancing properties. Now, a year later, Sandy experiences only minor, occasional arthritis flare-ups.

Natural Cures for Psoriasis

April Abernethy, ND, a naturopathic physician and interim chief scientific and medical officer at the National Psoriasis Foundation in Portland, Oregon. She is also a member of the board of directors at International Dermatology Outcome Measures, an organization working to establish common measurements of treatment effectiveness and outcomes.

Living day in and day out with psoriasis—known for its silvery scales and itchy, painful red patches (plaques) on the skin—is hard enough for the more than 7.5 million Americans who have the disease.

But researchers are now finding that people with psoriasis also may be more likely to develop other inflammation-based conditions such as diabetes and cardiovascular disease. People with psoriasis should be screened for these conditions and talk to their doctors about ways to reduce other risk factors they may have for these diseases.

Problem: Even though drugs, such as *apremilast* (Otezla) and *adalimumab* (Humira), that inhibit parts of the immune system involved in psoriasis are now available, any therapy that suppresses immunity can increase the risk for infections, gastrointestinal upset and other conditions.

Solution: There's mounting evidence that natural therapies can be used to reduce overall inflammation and help support the immune system. These drug-free approaches can improve the effectiveness of psoriasis medication and sometimes even eliminate the need for it (with your doctor's approval). First, try the dietary approaches in this article—they should result in improvements that increase over time. Supplements also can be used.

PUTTING YOUR DIET TO WORK

Eating the right foods (and using supplements when needed) can increase your ability to fight psoriasis on a systemic level by reducing inflammation and helping regulate your immune system—two key factors linked to psoriasis. *My advice...*

- **Go for anti-inflammatory foods.** Americans eat lots of processed foods—most of which promote inflammation in the body. Meanwhile, whole, nutrient-packed foods such as fresh fruits and vegetables help attack the inflammatory process that is increased in psoriasis.

Good choices: Beets, blueberries, kale or other leafy greens, salmon, garbanzo beans, quinoa, lentils, nuts and ginger. For other food choices, go to Psoriasis.org, and search "anti-inflammatory diet."

- **Get more vitamin D.** People with psoriasis, like many Americans, are often deficient in vitamin D, which is known to help regulate immune function and inhibit inflammation. That's why it's important to consume foods that contain vitamin D, such as oysters, shrimp, salmon, sardines and any fortified milk. Vitamin D supplements also may be needed. If you have psoriasis, ask your doctor for a blood test to check your vitamin D level.

- **Spice things up.** Turmeric, which gives mustard its bright yellow color and curry its distinctive flavor, contains the medicinal compound curcumin.

A 2013 study published in the journal *BioFactors* showed that turmeric helps healthy, new skin cells form more quickly. If you don't like curry or mustard (you would need to eat 1 g to 3 g a day to get the therapeutic effect), you can try turmeric in supplement form—400 mg to 600 mg two to three times a day.

Talk to your doctor first if you take antacids, diabetes drugs or blood thinners, since turmeric may interfere with these medications—and if you have a history of gallstones (turmeric may cause stomach upset in these people).

• **Load up on omega-3s.** Get lots of anti-inflammatory omega-3 fatty acids.

Daily amounts needed to fight psoriasis: Seven ounces of salmon…a small avocado…or two tablespoons of ground flaxseed (store in the refrigerator to prevent spoilage). If you don't like fish and other omega-3—rich foods, consider taking 2 g to 3 g daily of a fish oil supplement. Choose one that has more EPA than DHA, and check with your doctor first if you take a blood thinner or diabetes medication—fish oil could interact with them.

A 2014 study published in the *Journal of the American Academy of Dermatology* found that among many common supplements taken by people with psoriasis, fish oil—which may reduce tumor necrosis factor-alpha (TNF-alpha), a protein associated with systemic inflammation—demonstrated the greatest benefit.

FOR CRACKED SKIN AND PLAQUES

Among the more troubling symptoms of psoriasis are dry, cracked skin (that may even bleed) and the red, scaly, itchy plaques that can develop on the elbows, scalp, torso and other areas.

What works best…

• **Oregon grape root.** When used topically, this powerful, little-known antibacterial herb (also called mahonia) helps reduce skin irritation and topical infections common to people with psoriasis.

A 2013 research review published in the *British Journal of Dermatology* showed that Oregon grape root reduced the development of red, raised psoriasis plaques and healed psoriasis-related cracked skin.

Oregon grape root is found in tincture form at health-food stores, and you can add two or three drops to your favorite skin cream. The herb also can be found in over-the-counter creams containing 10% mahonia, which has been shown to help control mild-to-moderate psoriasis plaques.

FOR ITCHING AND FLAKING

Soaking in the high concentration of mineral salts found in the Dead Sea in Israel is a centuries-old remedy for the itching and flaking associated with psoriasis.

What helps: Adding one-quarter to one-half cup of Dead Sea (or Epsom) salts to a warm (not hot) bath has been shown to ease itching skin and remove dead, flaking skin cells. Dead Sea salts have a higher concentration of minerals than Epsom salts and are available online and at health-food stores and spas.

A substantial body of research, including a study published in the *Journal of Dermatological Treatment*, has shown that psoriasis patients who regularly take such baths report significant improvements in itch and irritation levels within three weeks.

For even greater benefits: Mix the salts with colloidal oatmeal, such as Aveeno. Take these baths two to three times a week.

CHAPTER 4

Backaches

Surprising Causes Of Back Pain

People blame all sorts of things for back pain. Maybe it started when you were lugging suitcases from the car or hauling boxes from the garage. *These may seem like obvious culprits, but most cases of back pain are caused by things that you would never suspect, including…*

A BIG WALLET

I'm sure that some men prefer streamlined billfolds, but in my experience, most men have wallets that are bulging with stuff—and they sit on those luggage-size lumps day after day.

What happens: When you sit on your wallet, one buttock is slightly higher than the other. Over time, this can cause pelvic misalignment and spinal twisting that can lead to chronic back pain and even sciatica.

My advice: Move your wallet to a front pocket. Even a thin wallet will cause problems if you sit on it long enough.

OVERSIZED BAGS

When you carry a heavy bag—a gym duffel, a purse, a computer bag—the working shoulder elevates and puts the spine out of alignment.

Another danger: "Bag jerk" occurs when a heavy bag abruptly falls off the shoulder, causing a jerk to the body. The resulting neck, shoulder and back strain can be comparable to a sports injury.

The best evidence that women's handbags have gotten too big comes from the American Chiropractic Association. It now advises women to limit the weight of their handbags to 10% of their body weight. But should a 150-

---

Todd Sinett, DC, chiropractor and founder/owner of Midtown Integrative Health & Wellness in New York City. He is author of *3 Weeks to a Better Back: Solutions for Healing the Structural, Nutritional and Emotional Causes of Back Pain*.

pound woman be carrying even 15 pounds over her shoulder? That's a lot of weight!

My advice: Put your bag on a diet—take out whatever you really don't need. When you're walking, shift the bag from shoulder to shoulder now and then. You also might consider a backpack.

FLIP-FLOPS

These casual slip-ons give almost no support. The thin soles are a common cause of heel and arch problems. The lack of heel support forces people to take shorter steps and to scrunch up their toes to keep the shoes on, both of which can lead to pain in the knees, hips and lower back. Walking in flip-flops is worse for you than walking barefoot.

My advice: Wear flip-flops only in the venues for which they were designed—at swimming pools, in locker rooms, at the beach, etc.

TOO MUCH SITTING

Sitting has been called the "new smoking" because it has been linked to type 2 diabetes, cancer and heart disease. It's also hard on the back because it exerts more pressure on the spine than standing. People who slouch when they sit—or hunch forward when watching TV or working on the computer—experience even more pressure.

My advice: Don't just sit when you're sitting. Shift your weight every few minutes. Arch your back. Lean back when you notice that you have been hunching forward. At least twice an hour, get up and walk around for a few minutes.

Also helpful: A reclining chair. Recliners lengthen the spine and cause less pressure than upright chairs.

CHEWING GUM

Too much jaw action stresses the temporomandibular (jaw) joint, which stresses the muscles throughout your back, leading to tension and pain.

Jaw-related problems may be accompanied by tightness all along the back and spine.

Possible signs of jaw problems: You can't open your mouth very wide...your jaw occasionally clicks or "sticks"...and you grind your teeth or clench your jaw a lot.

My advice: Give up chewing gum altogether. It's also helpful to stretch the jaw muscles. Place your hand under your jaw. Push with just a little resistance while you open/close your mouth. Repeat the stretch 10 times, three times a day.

Also helpful: Wearing a mouth guard when sleeping reduces pressure on the jaw from clenching. If an over-the-counter mouth guard doesn't fit properly, ask your dentist for a customized one.

CONSTIPATION

Believe it or not, constipation is a common cause of back pain. A lack of regular bowel movements causes buildups of inflammatory wastes that irritate the large intestine, which in turn irritates muscles in the back.

My advice: When you notice that "things aren't moving," drink a big glass of cold water. It will stimulate the urge to have a bowel movement.

Also important: Regular exercise and plenty of beans, fruits, vegetables and other high-fiber foods.

Caution: Don't depend on high-powered "digestive cleanses"—colonics, supplements, extreme fasts, etc.—for regular bowel movements. They can trigger irritation that is just as hard on the back as constipation.

STRESS BREATHING

Taking rapid, shallow breaths is part of the body's fight-or-flight response. People with stressful lives breathe this way often or even all the time, and they aren't really aware of it. Rapid breathing can't deliver all the oxygen your body needs. Muscles that are deprived of oxygen get tight and sore...and the stress that causes rapid breathing makes muscle tension even worse. Back pain can result.

Self-test: Turn your head all the way to the right or left—and see how far it goes. Then, take slow, deep breaths for about 30 seconds. Turn your head again. Did it go farther this time? If it did, you need to relax and get more oxygen.

My advice: Every day—particularly when you're stressed—take a few moments to breathe deeply. Inhale all the way for about four seconds, then exhale just as slowly. Do it for a few minutes, several times a day.

How to Wreck Your Back: 6 Little Mistakes That Cause Big Pain

David Borenstein, MD, clinical professor of medicine at The George Washington University Medical Center in Washington, DC, and a partner at Arthritis and Rheumatism Associates, the largest rheumatology practice based in Washington/Maryland. He is the author of *Heal Your Back* and the host of several podcasts. DrBhealth.org

As many as 80% of Americans will suffer an episode of back pain at some time in their lives. Back problems are among the main reasons for doctor visits, and they can be excruciatingly slow to heal.

What people don't realize is that most back injuries are predictable, and how to avoid them might surprise you. *Here are the six worst mistakes that people make that hurt their backs...*

WEIGHT AND EFFORT MISMATCH

I see this all the time. Suppose you lift a box that is heavier than you expected. You get it a few inches off the floor and then realize that it's really heavy. It's going to crash back down if you don't bring all of your strength into play. The sudden contraction of unprepared back muscles can cause an instant strain.

Or maybe you're lifting a box that you think is heavy but turns out to be as light as a feather. All of the muscle force that you generated causes a "snap" in the muscles (and the box goes flying).

Self-protection: Before you lift something, test the weight. Slide it a few inches, or lift just a corner. You have to know what you're dealing with. If it's heavy, get your legs under you...use the muscles in your legs more than the muscles in your back. If it's light, lift with a smooth motion—you won't need that initial hard jerk to get it moving.

OVERHEAD BIN REACH

If you think that the cramped, knees-to-chest seating in today's airplanes is hard on your back, wait until you use the overhead bins. You will pay in pain what you saved on checked luggage.

Travelers often overstuff their carry-ons. A 20-pound bag that's easy to carry (or wheel) can feel like 50 pounds when you're off-balance and reaching overhead. Unloading also is a hazard. You probably had to angle, wedge and stuff your bag to get it to fit. You will have to give it a hard yank to get it out, a motion that is very hard on the back.

Self-protection: Pack light. If you're in reasonable shape, you probably can manage, say, a 10-pound bag when your arms are extended and you're standing on tiptoe. Use both hands to place the bag in the bin...don't swing it up with one arm. Store it with the handle facing out. That way, you can grip the handle with one hand and use your other hand for support. For anything much heavier, put it in checked baggage—it's worth it even if you have to pay.

SUPER-SOFT CHAIR RECLINE

It feels good to sink into a soft chair or sofa—but it is hard to extricate yourself from the pillowy depths.

Surprising fact: Sitting in a soft chair is hard work.

When you sit in a firm chair, your back is supported, so it relaxes. But a soft chair doesn't provide the same sensory input, so the muscles stay contracted. After an hour or so, you might notice that your back is hurting even though you haven't done anything more strenuous than read a book or work the TV remote.

Self-protection: When you're settling in, choose a chair that provides a decent amount of back support. It doesn't have to be hard, but it should be firm.

Also helpful: If you have a history of back problems, you probably will do better if you stand up for one to two minutes now and then—say, every 15 or 20 minutes.

THE CAR TRUNK LEAN

How many times have you felt a "pinch" when you lift a suitcase or a sack of groceries from a car's trunk or cargo area? It's not so much the weight that causes problems but your position. When you bend over and lift, you are at a mechanical disadvantage. You are not using the big muscles in your legs. Your back muscles aren't very strong. Their job is to stabilize your spine, not help with heavy lifting.

Self-protection: Get as close to the vehicle as you can before pulling the item to the front of the trunk and taking it out. This allows you to bring your leg muscles into play. Most people stand back from the rear of the car because they don't want to get their clothes dirty. Step in closer. It's easier to clean your clothes than to deal with a month or two of back pain.

TWIST AND SHOUT

"Twist and shout" is what I call the stab of pain that occurs when people use a twisting motion to bend over. Suppose that you're picking something up off the floor that's a little bit off to your side. You might pivot at the hips and swing one hand down to snag it. Don't! This is an unnatural motion because the spinal joints are designed to shift from front to back, not side to side. Twisting strains the soft tissues and can lead to sprains and spasms.

Self-protection: Before you pick something up, take a fraction of a second to move into a position of strength. With both feet facing the object, squat down and pick it up. Face it square, and use your legs more and your back less.

SHOVELING ANYTHING HEAVY

Back specialists see a lot of new patients in the spring after they have been working in the yard shoveling mulch, dirt or gravel. The same is true after snowstorms. Even when snow looks light and fluffy, each shovelful packs a lot of weight—and you never move just one shovelful.

Self-protection: Warm up before picking up the shovel. Walk around the house for a few minutes. Stretch out the muscles in your back, legs and arms.

Once you're outside, let your legs do the work. Bend your knees when you load the shovel, then straighten them when you lift. Don't bend your back any more than you have to. And don't take the heaviest shovelfuls that you can manage—if you're grunting, it's too much.

Also helpful: Home-supply stores stock a variety of ergonomic shovels that make it easier to stand upright when you're shoveling.

Best Non-Drug Treatments For Back Pain

Richard A. Deyo, MD, MPH, Kaiser-Permanente Endowed Professor of Evidence-Based Medicine, department of family medicine at Oregon Health & Science University, Portland. He also is author of *Watch Your Back! How the Back Pain Industry Is Costing Us More and Giving Us Less—And What You Can Do to Inform and Empower Yourself in Seeking Treatment.*

Have you ever had an aching lower back? Most likely, your answer is yes—four out of five Americans have experienced low-back pain.

For some, acute low-back pain—lasting one to three months—turns into chronic low-back pain, a long-term problem that can limit activity and interfere with sleep. Back pain is the number-two symptomatic reason for doctor visits, right behind colds.

Problem: The help that most doctors offer is pills—either over-the-counter painkillers, powerful muscle relaxants such as *diazepam* (Valium) or even addictive opioid painkillers such as *oxycodone* (OxyContin). In fact, guidelines from the American College of Physicians, the main medical society for internists, previously had recommended drugs as the first step in treating low-back pain. But drugs usually are not best!

Surprising development: In February 2017, the American College of Physicians issued new guidelines for treating low-back pain—recommending nondrug treatments as the first choice for acute pain and often for chronic pain, too. ***Here's why, plus the nondrug treatments that scientific evidence shows are the most likely to provide real relief...***

MANY DRUGS DON'T WORK WELL

Research shows that many medications commonly prescribed or recommended by doctors for low-back pain don't work to relieve the pain—including *acetaminophen* (Tylenol) and oral steroids. As for opioid medications—they're dangerously addictive, and more than 16,000 Americans die yearly from overdoses.

That said, some medications can help a bit. *Ibuprofen* (Advil, Motrin), *naproxen* (Aleve) or aspirin provide some relief for low-back pain. Muscle relaxants such as *cyclobenzaprine* (Flexeril) also are moderately effective. In my experience, ibuprofen has the fewest side effects. But the truth is, if you have a classic case of low-back pain, you often don't need medication.

MISLEADING IMAGING

Getting an imaging test such as an MRI, a CT scan or an X-ray usually is not a good strategy for diagnosing acute low-back pain. Yes, the imaging may detect an abnormality such as a bulging disk in the spine. But such abnormalities are common and rarely are the cause of low-back pain—and treating them may lead to unnecessary tests and invasive procedures, even surgery, that are not needed.

When imaging is essential: There are several serious problems that can cause back pain and are considered medical emergencies that require imaging. A new episode of back pain could be caused by a tumor. If you have unexplained fever or weight loss and back pain, you may have a rare infection of the bones of the spine or the outermost part of the spinal canal. If you have muscle weakness in the foot or the leg and back pain, you may have a disk problem that requires further treatment.

Bottom line: It is not useful to do imaging in most people who don't have any of the above symptoms or situations. As I tell my patients—if you don't have imaging now and your pain persists, you can always have imaging later. There usually is no rush.

BEST NONDRUG TREATMENTS

The American College of Physicians now recommends the following nondrug treatments as among the best for low-back pain, and I agree...

- **Wait it out.** The little-used but effective strategy for most cases of acute back pain is... don't go to the doctor (and save $150 or more)! That's because low-back pain almost always improves substantially on its own within a month or so. *Instead, try one or more of the following nondrug treatments...*

- **Exercise.** There's good scientific evidence that exercise can help relieve chronic low-back pain—and there's little evidence that one type of exercise works better than another.

Beneficial types of movement include aerobic exercise, such as brisk walking or bicycling...yoga or stretching...and exercises that strengthen your abdominal and spinal muscles, such as Pilates.

Best: A physical therapist can tailor and guide an exercise program to get you started. For the long term, find an exercise that you enjoy and that you'll stick with.

For acute back pain, specific back exercises may not be helpful, but it's wise to keep walking and maintain normal activities as much as possible. It's when pain becomes chronic that exercise seems most helpful.

- **Cognitive behavioral therapy (CBT) or mindfulness-based stress reduction (MBSR).** I think the most effective regimen for chronic low-back pain often is a combination of exercise and a mind-body approach such as CBT (a psychological therapy that helps you identify dysfunctional patterns of thinking and behavior that increase your pain) or MBSR (which combines the nonjudgmental acceptance of experience with relaxation techniques). By helping you pace yourself in daily life, these techniques ease muscle tension, relieve depression (common in people with chronic pain) and improve sleep.

- **Heat.** Locally applied heat can soothe acute or chronic back pain. Use a heating pad, a hot-water bottle or an over-the-counter heat wrap such as ThermaCare.

Caution: A temperature that's too hot or an application that's too prolonged could burn your skin.

- **Hands-on professionals.** Research shows that spinal manipulation (most often performed by chiropractors but sometimes by osteopathic physicians or physical therapists), acupuncture, massage therapy and other hands-on healing techniques can help relieve both acute and chronic back pain.

• **Optimism.** A recent study I coauthored, published in *Spine*, shows that seniors with low-back pain are more likely to get better if they are confident that their treatment will work. Optimism helps healing!

IF PAIN PERSISTS

If your back pain persists for more than a month without significant improvement, it's wise to see a doctor. (Of course, see a doctor immediately if you have any of the serious symptoms mentioned above.) A physician can create a treatment program that is tailored for you.

If your doctor says that you need medication, you should ask, "What are the relative risks and benefits of this choice? What will happen if I don't take this medication? What are the alternatives?"

And if surgery is recommended, you should probably get a second opinion. The most common surgery for back pain alone is spinal fusion, which is invasive and extensive with a long recovery period.

Even worse: Research shows that the surgery is of questionable effectiveness for many back problems. It also shows that a rigorous rehabilitation program—involving physical therapy and training in pain management—works just as well.

Another Reason to Quit

Surprising link to chronic back pain. An analysis of 160 people found that smokers are three times more likely than nonsmokers to develop chronic back pain.

Possible reason: Smokers have a stronger connection between two brain regions that play a role in addictive behavior and chronic pain.

Good news: Study participants who quit smoking showed a drop in this brain circuit activity, decreasing their vulnerability to chronic pain.

A. Vania Apkarian, PhD, professor of physiology, Northwestern University Feinberg School of Medicine, Chicago.

Back Pain Relief from Plasma Shots

Gordon Ko, MD, medical director of the Physiatry Interventional Pain Clinic at the Sunnybrook Health Sciences Centre and an assistant professor in the department of medicine at the University of Toronto in Ontario. He also is medical director of the Canadian Centre for Integrative Medicine in Markham, Ontario. DrKoprp.com

Prolotherapy involves injecting a mildly irritating agent directly into the painful area in order to provoke an acute inflammatory response. This causes an increase in the flow of blood, nutrients and stem cells to the affected tissues, and these in turn stimulate the body to heal itself.

Since the inception of prolotherapy, various substances have been injected (for instance, a sugar solution or cod-liver oil extract)—but foreign substances such as these sometimes created too much inflammation and/or caused extreme discomfort.

Breakthrough: Recently, researchers discovered that better results occur when the injection consists of the patient's own blood, because the platelets are well tolerated and excessive inflammation is avoided.

PRPP can help cure or significantly relieve long-term chronic low-back pain for more than 80% of patients whose problems stem from injury or laxity in ligaments and/or tendons of the sacroiliac joint (where the base of the spine meets the pelvis). In addition, PRPP has been used successfully to treat other areas of the body where ligament or tendon problems lead to chronic pain, such as occurs with tennis elbow or Achilles tendinitis. PRPP injections also can help resolve muscle tears.

People with certain nutritional deficiencies may need to have these addressed before PRPP can work to best effect. Patients who have a low blood platelet count, a blood-clotting disorder or an inflammatory disorder (such as rheumatoid arthritis or psoriatic arthritis), or who take a blood thinner such as *warfarin* (Coumadin), may not be appropriate candidates for PRPP.

WHAT HAPPENS DURING PRPP TREATMENT

About one to four tablespoons of the patient's blood is drawn and then spun in a centrifuge for 14 minutes to separate the liquid plasma, platelets and white blood cells from the other blood components. This platelet-rich plasma contains about five times as many platelets as normal blood. The platelets are the primary healers, because they release growth factors that promote mechanisms called the healing cascade and stem cell migration.

After the patient is given local anesthesia, the platelet-rich plasma is injected directly into the painful tissues. While the number of injections given depends on the patient's condition, a typical session would include about 10 injections. Each injection is done using ultrasound guidance to ensure exact placement of the needle—because even a tiny slip might damage surrounding tissues, which can be very dangerous. As with any type of injection, PRPP carries a small risk for infection, bruising and bleeding.

Recovery: The injection site may be painful for a few days following treatment. *Acetaminophen* (Tylenol) can relieve this discomfort, but aspirin and other NSAIDs (*ibuprofen*, *naproxen*) should be avoided for at least two weeks (preferably longer) because they would diminish the inflammatory response needed for PRPP to work. To reduce swelling, an ice pack can be applied for 20 minutes three to five times a day as needed.

Many patients find that their chronic back pain improves after just one or two sessions. Injection sessions typically are given two to three months apart to allow time for healing to occur between visits.

Cost: About $750 per session. Since PRPP is still considered experimental, most insurance companies don't cover it.

PRPP is very specialized work that requires specific training.

Recommended: Seek treatment from a doctor of medicine, naturopathy or osteopathy who has been practicing prolotherapy for at least 10 years. Get a referral from your primary care doctor or from the American Association of Orthopaedic Medicine (AAOMed.org) or the Canadian Academy of Orthopaedic Medicine (CAOM.ca)...then contact the practitioner you are considering to inquire about his or her experience.

Important: After PRPP, patients should get physical therapy to help rehabilitate dysfunctional muscles and improve core strength...but should avoid any aggressive manipulation treatment that could undo the beneficial effects of the PRPP.

When You Need Antibiotics for Back Pain

Bacterial Infection—Nearly half the people whose pain is caused by a herniated disk later develop a bacterial infection. For those people, a 100-day course of the antibiotic amoxicillin reduced pain by up to 80% in a recent study. If you have had severe low-back pain for at least three months...have a damaged vertebra and swelling...and other treatment options have failed, ask your doctor whether an extended course of antibiotics is worth trying.

Study of 61 people with back pain by researchers at University of Southern Denmark, Odense, published in *European Spine Journal*.

Kidney Infection—Constant back pain may be a kidney infection, especially when accompanied by other symptoms. If you feel pain only when you move, it is most likely a back injury from strained muscles and ligaments when you work around your house or in your garden, for example, participate in sports or suffer a sudden jolt, such as from a car accident. A kidney infection, on the other hand, may cause fever, pain when you urinate, shaking, chills, blood in your urine and deep back pain that hurts with or without movement. If you have any of these symptoms, contact your doctor immediately. If you have an infection, antibiotics are typically prescribed.

Leslie Spry, MD, kidney specialist, Lincoln Nephrology and Hypertension, Lincoln, Nebraska.

Scoliosis Can Strike At Any Age

R. Douglas Orr, MD, director of the Cleveland Clinic Spine Institute at Lutheran Hospital and staff physician at the Cleveland Clinic Center for Spine Health. An orthopedic surgeon, Dr. Orr specializes in adult spinal surgery and deformity surgery. His research interests include spinal biomechanics and biomaterials.

It may have been years since you've heard anyone mention scoliosis. We tend to think of it as an ailment that strikes only children and adolescents.

What most people don't realize: Scoliosis, marked by an abnormal curvature of the spine, also affects adults, including those who have no history of the condition.

Why this is important: For adults, in particular, scoliosis can be an undiagnosed cause of pain in the back, legs or buttocks. Numbness or weakness in a leg or foot also may occur.

And these symptoms can go on for years without scoliosis being discovered as the culprit! In fact, the telltale "S" curve of adult scoliosis is sometimes severe enough that it's quite easy to see when the person is unclothed and viewed from behind, but in other cases, the curve is barely noticeable to the untrained eye.

WHAT HAPPENS TO THE SPINE

When scoliosis is discovered in an adult, it could have started in childhood but was never diagnosed…or the condition may have first developed in adulthood. If you're over age 40 and develop scoliosis for the first time, then you probably have degenerative scoliosis.

Here's what happens: As we grow older, the disks and facet joints (located between the vertebrae) of our spines degenerate. Over time, the degeneration can lead to scoliosis.

Important: If you have osteoporosis (bone thinning that is worse than the degeneration that naturally occurs with age) and develop scoliosis, the scoliosis will progress more rapidly than it would in a person without osteoporosis.

In some adults who had scoliosis as children, the degenerative process can cause the condition to worsen with age. If this occurs, the curve generally progresses by about one degree per year (scoliosis is diagnosed when the spine is curved vertically by more than 10 degrees).

In addition to the degenerative process that puts adults at increased risk for scoliosis, genetics may also play a role. The condition tends to run in families. The good news is that most adults with scoliosis have no symptoms.

HOW TO HAVE A HEALTHY SPINE

If you know that you had scoliosis as a child or think that you may have it as an adult, see your doctor for advice. If your childhood curvature was more than 30 degrees, you should go to a spine specialist every three to five years to monitor whether the curve is progressing.*

If you suspect that you have adult scoliosis, there are red flags that may signal the condition (see page 118). Scoliosis is relatively easy for a spine specialist to diagnose with a physical exam and spine imaging tests, such as X-rays and/or CT or MRI scans.

It's important for anyone who has scoliosis to keep a close eye on his/her body weight (being overweight puts additional stress on your spine)…and to stay physically active (inactivity can worsen symptoms by allowing trunk muscles to weaken, which can increase the muscle pain associated with scoliosis).

*For a referral to a spine specialist or a scoliosis support group near you, contact the National Scoliosis Foundation, Scoliosis.org.

No Surgery for Stenosis

You may not need surgery for stenosis. According to recent research, physical therapy worked as well as surgery to relieve the pain, numbness and weakness of lumbar spinal stenosis (age-related narrowing of the spinal cord). The two-year study followed 169 patients over age 50 after they had surgery or received twice-weekly physical therapy for six weeks. Physical therapy also helps patients avoid potential surgery-related complications, such as nerve injury and infection.

Anthony Delitto, PhD, PT, professor and chairman of physical therapy, University of Pittsburgh School of Health and Rehabilitation Sciences.

EASY WAYS TO HELP YOURSELF

Once you have scoliosis, exercise won't straighten your spine—nor will it stop the disorder from progressing. But it will help you keep your spine as supported as possible, reduce pain and keep you feeling strong.

While cardiovascular exercise (such as walking, swimming and biking) is a good idea for most people, a core-strengthening program is crucial for anyone with scoliosis. If you think of your spine as a flagpole with the muscles as guy wires, it's easy to visualize how the muscles help support the spine. The goal of core exercises is to strengthen the muscles of the abdomen, back and pelvis.

Depending on your overall fitness and agility, a core workout might include abdominal exercises as well as an exercise called the plank, which strengthens the abdominal and back muscles.

How to do the plank: Start in a raised push-up position with your toes perpendicular to the floor, then bend your elbows and rest your weight on your forearms. Keep your body in a straight line from your shoulders to your ankles. Stay still in this position—that is the exercise. If you can, begin by doing the plank for about 20 seconds and work up to about a minute daily. Because scoliosis can limit movement of the spine, stretching also can help ease stiffness.

Helpful: Many people with scoliosis are able to curb pain if they work with a physical therapist, who can help them design an exercise program that targets their specific issues.

IF YOU NEED MORE HELP

Because the severity of adult scoliosis varies so much from person to person, there is no one-size-fits-all treatment for the condition.

In addition to exercise, here's what often helps...

• **Nondrug therapies.** Chiropractic care (especially for acute episodes of pain), massage and acupuncture seem to help some people with scoliosis.

Note: Bracing, which is often prescribed for young scoliosis patients (whose skeletons are still growing), is rarely offered to adults, since it weakens the core muscles and can increase symptoms.

• **Medication.** A nonsteroidal anti-inflammatory drug (NSAID), such as *ibuprofen* (Motrin), sometimes helps control pain.

Note: If you take an NSAID for long periods, be sure that your doctor supervises your use to help you avoid side effects such as stomach irritation.

If your scoliosis pain is caused or worsened by narrowing or pressure on nerve roots, you may benefit from a steroid injection. The frequency and timing will depend on symptoms, but you should get no more than a few injections per year.

• **Surgery.** Contrary to what you might assume, the degree of your spinal curve is not used to determine whether surgery is needed. Instead, surgery is an option when pain—regardless of the severity of the curve—interferes with your ability to go about your daily activities.

Decompression surgery helps ease the pressure that is placed on nerves where the spine has weakened. This type of surgery usually involves removing (totally or partially) a bony structure or ligament that is applying pressure.

Another option is spine-stabilization surgery, which is performed to help straighten the spine. With this procedure, bones of the spine are fused together with bone grafts to stabilize the spine and eliminate as much of the spinal curve as possible. In most cases, a combination of both surgeries may be needed. The extent of surgery also varies. Major surgery is sometimes done to correct and stabilize the spine. In other cases, a small part of the curve can be addressed with a less extensive, lower-risk surgery.

The risk for complications, such as subsequent pain, increases with the magnitude of the surgery and can be as high as 30% in major reconstructions. There is a small (one in 3,000) risk for paralysis with major spine surgery. The patient's age and the presence of other conditions (such as diabetes) also affect risk for complications. Recovery times range from six weeks up to a year. A spine surgeon is best qualified to perform these procedures.

DO YOU HAVE SCOLIOSIS?

Signs that you may have scoliosis...

- **You have lost more than one inch of height.**
- **One shoulder appears higher than the other.**
- **One hip is higher than the other.**
- **If you find it more comfortable to stand or walk leaning forward,** or if you like to lean on a shopping cart in the grocery store, you may have spinal stenosis (a condition that causes narrowing in the spine), which is associated with adult scoliosis.

Could Your Back Pain Be Arthritis?

John D. Reveille, MD, professor of medicine, director of the division of rheumatology and clinical immunogenetics and vice chairman of research in the department of medicine at The University of Texas Medical School at Houston. He is on the board of directors of the Spondylitis Association of America, Spondylitis.org.

Nearly everyone experiences low back pain at one time or another. For many people, the pain is brought on by heavy lifting, a bad sleep position or twisting the wrong way. For others, it may be age-related osteoarthritis.

But for a significant number of back pain sufferers, the pain becomes chronic (occurring daily for months to years) and can be due to a condition known as ankylosing spondylitis (AS), a form of arthritis that causes painful inflammation of the spinal joints (vertebrae). Less often, pain also occurs in other parts of the body, such as the shoulders and hips—or even the jaw or small joints of the hands.

AS—most often referred to simply as spondylitis—is typically diagnosed before the age of 40, but the condition may go undetected or misdiagnosed until the patient is much older.

If spondylitis progresses, the inflammation can lead to new bone formation that causes the spine to fuse (a condition known as ankylosis) in a forward-stooped position. This occurred in Pope John Paul II, who suffered from AS.

Why do so many cases of spondylitis escape notice? For some patients, the back pain and stiffness caused by spondylitis are so mild or intermittent that the condition doesn't become a problem until later in life. For example, I recently diagnosed a man in his 70s who had spondylitis, but his back pain had become severe only recently.

Spondylitis also can go undiagnosed because most patients—as well as many health-care professionals—are unfamiliar with the condition. Few people know that back pain (often accompanied by fatigue and morning back stiffness that gets better with activity) can be due to spondylitis, but estimates show that the condition affects at least one in every 500 adults, making it nearly as common as rheumatoid arthritis.

What you need to know...

MORE THAN JUST BACK PAIN

The chronic inflammation caused by spondylitis can lead to other potentially serious complications. For example, up to 40% of people with spondylitis suffer from inflammation of the eye (iritis), which can result in pain and sensitivity to light. The condition is treated with corticosteroid eyedrops to ease the inflammation.

In addition, some people with spondylitis develop inflammation just below the aortic valve (the aorta transports blood from the heart to the rest of the body). This chronic inflammation can interfere with the heart's rhythm and/or cause the aortic valve to become leaky (aortic insufficiency), a condition that may require surgical valve replacement.

Recent research: Patients with spondylitis have more aortic stiffness (due to inflammation) than those without the back condition, according to a recent study. Stiffness in an artery raises the risk for high blood pressure and blood vessel damage.

In other spondylitis cases, the cartilage around the ribs may become inflamed, causing a painful condition known as costochondritis. The ribs may eventually fuse to the spine, which limits the chest's ability to expand and may aggravate an existing lung disease, such as asthma or bronchitis, and raise the risk for spinal fracture.

GETTING THE RIGHT DIAGNOSIS

Spondylitis is difficult to diagnose—primarily because it progresses so slowly. It often takes up to 10 years from the time a patient first feels the twinges of back pain before the inflammation shows up on an X-ray.

Ask your doctor about: Getting a magnetic resonance imaging (MRI) scan if spondylitis is suspected. A telltale sign of spondylitis is inflammation of the sacroiliac joints, located in the low back. But X-rays do not always detect this inflammation in the early stages of the condition.

Spondylitis is primarily caused by hereditary factors, especially a genetic marker known as HLA-B27, which is present in more than 90% of people who have spondylitis. However, only about one in 20 people with HLA-B27 develop spondylitis or a related disease.

Certain gastrointestinal conditions, such as Crohn's disease and ulcerative colitis, also have been associated with spondylitis.

Although no cure is yet available, recent advances in treatment have been successful in reducing the pain and inflammation associated with the disease.

BEST MEDICATION OPTIONS

Many people with spondylitis are able to control the pain with over-the-counter nonsteroidal anti-inflammatory drugs, such as *ibuprofen* (Advil) or *naproxen* (Aleve). Others may require the use of a prescription drug known as a TNF-alpha inhibitor, such as *infliximab* (Remicade), *etanercept* (Enbrel) or *adalimumab* (Humira).

Caution: The FDA recently issued a warning about increased risk for fungal infection in people who take these TNF-alpha inhibitors.

These medications, which often are used for rheumatoid arthritis, can eliminate the inflammation of spondylitis but won't prevent the spinal fusion associated with ankylosis.

Latest treatment advances: The FDA recently approved the use of *golimumab* (Simponi), another TNF-alpha inhibitor, for the treatment of spondylitis. Studies show that the drug works at least as well as other TNF-alpha inhibitors, and it is taken less often than those other drugs. *Certolizumab* (Cimzia), another drug in the same class, was recently approved for treatment of rheumatoid arthritis and is expected to be studied as a treatment for spondylitis.

GET SERIOUS ABOUT EXERCISE

Daily exercise—even if it's only five to 10 minutes of gentle stretching—is crucial in the treatment of spondylitis. Many studies have shown that spondylitis patients who exercise regularly experience less pain and better functioning than patients who do not get regular exercise.

Best types of exercise include...

- **Conditioning.** Aerobic workouts, such as swimming, are especially effective at decreasing pain and stiffness.

Helpful: If you have trouble turning your head to breathe while swimming, try a snorkel and mask. (To read about the benefits associated with other forms of water exercise, see page 105.)

- **Spinal extension.** These exercises loosen up the spine and prevent stiffness.

One to try: While on all fours, arch your back like a cat and hold until you feel a good stretch. Then let your back sway or sag downward toward the floor, while lifting up your head and buttocks. Repeat three to five times daily.

- **Range-of-motion for the neck.** Moving the neck can help guard against the stiffness caused by spondylitis.

What to do: Pull in your chin and shift your gaze to your chest. Return to the starting position, then tip your head backward as far as you comfortably can. Repeat three to five times daily.

Stabilize Your Sacroiliac

Jo Ann Staugaard-Jones, MA, advanced Pilates and Hatha yoga instructor and trainer based in Andover, New Jersey. She is a former professor of kinesiology, exercise science and dance at County College of Morris in Randolph, New Jersey, and the author of *The Vital Psoas Muscle* and *The Concise Book of Yoga Anatomy*. Move-Live.com

It's easy to blame nagging low-back pain on a muscle strain or even a disk problem. But that's not always the real cause.

A surprising culprit: Up to one-third of chronic low-back pain can actually be traced to pelvic instability. The sacroiliac (pronounced sak-ro-il-ee-ak) joints, commonly called the SI joints, are located on both sides of the pelvis, connecting it to the lower part of the spine (sacrum).

If this little area of the body gets out of whack, that is when the trouble begins. Unlike other joints throughout the body, a healthy SI joint doesn't flex and extend. Instead, it's considered a "gliding" joint, meaning that the ligaments holding it together can shift, but that shifting is ideally kept to a minimum. The SI joint's main job is to hold the lower spine and pelvis together to increase stability.

Certain life events can cause excess movement in the SI joint, however. Pregnancy is a big one—the SI joints can be affected when ligaments and joints in the pelvic area loosen before giving birth.

For women who are years beyond childbearing age—and men, too—SI joint pain is slightly different. Usually affecting only one side of the pelvis, this type of SI joint trouble leads to a chronic, nagging pain in the lower back, which typically worsens when bending over from a standing position. Sitting, which the average American does for up to 13 hours per day, is another risk factor for SI joint pain—it weakens these joints and promotes inflammation.

EASY STEPS THAT HELP

If you have SI joint pain (marked by a consistent ache on either side of the base of your spine) or suspect that your SI joints may be contributing to low-back pain, see an orthopedic specialist to confirm your diagnosis. Movement tests and an X-ray or a CT scan will be performed.

A clue to watch for: If your pain improves when lying down, this is a sign that the SI joints may be involved. (This can also be a sign of spine degeneration, which can affect the SI area.)

In addition to the exercises on the next page, most doctors recommend the following to help relieve pain due to one or both SI joints...

- **Ice.** It reduces inflammation and produces a brief numbing effect that temporarily relieves pain. Ideally, ice the affected area for 15 minutes three times a day.

What to do: Lie on your belly with an ice bag on the painful area. You can alternate ice packs with a heating pad after the first 24 hours of treatment, when inflammation has subsided, to increase blood flow to the area.

- **Massage.** For some people, this helps...for others, it can aggravate the problem. If you would like to try massage, ask the therapist to use gentle pressure to promote circulation but avoid deep tissue work.

- **SI belt.** It is designed to relieve overtaxed ligaments by decreasing motion in and around the pelvis. The research on these belts is mixed. One study reported significant pain reduction in those wearing the belt, while other research found no such benefit or a worsening of pain for a small number of people.

If you want to try an SI belt, a good product is the New Serola Sacroiliac Hip Belt (about $45, depending on size). But if pain seems to worsen with a belt, stop using it.

- **Pain-relief medication.** If the therapies described above and exercise routine below don't give you adequate relief, you may need to add pain medication such as *ibuprofen* (Advil) or topical arnica gel.

EXERCISE FOR YOUR SI JOINTS

The main goal of a workout to relieve SI pain is to balance the strength of the muscles and tendons surrounding the joints so they can provide stability. Exercises that work the transverse abdominis (the deep ab muscles that support internal organs)...the deep external hip rotators that connect the sacrum to the thighbone...and the gluteus muscles will also help the SI joints remain strong yet supple. If you're in pain, relax the muscles and do these exercises when pain has lessened. *Try the following 10-minute routine three times a week—you should get relief within three to six weeks...**

• **Squats.** *What to do:* While holding a light weight (five pounds to start, working up to 10) or a 10-pound bar overhead (keep your shoulders down), stand in front of a mirror with a chair behind you to assist with the exercise.

(Holding a bar or weights overhead helps keep the body in correct alignment.) Engage your abdominal and back muscles as you bend your knees, lowering yourself toward a sitting position. (If your lower back begins to sway, you have gone far enough and need to pull your navel in toward your spine.) Allow your hips to fall back toward the chair until your buttocks lightly touch the chair, but do not sit down. Aim for your upper thighs to be parallel to the floor. Hold the squat for 10 to 20 seconds, while breathing deeply, then slowly return to a standing position. Repeat three to five times.

• **Hand/knee balance.** *What to do:* Get down on all fours in a tabletop position with your back as level and flat as possible. Your hands should be directly under your shoulders and your knees under your hips. Begin by stretching your right leg back and lifting it to hip height, then slowly lift your left arm forward in line with your ear. Keep your pelvis stable and centered and your core muscles tight. Hold for 10 seconds. Then return to the tabletop position and repeat on the other side. Alternate sides for one minute.

• **SI stretch.** *What to do:* Lie on your back on an exercise mat or carpeted floor with your legs straight and your arms outstretched to your sides. Bend your right knee toward your chest, then let it fall across your body to the left, letting your hips roll with it. (Keep both your shoulders on the floor.) Relax and breathe in and out for a minute before repeating on the other side.

*As with any exercise program, check with your doctor first.

Inversion Therapy for Back Pain

David Hanscom, MD, board-certified orthopedic spine surgeon, Seattle Neuroscience Specialists, Swedish Medical Center, Seattle. He is the author of *Back in Control: A Spine Surgeon's Roadmap Out of Chronic Pain, Second Edition.* BackInControl.com

Inversion therapy is a form of traction that uses the force of gravity to stretch the spine. Your feet and ankles are securely strapped to a special table or chair, which you then tilt backward until your head is lower than the rest of your body. While inversion therapy hasn't been shown to provide long-term relief for back pain, many people do feel better for a short time while they are doing it and immediately afterward. That brief respite may be enough to allow a long pain-free walk or give you a break from the over-the-counter pain meds that you're taking.

The first thing you should know, though, is that you don't need to literally hang upside down with the soles of your feet pointing toward the ceiling! That's not necessary and isn't even a good idea for most people...at least not when you first try inversion therapy. I'll explain a safer approach below.

First, though, let's look at the potential benefits—and risks.

HOW INVERSION THERAPY CAN HELP

Inversion therapy can work in two very different ways...

• **Mechanical relief.** If pain is being caused by a compressed disc, removing stress on the disc by lying or sitting in an inverted position can reduce the pain.

• **Gravity creates a traction force to muscles and ligaments around the spine,** which temporarily releases muscle spasms. When that tightness disappears, you will feel more relaxed. Relaxation isn't just a nice extra—it's an integral part of treatment. That's especially true if you have back pain that has lasted 12 or more weeks.

Here's why: Living with pain for so long can make you frustrated and anxious, feelings that can become so ingrained that they form new pain pathways. Even after the original source of the pain—say, a pulled muscle—has dissipated, the new pathway still continues to send pain signals. Inversion therapy can relieve your pain so that as you relax, you can begin to "unwind" this nervous system response and break this painful pattern.

While short-term pain relief and relaxation can go a long way, they are rarely enough. Treating chronic pain is like fighting a forest fire—it must be attacked from all angles. Staying active is the top recommendation. Getting enough good-quality sleep is key. Nondrug treatments such as yoga, Pilates, tai chi and hypnosis can help.

By itself, then, a few minutes on the inversion table won't help much if you're not also staying active and getting your best sleep. On the positive side, combining inversion therapy with other nonpharmacologic treatments can further reduce pain. For example, hypnosis by itself, or inversion therapy by itself, may each provide only a modest amount of relief, but when you try them both, you may see big improvements in your back pain—without drugs.

WHO SHOULDN'T TRY INVERSION THERAPY

Inversion therapy is not for everybody. When your head is lower than the rest of your body, your heart rate slows but your blood pressure rises—and so does the pressure inside your eyes. If you have heart disease or any cardiovascular problem, including high blood pressure...or glaucoma, retinal detachment or any other eye condition...do not try inversion therapy. Pregnant women and people with hiatal hernia should also avoid it. (If you have any questions about whether it's safe for you, talk to your health-care provider.)

Even if you don't have any of these conditions, you could hurt yourself by being too gung-ho in your approach. If you hang upside down the first time out, you might hurt your ankles or knees. If you stay inverted too long, you might even pull a muscle, which will just make your pain worse.

That's why I recommend a go-slow approach. If you're healthy and you're interested in inversion therapy, speak with your health-care provider about first trying it under supervision at a physical therapist's office. You will most likely start gently and slowly by reclining at a slight angle (15 degrees below horizontal is a good start) for just a few minutes. If you feel better, periodically increase the angle and duration of the treatment (be careful not to overdo it). If you find it's really helping you after several sessions at the physical therapist's office, you might want to consider purchasing an inversion table—or an inversion chair, which provides a gentler angle for your body.

Steroid Shots May Raise Fracture Risk

You may want to think twice before getting an epidural steroid injection for back pain. A single shot increased risk for spinal fracture by up to 21% in a study of adults age 50 and older.

Why: Steroids are believed to hinder new bone formation and increase bone breakdown.

What to do: Ask your doctor about alternative ways to treat back pain, such as gentle exercise.

Shlomo Mandel, MD, MPH, orthopedic spine surgeon, Henry Ford West Bloomfield Hospital, Michigan.

Back Pain and Surgery: When You Need It... When You Don't

Jack Stern, MD, PhD, a surgeon who specializes in spine neurosurgery and is on the clinical faculty at Weill Cornell Medical College in New York City. He has a private practice in White Plains, New York, and is the author of *Ending Back Pain: 5 Powerful Steps to Diagnose, Understand, and Treat Your Ailing Back.* SafeSpineSurgery.com

Studies show that far too many people are now having surgery in an attempt to relieve back pain.

But only about 10% of all back pain sufferers actually need surgery. Even when pain is severe, the overwhelming majority of back patients will make a full recovery within two to three months with nothing more than painkillers, exercise, physical therapy or other conservative treatments.

Most people get their first episode of back pain in their 30s. But as we age, the incidence of back pain increases. With wear and tear, the spinal discs, which act as shock absorbers and allow the spine to flex, start to dry out and weaken (a condition called disc degeneration). This can result in painful back conditions such as a herniated disc, facet joint syndrome or spinal stenosis.

More about these back problems and the best treatments for them...

HERNIATED DISC—DON'T RUSH TO HAVE SURGERY!

About 20% of adults have one or more herniated discs without symptoms, but others aren't so lucky. A herniated disc is among the main causes of low-back pain and the "shooting" pain of sciatica.

As we age, the spinal discs lose some of their water content, which makes them more prone to tearing or rupture (a herniated disc). An MRI is used for diagnosis.

My advice: Unless you're having serious neurological symptoms—foot or leg weakness, for example, or a loss of bowel or bladder control—wait at least six weeks before considering surgery.

The surgery for herniated disc, called a microdiscectomy, is frequently performed on an outpatient basis, is very safe and has a high success rate. But research has shown that about 90% of patients with a herniated disc will get better without surgery. There's a good chance that the body's natural healing mechanisms will break down the damaged portion of the disc, and the pain will clear up on its own. The catch is that it can sometimes take up to a year or more to recover.

Even though doctors often recommend steroids (oral or as an injection), many patients prefer a nondrug approach to pain relief.

A therapy that's underutilized...

- **Alexander technique.** This is an especially good treatment choice for back pain or sciatica that is caused in part by poor posture or other issues involving body mechanics. It can also help some patients with spinal stenosis (see below).

With the Alexander technique, named after its inventor, Frederick Alexander, a patient's body movements are analyzed and then specific recommendations are made to relieve tension in the body and improve posture and movement.

Important finding: A study in *BMJ* involving 579 patients with chronic or recurrent low-back pain found that those who had six to 24 instructional sessions and practiced the technique had less pain than those given conventional treatments, such as massage and exercise.

FACET JOINT SYNDROME—WAIT IT OUT?

Facet pain affects at least 15% of all people with back pain—and nearly 45% of back pain sufferers ages 50 to 60. It can be caused by trauma—twisting too hard during a round of golf or a tennis serve, for example—but it's usually due to osteoarthritis in the spine. The facet joints are the round protrusions that you can feel when you touch your spine. Arthritis in these areas can cause pain and/or stiffness, just as it does in the knees or other joints.

Clues for facet pain: The pain usually comes on quickly...can make it difficult to stand up straight or get out of a chair...and may also cause pain in the buttocks or thighs.

If you have mild/occasional facet pain: I advise you to wait it out. Many people get better on their own within four to six weeks. While you're waiting for the issue to resolve, you can take *ibuprofen* (Motrin) or other painkillers...avoid stressing the area...and try chiropractic treatments (they're safe and can realign the facet joints to reduce pressure but avoid if you have severe osteoporosis or spinal cancer).

If you have severe/lasting pain: Ask your doctor about radiofrequency nerve ablation. It's a simple surgical procedure that uses a microelectrode to destroy the affected nerve. In one important study, the procedure was found to reduce pain by 50% to 80% in most people. Nerve ablation is unlikely to cause complications, although the nerve sometimes grows back—and could cause pain in the future. Insurance usually covers the procedure.

SPINAL STENOSIS—SURGERY IS TYPICALLY NEEDED

With spinal stenosis, there is a narrowing of the spinal canal (the open space in the spine that holds the spinal cord), which can exert pressure on spinal nerve roots, resulting in pain. Some people are born with a narrow spinal opening, but most often it's caused by age-related changes such as arthritis or the growth of bone spurs in the spinal canal. Some people with spinal stenosis have low-back pain while others have pain that radiates down the leg (it can be similar to the pain that's caused by sciatica).

Clues for spinal stenosis: Pain increases when you walk and quickly gets better with rest. With sciatica, pain is sometimes relieved by walking. Also, if there is pain relief when bending forward (this movement "opens up" spinal spaces and reduces pressure), this points to stenosis. A diagnosis can be confirmed with a CT scan or MRI of the lumbar spine.

My advice: I almost always recommend surgical decompression for patients with spinal stenosis. One large study showed that people who have surgery recover more quickly and stay pain-free longer than those who have physical therapy or undergo other treatments for spinal stenosis. The procedure is usually covered by insurance.

With surgical decompression, the surgeon removes the excess bone and overgrowth of ligaments that's causing the pressure. It takes about three months for full recovery—but it's one of the most successful spinal operations, with more than 80% of patients reporting good improvement. However, surgery can't correct arthritis, so symptoms may eventually return. Risk for side effects is low but includes nerve injury and infection.

Stop Chronic Back Pain Without Surgery

David Hanscom, MD, board-certified orthopedic spine surgeon, Swedish Medical Center, Seattle. He is the author of *Back in Control: A Spine Surgeon's Roadmap Out of Chronic Pain.* DrDavidHanscom.com

It hurts just to read the latest statistics on back pain. Every year, Americans spend an estimated $86 billion on back pain treatments, including pain pills, injections and surgery. And although about 800,000 surgical procedures are performed each year for back pain, in about 75% of those cases, the surgery doesn't help.

That's why David Hanscom, MD, an orthopedic spine surgeon at Swedish Medical Center in Seattle, does something that few surgeons would dream of—he talks most of his patients out of having surgery. Instead, he recommends a new six-step approach to treating chronic back pain that he finds far more effective than surgery for most people.

WHY SURGERY USUALLY WON'T HELP

The main reason why spine surgery so often doesn't work, Dr. Hanscom said, is that an operation can relieve back pain only if there is a structural abnormality, such as a ruptured disk or pinched nerve. But the vast majority of chronic, severe back problems don't fall into that category. Instead, the back pain is nonspecific, rooted in inflammation in the body's soft tissues (ligaments, tendons, fascia, muscles). "These types of problems cannot be seen on imaging tests—and if you can't see it, the best surgeon in the world won't be able to fix it," said Dr. Hanscom.

So when the problem is a soft-tissue issue, whether or not the patient undergoes surgery, his pain is likely to go on and on. Understandably, this leads to a lot of frustration (because nothing is helping) and fatigue (because pain is exhausting). A vicious cycle is created—pain leads to frustration and fatigue, and frustration and fatigue exacerbate pain.

The longer the pain continues, the worse the situation gets. "Long-lasting pain creates neurologic pathways that outlast the root cause," Dr. Hanscom explained. "Once these pain pathways are formed and remembered, the cycle is established and the pain becomes chronic. So even after the soft-tissue problems are gone, the pain often isn't. The only way to fix this type of chronic pain is to tackle the central nervous system's response to pain."

TAKING CONTROL

Dr. Hanscom knows firsthand whereof he speaks. His book *Back in Control: A Spine Surgeon's Roadmap Out of Chronic Pain* describes his own battle with chronic pain—from tennis elbow, migraine headaches, burning feet syndrome and more—and the surprising strategy that he used to overcome it. Based on his personal and professional experience, he has developed a program—called Defined, Organized, Comprehensive Care (DOCC)—that he uses in treating his own patients and in training other surgeons. Its premise is that pain is a perception...and that understanding it gives you greater power to gain control over it. "Freedom from pain is not only possible, with the right tools it is probable," he said.

Basically, the DOCC approach works by calming down the nervous system and allowing it to heal while also laying down new neurological pathways so the nervous system isn't trapped in the endless loop of pain signals. Dr. Hanscom explained, "It's not that you simply learn to live with the pain. Instead, your brain stops responding to the pain—so you literally do not feel it." *The DOCC program involves six basic steps...*

- **Sleep.** Getting at least eight hours of sleep per night is a cornerstone of the program. "If sleep issues aren't addressed, nothing else will work," Dr. Hanscom said. For people who have trouble sleeping due to their pain, prescription sleep medications are an option.
- **Stress management.** Chronic stress creates a cascade of biological events that exacerbate inflammation and sleeplessness, which in turn perpetuate chronic pain. Managing stress requires a two-pronged approach—making time for activities that build up your energy reserves (exercise, hobbies, socializing, spending time alone)...and learning to deal more effectively with aspects of your life that drain your energy (things that make you anxious, angry or unhappy).
- **Pain medication.** If you (or your doctor) have been leery of using pain medication for fear of its potential side effects, it is worth reconsidering this issue. Taking pain medication to achieve short-term relief while you work to resolve your chronic pain problem can help you halt that vicious cycle through which pain begets more pain, Dr. Hanscom said.
- **Physical therapy.** Rehabilitation of soft tissues soothes inflammation and facilitates true healing.
- **Goal setting.** Creating a detailed picture of what you are trying to achieve and devising a plan to work toward that goal helps you decrease anxiety, frustration and depression. This, in turn, calms the central nervous system and eases physical pain.
- **Retraining the brain.** The DOCC program moves people from being reactive to being creative in their lives. Meditation, visualization and creative play are among the primary tools Dr. Hanscom recommends. Particularly helpful is writing, he said.

Example: Write down a situation that bothers you (for instance, "My spouse is always late and it stresses me out"). Then, on paper, examine your thought processes about this situation (such as, "When she's late, I imagine that she's been in a terrible accident...or that she just doesn't care enough about me to be on time"). Next, look for errors in your thinking ("It's highly unlikely that she's had an accident...and she shows me in many ways every day that she loves me"). Finally, write about more rational ways in which to view the situation ("She's just not good at budgeting her time. I'll ask her to meet me 15 minutes earlier than necessary so that, by the time she arrives, we'll be right on schedule"). Even though the problem or problems you write about might not seem to be related to your back pain, the writing exercises essentially help reprogram your nervous system to undo the old pain pathways, allowing your brain to lay down new, positive, pain-free neural pathways.

Helpful: To access the online content of the publication called *STOMP* (*Structuring*

Your Own Management of Pain), which Dr. Hanscom coauthored, go to Swedish.org/services/pain-services/pain-management-guide. It describes in more detail many of the concepts and pain-relieving strategies discussed above—so that you can take control of your pain instead of having it control you.

Soothing Supplements for Back Pain

Mark A. Stengler, NMD, naturopathic doctor and founder of the Stengler Center for Integrative Medicine in Encinitas, California. He is author or coauthor of numerous books, including *The Natural Physician's Healing Therapies* and *Bottom Line's Prescription for Natural Cures,* and author of the newsletter *Health Revelations.* MarkStengler.com

Various natural substances can alleviate back pain. All are sold at health-food stores and, unless otherwise noted, generally are safe and can be taken until symptoms are gone. Use the lower end of each dosage range if you weigh less than 200 pounds, and the higher dosage if you weigh more or if relief has not been achieved within one week. Depending on the aggressiveness of the treatment you desire, these supplements can be used individually, in any combination or even all together. *To reduce muscle pain and inflammation...*

• **Devil's claw,** an African root.

Dosage: For acute pain, take 800 mg three times daily of concentrated extract capsules (standardized to 1.5% to 3% harpagosides) for up to two weeks. For chronic pain, take 200 mg to 400 mg three times daily for up to eight weeks. Consult a doctor before using if you have diabetes. Do not use if you have an ulcer, heartburn, gastritis or gallstones...are pregnant or nursing...or take a blood thinner, such as aspirin or *warfarin* (Coumadin).

• **Protease (protein-digesting) enzymes.**

Dosage: Bromelain at 1,000 mg three times daily between meals.

Alternative: A combination enzyme formula, such as Wobenzym from Naturally Vitamins (888-766-4406, Wobenzym.com). Take five to 10 tablets three times daily on an empty stomach. Do not use if you take a blood thinner or have an ulcer.

• **B vitamins.**

Dosage: Vitamin B-1 and vitamin B-6, each at 50 mg to 100 mg three times daily...plus vitamin B-12 at 250 micrograms (mcg) to 500 mcg three times daily.

To ease muscle spasms...

• **Methylsulfonylmethane (MSM),** an organic sulfur compound.

Dosage: 4,000 mg to 8,000 mg daily.

• **Magnesium.**

Dosage: 250 mg twice daily.

• **Calcium.**

Dosage: 500 mg twice daily.

To alleviate stiffness...

• **Rhus tox,** a homeopathic remedy derived from poison ivy.

Dosage: Two pellets four times daily of a 30C potency.

To soothe nerve pain...

• **St. John's wort oil.** Rub a bean-size amount of this herbal oil over the affected area twice daily.

Natural supplements may take 24 hours or more to provide relief. In the interim, if pain is severe, also take an over-the-counter nonsteroidal anti-inflammatory drug (NSAID), such as aspirin, *ibuprofen* (Advil) or *naproxen* (Aleve). Or ask your doctor about prescription pain medication, such as *hydrocodone* with *acetaminophen* (Vicodin)...and/or a prescription muscle relaxant, such as *cyclobenzaprine* (Flexeril). Take these medications as briefly as possible to minimize the risk of side effects, such as ulcers, kidney disease and/or liver damage.

Back Pain Remedy: Walking—On Hills

Jamison Starbuck, ND, naturopathic physician in family practice in Missoula, Montana. She is a past president of the American Association of Naturopathic Physicians and a contributing editor to *The Alternative Advisor: The Complete Guide to Natural Therapies and Alternative Treatments.* DrJamisonStarbuck.com.

Recent research tells us that walking regularly is as effective as physical therapy, chiropractic care and medication for many types of low-back pain. That's because walking uses and strengthens muscles in the back and abdomen but doesn't overwork them. As these muscles are gently worked, circulation improves, tissues repair and spasms relax.

Here's a little secret that will make walking even more effective for low-back pain: If possible, do hill walking. Why is this better? Walking uphill requires you to lift your leg more than flat walking does. In doing this, the muscles along the spine are elongated, stretched and strengthened more effectively than with flat walking. Downhill walking is less helpful than walking uphill, though it does generally help and strengthens thigh muscles.

Important: Hill walking does not mean climbing up mountains or steep hills. If you want to try hill walking for back pain, look for rolling hills and choose a route with more up than down if possible. Walk a minimum of 20 minutes per day, four times a week. If this is painful, start with five-minute walks, spread throughout the day, and work up to 20 or more minutes per walk when you are able.

Practice deep breathing as you walk. Take deep breaths to increase oxygen intake and help relax back muscles. Imagine your back muscles relaxing with each inhalation, strengthening and healing with each exhalation.

Back Pain Linked to Lack of Vitamin D

Gregory E. Hicks, PT, PhD, assistant professor, department of physical therapy, University of Delaware, Newark, and leader of a study of 958 people, published in *Journal of the American Geriatrics Society.*

Women with low blood levels of vitamin D were more than twice as likely to have low-back pain, perhaps due to bone softening.

Best: Ask your doctor about taking vitamin D supplements.

The Right Bed Can Ease Back Pain

Baljinder Bathla, MD, cofounder of Chicago Sports & Spine, a pain-management practice. He is certified in physical medicine, rehabilitation and pain management. ChicagoSportsSpine.com

People with back pain often think that a very firm mattress is best. Not true. In a study published in *The Lancet*, 313 individuals with low-back pain slept on either a firm or a medium-firm coil mattress. After 90 days, the participants with the medium-firm mattresses had less pain in bed, upon rising and during the day than those with firm mattresses. *Other misconceptions about beds and back pain...*

Misconception: Everyone with back pain feels the pain when he/she first wakes up—so you can't tell if the mattress is a problem or not.

Fact: Most back pain is mildest in the morning, before you get out of bed and begin moving. If you wake up stiff and sore, your mattress may be to blame. Try sleeping on a different mattress—in the guest room, at a friend's, in a hotel—and see if you notice an improvement when you get up.

Misconception: Heavier people with back pain need soft beds.

Fact: Everyone needs enough support during the night to keep the spine in a normal position. If the spine sinks into a sagging bed, the muscles are strained. Heavier people and those who sleep on their backs tend to need firmer mattresses. Side and stomach sleepers need softer beds.

Misconception: A foam pad or an entire mattress made of foam helps relieve back pain.

Fact: There are two kinds of foam generally available—egg-crate and memory foam. Egg-crate foam creates a layer of softness but does not change the support beneath. Memory foam is sensitive to temperature and conforms to the body. However, there is no scientific evidence that either kind of foam reduces back pain.

Misconception: You can't tell in the store if the mattress is right for you.

Fact: Trying out a mattress in the store can help you determine if it's comfortable. Lie on each mattress for at least five minutes. Start on your back, without a pillow. Your hand should fit snugly in the small of your back. Lying on your side, you shouldn't notice significant pressure on your hips or shoulders. Choose a retailer that will allow you to return a mattress if it isn't comfortable. These include Sleepy's and 1800Mattress.com. (You may have to pay an exchange fee.)

Simple Supplement for Back Pain Relief

Joseph C. Maroon, MD, professor, and vice-chair, department of neurological surgery, University of Pittsburgh School of Medicine, and lead author of a study of 250 people, published in *Surgical Neurology.*

Omega-3s, found in fish and fish oil supplements, block inflammation and accompanying pain.

Study: 60% of participants with neck or back pain who were given 1,200 milligrams (mg) of fish oil per day reported relief after two to four weeks, and almost all of that group were able to discontinue their use of nonsteroidal anti-inflammatory drugs (NSAIDs). The study also found that most patients taking fish oil had no significant side effects.

Wool Underwear Can Help Your Back Pain

Study by researchers at Atatürk University, Erzurum, Turkey, published in *Collegium Antropologicum.*

Men with lower back pain who wore merino wool underwear for two months reported 89% less pain and needed fewer pain medications than men who wore cotton underwear. Wool's heat-retaining properties help keep back muscles flexible, reducing pain. Merino wool is comfortable to wear.

How to Get Rid of That Knot in Your Back

Donald O. Miles, PhD, LMT, CNC, is a licensed massage therapist with Fitness Plus, a service of Saint Francis Medical Center in Cape Girardeau, Missouri, and with Caring Touch Center in Jackson, Missouri. FitnessPlus.sfmc.net

Don't you hate it when a muscle in the middle of your back cramps up, creating a knot of hot pain? You long to rub away the agony, but unless you're as flexible as an acrobat, the tender spot is impossible to reach.

Such cramps often are the result of muscles overreacting to try to protect you from whatever stress you are under—whether that stress is emotional or physical (for instance, the result of sitting too long in one position). The muscle fibers, which normally are stretchy, temporarily lose their pliability and clench up. This cuts off circulation, depriving the tissue of needed nutrients and oxygen and leading to pain.

Massage techniques and other tactics can help disperse tension from muscle fibers and promote healing by restoring circulation to the affected area. *To release a hard-to-reach knot in your back, try the following...*

Tennis-ball tip: Place a tennis ball inside the toe end of a long sock. Grasping the open end of the sock, toss the ball over one shoulder and stand with your back close to a wall. Lean backward so the ball is pressed between you and the wall, positioned directly against the sore spot. Maintain as much pressure as possible for as long as you can stand it—though that may be only a few seconds to start. Rest for a moment, then repeat several times. Use the technique as needed throughout the day.

Candy-cane cure: For more precise control, try the Thera Cane Deep Pressure Massager (Theracane.com, $39.95), which is shaped like a two-foot-long candy cane with several projections that allow for a firm grip and various self-massaging options. Experiment to determine the specific positions and degrees of pressure that bring the most relief.

Hot-and-cold healing: Between your self-massage sessions, wrap an ice pack in a towel and lie on top of it so that the sore spot is in contact with the ice pack (but don't let your skin get uncomfortably cold). Or try alternating the ice pack with a warm pack, such as a hot water bottle or heating pad, at intervals of 15 minutes or less. The ice brings relief by numbing the area, while the heat relaxes the contracted muscle and improves circulation. Repeat the sequence three times throughout the day.

Get-up-and-go: You probably don't feel like moving much when your back is causing you pain, but staying stationary may only exacerbate the muscle cramp. So rather than sitting (or lying) around for hours on end, get up at least every hour and walk around...shrug and roll your shoulders...and gently stretch your neck and arms.

If symptoms persist: See a professional massage therapist. Ask your doctor for a referral or check the website of the American Massage Therapy Association at AMTAmassage.org.

Morton's Toe and the Simple 25¢ Remedy for Back and Leg Pain

Burton S. Schuler, DPM, podiatrist and director of the Ambulatory Foot Clinic at the Podiatric Pain Management Center in Panama City, Florida. He is author of *Why You Really Hurt.* FootCare4u.com

Do you have back pain you can't fix? Take off your socks and look at your toes. If the second toe is even slightly longer than the big toe, you might have Morton's toe, a condition that disrupts normal alignment and can cause pain throughout the body, particularly in the back, legs and feet.

The condition is named after Dudley J. Morton, MD, of Yale Medical School, who first wrote about it causing foot problems. Janet Travell, MD—White House physician to former presidents Kennedy and Johnson—took the concept further by explaining that Morton's toe could cause pain all over the body.

It's estimated that up to 15% of Americans have Morton's toe. Among those with chronic musculoskeletal pain, the prevalence might be as high as 80%. People are born with Morton's toe, but it usually takes decades of accumulated stress and the age-related loss of tissue elasticity to start producing symptoms that can develop into chronic pain.

WHY IT HURTS

When we walk and our feet push off from the ground, the big toe typically touches before the other toes. For a fraction of a second, it absorbs virtually all of the body's weight. Then as the foot rolls forward, some of the pressure is shifted to the adjoining, weaker toes.

In patients with Morton's toe, the first metatarsal bone (in the big toe) is abnormally short and the longer second metatarsal bone typically touches the ground first and absorbs most of the body's weight. The second metatarsal bone isn't strong enough for this much pressure. To compensate, the foot overpronates—it rolls in the direction of the big toe to support the excess weight.

Overpronation makes the foot unstable. It also prevents the big toe from pushing your weight upward. This means that other muscles and joints have to compensate.

The result: Decades of abnormal stress that can disrupt your posture and potentially damage joints throughout the body, causing pain.

THE 25¢ FIX

The simple, inexpensive remedy for Morton's toe is a toe pad. It will act like a shim under the first metatarsal bone and cause the big toe to meet the ground a fraction of a second sooner. This will prevent overpronation and help keep the foot stable. It often relieves symptoms within a few weeks—and sometimes right away.

Exception: Because a toe pad changes the body's alignment, some people experience a temporary increase in pain. This usually diminishes within a few days.

Once the pain goes away, you still will need to wear a toe pad every day, just as someone with sight problems needs to wear glasses or contact lenses every day. *To make a toe pad...*

- **Buy a package of inexpensive foam shoe inserts.** I have found that Dr. Scholl's Molefoam is a good product for making a toe pad (one pack provides six to eight toe pads). Just about any product will work—even no-name brands available at most pharmacies and discount stores, usually for less than $2.

Cut out a rectangle about one-inch wide and two-and-a-half inches long. That's about the size of a stick of chewing gum or a Band-Aid. Put it over the first metatarsal head, the bulge on the bottom of the foot that is below the point where the big toe joins the foot. Position the pad so that the longer dimension runs lengthwise with the foot. If the insole doesn't have an adhesive backing, tape it to the foot with duct tape, electrical tape or even Scotch tape. It does not have to look pretty.

You can take the toe pad off at night and put it back on the foot in the morning. One toe pad usually lasts two to four days.

Helpful: If you don't have a foam insert, a quarter can work. Anything that adds thickness to the first metatarsal head will help restore proper alignment.

Acupuncture Relieves Back Pain

In a study of 1,162 people with chronic low-back pain, one group received acupuncture and another group received conventional therapy using painkillers, physical therapy and exercise. Those who had 10 half-hour acupuncture sessions over six weeks were nearly twice as likely to report improvements in pain as patients given conventional therapy.

In other research, after receiving acupuncture for chronic back pain for eight weeks, 60% of study participants experienced significant improvement in their levels of functioning, compared with 39% who continued usual care, including medications and doctor visits.

Theory: Acupuncture triggers a pain-dulling response by the central nervous system.

Heinz G. Endres, MD, clinical epidemiology specialist, Ruhr-University Bochum, Germany.

Daniel C. Cherkin, PhD, senior scientific investigator, Group Health Research Institute, Seattle.

APPLY HEAT

If a toe pad doesn't eliminate the pain right away, you might want to apply heat. Rest your feet on a heating pad or soak them in warm water for about 15 minutes, once or twice a day.

If after two to three weeks you still have pain, see your physician.

For Back Pain, Massage Your Hand and Foot

Deborah Flanagan, certified reflexologist and founder of the Center for True Health in New York City.

If you have back pain, relief may lie in the palms of your hands...or sole of your foot. Reflexology involves applying mild pressure to specific spots on the hands and feet that are believed to correspond with different body organs. While it hasn't been extensively studied, there is scientific evidence that reflexology can help with chronic back pain.

HELPING HAND

This move is one that you can perform for yourself—any time, anywhere—to get speedy relief.

How it works: Relieve a tense, aching back by stimulating the spine reflex. This is the area on each thumb that extends down the outside, along the base to the wrist.

What to do: Press with the pad of your left thumb along the outside edge of your right thumb, inching from the top of the thumb, down across the base and across to the middle of your wrist. Then use your right thumb to do the same thing to the outer edge of your left thumb.

Repeat this exercise three or four times on each hand, several times a day. Spend a little more time on any spot that feels tender.

SOLE-SEARCHING PAIN RELIEF

Here's another way to relieve pain-causing stress (most back pain is caused by stress)—trigger the reflexology point that connects to your spine. It's located in the soles of your feet. Starting with your left foot, use your thumbs to apply firm pressure along the inner sole from the big toe to the heel. Massage for a good five minutes. Then do the same with your right foot. If relief isn't instant, repeat the procedure again. Ahhhh...that feels good.

A Simple 5-Step Plan to Get Rid of Back Pain...for Good

Miriam E. Nelson, PhD, associate professor and director of John Hancock Center for Physical Activity and Nutrition at the Gerald J. and Dorothy R. Friedman School of Nutrition Science and Policy at Tufts University, Boston. A fellow of the American College of Sports Medicine, she is author, with Lawrence Lindner, of *Strong Women, Strong Backs.*

As many as 90% of all adults suffer back pain at some point in their lives. Back pain—lower back pain, in particular—ranks fifth among the most frequent reasons for hospitalizations.

Worse for women: Their musculoskeletal systems—ligaments, vertebrae, spinal disks, etc.—are more delicate than men's and more vulnerable to injury. Women also tend to be less active, on average, than men, and a sedentary lifestyle is a common cause of back pain.

Most back problems are caused by prolonged sitting or by lifting heavy objects the wrong way, but other factors contribute to back pain, including excess body weight, stress and depression. Even smoking is a factor for reasons that aren't exactly clear.

Simple lifestyle measures—maintaining a healthy weight, not smoking and controlling stress and depression—can prevent many cases of back pain. Most important, though, are exercises that strengthen muscles in the back, chest, abdomen, hips and sides. These are the core muscles—the scaffolding that supports the spine and enables the back to flex and twist without injury. Strengthening these muscles can relieve pain and also prevent it.

A FIVE-STEP PLAN

The following workout, which takes no more than 20 minutes, targets all of the core muscles. It can be done three to five times weekly (unlike most strength-training workouts, which should be done no more than three times a week, because muscles need time to recover between sessions). These exercises can be done more often because the intensity is lower—and they're less likely than traditional workouts to cause back pain or other injuries.

For each of the following exercises...

- **Complete 10 repetitions,** rest for one minute, then complete another 10 reps. If you can complete only five or six reps, the intensity is too high and you should do only what you can comfortably manage.
- **Work up to an advanced progression.** This is a way to increase the exercise intensity by making the movements more difficult.
- **Always warm up**—by taking a brisk walk around the block or stepping quickly in place—for five minutes before doing the exercises.

Step 1: **Abdominals.**

Most people's abdominal muscles are weaker than they should be. Strengthening the abdominals is among the best ways to prevent back pain.

Starting position: Lie on your back on the floor with your knees bent and the soles of your feet flat on the floor. Lightly rest your hands on the lower part of the stomach.

The movement: Contract the abdominal muscles until you feel the small of the back pushing toward the floor. Imagine that you're pulling your belly button downward. Hold the "tense" position for three seconds, then relax.

Progression: Do almost the same exercise as above, with this difference. While the abdominal muscles are tight, raise the still-bent right leg a few inches off the floor and hold it up for three seconds, then place that leg down and raise the left leg for three seconds. The entire move will take 10 to 12 seconds.

Step 2: **Chest muscles.**

Along with abdominal exercises, chest workouts protect the back by strengthening the "front" of the core muscle groups.

Starting position: Stand facing a wall or a counter, about an arm's length away, with your feet hip-width apart and knees slightly bent. Put your palms on the wall (or lightly hold the edge of the counter).

The movement: Holding your body straight, bend at the elbows until you are leaning forward toward the wall or counter about 30 degrees. Pause in this position for a moment, then push with your arms until you're back in the starting position.

Progression: Work the same muscles with more intensity with a modified push-up. Lie facedown on the floor, with your palms directly next to your shoulders, elbows bent.

Keeping your knees on the floor, slowly push up only your chest. Keep your trunk in a straight line from your head to your knees. Push up until your shoulders are over your hands, but don't lock the elbows. Pause for a moment, then lower back down until your nose is about four inches from the floor. Keep your trunk in a straight line throughout the movements.

Step 3: **Mid-Back.**

Many exercises target the upper/lower back, but relatively few target the middle back—a common area for problems.

Starting position: Lie facedown on an exercise mat or carpet, with your arms straight out to the sides, perpendicular to the body.

The movement: Contract your shoulder blades to lift the arms up and slightly back. Hold the arms in the lifted position, and make four figure-eights with the hands. Then lower your arms to the starting position.

Progression: Make the figure-eights with the thumbs down or up...or while holding a balled-up sock in each hand...or with the little finger up or down. Varying the movement works different parts of the muscles.

Step 4: **Upper Back.**

This exercise increases shoulder strength as well as back strength.

Starting position: Tie a knot in the middle of an elastic exercise band (available at sporting-goods stores for $4 to $15). Place the knot over the top of a door, and then close the door to anchor the band in place. The two ends should be hanging down on the same side of the door. Sit in a chair facing the door, with your toes against the door. Hold one end of the band in each hand.

The movement: Slowly pull your hands down and in toward your chest. Keep your elbows pointed down and close to your body. Pause for a moment, then slowly let your arms extend back to the starting position.

Progression: When the exercise starts feeling easy, change to a higher-resistance band.

Step 5: **Lower Back.**

This is the area that gives most people problems.

Starting position: Lie facedown on an exercise mat or carpet. Reach your right hand in front of you, palm down. The left arm should be down alongside your body, with the palm up.

The movement: Slowly raise your right arm, chest and left leg about five inches off the floor. Keep your face down, so your spine is in a straight line. Keep your right leg and left hand on the ground. Pause for a moment, then return to the starting position.

Reverse the movement, raising your left arm, chest and right leg, and keeping the left leg and right hand on the floor.

Progression: Kneel on all fours. Raise your right arm straight in front of you while simultaneously raising the left leg straight behind. Keep the abdominal muscles contracted. Pause, return to the starting position. Then reverse the movement.

***Optional exercise:* Thighs, Hips and More.**

This optional exercise is a complex move that targets the upper legs as well as the trunk. It is good for improving stability and balance. The exercise requires the use of a stability ball, available at sporting-goods stores for about $20.

Starting position: Stand with your back to a wall, with the stability ball positioned between your back and the wall. Lean back against the ball, with your feet a bit more than hip-width apart. Hold your arms straight in front of you or crossed over your chest.

The movement: While keeping light pressure on the ball with your lower back, bend at the knees and slowly squat down—the ball will roll with the movement. Squat down as far as you comfortably can. The ball will then be positioned at about the midback.

Keeping pressure on the ball, contract the buttocks and slowly "roll" yourself up and back to the starting position.

The "Hidden Core" Workout You're Probably Missing

Patrick A. Roth, MD, FACS, chairman of the department of neurosurgery and director of the neurosurgical residency training program at Hackensack University Medical Center in Hackensack, New Jersey. He is also the founder of the North Jersey Brain & Spine Center in Oradell, New Jersey, and author of *The End of Back Pain.*

You're lucky if you haven't suffered a backache recently. It's common...make that very common.

In any three-month period, 25% of adults will suffer at least one day of back pain. Over the course of a lifetime, about 85% of us will experience back pain at some point.

My story: As a spinal surgeon and a former back pain sufferer, I've examined this malady from all angles. What I have discovered is that contrary to our culture of "pop a pill" or "go under the knife," the best course of action starts with discovering your "hidden" core.

FINDING YOUR HIDDEN CORE

If I told you that you needed to strengthen your core, you might assume that means doing crunches to work on your abdominal muscles, or abs. While washboard abs are the most visible and easily trained part of your core, they are only part of a larger muscle group that makes up the core.

In fact, strengthening your abs without also working on your hidden core can make back pain worse. That's because unbalanced core muscles cause an unstable spine.

The muscles you don't see: Your core is a group of muscles that encircles your midsection—front, sides and back. And most of the muscles lie deep inside your body—hidden from view. Taken together, these muscles form an internal brace around your spine, holding it erect, protecting it from damage. In order to reduce or limit back pain, you need to strengthen all your core muscles equally.

THE HIDDEN CORE WORKOUT

The workout I've developed targets all the inner muscles that make up your body's natural support system. Don't worry—even if you're not in great shape, you can start by doing the exercises at your own pace. However, do each of the exercises below so that you'll strengthen all the muscles equally to keep your spine in balance.

Here's the drill: Perform the exercises three times a week...and focus on maintaining proper form. Even if your back is aching, do the exercises if you can—they often give some immediate relief and help prevent future flare-ups.

Give it time: It may take three to four weeks before you notice significant pain reduction.

Important: These exercises can be safely done by most people, but check with your doctor first. See your doctor right away if you have back pain and severe leg pain (a sign of sciatica) or you have a history of cancer (back pain could be a sign that cancer has spread).

***Exercise 1:* Front plank.** This exercise focuses on the muscles at the front of the core—the rectus abdominis (the abs) and the transverse abdominis—and the obliques, which are on the sides of the core.

What to do: Start by lying on your stomach on a carpet or mat. Place your hands on the floor at about the level of your ears, with your elbows bent and close to your sides.

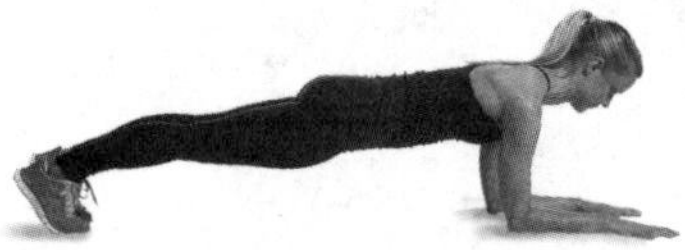

Slowly lift your body off the floor using just your forearms and rising up on your toes. Your elbows and hands should remain on the floor. Keep your back straight by contracting your front abdominal muscles. (If you cannot lift your body as described, try supporting your lower body from your knees rather than your toes.)

Breathe normally...and hold the position for 10 seconds. As you are able, increase the amount of time you hold the position. A minute is a good goal for most people.

***Exercise 2:* Side plank.** This strengthens the sides of your core—the internal and external obliques.

What to do: Start by lying on the floor on your right side, with your feet together. Prop yourself up on your right elbow, with your right hand and forearm flat on the ground and your forearm perpendicular to your body. Put your left hand on your left hip. Contract your abdominal muscles, and raise your hips off the floor until your back is straight.

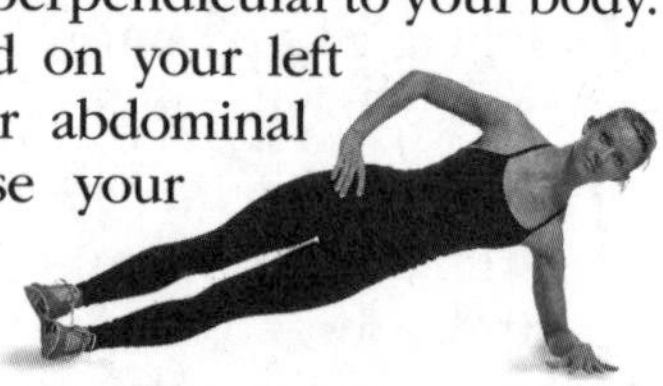

Breathe normally, and hold the raised position for 10 seconds. As you are able, increase the amount of time you hold the position to 60 seconds. Repeat on your left side.

***Exercise 3:* Bird-dog.** This exercise strengthens the back muscles that support your spine, including the multifidus muscles and the erector spinae muscles.

What to do: Start on your hands and knees, with your wrists below your shoulders (hands facing forward) and your knees below your hips. Stabilize your spine by tightening your abdominal muscles.

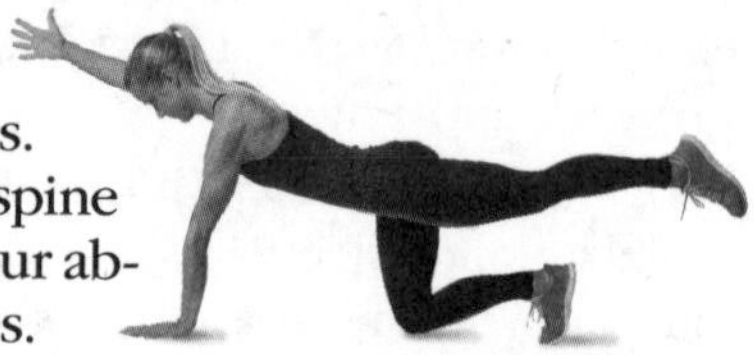

Simultaneously extend your right arm straight forward and your left leg straight back until both are parallel to the ground. Remember to keep your back and neck straight, without sagging or arching.

Hold this position for two seconds, then return to the starting position. Repeat, using the other arm and leg. Do the cycle five times. As you are able, increase the amount of time you hold the position each time for up to 10 seconds.

START RUNNING

If you have back pain, you've likely been advised to do only low-impact aerobic exercises and avoid running. I disagree. After years of examining runners, I noticed that their disks (and spines) tend to be healthier than those of nonrunners. Unexpected, right? But it makes sense.

All weight-bearing exercises stimulate bone cells so that the bones themselves become stronger. Similarly, disks also improve with high-impact exercise—the cells that make up the gel of a disk proliferate, retaining more water and becoming "fuller," which cushions the bones of the spine, reducing pain.

If you want to try running (and it doesn't cause you knee or hip pain), start slowly. Walk for one mile—and three times during that walk, run for 20 to 30 seconds. Thereafter, double the number of times you run until you're running more than walking. Try to work up to at least 30 minutes, three times a week.

Stretch Away Your Back Pain: A Surgeon's 7-Minute Strategy

Gerard Girasole, MD, orthopedic spine surgeon at The Orthopaedic & Sports Medicine Center in Trumbull, Connecticut. He is coauthor, with Cara Hartman, CPT, a Fairfield, Connecticut–based certified personal trainer, of *The 7-Minute Back Pain Solution: 7 Simple Exercises to Heal Your Back without Drugs or Surgery in Just Minutes a Day.*

For the overwhelming majority of back pain sufferers, the culprit is tight, inflamed muscles.

Surprising: This inflammation usually is not caused by strain on the back muscles themselves, but rather a strain or injury to the spine—in particular, to one of five "motion segments" in the lower back.

Each segment, which is constructed to bend forward and back and side to side, consists of a disk (the spongy cushion between each pair of spinal vertebrae)...the two vertebrae directly above and below it...and the facets (joints) connecting the vertebrae to the disk.

Unfortunately, the segments' disks or facets can be injured in a variety of ways—by lifting something the wrong way, twisting too far, sitting too long or even sneezing too hard—causing the surrounding muscles to contract in order to protect the spine from further damage.

This contraction and the muscle inflammation that it produces is what causes the intense lower back pain that so many Americans are familiar with.

WHEN BACK PAIN STRIKES

Low-back pain caused by inflammation usually subsides on its own within three to six weeks.* However, the healing process can be accelerated significantly by taking over-the-counter *ibuprofen* (Motrin) for several days after injury to reduce inflammation if you don't have an ulcer (follow label instructions)...and getting massage therapy to help loosen knotted muscles and increase healing blood flow to them.

Also important: Perform the simple stretching routine described in this article. In my more than 16 years of practice as an orthopedic spine surgeon, it is the closest thing I've found to act as a "silver bullet" for back pain.

How it works: All of the muscles stretched in this routine attach to the pelvis and work in concert to stabilize the spine. Stretching increases blood flow to these specific muscles, thereby reducing the inflammation that leads to painful, tightened back muscles.

GETTING STARTED

In preparation for the back stretch routine described here, it's important to learn a simple approach that systematically stimulates and strengthens your core (abdominal, back and pelvic muscles). This is one of the best ways to protect your spine. Although there are many types of exercises that strengthen the core, abdominal contractions are the easiest to perform.

What to do: Pretend that you have to urinate and then stop the flow—a movement known as a Kegel exercise. Then while lying on your back, place your hands on your pelvis just above your genitals. Now imagine that someone is about to punch you in the stomach, and feel how your lower abdomen tightens protectively.

To do a full abdominal contraction, combine these two movements, holding the Kegel movement while tightening your lower abdomen. Then, continuously hold the full abdominal contraction during all of the stretches described on this page.

7-MINUTE STRETCHING ROUTINE

Do the following routine daily until your back pain eases (start out slowly and gently if you're still in acute pain). Then continue doing it several times a week to prevent recurrences. Regularly stretching these muscles makes them stronger, leaving your lower spine less prone to painful, back-tightening strains.

1. Hamstring wall stretch. Lie faceup on a carpeted floor (or on a folded blanket for padding), positioning your body perpen-

*If you suffer from severe back pain or back pain accompanied by fever, incontinence or weakness or numbness in your leg, see a doctor right away to rule out a condition that may require surgery, such as serious damage to disks, ligaments or nerves in the back.

dicular inside a doorframe. Bend your right leg and place it through the door opening. Bring your buttocks as close to the wall as possible and place the heel of your left foot up against the wall until it is nearly straight. Next, slide your right leg forward on the floor until it's straight, feeling a stretch in the back of your left leg. Hold for 30 seconds. Repeat twice on each side.

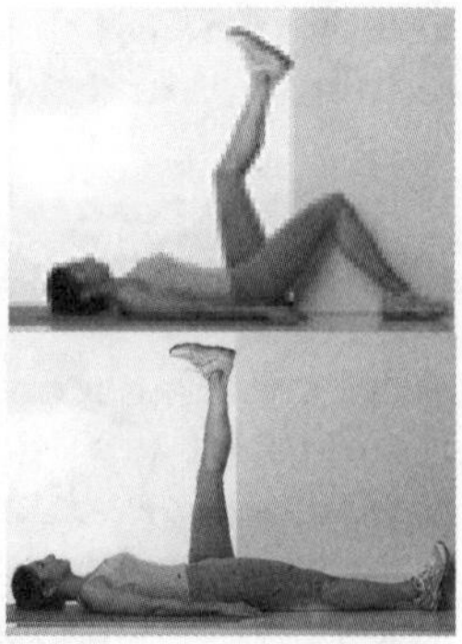

2. Knees to chest stretch. Lie on your back with your feet flat on the floor and your knees bent. Use your hands to pull your right knee to your chest. Next, try to straighten your left leg on the floor. While keeping your right knee held to your chest, continue the stretch for 20 seconds, then switch sides and repeat. Finally, do the stretch by holding both knees to your chest for 10 seconds.

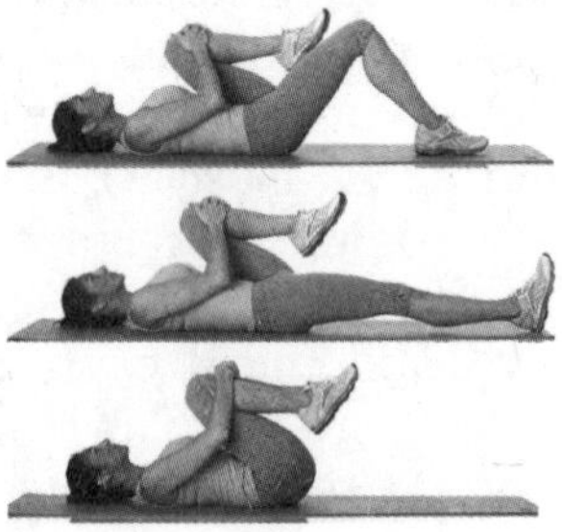

3. Spinal stretch. While on the floor with your left leg extended straight, pull your right knee to your chest (as in stretch #2), then put your right arm out to the side. Next, use your left hand to slowly pull your right knee toward your left side so that your right foot rests on the back of your left knee. Finally, turn your head toward your right side. Hold for 20 seconds, then reverse the movements and repeat.

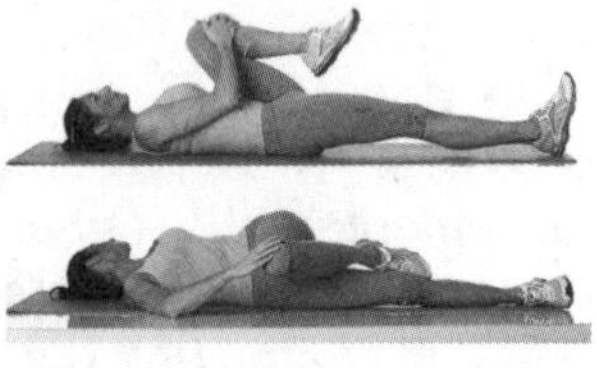

4. Gluteal (buttocks) stretch. Lie on your back with your feet flat on the floor and your knees bent. Cross your right leg over your left, resting your right ankle on your left knee. Next, grab your left thigh with both hands and bring both legs toward your body. Hold for 30 seconds, then switch sides and repeat.

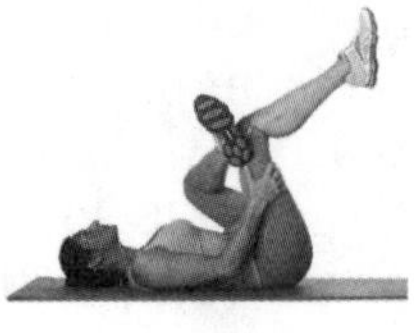

5. Hip flexor stretch. Kneel on your right knee (use a mat) with your left leg bent 90° in front of you and your foot flat on the floor. Place your right hand on your waist and your left hand on top of your left leg. Inhale and then, on the exhale, lean forward into your right hip, feeling a stretch in the front of your right hip. Hold for 30 seconds, then switch sides and repeat.

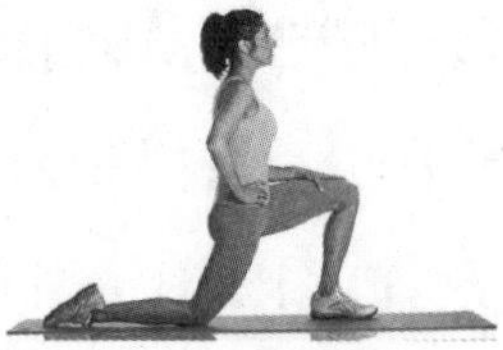

6. Quadriceps stretch. While standing, hold on to the back of a sturdy chair with your left hand for balance. Grasp your right foot with your right hand and gently pull your right leg back and up, with your toes pointing upward. Be sure to keep your right knee close to your left leg. Hold for 30 seconds, then switch sides and repeat.

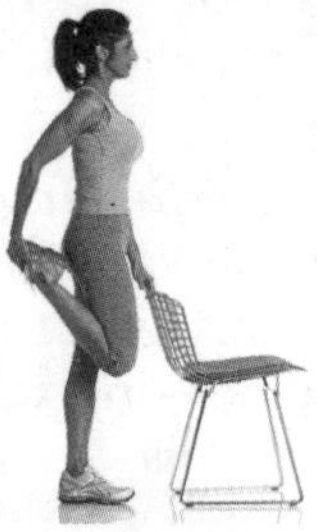

7. Total back stretch. Stand arm's length in front of a table and lean forward with knees slightly bent so that you can grasp the table edge. Keep your arms straight and your head level with your shoulders. Hold for 10 seconds.

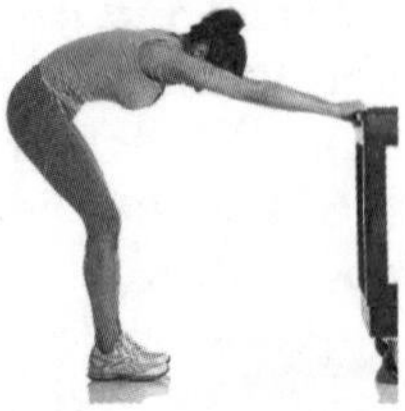

Next, stand up straight with your left hand in front of you. Bring your right arm over your head with elbow bent, then bend your upper body gently to the left. Hold for 10 seconds, then switch sides and repeat.

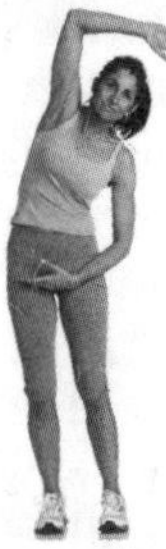

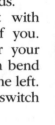

Ease Low-Back Pain By Realigning Your Body

Mark A. Stengler, NMD, naturopathic doctor and founder of the Stengler Center for Integrative Medicine in Encinitas, California. MarkStengler.com

When patients have chronic low-back pain, one effective therapy is the Egoscue Method, a nonmedical technique that incorporates stretches and exercises that realign the body and restore proper muscle and joint function. The technique is based on the concept that musculoskeletal discomfort occurs when biomechanical imbalances place abnormal stress on the muscles and ligaments. To give you an idea of how this method can help reduce low-back pain, we spoke to Brian Bradley, vice president of education and therapy protocol at Egoscue, Inc., in San Diego (800-995-8434, Egoscue.com).

ALIGN YOUR SHOULDERS, HIPS AND PELVIS

You may feel pain in your lower back, but that may not be the area of the body that needs attention. Shoulder misalignment, uneven hips or a tilted pelvis often is the cause of low-back pain. When you correct imbalances in the shoulders, hips or pelvis, back pain eases.

When Egoscue practitioners work one on one with patients, they look very carefully at the individual's anatomy to determine why the imbalances—and the resulting pain—occur. The three exercises below are most often recommended to help ease low-back pain. You may be surprised to find that you experience some pain relief the very first time you do these exercises. Most people experience less pain in a few weeks (the amount of time varies by individual). You can incorporate all three of these exercises into your regular fitness regimen—and you can do them indefinitely to keep your body aligned.

THE UPPER BACK AND SHOULDERS

Standing Arm Circles. This exercise engages the shoulder muscles, which, in turn, helps to stabilize and strengthen the muscles of the mid-spine, resulting in less low-back pain.

Stand up straight, feet hip-width apart. Raise your arms so they are extended out to your sides at shoulder level. Palms up, place the fingers into the pad of each hand, thumbs pointed behind you. Squeeze the shoulder blades together. Keeping the shoulder blades squeezed and your arms raised at your sides, rotate both of your arms backward in a circle of about a six-inch circumference.

Goal: One set of 40 circles. Then, palms down, thumbs pointed forward, rotate both arms forward in a six-inch circle.

Goal: One set of 40 circles.

THE MID-SPINE

Static Back Knee Pillow Squeeze. This exercise promotes pelvic stability by supporting the shoulders and spine as you engage the pelvic muscles and extend the mid-spine.

Lie on your back with your legs up over the seat of a chair. Place a pillow between your knees, and hold it with your inner thighs. Extend your arms out to the sides at a 45° angle, palms up. Gently squeeze the pillow with your knees and hold for a count of one second, keeping the upper body and abdomen relaxed. Release the squeeze (although your legs continue to hold the pillow in place). With this movement, the inner thigh and primary hip flexor do the work that they are supposed to do, allowing the back muscles to let go of tension.

Goal: Three sets of 20 squeezes.

THE PELVIS

Airbench. This exercise promotes proper function of the hips and stabilizes the pelvis. Be sure to wear nonskid shoes when performing this exercise.

Stand with your back against a wall with your feet and knees hip-width apart. Walk your feet away from the wall about one-and-a-half feet while sliding your body down to a "seated position"—work toward achieving a 110° angle at the knee, with the hips slightly higher than the knees and the ankles slightly ahead of the knees. Press the lower back flat against the wall. Allow the arms to hang down at your sides or rest your hands gently on your lap. It's important to keep your weight in your heels. This enables you to engage the quadriceps and hip muscles—and relieves stress in the back.

Goal: Hold the "seated" position for one to two minutes.

100-Year-Old Solution to Back Pain: Alexander Technique Body Movement

Hope Gillerman, certified teacher of the Alexander technique, and founder and creator, H. Gillerman Organics, New York. HGillermanOrganics.com

If you suffer from chronic back pain, you may want to consider a century-old, noninvasive, drug-free treatment method called the Alexander technique, which reeducates people on how to support and move their bodies. Recently an English study involving 579 patients with back pain put the Alexander technique to the test and demonstrated that it was effective and provided sustainable relief.

THE STUDY

Researchers established four groups of patients—one took six Alexander technique lessons...another took 24 lessons...a third group had massage therapy only...and the fourth group had what the study team called "normal care." (Normal care was defined as care that would be offered by a general practitioner, and could include pain medications, non-mandatory referral to physiotherapy, etc.) All four groups were further divided in half, with one half walking briskly for 30 minutes a day and the others not exercising at all. Participants answered questionnaires about pain and function improvement at three months and one year.

Results: The two Alexander technique groups reported significantly reduced back pain and improved functioning, including after 12 months, while there was little change in the massage and normal care groups. Among those who took just six lessons but who also did brisk walking, improvement was almost as great as those who took 24 lessons but did not exercise.

Methods like acupuncture can offer immediate pain relief, but people with back pain also need a long-term, self-healing regimen—and that is what the Alexander technique is. Most back pain comes from incorrect posture, poor body mechanics and excessive muscle tension, which increases when people are fatigued, angry, upset or in one position for a long time. Under duress, tension automatically builds in the back of the neck and the shoulders, pulling the heavy head downward into the spine, which causes compression. The fact that the pain becomes chronic further exacerbates all of these problems...since pain is upsetting and stops people from doing things and moving as they normally would, people develop more harmful habits. The Alexander technique can be effective because it addresses and helps to correct not only the cause of the injury, but also those harmful habits brought on by the pain.

If You Sit a Lot

If you sit a lot, stand up every hour, put your hands on your hips, bend backward as far as feels comfortable and hold for three seconds. Repeat five times. This helps extend the spine and relieve stiffness.

Anthony Delitto, PhD, professor of physical therapy and dean of the School of Health and Rehabilitation Sciences at University of Pittsburgh.

HOW IT WORKS

At the heart of the Alexander technique is learning to keep the spine erect and properly supported. Most people are unstable and "collapsed" through their torso, and hold and move their limbs in a rigid and stiff pattern. Without proper muscular support, the spine compresses, harming joints and tissues.

Here are three ways Hope Gillerman, a certified teacher of the Alexander technique, helps her students envision what to do...

- **Envision your body as a tree**—with the trunk (the torso) rooted and stable, freeing the limbs to move easily. Students learn how different it feels to move with the torso thus stabilized and supported, with posture that lengthens the spine and opens the spaces between the vertebrae, enabling discs to function as shock absorbers.

- **For further illustration of what proper posture and body mechanics looks like, study elite runners**—their torsos don't move but their legs and arms move constantly, in a powerful yet flowing fashion.

• **To better understand the degree of tension you need for proper back support, tightly grip a spoon.** Then release your grip slowly until you can comfortably hold the spoon...but not loose enough to let it slip from your grasp. This helps you understand how much tension to hold in your back.

HELPFUL TIPS

Regular exercise fits well with lessons in the Alexander technique, but the kind most people do at the gym, working on one muscle at a time, may not be effective. Abdominal strength is key, but workouts should include the muscles in the back and legs, not just pelvic muscles. Crunches, for example, train the abdominal muscles to flex the torso—this is useful when you get out of bed in the morning, but does not train the abdominal muscle to keep the spine lengthened. Instead, people should exercise to train their muscles to lift and stabilize the spine, not crunch. Vigorous walking, with arms swinging, abdominals pulled in, is great for this and is an excellent way to practice the new body mechanics students learn through the Alexander technique.

Gillerman says that many students find Alexander technique lessons so pleasurable and relaxing, they take them for months or even years—but the real purpose of the technique is as a tool for change. People often feel better after just one lesson, but it is important to take a full introductory course of about 10 lessons over two to three months. Those who need yet more pain relief should take an additional six months of lessons. The technique works by changing neuromuscular patterns—the bad habits you have formed—and that takes time. "In the beginning students don't feel like themselves because we take away their familiar habits," says Gillerman. "When students get to the place that the old habits are the ones that feel wrong, they are ready to self-regulate."

Gillerman suggests doing at-home exercises to help make the subtle adjustments that correct posture and change habits and reinforce new self-care techniques. *Here is one to try that may soothe your back pain...*

• **Lie down on your back on a mat or carpet,** with your head resting on a telephone book.

• **Bend your knees,** bringing your feet close to your hips.

• **Place your hands on your rib cage,** elbows pointing out to the sides of your body.

• **Notice your breathing.** Practice making your exhalation longer than your inhalation.

• **Visualize images that help you release muscle tension**—for instance, your back melting into the floor...or the crown of your head sliding away from the shoulders. These are excellent ways to help correct the common problem of letting your skull sink into your neck.

• **Do 10 to 15 minutes every day, or more often if you need to relax.**

You can find a qualified Alexander technique trainer by going to the American Society for the Alexander Technique (AlexanderTech.org). Costs vary greatly according to where you live and lessons are generally from 30 minutes to one hour. Though insurance does not cover these, Gillerman says that employee flexible spending accounts can be used to pay for them.

Banish Back Pain with 7 Easy Yoga Poses

Kimberly Williams, PhD, research assistant professor, department of community medicine, West Virginia University School of Medicine, Morgantown, and leader of a study on yoga and low-back pain.

Low-back pain makes almost everything more difficult.

Good news: Recent research shows that simple Iyengar-style yoga poses reduce pain and increase the ease of daily activities—without drugs.

Props: A mat, folding chair, blanket, towel, bolster (or two blankets rolled together) and strap. Breathe slowly and deeply...never push to the point of discomfort. Practice the poses below (which have been modified for people with back pain) in the order given three to seven days per week.*

• **Savasana (corpse pose).** Place chair at end of mat, a folded blanket on seat. Lie on your back, head on folded towel. Rest calves on chair seat, knees comfortably bent and tailbone tucked under so back is not arched. Place bolster across abdomen. Let arms rest at sides, palms up. Relax completely. Hold for five minutes.

• **Supta Tadasana (reclining mountain pose).** Place short edge of mat against wall. Lie on your back, head on folded towel, feet hip-width apart, toes pointing up, soles pressed against wall. Hold edges of mat, elbows straight, outer arms pressed down. Hold for one minute.

• **Supta Padangusthasana I (supine big toe pose, bent knee).** Start in supta tadasana pose (above). Keeping left leg pressed to floor and left sole against wall, bend right knee toward chest and clasp shin with both hands. Hold for 20 seconds, then switch legs. Do three times per side.

Straight-leg variation: Instead of clasping shin, place center of a strap across right sole and hold ends of strap. Straighten leg and flex foot, so sole faces ceiling.

• **Supta Pavanmuktasana (wind-releasing pose).** Lie on your back, head on a folded towel. Bending both knees, bring knees toward chest. Grasp shins with hands, keeping knees hip-width apart. Hold for 30 seconds.

• **Adho Mukha Svanasana (downward-facing dog).** Place short edge of mat against wall. Come to hands and knees, hands shoulder-width apart, tips of thumb and first two fingers touching wall. Curl toes under and lift knees off floor, straightening legs and raising buttocks toward ceiling. Pushing down and forward with hands, stretch shoulders back and away from wall while stretching heels toward floor. Hold for 30 seconds.

• **Bharadvajasana (seated twist on chair).** Place folded blanket on chair seat, then sit backward with hips close to front edge of seat. Spread knees and place feet on outside edges of back chair legs. Place right forearm on top of chair back and grasp front edge of seat with left hand. Keeping chest lifted, turn chest to the left, twisting gently. Hold for 20 seconds, then switch sides. Do three times per side.

• **Adho Mukha Virasana (downward-facing hero).** Place a bolster on mat. Kneel at one end of bolster, knees apart and toes together. Sit back on heels (tuck folded blanket under buttocks, if necessary). Place rolled towel in hip crease. Bending forward at hips, place hands on either side of bolster for support while lowering torso and forehead onto bolster. Rest forearms on floor. Relax completely. Hold for five minutes.

*Check with a health-care professional before beginning any new exercise routine.

Simple Exercise to Strengthen Your Back

Stand, sit or lie on your back, and exhale all your breath while pulling your navel in and up toward your head. Hold for 10 seconds, and release. Repeat 12 times.

Todd Sinett, DC, chiropractor and founder/owner of Midtown Integrative Health & Wellness in New York City. He is author of *3 Weeks to a Better Back*.

When Lower Back Pain Is Really in Your Butt

Mitchell Yass, DPT, a Florida–based physical therapist and creator of the Yass Method for treating chronic pain. He is the author of *Overpower Pain: The Strength Training Program That Stops Pain Without Drugs or Surgery* and *The Pain Cure Rx: The Yass Method for Diagnosing and Resolving Chronic Pain* and host of the PBS special *The Pain Prescription*. MitchellYass.com

The lower back is the most common area where people suffer from pain. The simple reason is that the back is a transition point between the upper and lower body. When performing activities with the upper or lower extremities, the lower back must work to create a solid plateau for the muscles of the extremities to work from. The funny thing about this area of the body is that most people don't know where the lower back ends and the gluteal (buttocks) region begins. This might seem like a simple case of semantics. But when talking about pain and how to resolve it, this is a critical issue and one that must be understood to treat the root cause of your pain.

I have treated thousands of patients who actually had pain in the gluteal region but were diagnosed with a herniated disc, stenosis or pinched nerve in the lumbar spine or lower back region. There is simply no way that a structural variation at the lumbar spine can lead to pain at the gluteal region. That is why these people never were able to get a remedy for their pain until they saw me. And that is when they understood the difference between the lower back and the gluteal (buttocks) region.

The way to differentiate the lower back from the gluteal region is to identify the pelvic rim (iliac crest). This is the bony surface that most people perceive to be their hips. It is the spot everybody reaches for when prompted to "put your hands on your hips" while playing the game Simon Says. And it is actually the top of the pelvis.

If you notice in the illustration, this level is generally in line with the bottom of the lumbar spine. So if you put your hand on the pelvic rim and the pain you are experiencing is above that line, your pain is in the lumbar region. If the pain you are experiencing is below this line you are experiencing pain in the gluteal region. The cause of the pain in this region is completely different.

Pain in the gluteal region is associated with hip dysfunction and has nothing to do with the spine. The muscles that exist in the gluteal region all attach to the hip joint and perform some type of hip motion. The most common muscle to strain in the gluteal region is the piriformis muscle. This muscle sits just below the gluteus medius muscle, which is responsible for creating balance and stability. If this muscle is to strain, the

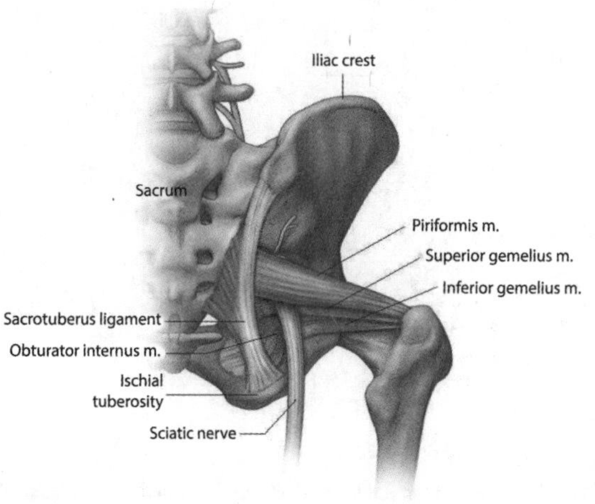

piriformis will try to compensate but ultimately will strain and cause pain in the gluteal region.

Resolution of pain in the gluteal region comes from strengthening the gluteus medius muscle, the hamstrings and gluteus maximus muscles. Perform these three exercises—hip abduction, hamstring curls and hip extension—on the side that is causing you pain. Do them three times a week, performing three sets of 10 repetitions each with a one-minute break between sets. Your goal is to continually increase the resistance until the muscles involved are strong enough to perform your functional activities without straining and creating symptoms. Once muscles are adequately strengthened and you can do the exercises pain-free, you can perform them on both sides to maintain equal strength.

Exercise 1: **Hip Abduction** (*gluteus medius*). This exercise can be performed either lying on your side or standing. To do this exercise correctly, make sure you do not go too far when moving your leg outward. People falsely belief that more range of motion is better, but in this case too much range of motion means you are using the lower back muscle to create the motion, not the gluteus medius (hip muscle). The gluteus medius muscle can only move the leg out to the point where it is parallel with the hip joint. Any outward motion beyond that is created by the lower back muscle.

To do the exercise lying down, lie on your side with the knee of the bottom leg bent and

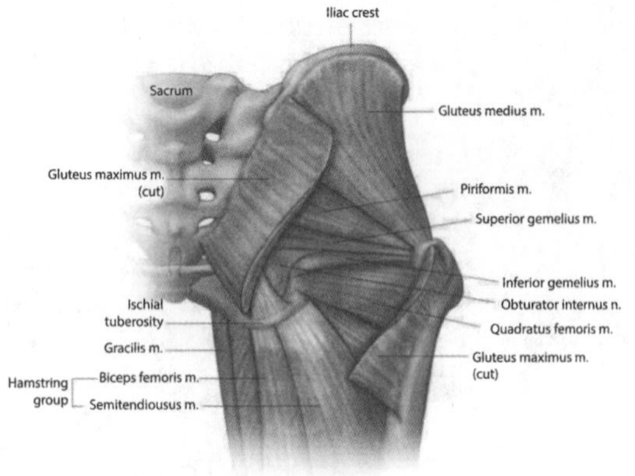

the top leg straight. The top leg should run in a continuous line from the torso—if the leg is angled in front of the torso, you would use the wrong muscle. Start to raise the top leg off the supporting leg until your top leg is parallel with the floor. As you lift, try to turn the leg in slightly so the heel is the first part of the foot that is moving. This puts the gluteus medius in the optimal position to raise the leg. Once your leg reaches parallel to the floor, begin to lower it back onto the supporting leg.

If you prefer to stand, the outward movement is similar to lying down—lead with the

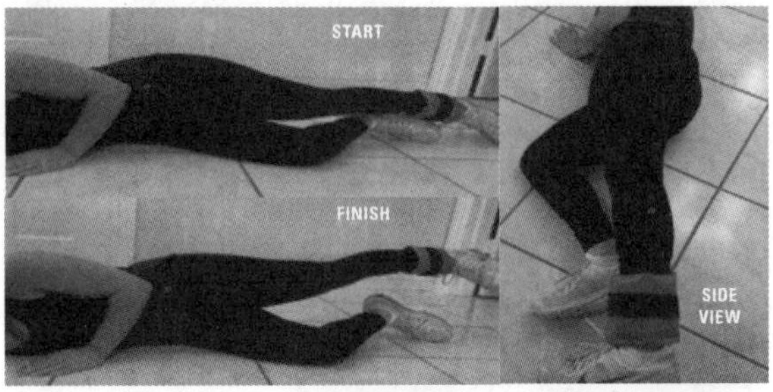

heel, and don't move your leg too far to keep the exercise focused on the gluteus medius. Holding on to a sturdy table or

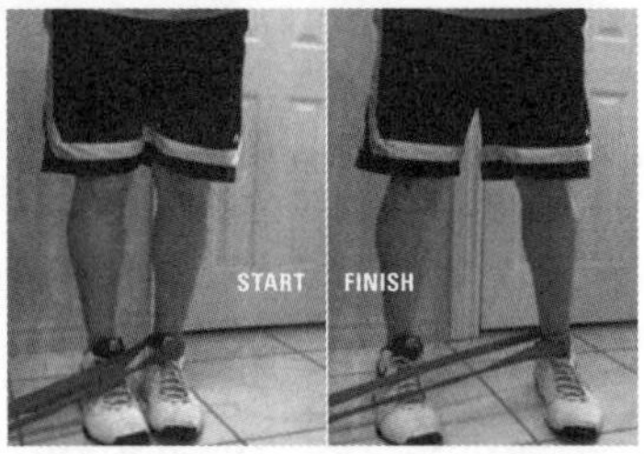

chair while you perform the exercise will make it easier to use proper form.

***Exercise 2:* Hamstring Curl** (*hamstrings*). In a seated position place the resistance at the back of the ankle. Make sure you are supported in the seat. Begin with the exercising leg

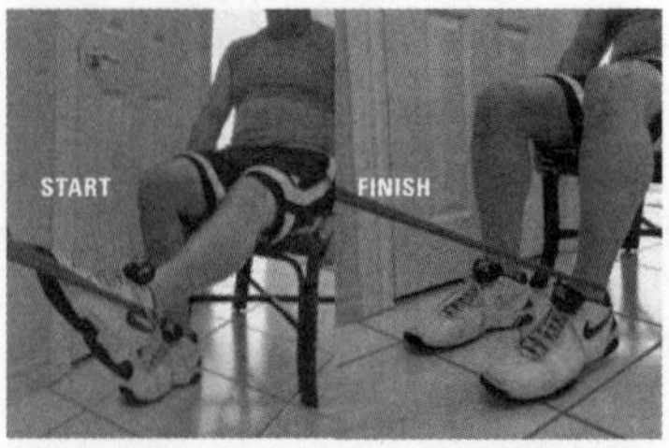

pointing straight out with the knee unlocked. Begin to bend the knee until it reaches 90 degrees. Then return to the start position. To isolate the hamstrings better, have the toes of the exercising leg pointing toward the face as the exercise is being performed. In the case of using a seated Hamstring Curl machine, make sure the pivot point of the machine is aligned with the knee joint.

***Exercise 3:* Hip Extension** (*gluteus maximus*). In a standing position, place the resistance behind your knee and hold on to the table or sturdy chair in front of you. Start with

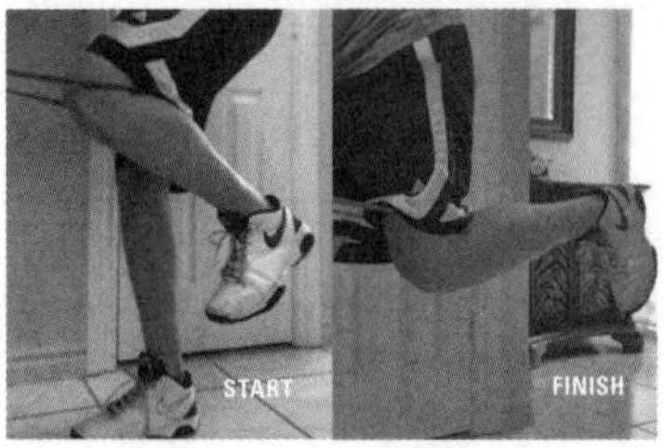

the hip flexed to about 60 degrees. Bring the knee about 10 degrees behind the hip. Then return to the start position. Make sure your back is rounded and the knee of the leg you are standing on is unlocked.

Exercise photos and medical illustrations: From *The Pain Cure Rx* by Dr. Mitchell Yass, by permission of the author.

Touch Here for Persistent Back Pain

Daniel C. Cherkin, PhD, senior investigator at Group Health Research Institute in Seattle and lead author of a study on lower back pain and massage published in *Annals of Internal Medicine.*

"Oh, my aching back!" If you have ever uttered this common lament then you will want to know about the surprising results of a recent study. Participants included 401 patients, mostly middle-aged women, who had been suffering for at least three months from chronic low-back pain with no identified cause.

Patients were randomly assigned to receive either "usual care" (the standard treatment doctors typically recommend, including painkillers, anti-inflammatories and/or muscle relaxants) or hour-long massages once per week for 10 weeks. Massage recipients got either the commonly available relaxation massage (also called Swedish massage)...or structural massage, which uses specialized techniques to alleviate musculoskeletal problems that can contribute to back pain.

Results: After 10 weeks, 36% to 39% of patients in the massage groups reported that their back pain was "much better or gone," versus only 4% of patients in the usual-care group. Also, massaged patients reported spending fewer days in bed, being more active and using less medication than usual-care patients.

Surprising: Contrary to expectations, researchers found that relaxation massage was just as effective as the more specialized structural massage at relieving pain and improving patients' ability to function normally. While the benefits of massage began to decrease after treatment ended, improvement was still evident six months later.

Bottom line: Massage is a generally safe therapy that can be used alone or as a supplement to other treatments for chronic low-back pain. Though relaxation massage typically is not covered by health insurance, some policies do cover structural massage, which is considered similar to physical therapy.

Ahhhhhh...Stretch for a Stiff Back

Arthur H. White, MD, retired orthopedic spine surgeon based in Walnut Creek, California, and author of *The Posture Prescription: The Doctor's Rx for Eliminating Back, Muscle, and Joint Pain.*

By the end of the day, after hours of hunching over a computer, what your back needs is a good stretch...

The draping stretch feels great—and promotes good posture—because it pulls the shoulders back and stretches the chest muscles. It requires a large inflated exercise ball, available at sporting-goods stores for about $20. (As with any new exercise, get your doctor's OK before beginning.)

Your goal is to lie backward over the ball so that your back is somewhat arched yet fully supported. To get into position, sit on the floor with your knees bent and the ball nestled against your rear end and lower back. Carefully raise your hips and step your feet away little by little until your mid-back, upper back and the back of your head are resting on the ball. Your feet should be flat on the floor, shoulder-width apart...knees bent at about 90 degrees...neck relaxed and tilted back (not too far)...and arms hanging out to the sides. Allow your body to relax as you drape over the ball. Hold for a minute or two...repeat daily.

Fix Your Back By Watching What You Eat

Todd Sinett, DC, chiropractor and founder/owner of Midtown Integrative Health & Wellness in New York City. He is author of *3 Weeks to a Better Back: Solutions for Healing the Structural, Nutritional and Emotional Causes of Back Pain.*

If you have persistent back pain, most doctors look for structural problems—a herniated disc, for example, or a misaligned spine. These can be real issues, but they point to a solution for only a small percentage of patients.

Surprisingly, back pain can be the result of poor nutrition and poor digestion, which causes chronic inflammation that irritates muscles, ligaments, tendons and/or nerves. A recent study in *Asian Spine Journal* found that nearly one-third of women and one-quarter of men with back pain also had food intolerances or other gastrointestinal complaints.

Dietary changes won't always eliminate back pain (although they might), but they often reduce pain significantly. *What to do...*

• **Get enough fiber.** If you're often constipated or have infrequent bowel movements, you'll have buildups of toxins that increase inflammation and back pain. A high-fiber diet can fix this and reduce your back pain.

My advice: Look at your stool. It should be more or less smooth (and should pass easily). If it is lumpy and hard, you probably need more fiber. Increase your water, fruit and vegetable intake.

• **Cut back on caffeine.** Caffeine is a stimulant that increases levels of cortisol, a hormone that triggers inflammation. People who drink a lot of coffee or other caffeinated beverages are more likely to have painful muscle cramps and spasms.

My advice: Eliminate caffeine for two to three weeks. If this makes a big improvement, give it up altogether. If it doesn't help, you can go back to it because caffeine isn't the culprit.

• **Stay well-hydrated.** Many of my patients don't drink water very often. This is a problem because you need water to improve digestion and reduce inflammation—and because people who don't drink much water often consume less-healthful beverages, such as sodas. Water also helps lubricate the spinal discs and can help prevent fissures, cracks in the discs that can allow the soft middle portion to bulge out and press against a nerve.

Everyone with back pain should drink between four and 10 glasses of water a day. Or about one-half ounce of water per pound of body weight. If you're not a fan of plain water, you can spruce it up with a squeeze of lemon or lime or substitute watered-down juice (half juice, half water).

• **Eliminate all added sugar.** The rapid rise in glucose (blood sugar) that occurs when you eat sweetened foods triggers the production of cytokines, proteins secreted by immune cells that increase inflammation. A high-sugar diet also irritates the digestive tract, which can lead to back pain.

My advice: Give up all added sugar for at least three weeks. This includes hidden sugar in processed foods. It takes about two weeks for existing inflammation to "calm." Staying off added sugar for an additional week will help reinforce the change in your usual habits. After that, you can reintroduce a small amount of sugar—by having an occasional dessert, for example, or adding a small amount of sugar to your morning coffee.

If you add back a bit of sugar and your pain doesn't increase, you'll know that you can enjoy some sugar. On the other hand, you might notice that you're having more back pain again, in which case you'll want to cut out sugar.

• **Look for sensitivities.** The healthiest diet in the world won't improve back pain if you're eating foods that trigger a reaction in you. Many foods (including foods considered healthy, such as broccoli) can trigger symptoms in some people. In addition to pain, these symptoms could include digestive irritation, sleepiness after a meal, fogginess, achiness and/or congestion.

To find out whether you're sensitive to one or more foods, use a journal to track what you eat. When you notice an increase in pain, you can review the journal and find the food(s) that might be responsible. In addition to the foods mentioned in this article, dairy and gluten are common offenders.

My advice: When you identify a likely food suspect—maybe you drank a beer on the day your back got worse—give it up for a few weeks. If your symptoms improve, test your conclusion by having a small amount of that food or beverage. If the pain increases again, you'll know that you have to avoid that food in the future. Or you can go to a gastroenterologist, allergist, nutritionist or integrative medical doctor for food-sensitivity testing.

CHAPTER 5

Cancer Pain and Discomfort

Cancer Prehab: The First Thing You Need After a Diagnosis

If you are facing a cancer diagnosis now—or if you ever face one in the future—cancer prehab could be your key to an easier, more complete recovery. From the minute you're diagnosed with cancer, you're considered a survivor of the disease. Survivors need to do whatever they can to improve their health from the very start. Prehab helps you use the time between diagnosis and treatment most effectively by preparing you physically and emotionally.

Cancer prehab services are provided by a range of specialists including physicians, psychologists, social workers, physical therapists, occupational therapists, speech therapists, nutritionists, exercise physiologists and others. The particular types of specialists assigned to your case will depend on your individual needs.

There are certain services that just about all patients can benefit from, regardless of the kind of cancer they have. *These include...*

- **Instruction in coping skills.** Taking classes in deep breathing, progressive muscle relaxation and/or meditation can provide skills that will be invaluable for pain management and for coping with the inevitable fear and anxiety that a cancer diagnosis brings.
- **Evaluation of caregiving needs.** Prehab personnel will advise you on the type of assistance you may need during your treatment and recovery and help you coordinate the practical aspects of your care.

You'll resolve questions such as: Will you be going home or to a rehab center after sur-

Julie Silver, MD, associate professor, department of physical medicine and rehabilitation, Harvard Medical School, Boston. She also is founder of Oncology Rehab Partners, creator of the STAR Program Certification and author of *After Cancer Treatment: Heal Faster, Better, Stronger.* JulieSilverMD.com

gery? Should any temporary changes be made in your home (such as setting up a ground-floor bedroom) to make it easier for you to navigate during your recovery? Who can help with meals, driving and other daily tasks during the weeks while you are healing? Addressing these issues now will save you a lot of stress and uncertainty later.

• **Targeted physical exercises.** These can be hugely beneficial not only for overall health and strength but for helping you survive cancer. Exercise may reduce the risk for recurrence in some types of cancer, so a prehab program that gets a patient to be more active may increase the length of his/her life. In some cases, improvements in physical well-being can expand patients' treatment options, too. For instance, one study showed that prehab improved the respiratory status of lung cancer patients, even making some patients strong enough for surgery that had previously been ruled out.

• **Help with smoking cessation, if needed.** Without a doubt, nonsmokers heal better than those who continue to smoke. Quitting even shortly before cancer treatment begins can make a significant difference in your recovery.

Your specific diagnosis and state of health determine what additional services you might need. That makes sense—a colorectal cancer patient has different concerns than, say, a breast cancer patient. *Examples include...*

• **Skin-protection counseling for patients** whose treatment will include radiation and/or chemotherapy (since both of these treatments can affect the skin).

• **Range-of-motion evaluation and exercises.** For instance, postsurgical breast cancer patients often have shoulder pain and limited shoulder movement—so in prehab, patients can work on increasing range of motion prior to surgery so that the aftereffects will be less severe.

• **Pelvic-floor strengthening. After surgery and/or radiation for prostate cancer or gynecological cancer,** many patients have trouble with urinary incontinence. Doing exercises to strengthen the muscles of the pelvic floor prior to treatment helps reduce the likelihood and severity of post-treatment incontinence.

• **Balance and gait evaluation and training.** Working with a physical therapist to improve strength, balance and gait skills before cancer treatment helps patients recover mobility more quickly afterward, especially for older people who may already have some subtle balance problems. Yet young cancer patients can benefit, too, because chemotherapy may cause nervous system problems that affect balance and walking.

HOW TO GET PREHAB

After recovering from cancer myself, I developed the STAR Program (Survivorship Training and Rehabilitation) Certification for hospitals and cancer centers, which involves a protocol for best practices in cancer rehab as well as cancer prehab. More than 100 hospitals and cancer centers nationwide have signed up for STAR Program certification so far, and it is offered at several hundred sites. For information and/or a referral to a STAR Program in your area, visit the website of Oncology Rehab Partners (OncRehab.com) an organization I founded that is dedicated to advancing survivorship care.

Alternative: Ask your oncologist about prehab and see if he has any suggestions. Fortunately, health insurance and Medicare often cover prehab services.

Is Early Breast Cancer Painful?

Benjamin O. Anderson, MD, professor and director, University of Washington Breast Health Clinic, and chair and director, Breast Health Global Initiative, both in Seattle.

Ironically, it would be good if pain were the first sign of breast cancer, because that would help us catch it earlier. However, malignant breast lumps usually are painless in the early stages. Rarely, a woman reports a tugging or pulling sensation in a breast and then a biopsy reveals cancer—but we seldom do biopsies based on breast pain. Usually the pain has some benign cause, such as cyclical hormonal changes, pulled ligaments or tenderness related to fibrocystic lumpiness. Discomfort that occurs in both breasts or at the same time every month is highly unlikely to signal cancer.

Cystic pain prevention: Try taking evening primrose oil capsules at 1,500 mg twice daily.

Also: Consider giving up caffeine. (For more on breast pain, see chapter 20, "Very Personal Pain.")

Stop Painful Breast Cancer Treatment Side Effects

Lyndsey Kilgore, MD, researcher and resident, department of surgery, University of Kansas Cancer Center, Kansas City, and leader of a study presented at the annual meeting of the American Society of Breast Surgeons.

Painful breast cancer treatment side effects can be reduced. The new technology Bioimpedance spectroscopy (BIS) is a noninvasive test that detects lymphedema—arm swelling that often results from standard treatment such as lymph node surgery or radiation. Early detection with BIS enables the use of home therapy, including compression sleeves and massage. In a study of 146 women, BIS identified 49 women with lymphedema—and home therapy greatly reduced symptoms in 40 of them.

Preventing Arm Swelling After Breast Cancer Surgery

Gwen White, PT, physical therapist and lymphedema specialist with Kaiser Permanente in Portland, Oregon, and coauthor of *Lymphedema: A Breast Cancer Patient's Guide to Prevention and Healing.*

If you have breast cancer you may already be familiar with the condition lymphedema. This condition—which involves mild to extreme swelling, usually in the arm—can cause significant pain, loss of arm function, disfigurement and emotional distress. Symptoms can develop soon after surgery or may appear months or even years later. According to the National Cancer Institute, as many as 56% of breast cancer patients experience it within two years after surgery.

Good news: A recent Spanish study suggests that physical therapy (PT) provided soon after breast cancer surgery can significantly reduce the risk of developing lymphedema. One group of breast cancer patients who did not have lymphedema received typical instruction on prevention strategies...a second group got instruction plus three sessions of PT per week for three weeks. After one year, 25% of the instruction-only group had developed lymphedema—compared with only 7% of the PT group.

LYMPHEDEMA LESSON

The lymphatic system, which is part of the immune and circulatory systems, helps clean the body's tissues and maintain its balance of fluids. It includes vessels that carry lymph fluid through the body, plus nodes that filter out waste. If part of the lymphatic system is damaged, lymph fluid can accumulate in nearby tissues, triggering severe swelling, increasing infection risk and eventually causing skin to thicken and harden. Breast cancer patients are at risk because one or more lymph nodes typically are removed during a mastectomy or lumpectomy and because radiation therapy can produce scar tissue—and both these factors can interrupt lymph flow.

WHAT HAPPENS IN PT

Specially trained physical therapists in the US use the same techniques to prevent and treat lymphedema as the Spanish researchers used. Many insurance policies cover PT—check with your carrier. *Generally therapy includes...*

- **Manual lymph drainage.** This gentle massage technique moves lymph fluid away from areas that are swollen or at risk for swelling and into areas where it can drain normally. During the 45- to 60-minute massage, the therapist presses no harder than she would on a newborn baby's head.

Caution: Deep-tissue massage must be avoided, as it can bring on lymphedema even years after surgery.

• **Scar tissue massage.** Surgery and radiation can leave inflexible scars that inhibit lymph flow. Massage techniques using heavier pressure stretch and soften scar tissue.

• **Lymph drainage exercises.** Specific exercises, done in sequence, help pump lymph fluid through the lymphatic pathways. A typical routine includes pelvic tilts, partial sit-ups, neck rotations, shoulder shrugs, elbow bends and wrist circles.

• **Self-care instruction.** PT patients learn lymphedema-minimizing strategies for home use, including self-massage...exercises...abdominal breathing (which acts as a pump to stimulate lymph flow)...hydration, diet and weight control...infection avoidance...stress reduction...use of a compression garment (a special sleeve that limits lymph accumulation)...and application of elastic Kinesio tape, which lifts the skin to promote lymph flow.

• **Prevention policy problem.** Given the Spanish study's findings about PT's effectiveness in preventing lymphedema, you would think that all breast cancer patients would get PT—but that's not happening. Ideally, patients would be referred for PT before or shortly after surgery...but doctors tend to send patients to PT only if signs of lymphedema occur.

Self-defense: Don't wait for lymphedema to develop. Even if you show no signs of it after breast surgery, ask your doctor for a referral to a physical therapist with expertise in lymphedema...or find one through the National Lymphedema Network (646-722-7410, Lymphnet.org). You also can download a PDF from the American Cancer Society called "Lymphedema: What Every Woman With Breast Cancer Should Know."

If any symptoms do appear, alert your physician without delay. Unless treated promptly, lymphedema can worsen quickly and eventually become chronic. The area may not look swollen at first, so watch for warning signs—a sensation of fullness, heaviness, heat, numbness or "pins and needles" in the arm, hand, breast or side of the torso.

Vitamin D Eases Breast Cancer Drug Pain

Antonella Luisa Rastelli, MD, assistant professor of medicine in the section of medical oncology at Washington University School of Medicine in St. Louis, and leader of a study of 60 breast cancer patients.

Drugs called aromatase inhibitors, which are used to treat breast cancer, can make muscles and joints so painful and stiff that some women taking the medications say that they feel like they're 100 years old...many users experience bone loss, too. Yet because the medication is effective at halting breast cancer cell growth, shrinking tumors and reducing recurrence risk when taken for several years or more, discontinuing its use prematurely often is inadvisable.

New study: Recognizing that many breast cancer patients have low blood levels of vitamin D, researchers tested a simple potential solution to the problem of drug side effects—vitamin D supplements. For details, we contacted study leader Antonella Luisa Rastelli, MD, an assistant professor of medicine in the section of medical oncology at Washington University School of Medicine in St. Louis.

Participants included 60 early-stage breast cancer patients with low vitamin D levels who had painful side effects from the aromatase inhibitor *anastrozole* (Arimidex). All received a standard daily dose of 400 international units (IU) of vitamin D-3 (the type typically found in supplements) and 1,000 mg of calcium. Half of the participants also received 50,000 IU of vitamin D-2 (a form that leaves the body more quickly than D-3) weekly for eight or 16 weeks, then monthly to the end of the six-month study period. The other half, serving as the control group, got a placebo weekly or monthly.

Results: After two months of weekly supplementation, the high-dose vitamin D groups reported significantly less musculoskeletal pain than the control group (though pain relief did not continue when participants switched to the monthly regimen).

Also: After six months, the high-dose vitamin D users showed no reduction in bone density, whereas the control group did have some bone loss.

Caution: Excessive vitamin D can have side effects of its own, including high levels of calcium in the urine that may increase the risk for kidney stones. Risks are thought to be lower with vitamin D-2 than with D-3—but even so, Dr. Rastelli cautioned that all patients taking high-dose vitamin D supplements must be monitored closely, as the study participants were.

Better Cancer Pain Relief

Giovambattista Zeppetella, MD, medical director, St. Clare Hospice, Hastingwood, England. His study of 393 cancer patients was published in *The Cochrane Library.*

Cancer patients who ordinarily used oral morphine for "breakthrough" pain (sudden moderate to severe pain that is not controlled by regular drug therapy) experienced 33% greater relief within 15 minutes of dissolving a lozenge containing the painkiller *fentanyl* (Actiq) in their mouths.

Theory: The fentanyl lozenge dissolves quickly, allowing it to pass into the central nervous system faster than oral pain medication, such as morphine.

Less Invasive Surgery Effective for Colon Cancer

Esther Kuhry, MD, PhD, Namsos Hospital, Namsos, Norway, and leader of a review involving 3,346 patients, published in *The Cochrane Library.*

Surgeons usually perform open surgery—making large incisions in the abdominal wall—to view and remove cancerous colon tissue.

New finding: An analysis of 12 studies found no differences in rates of surgical complications, cancer recurrence or survival between open surgery and laparoscopic surgery, which involves much smaller incisions and the use of tiny cameras.

Bottom line: Consider a surgeon trained in laparoscopic surgery—it involves less pain and quicker recovery.

Too Much Radiation For Bone Pain?

Justin E. Bekelman, MD, assistant professor of radiation oncology at Perelman School of Medicine at University of Pennsylvania, Philadelphia, and leader of a study published in the *Journal of the American Medical Association.*

Radiation may be administered to patients with advanced prostate cancer who are experiencing pain because the cancer has spread to the bone. This type of treatment is different from radiation to treat prostate cancer and prolong survival. The majority of patients get pain relief from just one radiation treatment.

But: More than half of patients studied received more than 10 treatments.

Patients should speak to their doctors about starting with just one treatment and monitoring their pain level.

Antidepressant Helps Nerve Pain and Numbness from Chemotherapy

Ellen M. Lavoie Smith, PhD, assistant professor, University of Michigan School of Nursing, and researcher, University of Michigan Comprehensive Cancer Center, Ann Arbor. Her study was published in *JAMA.*

About 20% to 40% of cancer patients receiving neurotoxic (nerve-damaging) chemotherapy develop a side effect known as peripheral neuropathy that leaves their fingers and toes, and often their hands and feet, numb or tingling. And this isn't a good kind of tingling—for some, the sensation is so uncomfortable or painful that their chemotherapy dosage must be reduced. Unfortunately, the discomfort can last for months or years after chemotherapy ends.

No medication or other known treatment has succeeded at relieving the discomfort—until now. According to a new study, a drug that is already on the market can relieve chemotherapy-induced peripheral neuropathy. It is duloxetine, better known as the antidepressant Cymbalta. Though it can have side effects of its own, cancer patients who are really suffering from neuropathy will want to be aware of this new option.

MEASURING THE DIFFERENCE

For this study, researchers decided to see whether duloxetine could help cancer patients with peripheral neuropathy because the drug had previously been shown to help diabetics who had a similar condition called diabetic neuropathy. Participants in the new study included 231 adult cancer patients who developed peripheral neuropathy after receiving neurotoxic chemotherapy.

Half of the participants took a placebo and the other half took duloxetine. Initially, the patients receiving duloxetine were given 30 mg per day, but after a week the dose was increased to 60 mg, which is a typical dose used to treat depression. In addition, each week for five weeks, all the study participants rated their pain severity on a scale from zero to 10.

Results: In the duloxetine group, 59% of patients reported a decrease in pain...in the placebo group, 38% reported a decrease in pain. The amount of the reduction was significant. At the start of the study, the average neuropathic pain score for patients receiving duloxetine was 6.1—and after five weeks of treatment, that score dropped by 1.06, on average. For placebo-treated patients, the baseline neuropathic pain score was 5.6—and that score dropped by an average of just 0.34 points after five weeks. (The study was not designed to determine whether patients experienced any mental health benefits from taking duloxetine, nor whether the neuropathic pain returned after patients went off the drug—more research is needed to answer those questions.)

HOW IT WORKS

Duloxetine is in a class of drugs knows as selective serotonin and norepinephrine reuptake inhibitors (SSRIs). These drugs work by upping the amounts of serotonin and norepinephrine, natural substances in the brain that interrupt pain signals to the brain.

Caveats: Not all chemotherapy drugs work the same way or have the same lasting effects on cancer patients' systems. For instance, study participants who had received the chemotherapy drug oxaliplatin got somewhat better pain relief from duloxetine than participants who had received the chemo drug paclitaxel. With yet other chemotherapy drugs, the effects also could vary.

In addition, duloxetine has its own possible side effects, such as nausea, dry mouth, constipation and sleep difficulties, although these generally are mild and some typically subside within a few weeks. Adverse psychological side effects from duloxetine, though uncommon, are possible—these can include anxiety, anger, aggression and, rarely, thoughts of suicide. In the new study, no participants reported any severe physical or psychological side effects from taking the medication.

As with all drugs, there are certain interactions to be aware of. For instance, taking duloxetine with warfarin (the blood thinner) or NSAIDs (such as aspirin or ibuprofen) may increase bleeding risk.

Bottom line: If you are suffering from peripheral neuropathy after being on chemotherapy, consider asking your doctor whether duloxetine is worth a try.

(For more help with neuropathy, see chapter 18, "Neuropathy and Other Nerve Pain.")

Feel Your Best After Cancer...

Sheetal Kircher, MD, oncologist and clinical director of the Cancer Survivorship Institute at the Robert H. Lurie Comprehensive Cancer Center of Northwestern University in Chicago. Dr. Kircher's research interests are focused on improving the quality of cancer care and cancer survivorship.

You beat cancer. Now what? For the 14 million cancer survivors in the US, this is no small question.

Once you've given that sigh of relief for having survived a possibly life-threatening illness, you're immediately confronted with a new set of concerns: How should you protect yourself against the dangerous aftereffects of cancer treatments? What about nagging emotional issues, including depression? And what can be done to keep cancer from coming back?

Recent development: Cancer survivors have traditionally lacked coordinated follow-up care by their physicians after completing their treatments. But there's now a new option for getting specialized aftercare. Hospitals and cancer centers across the US are offering survivorship-care programs* that give patients state-of-the-art methods for keeping tabs on their health and reclaiming their emotional equilibrium after battling cancer.**

GETTING ON WITH YOUR LIFE

At a cancer-survivorship program, a team of medical doctors, physical therapists, psychologists, nutritionists and other health professionals focus exclusively on the individual needs of each cancer patient. This includes monitoring for complications that can result from cancer treatment. *Among the most important to watch for...*

- **Heart damage.** Chemotherapy and radiation can harm any organ, notably the heart. It doesn't necessarily happen right away—a potent class of drugs called anthracyclines, commonly used to treat some lymphomas, breast cancer and certain rare types of cancer like sarcoma, can cause cardiomyopathy (weakening of the heart) decades after treatment is completed.

Radiation that reaches the heart, as often occurs, for example, with lung cancer, can cause damage, too. Similarly, a study appearing in the *Journal of Clinical Oncology* attributed up to 25% of the deaths of former Hodgkin's disease patients to heart disease caused in some part by radiation.

Best self-defense: Depending on the treatment you received, your doctor may recommend one or more tests, such as MRI, ultrasound and/or electrocardiogram, to closely monitor your heart health.

- **Infection.** Chemo, radiation and stem cell transplants used to treat cancer suppress the immune system, increasing risk for infection.

Best self-defense: Vaccines must be used carefully in cancer survivors. For example, "live" vaccines (such as Zostavax for shingles) should not be used in cancer patients with weakened immunity—they are at increased risk of contracting the infectious disease from the live organism in the vaccine. Cancer patients should talk to their doctors about the vaccines they need.

- **Fatigue.** Up to 82% of cancer survivors are affected by persistent fatigue, brought on by chemo and/or radiation or as a result of stress or chronic pain.

Best self-defense: It's common for individuals who have received chemo and/or radiation to suffer mild-to-moderate fatigue for up to a year. However, other conditions not directly related to the cancer itself—for example, an underactive thyroid, anemia, arthritis or insomnia—or even the use of pain medication may be partially to blame.

If these possibilities are ruled out, the best defense is often a carefully designed exercise program. A physical therapist on staff at a cancer-survivorship program will be knowledgeable about the issues that cancer survivors confront.

*To find a cancer-survivorship program near you, go to the National Cancer Institute (NCI) Web site, CancerCenters.Cancer.gov. Cancer-survivor programs are often used in conjunction with care from one's primary care doctor and are covered by most health insurers.

**To find a medical center near you that offers cancer rehab services, consult Oncology Rehab Partners, OncologyRehabPartners.com.

For best results: Pace yourself! Start with just 20 minutes of brisk walking and/or resistance training one to three days a week…and gradually increase to 20 to 60 minutes up to five days a week.

• **Pain.** More than one-third of cancer survivors experience chronic pain—often due to chemotherapy, radiation or surgery.

Best self-defense: Don't rely on just one pain-fighting strategy. A combination of approaches, such as physical therapy, exercise, oral painkillers, lidocaine (injections, creams or patches) and massage, may be recommended.

• **Depression.** This is also common after cancer treatment.

Best self-defense: Don't shrug off worrisome symptoms, such as trouble sleeping, an inability to focus, lingering feelings of sadness and anger or an overwhelming sense of isolation or fear. These are all red flags that depression may have taken hold.

The psychologists, social workers and other mental health professionals at survivorship programs are trained to identify and treat cancer-related complications, such as fatigue and pain, that may contribute to depression. In addition, therapy and/or medication may be needed to treat the depression.

• **Additional postcancer issues.** Cancer-survivorship programs also treat sexual dysfunction…cognitive decline…and sleep problems.

RISKS FOR RECURRENCE

Up to 70% of cancer survivors report having significant fear of a cancer recurrence. If you have survived cancer, the best way to catch a recurrence early—when the malignancy would be most treatable—is to stay on top of follow-up visits to your doctors.

How often? Follow-up visits are generally recommended every three to four months for the first few years following treatment and once or twice annually after that. However, the exact schedule depends on such factors as the type of cancer you had, the treatments you received and your age.

Which tests? It's crucial to have an after-cancer screening plan that may include specific tests (such as blood tests and MRI and/or CT scans) that are sometimes used to help detect cancer recurrences.

Best resource: Guidelines from the National Comprehensive Cancer Network. Go to NCCN.org. Under "NCCN Guidelines," click on "NCCN Guidelines for Patients."

Get the Very Best Cancer Care—Complementary Therapies That Work

Barrie R. Cassileth, PhD, former Laurance S. Rockefeller Chair and chief of the integrative medicine department at Memorial Sloan Kettering Cancer Center in New York City. She is also the author of *Survivorship: Living Well During and After Cancer.*

A cancer diagnosis is always fraught with fear and anxiety—not to mention nagging questions about the best possible treatments.

Bridging the gap: While surgery, chemotherapy and radiation have long been the mainstay treatments for cancer, major cancer centers throughout the US now offer a variety of additional "complementary" therapies that help patients cope with a wide range of cancer-related problems.

Latest development: Recent studies continue to be added to the growing body of evidence supporting the use of such nondrug and nonsurgical therapies, which are used along with conventional cancer treatment.

LOOK FOR PROVEN BENEFITS

Only a small number of complementary therapies have been thoroughly tested with randomized, placebo-controlled clinical trials—the gold standard of scientific research. Some of these approaches have now been proven to work.

Common cancer symptoms that can be relieved with complementary approaches—some services may be covered by insurance, so check with your health insurer…

• **Less nausea.** Nausea and/or vomiting are among the most common symptoms cancer patients have—and among the most feared. Antinausea medications help, but they're not a perfect solution. That's why they're sometimes used in tandem with acupuncture, a complementary therapy that has been shown to be particularly effective.

Scientific evidence: When acupuncture was tested in a group of breast cancer patients being treated with a form of chemotherapy that's notorious for causing nausea, those who were given acupuncture for five days had one-third fewer episodes of nausea than those who were treated only with medications that were used for nausea, such as lorazepam and diphenhydramine. Self-acupressure, in which patients merely press on certain points, such as the PC6 point on the wrist (without using needles), can also help.

To find the PC6 point: Turn your hand so your palm is facing up and locate the area, which is between the tendons three finger widths from the base of the wrist. Massage the area for four to five seconds…or longer, as needed.

• **Pain relief.** Both gentle massage and acupuncture can reduce the pain that's caused by cancer (such as bone cancer) and cancer treatments (such as radiation)—and sometimes allow patients to take lower doses of medication, which can help reduce troubling side effects, including constipation.

Scientific evidence: A study that looked at nearly 1,300 cancer patients found that massage improved their pain scores by 40%…and the improvements lasted for hours and sometimes days after the massage.

Imaging studies show that acupuncture also helps by deactivating brain areas that are involved in pain perception. In one study, patients with chronic cancer pain were treated with either auricular acupuncture (needles placed in the ear) or with sham treatments. After two months, patients in the acupuncture group reported reductions in pain intensity of 36% versus 2% in the placebo group.

• **Less fatigue.** Only about 10% of cancer patients are physically active during treatment. But the vast majority can safely exercise before, during and after treatments…and exercise is among the best ways to reduce treatment-related fatigue.

Scientific evidence: When researchers at the University of Connecticut analyzed 44 studies focusing on patients with cancer-related fatigue, they found that those who exercised had more energy than those who were sedentary.

Any form of exercise seems to help. Yoga that focuses on gentle postures and breathing is good because it's easy on the body and has been shown to reduce anxiety and other stress-related symptoms.

Bonus: Cancer patients who exercise tend to live longer than those who don't stay active. A study of more than 900 breast cancer patients found that those who engaged in brisk walking for two and a half hours a week—the same level of exercise that's recommended for the general population—were 67% less likely to die during the nine-year study period than those who were sedentary.

• **Fewer hot flashes.** Both men and women who have hormone-dependent cancers (such as breast and prostate cancers) often experience hot flashes when they're given hormone-based treatments. Once again, acupuncture seems to help.

Scientific evidence: One study found that nearly 90% of patients with breast or prostate cancers who were given acupuncture had a reduction in hot flashes of nearly 50% that lasted at least three months.

HOW TO STAY SAFE

Virtually all oncologists and respected cancer centers in the US now support the use of complementary therapies, such as acupuncture and massage, to help cancer patients cope with nausea, pain, anxiety and other symptoms. These and other complementary therapies are used in addition to conventional treatments.

To find an evidence-based complementary oncology program: Look for a comprehensive cancer center at the National Cancer Institute's website, Cancer.gov/research/nci-role/cancer-centers/find.

Very important: When seeking complementary care, it's vital that the practitioner (including massage therapists, acupuncturists, etc.) be properly trained to work with cancer patients. Getting therapy at a comprehensive cancer center helps ensure that.

Also crucial: Cancer patients should always talk to their doctors before taking any supplements (herbs, vitamins, etc.). They can sometimes interfere with chemotherapy and other cancer treatments. For more on specific supplements, go to Memorial Sloan Kettering's website, MSKCC.org/aboutherbs.

Natural Ways to Fight Side Effects of Cancer Treatment

Mark A. Stengler, NMD, naturopathic doctor and founder of the Stengler Center for Integrative Medicine in Encinitas, California. He is author or coauthor of numerous books, including *The Natural Physician's Healing Therapies and Bottom Line's Prescription for Natural Cures,* and author of the newsletter *Health Revelations.* MarkStengler.com

The vast majority of cancer patients will choose to be treated with conventional therapies, such as chemotherapy, radiation, surgery or a combination. I often advise patients who are undergoing these treatments and want to reduce their risk of side effects and optimize their outcome. It is gratifying to help these people who are in physical and emotional turmoil. An example is Yolanda, a 62-year-old woman who was diagnosed with a form of lymphoma (cancer of the lymphatic system). A program of nutrition and dietary supplements gave her more energy, promoted bowel regularity and boosted her immunity. Her oncologist was quite surprised with how well she tolerated her chemo treatments and remarked on her quick recovery.

UNDERSTANDING CHEMOTHERAPY AND RADIATION

Chemotherapy involves the use of one or more drugs to destroy cancer cells. The treatments are given intravenously (IV) through a vein, orally or by injection into a muscle. These medications not only attack cancer cells but also harm healthy cells. This causes a variety of side effects, depending on the chemotherapeutic agents being used and the individual's response. Examples of short-term side effects include loss of appetite, memory impairment, constipation, diarrhea, hair loss, nausea, mouth sores, easy bruising, fluid retention and pain in muscles, bones, nerves and joints. It also can result in bone marrow suppression, which can lower white and red blood cell counts, causing fatigue and increasing a patient's susceptibility to infection. Long-term side effects can include infertility, chronic fatigue and continued bone marrow suppression. In addition, chemotherapy can result in secondary cancers—for example, a breast cancer patient might develop acute leukemia.

Radiation therapy also kills cancer cells and shrinks tumors. It is mainly used to attack localized cancers as opposed to cancer that has spread. Radiation treatments can be administered externally by a machine, internally through radioactive material placed in the body near cancer cells or via radioactive substances that are injected and circulate throughout the body. Side effects can be similar to those caused by chemotherapy, but symptoms such as redness, swelling and a burning sensation often are specific to the region being treated. Burned or reddened skin also can develop at the treated area.

SUPPLEMENTS THAT HELP

The following supplements are recommended for people undergoing chemotherapy or radiation therapy. You can take all of them at once—with the exception of the mushrooms listed, which are typically taken one at a time, as directed. Always consult with your oncologist before taking any supplement. Supplements work best in conjunction with a healthful diet and lifestyle.

DETOXIFICATION THERAPIES

Toxic by-products are formed by cancer treatments. You can help eliminate these toxins from your body by supporting liver and kidney detoxification.

- **Milk thistle** is an excellent herb that supports liver detoxification and protects against liver and kidney cell damage. Studies show

Melatonin for Chemo Pain

The popular supplement for jet lag appears to ease chemotherapy side effects. Animals given melatonin prior to treatment had less chemotherapy-induced nerve pain.

Important: Melatonin works only for prevention, not for pain that's already under way.

Universities of Edinburgh and Aberdeen.

that it actually helps liver cells regenerate. I recommend a 175-mg to 250-mg capsule of standardized extract (70% to 85% silymarin) taken three times daily. It can also be taken in liquid form. An excellent product is Thisilyn by Nature's Way, available in capsule form at most health-food stores, or you can contact the manufacturer to find a retailer (800-962-8873, NaturesWay.com).

- **Chlorella,** spirulina, wheatgrass and other "super greens" are nature's great detoxifiers. You can take chlorella by itself—it contains chlorophyll and a host of other detoxifying nutrients. A good choice, SunChlorella A, is available at health-food stores or from Sun Chlorella USA (800-829-2828, SunChlorella USA.com). Follow label instructions. Kyo-Green Energy by Kyolic is a good formula that contains a mixture of greens. It is available in tablet or powder form. To locate a store or mail-order company, contact Wakunaga (800-421-2998, Kyolic.com).

BOOSTING IMMUNITY

Because cancer treatments, especially chemotherapy, have a suppressive effect on the immune system—which makes you more vulnerable to infection—immunity boosting is critical. The following natural therapies can be used to support normal immune function without interfering with treatment.

- **Coriolus versicolor mushroom extract** is routinely used in Japan and China to support the immune function of people with cancer. It also is helpful in reducing the side effects of chemotherapy and radiation.

A 1994 study published in *The Lancet* examined the effects of coriolus on patients undergoing chemotherapy after surgical removal of stomach cancer. The 262 patients were randomly assigned chemotherapy alone or with coriolus extract. The survival rate of the group using the combination was 73% after five years, while the chemotherapy-only group had a survival rate of 60%. Researchers concluded that coriolus had "a restorative effect in patients who had been immunosuppressed by both recent surgery and subsequent chemotherapy." The recommended dose is 2,000 mg to 3,000 mg daily. The Mushroom Science brand of coriolus duplicates the formula that was used in the study and is available at health-food stores or by contacting Mushroom Science (888-283-6583, MushroomScience.com).

Maitake mushroom extract is one of the most-studied mushroom extracts. Since the 1980s, Hiroaki Nanba, MD, a professor of microbiology at Kobe Pharmaceutical University, Kobe, Japan, has been researching maitake extract. It has been shown to enhance the activity of the body's natural killer cells against cancer cells. In addition, maitake extract has been shown to reduce the side effects of chemotherapy. A survey of 671 patients showed that the use of maitake during chemo reduced adverse effects such as hair loss, pain and nausea. Maitake Gold 404 is the form recommended by Dr. Nanba. Typical dosage is 1 mg per two pounds of body weight daily. It is available in capsule or liquid form at health-food stores. For a store locator, consult Natural Factors (877-551-2179, NaturalFactors.com). Or you can buy Cellular Essentials NK-5 from Swanson Health Products (800-824-4491, SwansonVitamins.com)—it contains Maitake Gold 404.

Note: Choose either coriolus or maitake based on the type of cancer being treated. Coriolus is a good general choice, especially for people with cancers of the throat, lungs and digestive tract. Maitake is better studied for cancers of the breast, prostate and liver.

- **Curcumin** is the yellow pigment found in turmeric, a prime ingredient in curry. It has been shown to have anticancer properties and to enhance the effectiveness of some chemotherapy drugs, such as *cisplatin* (Platinol). It has no known side effects. The recommended supplement dose is 400 mg twice daily. Many brands are available at health-food stores.

• **Whey protein,** derived from cow's milk, supplies all the essential amino acids the body needs for repair, including the amino acid glutamine, which prevents mouth sores and strengthens immunity. Take 20 g of whey protein powder twice daily, in water or a shake.

DIGESTIVE HELP

Digestive function often is compromised by cancer treatments, particularly chemotherapy and radiation for cancers in the abdominal area. These treatments destroy "friendly" bacteria, which are important for digestion, detoxification and immune function.

• **Probiotics contain beneficial bacteria,** such as *Lactobacillus acidophilus* and *Lactobacillus bifidus*. Take a daily dose of 10 billion or more active organisms. Good products include DDS Plus by UAS Laboratories (800-422-3371, UASlabs.com) and Bio-K Plus by Bio-K Plus International (for a store locator, go to BioKplus.com or call 800-593-2465).

• **Ginger** helps relieve indigestion, nausea, bloating and diarrhea. Sip ginger tea throughout the day, or take two 300-mg capsules twice daily.

• **Homeopathic Nux vomica,** derived from the poison nut tree, combats nausea and constipation. Take two pellets of a 30C potency twice daily until symptoms subside, usually within two to three days.

SKIN SOOTHER

Aloe vera gel can be applied topically to areas irritated or burned by radiation therapy. Choose a product that is 95% to 100% pure aloe vera. Aloe vera gel is available at health-food stores and pharmacies.

ANTIOXIDANTS MAY HELP

Antioxidants—such as vitamins A, C and E, selenium and coenzyme Q10—are controversial cancer treatments. Because conventional cancer treatments work in part by producing free radicals, and because antioxidants attack free radicals, the fear is that antioxidant supplements may neutralize the effects of chemotherapy or radiation. This is an area that needs to be better studied. I recommend consulting your oncologist on this issue. Certainly, multivitamins and an antioxidant formula (containing CoQ10, mixed vitamin E, green tea extract and vitamin C) should be used after the completion of treatment for optimal recovery.

Jin Shin Jyutsu Touch Therapy Relieves Cancer Pain and Stress

Jennifer M. Bradley, Jin Shin Jyutsu integrative practitioner at the University of Kentucky Markey Cancer Center in Lexington. JSJHarmony.com

It hurts so much to know that someone you love is ill and in pain and yet you are powerless to help. There's a unique hands-on technique that can bring significant comfort to patients—and to caregivers, too.

Called Jin Shin Jyutsu (pronounced jin shin jit-su), it's an ancient form of touch therapy that is simple and safe...often provides immediate relief...and can be performed at a basic level by people with no formal training. It's completely natural and noninvasive, involving only your hands—no pills, potions, side effects or equipment.

Jin Shin Jyutsu is an energy healing technique that utilizes the same principles of Eastern medicine as acupressure, except that little or no pressure is applied. It is based on the premise that energy flows through our bodies along certain pathways, and when that energy is blocked, we experience disharmony, including pain. Like jumper cables for a car, Jin Shin Jyutsu sparks the flow of energy to help restore proper functioning.

Exciting research: A recent pilot study involved 159 cancer patients who ranked their pain, nausea and stress on a scale of zero (no symptoms) to 10 (extremely severe symptoms) before and after receiving Jin Shin Jyutsu therapy.

Results: Participants reported an average two-point reduction in pain and nausea and three-point reduction in stress after their first and subsequent Jin Shin Jyutsu sessions. Benefits typically lasted for many hours or days, depending on the individual.

The technique provides a means of maintaining a deep connection at the end of life, when a person is no longer able to communicate verbally. Family members can be taught some simple Jin Shin Jyutsu holds, so they can bond with their loved ones in a profound way during what can often be a difficult transition for everyone.

WHAT A PROFESSIONAL PRACTITIONER DOES

Jin Shin Jyutsu uses 52 energetic points, or safety energy locks, on the body (similar to acupressure points). These energy locks can be thought of as small breaker boxes that keep the energy system in check, like the fuse box in a home. These points are stimulated in predetermined orders called flows. The specific hand and finger positions the practitioner uses are called holds, though this word applies only in the most passive sense because there is no gripping, grasping or manipulation at all—instead, a very light touch is used.

During a Jin Shin Jyutsu session, the patient lies comfortably on a padded surface, fully clothed except for shoes...watches and jewelry also may be removed from the wrist. First the practitioner places her hands on the patient's wrists in a technique called pulse listening, to sense the energetic pulse and determine which procedures are needed to promote balance. Then she works her way through various safety energy locks, moving from one to the next as she senses that harmony is being restored.

A session with a professional typically lasts about an hour. The cost is similar to the charge for a massage, depending on the location, practitioner and years of experience. To find a practitioner near you, go to JSJinc.net/locatorsearch.php.

TECHNIQUES YOU CAN DO FOR A LOVED ONE

Here are some basic holds that anyone can do to ease a loved one's suffering. You can do any or all of them, in any order. Use whichever holds feel good to your loved one.

The patient may sit in a chair or couch with feet propped up or may lie in bed, whatever is comfortable for her or him. For techniques that involve the toes, the patient's feet can be bare or in socks. In each case, maintain a gentle hold without squeezing or rubbing for several minutes per position or until you feel a gentle rhythmic pulsation. If possible, do the holds once or more daily—there is no limit on the amount of time or number of times the techniques can be performed. *What to do...*

To reduce fatigue: Wrap the fingers of your right hand around the patient's right thumb and the fingers of your left hand around his/her left thumb...hold...then reverse your hands and repeat.

To lessen anxiety: Place one hand under the back of the head just above the neck area. This can be done underneath the pillow if necessary. At the same time, gently wrap the fingers of your other hand around the patient's fingers, one by one. If it is not possible to hold the back of the head, gently hold the patient's palm with one of your hands while using your other hand to hold each finger individually. Then repeat for the patient's other hand.

To ease back pain and trauma (including spinal paralysis) or to relax the body overall: You will use one hand to hold each of the patient's fingers (one after the other) while at the same time using the other hand to hold each of his/her toes. *Going in the following order, hold the patient's...*

- **Right pinkie at the same time as the left big toe**
- **Right ring finger at the same time as the left second toe**
- **Right middle finger at the same time as the left middle toe**
- **Right index finger at the same time as the left fourth toe**
- **Right thumb at the same time as the left pinkie toe.**

When finished, repeat the same sequence, holding each left finger at the same time as each right toe. It is also fine to begin with the left fingers/right toes sequence first, followed by the right fingers/left toes sequence.

- **To help clear anesthesia from the body after surgery.** Stand at the end of the bed or sit at either side of the bed. With your palms facing up, place your left palm under the patient's right calf and your right palm under his/her left calf, gently cradling the legs...hold...then reverse so your right palm cradles the right calf and your left palm cradles the left calf.

• **To soothe radiation treatment side effects (burning pain, skin sensitivity, skin damage).** This can be done any time after treatment. Place the palm of your left hand on or just above the irradiated area, then place your right hand atop the left...hold for 20 minutes, repeating as much as requested.

Intrigued? You can view several videos demonstrating Jin Shin Jyutsu on Youtube.com.

To Ease Chemo Pain, Walk This Way

Abstract titled "A URCC NCORP Nationwide Randomized Controlled Trial Investigating the Effect of Exercise on Chemotherapy-Induced Peripheral Neuropathy in 314 Cancer Patients," by Ian Kleckner, PhD, research assistant professor, University of Rochester Medical Center, New York, and colleagues, presented at the 2016 American Society of Clinical Oncology meeting.

A whopping 38% of people being treated with multiple drugs for cancer develop nerve pain—resulting in tingling, shooting pains, movement problems and/or numbness. It's called chemotherapy-induced peripheral neuropathy (CIPN), and it's so painful that some people drop out of lifesaving chemo, and the pain can last for years. There are no FDA-approved drugs to prevent it—or treat it.

But there is something incredibly simple that you can do yourself that makes a real difference. It's a gentle exercise program that's easy to do at home.

A WAY TO EXERCISE WHILE YOU ARE IN CHEMO

The program is called Exercise for Cancer Patients (EXCAP), and it's the brainchild of Karen M. Mustian, PhD, MPH, at the University of Rochester Medical Center. She has conducted trials on the effect of exercise on cancer patients since 2007.

EXCAP is deceptively simple, especially for something that can transform cancer patients' lives. It's daily walking plus a set of exercises using stretchy elastic resistance bands to build muscle strength. That's all—but it's tailored to each individual's fitness needs...it's based at home...and it includes coaching by a trained instructor who can help each patient progress (and overcome any obstacles encountered). The goal is to slowly build endurance and strength with daily exercise—by increasing the number of steps walked and with progressively challenging resistance band exercises. It lasts six weeks, although it's easy to continue on your own after the official program ends.

FIGHTING NEUROPATHY WITH YOUR OWN TWO FEET (AND ARMS)

In this study, researchers identified 314 patients in the ongoing clinical trials on EXCAP who were getting chemo drugs known to contribute to nerve pain, including platinum, vinca alkaloid and taxane. (If you are being treated with one of these drugs, the chance that you'll get CIPN is 60%.) These drugs often are used to treat breast cancer, and indeed three-quarters of the patients were being treated for breast cancer. Everyone got chemo, but about half of the patients were also enrolled in EXCAP.

Results: Exercisers had significantly less chemo-induced nerve pain—especially older ones.

How does exercise help? The exact mechanisms aren't known, but other EXCAP studies have shown that the program reduces chronic inflammation. It has other benefits, too, such as reducing cognitive impairment—aka, "chemo brain"—in people being treated with drugs for cancer. Plus, regular exercise reduces the risk for cancer recurrence and it even may make cancer treatments more effective.

How much exercise is enough to minimize cancer treatment side effects such as nerve pain? There aren't any official guidelines yet, so your best bet is to discuss an exercise plan with your doctor, who may be able to recommend a physical therapist or exercise trainer you can work with. Use common sense—start slowly

Hypnosis Eases Cancer Surgery Pain

Hypnosis eases cancer surgery pain. Breast cancer patients who were hypnotized within one hour before surgery required less anesthesia and reported less postsurgical pain, nausea, fatigue and emotional upset than women who spoke with a psychologist before surgery.

Guy Montgomery, PhD, associate professor, department of oncological sciences, Mount Sinai School of Medicine, New York City, and lead author of a study of 200 women, published in *Journal of the National Cancer Institute.*

and build up very gradually. Don't overdo it. Chemo is taxing and exhausting, but the good news is that this very mild exercise program, tailored to your energy level, may help you get through the process with less pain now—and in the future—and will also improve your circulation so that toxic compounds that result from chemotherapy move out of your body faster. (And if you haven't started cancer treatment yet, make sure that exercise is part of your cancer prehab program.) (For more on painful neuropathy, see chapter 18, "Neuropathy and Other Nerve Pain.")

If Your Loved One Has Cancer, Offer Your Touch

William Collinge, PhD, director of Collinge Associates, an independent research and consulting organization in Kittery, Maine. He is author of several books, including *Partners in Healing: Simple Ways to Offer Support, Comfort, and Care to a Loved One Facing Illness,* and executive producer of the Touch, Caring, and Cancer DVD program. Collinge.org, PartnersInHealing.net

Research sponsored by the National Cancer Institute has discovered a powerful treatment for people with cancer that can decrease stress, anxiety and depression...reduce fatigue...relieve pain...and ease nausea.

THE LOVING TOUCH OF A CAREGIVER'S HANDS

Striking research finding: The study looked at 97 cancer patients and their caregivers (spouse or family member), dividing them into two groups.

Half the caregivers watched a DVD called Touch, Caring and Cancer and read the accompanying manual—and then gave three massages a week for four weeks to the cancer patients. The other half read to the cancer patients three times a week from a book the patients said they would enjoy.

Those receiving the massages had less...

- **Stress/anxiety** (44% less, compared with 28% less for the reading group)
- **Pain** (34% less, compared with 18%)
- **Fatigue** (32% less, compared with 20%)
- **Depression** (31% less, compared with 22%)
- **Nausea** (29% less, compared with 12%).

The results were in the *Journal of the Society for Integrative Oncology.*

"It appears that caregivers receiving video instruction can achieve some of the same results as professional massage therapists," says William Collinge, PhD, the study leader, director of Collinge Associates in Kittery, Maine, which provides consultation and research in integrative health care, and author of *Partners in Healing: Simple Ways to Offer Support, Comfort, and Care to a Loved One Facing Illness.*

"This has important implications for the quality of life of cancer patients, helping them feel better," says Dr. Collinge. "But it's also important for caregiver satisfaction. Cancer caregivers are at risk of distress themselves—they can feel helpless and frustrated at not being able to help. This gives them a way to help the patient feel better and increase their own effectiveness and satisfaction as a caregiver. It also appears to strengthen the relationship bond, which is important to both caregiver and patient."

THE NEW CAREGIVER

"About one-third of adults have been in a caregiving role in the past year for a loved one with cancer or another chronic illness," says Dr. Collinge. "Caregiving is becoming a universal dynamic in relationships. And there are very simple complementary therapies—such as touch—that can make a big impact on both the person with the illness and the caregiver."

If you're a caregiver, here is what Dr. Collinge says you need to understand and do to help your loved one (and yourself) with the caring power of touch...

• **Know the benefits.** "A caring touch introduces so many dimensions of healing," says Dr. Collinge. "Skin to skin contact is so comforting by itself. It improves emotional intimacy between the person with cancer and the caregiver—it reassures the person with cancer of the presence and caring of the other person."

And then there are all the physiological benefits of touch—the relaxation from touch triggers the release of mood-boosting endorphins that can counter stress, anxiety and depression, and reduce pain, nausea and fatigue.

"Touch is unique. You won't find a single drug or other treatment that can yield all of its simultaneous benefits."

• **Be reassured about safety.** "The brief training of the Touch, Caring and Cancer video and manual can overcome some of the historical fears and misunderstandings about touch and cancer," says Dr. Collinge.

"It reassures the caregiver that touch and massage can't spread the cancer, or that cancer is somehow contagious.

"The manual also provides a precaution checklist to discuss with the cancer patient's doctors, so that the caregiver can simply and easily avoid any type of touch or area of touch that would cause pain or discomfort."

• **Understand that even simple touch works.** "For example, you can relax a person's whole body just by massaging their hand," says Dr. Collinge, "and you can do that while sitting in a waiting room or watching TV at home. Just lightly resting your hand on a loved one can provide comfort and relaxation."

• **Realize that you might offer more benefits than a massage professional.** "Some of the people in this study—such as older caregivers who were at home all day—would give short massages six or seven times a day," says Dr. Collinge. "When we asked them why, they'd say, 'We just enjoy it so much that we do five minutes here and five minutes there several times a day.' That means some people were giving 50 mini-massages a week—for enduring impact, that's so much greater than could be achieved by the patient seeing a massage therapist once a week."

• **Attitude matters more than technique.** "The bottom line is not how you touch, but receiving the permission and encouragement to touch," says Dr. Collinge. "The technique is really of minimal importance. What's important is the actual touching, and the compassionate presence of the caregiver."

• **Expand your concept of caregiving.** "We have the notion in our culture that caregiving is about changing the linens, monitoring medications, bringing good food, bathing, taking the patient to appointments and other similar tasks," says Dr. Collinge. "But we can expand the notion of home caregiving to include some simple complementary therapies such as touch that are deeply satisfying both to the person being cared for and the person doing the caring."

• **Watch the video and read the manual.** The DVD and manual used in the study—Touch, Care, and Cancer—is available at PartnersInHealing.net.

Massage Therapy for Cancer

Barrie R. Cassileth, PhD, chief, Integrative Medicine Service, Memorial Sloan-Kettering Cancer Center, New York City.

In a three-year study of the effect of massage on more than 1,000 cancer patients—the largest study to date of massage used for cancer patients—patients rated their symptoms immediately before and after a single treatment of massage therapy.

Result: Anxiety declined by 52%...pain, 40%...fatigue, 41%...depression, 31%...and nausea, 21%. Massage was as effective as standard drug therapy for these symptoms.

Helpful: Insurance companies are more likely to pay for massage therapy if a doctor writes a referral to a certified therapist or if treatment is part of a hospital in-patient therapy. To locate a massage therapist in your area, contact the American Massage Therapy Association, 888-843-2682, or visit AMTAmassage.org.

Rebuilding Your Body After Cancer Treatment

Mark A. Stengler, NMD, naturopathic doctor and founder of the Stengler Center for Integrative Medicine in Encinitas, California. He is author or coauthor of numerous books, including *The Natural Physician's Healing Therapies* and *Bottom Line's Prescription for Natural Cures,* and author of the newsletter *Health Revelations.* MarkStengler.com

Cancer survivor is the title everyone diagnosed with this terrible disease hopes to own—and many do. Once treatment is over, however, many people feel alone, no longer getting the close attention, advice and support they've received from their oncology team. *Specific challenges include...*

- **Peripheral neuropathy,** which causes tingling, burning pain and numbness in the feet and sometimes hands.
- **A build-up of cellular waste in remaining tissue,** due to the extreme toxicity of chemotherapy drugs. These powerful drugs kill healthy cells right along with the cancerous ones, leaving a residue that needs to be removed from the body.
- **Chemo depletes many important nutrient levels,** often causing digestive problems as the drugs destroy much of the good flora in the gastrointestinal tract in addition to the lining of the tract itself.
- **"Chemo brain" is a catch-all term for the common memory glitches,** lack of focus, mild cognitive impairment and fatigue that follow cancer treatment.

DIET AND SUPPLEMENTS TO DETOX, BUILD STRENGTH

You can take control with both diet and natural supplements. These can help create a healthier cellular environment, clean out the damage done by treatment and rebuild digestive health. *Dietary recommendations...*

- **Fermented foods.** Eat lots of miso, sauerkraut (the kind you buy at the health food store, not the deli), kefir and yogurt.
- **Water.** Drink 60 to 70 ounces daily to flush toxins from your system. (*Note*: Limit water with meals to eight ounces as more can dilute the effectiveness of stomach acid.)
- **Fruits and vegetables.** Enjoy these every day. If possible, buy organic, especially for soft fruits such as peaches, nectarines, strawberries and pears.
- **Avoid processed foods—including sugar and white flour.** This will eliminate refined sugars and unhealthy fats (trans fats, partially hydrogenated or hydrogenated fats and interesterified fats), all of which can be harmful to health.
- **Eat plenty of healthy fats.** These are omega-3s, (found in flaxseed, walnuts and fatty fish including salmon, herring and sardines), balanced by some omega-6s (in corn and soybeans).
- **Avoid tuna, king mackerel, shark, swordfish and others with potentially high levels of mercury.** You don't need to add yet more toxins to your system.

Many tissues in the body are challenged by chemotherapy. Supplements are helpful to strengthen health overall and detoxify the liver—which often endures the greatest insult. *I often prescribe the following...*

- **Antioxidants.** These help rebuild health, potentially improve chemo outcomes and help to heal tissue damaged by radiation treatment. Among the supplements I may prescribe—CoQ10...vitamin C...vitamin E mixed with tocopherol/tocotrienols and a carotenoid complex...vitamin D...lycopene and selenium.
- **Probiotics.** These can help balance the digestive system. I typically prescribe one with a blend of *Lactobacillus acidophilus* and *Bifidobacterium bifidum.*

• **Greens-chlorella.** These deliver phytochemicals, which can be helpful to a system damaged by chemotherapy. Sun Chlorella is a trusted brand I prescribe.

• **Wheatgrass.** It contains helpful vitamin K and chlorophyll antioxidants.

• **Milk thistle.** This herb helps support the liver and kidneys by protecting cells against damage caused by breakdown products of the cellular debris and chemo drugs.

• **NAC.** N-acetylcysteine, derived from a protein amino acid derivative L-cysteine, aids in the breakdown of drug and cellular wastes.

OTHER STRATEGIES TO BOOST HEALTH

Systemic inflammation is, not surprisingly, a problem that lingers long after cancer treatment. Patients who follow an improved diet and take many of the above supplements, along with getting regular exercise, often note reduced inflammation.

I usually recommend an aerobic form of exercise for 30 minutes five times weekly and strength training for 15 minutes twice weekly. If you haven't already been exercising, go slowly in establishing a routine—fighting cancer and taking chemo or radiation exhaust many energy reserves in the body. Rest and recuperation are more important than pushing your workout to a higher level.

It can be challenging to keep your stress levels under control after dealing with cancer, but this too is important to strengthen your health. If you are having trouble with lack of focus, depression or anxiety, counseling may help you regain your physical and mental strength. Certain natural substances can also be helpful—such as phosphatidylserine for cognitive dysfunction…S-adenosylmethionine (SAMe) for depression… and 5-hydroxytryptophan (5-HTP) for anxiety and depression.

KICK-START IMMUNE SYSTEM TO PREVENT RECURRENCE

Immunity levels may need a push after the challenges of treatment. There are several substances that may be supportive. These include Beta Glucan Formula, and mushroom extracts such as *Grifola frondosa* (maitake), *Lentinula edodes* (shiitake) and Coriolus versicolor. Fermented wheat germ extract in powder form (mixed in water or juice) may also be prescribed. Under your doctor's supervision, it is okay to use these supplements in combination, but your bank account may feel the pain. Ask your doctor what your priorities should be and choose a regimen accordingly.

Cancer-Fighting Superfoods

Rebecca Katz, MS, senior chef-in-residence and nutrition educator at Commonweal Cancer Help Program in Bolinas, California. She is author, with Mat Edelson, of *The Cancer-Fighting Kitchen: Nourishing, Big-Flavor Recipes for Cancer Treatment and Recovery.* RebeccaKatz.com

---

Some people experience virtually no side effects from cancer chemotherapy, but this is rare. Most patients report at least some problems, including nausea, fatigue and pain during the treatment.

Reason: The drugs that are used in chemotherapy are designed to kill fast-growing cancer cells. But they also damage fast-growing healthy cells, particularly in the mouth, digestive tract and hair follicles.

Good nutrition is critical if you're undergoing chemotherapy. It's estimated that up to 80% of cancer patients are malnourished. People who eat well before and during chemotherapy tend to have fewer side effects. They also are more likely to complete the full course of therapy than those who are poorly nourished and may feel too sick to continue. *What to do…*

• **Load up on nutrient-rich foods.** In the weeks before chemotherapy, patients should emphasize nutrient-dense foods, such as whole grains, vegetables and legumes. The high nutrient load of a healthy diet helps strengthen healthy cells so that they're better able to withstand—and then recover from—the effects of chemotherapy. *Good choices…*

• **Dark leafy greens, such as spinach, kale and Swiss chard.** They're high in antioxidants, such as beta-carotene, lutein and other phytonutrients. These compounds help minimize the damaging effects of free radicals, tissue-damaging molecules that are produced in large amounts during chemotherapy. Kale is particularly good because it contains indole-3-carbinol, a compound that has anticancer properties.

- **Olive oil, like green vegetables, is high in antioxidants.** It's one of the best sources of oleic acid, an omega-9 fatty acid that strengthens cell membranes and improves the ability of the immune system to fight cancer cells. I like extra-virgin olive oil because it has been exposed to the least heat.

- **Garlic.** The National Cancer Institute reports that people who eat garlic regularly seem to have a lower risk for intestinal and other cancers, including breast cancer. The strong-tasting sulfur compounds in garlic, such as allicin, have strong antiviral and antibacterial effects—important for chemotherapy patients because they're susceptible to infection. In my recipes, I use fresh garlic. I smash it and let it sit for 10 minutes to allow the antiviral properties to become more accessible—then chop and cook. (To smash garlic, set the side of a chef's knife on the clove, place the heel of your hand on the flat side of the knife and apply pressure.)

- **Increase protein.** It's the main structural component of muscle and other tissues. People who undergo chemotherapy need large amounts of protein to repair tissue damage that occurs during the treatments.

Recommended: About 80 grams of protein daily. That's nearly double the amount that healthy adults need. Cancer patients who increase their protein about a week before chemotherapy, and continue to get extra protein afterward, recover more quickly. They also will have more energy and less fatigue.

Try this: Two or more daily smoothies (made in a blender with juice or milk, a variety of fresh fruits and ice, if you like) that are supplemented with a scoop of whey powder. The protein in whey is easily absorbed by the intestine. And most people can enjoy a nutrient-rich smoothie even when they have nausea or digestive problems related to chemotherapy.

- **Drink to reduce discomfort.** Stay hydrated both before and after chemotherapy sessions to reduce nausea. Drink liquids until your urine runs clear—if it has more than a hint of yellow, you need to drink more.

Helpful: Soups and broths provide water, as well as protein, minerals and vitamins.

- **Avoid your favorite foods two days before treatments.** It's common for chemotherapy patients to develop food aversions when they get nauseated from treatments and then to associate the nausea with certain foods. It's sad when people develop aversions and can never again enjoy their favorite foods.

- **Eat lightly and frequently.** People tend to experience more nausea when the stomach is empty. During and after "chemo days," keep something in your stomach all the time—but not too much. Patients do better when they have a light snack, such as sautéed vegetables or a bowl of broth, than when they go hungry or eat a lot at one sitting.

- **Treat with ginger.** When your stomach is upset, steep three slices of fresh ginger in a cup of simmering water for 10 minutes, then drink the tea. Or grate fresh ginger with a very fine grater, such as a microplane, and put the shavings under your tongue. Ginger alleviates nausea almost instantly.

- **Overcome "metal mouth."** The drugs used in chemotherapy can damage the nerves that control the taste buds. Some people complain about a metallic taste in their mouths after treatments. Others notice that foods taste "flat" or that their mouths are extremely sensitive to hot or cold.

These changes, known as transient taste changes, usually disappear a few weeks (or, in some cases, months) after treatments, but they can make it difficult for people to eat in the meantime.

Helpful: The FASS method. It stands for Fat, Acid, Salt and Sweet. Most people will find that it's easier to enjoy their meals, and therefore ingest enough nutrients, when they combine one or more of these elements in every meal.

For fat, add more olive oil than usual to meals...lemons are a good source of acid...sea salt has less of a chemical aftertaste than regular salt...and maple syrup gives sweetness with more nutrients (including immune-building manganese and zinc) than table sugar.

• **Try kudzu root.** Used in a powder form to thicken sauces, puddings and other foods, it soothes the intestine and can help prevent diarrhea. You also can dissolve one teaspoon of kudzu root in one teaspoon of cold liquid and drink that. Drink after meals, as needed. Kudzu root is available in most health-food stores.

• **Soothe mouth sores** with soft, easy-to-eat foods, such as granitas (similar to "Italian ices") or smoothies. The sores can be intensely painful, which makes it difficult to eat.

Recommended: Watermelon ice cubes. Purée watermelon, and put it in a tray to freeze. Then suck on the cubes. The cold acts like a topical anesthetic—you can numb the mouth before eating a regular meal. And the juice from the melon is just as hydrating as water but provides extra nutrients, including the antioxidant lycopene.

• **Sautéeing Swiss chard**—or any green—in olive oil makes the flavor and consistency much more palate-friendly for chemo patients. And that's a great thing because greens are a must-have for health. The other ingredients, such as cranberries and orange juice, are high in antioxidants...pepper flakes (optional) are anti-inflammatory.

The flavor of this dish is greatly intensified by reducing the liquid in the pan. Take the time to perform this step. Your taste buds will be rewarded. *Another trick...*

Rip the leaves of the greens off their tough stems and discard the stems. This makes the dish easier to eat and digest.

EMERALD GREENS WITH ORANGE

2 Tablespoons extra-virgin olive oil
1 teaspoon minced garlic
Pinch of red pepper flakes
2 Tablespoons dried cranberries
¼ cup freshly squeezed orange juice
6 cups stemmed and chopped Swiss chard, in bite-size pieces
¼ teaspoon sea salt
½ teaspoon orange zest
¼ teaspoon maple syrup

Heat olive oil in a large sauté pan over medium heat, then add the garlic, red pepper flakes, cranberries, and orange juice, and sauté for 30 seconds, just until aromatic. Add the chard, salt, and zest, and sauté until the color of the chard begins to darken and intensify. Use a slotted spoon to transfer the greens to a bowl, then bring the liquid in the pan to a boil. When the liquid shrinks in from the sides of the pan and thickens a bit, stir the greens back in, then stir in the maple syrup. Serve immediately. Serves four.

Reprinted with permission from *The Cancer-Fighting Kitchen: Nourishing, Big-Flavor Recipes for Cancer Treatment and Recovery.* Copyright © 2009 by Rebecca Katz with Mat Edelson, Celestial Arts, an imprint of the Crown Publishing Group, Berkeley, California.

CHAPTER 6

Chest Pain

Don't Ignore Chest Pain

Virtually everyone feels chest pain at some point—and for good reason. Any of the organs in the chest, as well as the chest wall itself, can cause pain.

While severe pain is clearly something that you should pay close attention to, lesser degrees of pain also can indicate trouble. Surprisingly, mild chest pain can signal a heart attack, while some severe pains may not always be serious (such as pains due to sore muscles).

Your health—and, in some cases, your life—depends on knowing when chest pain indicates a serious condition that needs immediate attention.

Important: If you experience any feeling in your chest that's new or that you don't understand—especially if it persists—consult a doctor.

Some possible causes of chest pain—and what each may mean...

IT'S THE HEART!

• **Heart attack.**

Typical symptoms: Pressure, squeezing or heaviness behind the breastbone in the center of your chest, often associated with nausea, sweating, light-headedness or shortness of breath.

This could signal a heart attack, caused when blood flow to the heart is cut off by a blood clot in a coronary artery. Many people mistakenly think the heart is located on the left side of the chest (because they feel their heartbeat there), but it's actually in the center—so pain in the mid-chest should be taken seriously.

What you may not know: It's common to have a history of milder chest pain in the center of the chest preceding (by up to two weeks in some cases) the more severe pain of a heart attack. Pain from a heart attack also can radi-

Albert Miller, MD, professor of clinical medicine (cardiology) at Northwestern University's Feinberg School of Medicine and a clinical cardiologist at Northwestern Memorial Hospital, both in Chicago. He is the author of *Chest Pain—When & When Not to Worry*.

ate to one or both shoulders and arms (especially the left) or to the neck or jaw.

If you suffer mid-chest pain, call 911 and get to a hospital emergency department as quickly as possible! Do not wait to see if the pain goes away. Prompt treatment will minimize damage to your heart muscle and may save your life.

• **Stable angina pectoris.**

Typical symptoms: A crushing pain or mild-to-moderate squeezing, tightness or heaviness in the middle of the chest brought on by physical exertion, emotional stress or cold weather—all of which can increase the work of the heart. Pain is relieved by rest and usually lasts five minutes or less.

The pain of angina pectoris indicates insufficient blood flow to the heart muscle, usually due to partial blockages from fatty deposits that narrow one or more coronary arteries. While this pain isn't a medical emergency like a heart attack, it's a sign that you need to schedule a doctor visit.

• **Unstable angina pectoris.**

Typical symptoms: Unexplained pain (not necessarily severe) in the middle of the chest, tightness, constriction, squeezing or heaviness...and/or pain in the neck, left shoulder or left arm. These symptoms persist and/or may occur while you're at rest or awaken you at night.

Associated with significantly impaired blood flow to the heart muscle, unstable angina pectoris frequently indicates an impending heart attack. If you experience these symptoms, go to a hospital emergency department immediately.

THE HEART IS NOT THE CULPRIT

• **Lung condition.**

Typical symptoms: A sharp pain in either side of the chest, made worse by breathing.

This may indicate a lung problem such as pneumonia...pleurisy (inflammation of the surface lining of a lung)...or a blood clot that formed elsewhere (usually in a leg vein), broke off and traveled to the lungs. A pulmonary blood clot is life-threatening and requires hospitalization and treatment.

• **Aortic dissection.**

Typical symptoms: Usually excruciating, tearing pain in the chest or between the shoulder blades.

This pain arises from "dissection" of the aorta (the large artery that carries blood from the left ventricle to the rest of the body) and occurs when blood from the aorta burrows between the layers of its wall. This condition is a major emergency requiring immediate medical care.

LESS SERIOUS CHEST PAINS

• **Acid reflux.**

Typical symptoms: A burning discomfort in the middle of the chest that may radiate to the throat, usually after eating spicy food or drinking alcohol or coffee. Acid reflux (in which stomach contents wash up into the esophagus) is not an emergency but warrants treatment if it is recurrent.

• **Musculoskeletal problem.**

Typical symptoms: Pain in the chest, shoulder or upper back that is aggravated by specific movements, such as reaching for an object or putting an item on a high shelf.

These pains are typically due to a musculoskeletal problem, such as a strained muscle or tendon or arthritis. Each merits medical attention, but none is a serious health threat.

Important: Sharp, shooting pains in the chest that last just a few seconds also can be musculoskeletal in origin. These transitory pains are usually insignificant.

• **Neck problem.**

Typical symptoms: Pain on the side of the neck and/or across the right or left shoulder, and sometimes also in the upper chest on the same side of the affected shoulder.

This can be caused by a ruptured spinal disk in the neck. Treatment depends on the severity of the problem.

• **Panic attack.**

Typical symptoms: Breathing problems (such as shortness of breath or hyperventilation), perhaps accompanied by chest discomfort. These symptoms should be evaluated by a doctor.

Heart Attack–The Red Flags That Too Often Get Overlooked

Antonio M. Gotto, Jr., MD, DPhil, dean emeritus, Lewis Thomas University Professor and cochairman of the board of overseers for Weill Cornell Medical College in New York City. He is also coauthor of *The Living Heart in the 21st Century*.

It's common for women and men to fail to tell their doctors about elusive heart disease symptoms that often precede a heart attack. If recognized, these symptoms often can be effectively treated to stop a heart attack before it occurs.

WHAT GETS MISSED

Most people do not realize just how important it is to report new symptoms during a doctor visit. With heart disease, in particular, there can be such a wide range of mild and/or fleeting changes in the heart, that the way you describe any possible abnormality to your doctor can mean the difference between an accurate diagnosis and a missed one. That's why you always should be sure to include details whenever you tell your physician about a symptom.

Examples: Don't just say that you're short of breath—do you feel this way all the time or just when you're climbing stairs? And don't just say that you've noticed changes in your heartbeat—is it too fast, too slow, fluttery, irregular, etc.?

Other important symptoms that should be discussed…

• **Intermittent chest pain.** The majority of heart attacks are preceded by the development of atherosclerosis, accumulations of fatty deposits in the arteries that inhibit the normal flow of blood and oxygen. When these deposits restrict blood flow to the heart, the result can be myocardial ischemia, a condition that typically causes chest pain due to a lack of oxygen.

Main symptom: Sharp chest pains or pressure that can last anywhere from a few seconds to about five minutes. This type of chest pain, known as angina, usually occurs during physical exertion, such as climbing stairs or working in the yard. It also can occur during cold weather, which causes blood vessels to constrict, or during stressful situations, which can increase demands on the heart and cause it to beat faster.

Exceptions: Angina isn't always painful, and you won't necessarily feel it in your chest. Patients with myocardial ischemia affecting the base of the heart might have abdominal discomfort instead of chest pain. (Some people mistake it for heartburn.) People with diabetes who have nerve damage, or those with a high pain threshold, might have no pain at all.

My advice: Suspect angina when you have chest and/or abdominal pain that occurs only during physical exertion. Rest if you experience pain in these areas. The pain should go away within five minutes if angina is the cause. In this case, call your doctor promptly to make an appointment. Call 911 if the pain isn't gone after five minutes.

• **Shortness of breath (dyspnea).** It is one of the main symptoms of heart disease, yet patients don't always mention it because they attribute it to other factors, such as smoking, advancing age and/or a lack of exercise.

Important: Shortness of breath can be caused by atypical angina. These angina patients do not experience pain as the main symptom. They are more likely to have episodes of breathlessness, weakness, fatigue and/or sweating. This is particularly common in older adults and those with diabetes.

My advice: To distinguish "normal" shortness of breath from a heart-related condition, ask yourself whether the dyspnea is out of proportion to what you're doing.

For example, people do not normally get winded from unloading the dishwasher or walking to the mailbox. If you do—and you haven't been diagnosed with a condition to explain it, such as lung disease—see your doctor. Also, any change in your tolerance for exercise could indicate a heart problem. If you experience unexplained shortness of breath or a significant change in your tolerance for exercise, see your doctor as soon as possible.

Call 911 if you have severe shortness of breath that comes on suddenly, especially if it's accompanied by chest pain, fainting or nausea—these could be signs of heart attack or pulmonary embolism.

• **Palpitations.** Everyone has occasional changes in the heart's pumping rhythm. You might notice that your heartbeat is rapid, pounding or fluttering, particularly during exercise or when you're stressed. The heart is probably still pumping blood effectively, but you'll want to talk to your doctor anyway.

The risk: Heart palpitations can indicate that you have arrhythmias, problems with the heart's electrical systems. A heartbeat that's too rapid (tachycardia), too slow (bradycardia) or irregular (atrial fibrillation, among others) can be life-threatening.

Example: Atrial fibrillation is common in older adults. The heart usually regains its normal rhythm within a few seconds, but not always. There's an increased risk for stroke if the irregular heartbeat continues for more than 24 hours.

My advice: Call 911 immediately if palpitations are accompanied by other symptoms, such as fainting, heavy sweating or extreme anxiety—all of which can signal a heart attack or an impending one. If you have palpitations without other symptoms, make an appointment to see your doctor as soon as possible.

• **Leg pain.** It's normal to experience occasional "charley horses," cramps in the muscles in your legs. It's not normal to have frequent pain in a foot, calf, thigh or buttock when you're walking or doing other activities. Leg pain that develops during exertion is often a sign of peripheral artery disease, a form of atherosclerosis that occurs in arteries in the leg. Patients with peripheral artery disease have a high risk of having (or developing) cardiovascular disease.

My advice: If you notice aching, cramping or pain in one or both legs during physical activity, see your doctor. Peripheral artery disease also can cause a sensation of "burning," tingling or numbness in the legs and/or feet. These symptoms indicate that the leg isn't getting enough oxygen-rich blood—and there's a good chance that your heart arteries are also at risk. With advanced peripheral artery disease, the symptoms occur even at rest.

• **Hair loss on the legs/feet.** Sedentary patients with peripheral artery disease might not notice leg pain or cramps. However, they might have other "silent" symptoms that indicate impaired circulation, including hair loss on the legs and/or feet.

My advice: See your physician as soon as possible if you notice hair loss on the legs or feet or one of the other possible signs of peripheral artery disease—one leg/foot that is colder than the other...sores that are slow to heal...a "shine" to the skin...or thick, slow-growing toenails. The symptoms may occur in both legs, but patients often report that only one leg is affected.

WHEN TO CALL 911

Severe chest pain (often described as "crushing" pain) is the heart attack symptom that everyone knows about—and fears. You most likely are having a heart attack if you have severe, unexplained chest pain that lasts longer than 20 minutes. But do not wait that long before getting help.

Call 911 even if your chest pain has lasted just a few minutes—or if you do not have chest pain but are experiencing other symptoms that could indicate a heart attack, such as unexplained nausea, breaking out in a cold sweat, dizziness, shortness of breath or extreme anxiety accompanied by a feeling of impending doom.

Emergency personnel may advise you to chew aspirin while you wait for help to arrive, so always keep a bottle of aspirin handy.

The Hidden Heart Disease Even Doctors Miss

Holly S. Andersen, MD, attending cardiologist and director of Education and Outreach at the Ronald O. Perelman Heart Institute of New York-Presbyterian Hospital in New York City and medical adviser to the Women's Heart Alliance. She is an expert in the field of heart disease in women.

It's hard to imagine that with all the technology available today, heart disease could be completely missed. But that's exactly what's frequently occurring with a tricky heart condition known as small vessel disease or coronary microvascular disease (MVD).

Here's what happens: Patients, most often women, have chest pain, other symptoms that suggest heart disease or even heart attacks. But when doctors examine their coronary arteries, they find no evidence of blockage and often rule out heart disease.

Result: Patients go without the vital treatment they need.

Mystery solved: The problem in these cases, researchers have recently discovered, often lies in the tiny blood vessels—which can't be seen with the naked eye or conventional heart disease testing—that branch off the larger coronary arteries in the heart.

Researchers still have much to learn about MVD, but here's what's known now and what you can do to protect yourself...

A DIFFERENT KIND OF HEART DISEASE

The most common variety of coronary heart disease (CHD) is caused by atherosclerotic plaques—cholesterol-containing deposits that pile up and narrow one or more of the large arteries that carry blood to the heart, restricting flow. When the heart gets too little blood to meet its needs—during exertion, for example—people with CHD have chest pain (angina). And if blood flow is restricted even further—usually due to a clot lodged in the narrowed artery—a heart attack and death may occur.

Plaque is often involved in MVD, too. But instead of accumulating in clumps that block off segments of specific coronary arteries, cholesterol is deposited more evenly inside whole areas of microscopic circulation. Additionally, in MVD the walls of the tiny arteries are injured or diseased—instead of opening wider to allow more blood to reach the heart during exercise or at times of emotional stress, they tighten up, constricting blood flow when it's needed most.

The reason for this is unclear, but it seems that at least some of the time, it's due to malfunction of the endothelial cells that line the blood vessels. The resulting symptoms can be indistinguishable from garden-variety CHD—and the risk for heart attack may be just as real.

DO YOU HAVE MICROVASCULAR DSEASE?

Diabetes and high blood pressure raise one's risk for MVD, as does CHD. High cholesterol, obesity, smoking and a lack of physical activity are risk factors, too, and like CHD, MVD becomes more common with advancing age.

Symptoms of MVD can be identical to the classic signs of CHD—pain, a squeezing sensation or pressure in the chest, usually during activity or emotional stress. The discomfort can also occur in the shoulders, arms, neck or jaw.

MVD tip-off: Painful episodes of MVD usually last longer—more than 10 minutes, and sometimes longer than 30 minutes—than those of classic CHD.

Other symptoms of MVD: Fatigue or lack of energy, trouble sleeping and shortness of breath. Women are particularly likely to have these vague manifestations rather than the kind of distinct chest pain that we usually associate with heart disease. Forty percent of women don't have chest pain even while having a heart attack, whether it's caused by CHD or MVD.

Another clue: With MVD, patients often notice symptoms during daily activities and/or during times of mental stress rather than during times of physical exertion as is more often the case with CHD.

GETTING A DIAGNOSIS

The standard tests for heart disease may not uncover MVD. If you suspect you have the condition, be sure to see a cardiologist with significant experience in treating MVD. An academic medical center is the best place to find such a doctor. *He/she may be able to diagnose it from your symptoms, medical history and earlier test results, or he may order additional tests...*

- **Nuclear imaging,** which uses a radioactive compound injected into the bloodstream to reveal a detailed image of the heart and blood flow through the arteries, including microcirculation.

• **Magnetic resonance imaging (MRI)** to produce a picture of the heart and its circulation without subjecting the patient to dye or radiation.

• **Positron emission tomography (PET),** which provides information on metabolism in the heart. This can uncover certain areas that aren't getting enough fuel and oxygen, suggesting MVD.

IF YOU HAVE MVD

If MVD is diagnosed, the goal is to keep it from progressing and to prevent heart attack and stroke. *Key strategies...*

• **Tweak your diet, and punch up your exercise routine.** A healthy eating plan, such as the Mediterranean diet, emphasizes fruits, vegetables, legumes, whole grains and nuts and fish, which contain healthy fats. Weight control and exercise reduce heart disease risk overall and also reduce blood pressure and help prevent diabetes, which are additional MVD risk factors. Beyond its general cardiovascular benefits, regular exercise appears to improve the function of the endothelial cells that line blood vessels and function poorly in MVD.

• **Get help from medication.** Doctors prescribe the same medications to treat MVD as for CHD—to reduce blood pressure and cholesterol. Aspirin or other drugs to reduce clotting risk are recommended as well.

Some evidence suggests that statins may be particularly useful because they not only reduce cholesterol but also improve endothelial function and relax the muscles around tiny blood vessels.

Similarly, calcium channel blockers, such as *amlodipine* (Norvasc), and ACE inhibitors, like *enalapril* (Vasotec), may be good choices for lowering blood pressure because they too help keep arteries open.

• **Get treated for anemia if you have it.** Anemia (low red blood cell count) may slow the growth of cells that help repair artery walls. This condition is treated with iron or B-12 supplements.

Note: If you have CHD and MVD (it's possible to have both) and have had angioplasty, a stent or bypass surgery, be aware that these procedures do not help MVD.

Better Treatment for Most Angina Patients

Harmony R. Reynolds, MD, cardiologist and the Saul J. Farber assistant professor of medicine, Leon H. Charney Division of Cardiology, NYU Langone Medical Center, New York City.

People with partly blocked coronary arteries may feel chest pain (angina) when walking or having a cardiac stress test, but the pain goes away if they stop and rest. For these stable angina patients, drugs—particularly statins—often are better than surgical stent insertion.

Important: Some patients with stable angina do need stents or surgery—talk to your doctor.

Gout Drug for Angina

Allan D. Struthers, MD, professor of cardiovascular medicine, Centre for Cardiovascular & Lung Biology, University of Dundee School of Medicine, Dundee, UK.

Angina sufferers may benefit from gout drug.

Study: Among 65 adults with heart disease and stable angina (chest pain that occurs with activity or stress), those who took 600 mg of the gout medication *allopurinol* (Aloprim) daily for six weeks could exercise longer before chest pain occurred than those who took a placebo.

Theory: Allopurinol blocks a crucial enzyme, reducing oxygen demand during exercise.

If you have stable angina: Ask your doctor about allupurinol. Side effects may include upset stomach, diarrhea and drowsiness.

"Massage" Therapy For Angina

C. Richard Conti, MD, professor of medicine, division of cardiovascular medicine, University of Florida, Gainesville, Florida.

If climbing stairs, walking fast or running brings on a crushing pain in your chest, you may be experiencing angina. You should not treat this lightly. Angina is a symptom of ischemia, which occurs when blood flow to your heart slows, starving the muscle of the oxygen it needs. Though the pain typically subsides when you rest, it's not safe to ignore it. Angina is almost always a symptom of coronary artery disease, and it should be evaluated by your physician.

A SAFE AND NONINVASIVE TREATMENT

First-line therapy for angina typically involves addressing the underlying problem, according to C. Richard Conti, MD, a professor of medicine at the University of Florida in Gainesville, which is usually high blood pressure, high cholesterol or diabetes. Some patients are found to have blocked arteries, which conventional Western medicine generally treats with angioplasty or stenting. Both of these can be effective, short-term solutions to open the arteries, but Dr. Conti said that some patients find they still experience angina. Also, there are some patients for whom such invasive treatments aren't advisable, due to underlying medical problems. Fortunately, there's another solution that is quite effective—external counterpulsation (ECP) therapy, which significantly reduces or eliminates angina about 70% of the time.

In contrast to the other treatments available, ECP isn't all that complicated or high tech. The technology itself resembles a large, comfortable reclining chair. The patient sits and a technician wraps three pressure cuffs—similar to but slightly larger than standard blood pressure cuffs—around the calves, lower thighs and upper thighs or buttocks. The cuffs inflate and deflate, compressing and releasing blood vessels in the limbs to move blood toward the heart. This "unloads" the heart by relaxing pressure in the arteries while the heart is pumping, Dr. Conti explains. As the cuffs inflate and deflate in harmony with your cardiac cycle, they encourage optimal coronary blood and oxygen flow. This action relieves chest pain and improves exercise tolerance, which means that you can begin to work out again without discomfort—another plus for heart health.

A standard course of ECP treatment consists of 35 one-hour outpatient sessions over a period of seven weeks. This is a big time commitment, Dr. Conti acknowledges, but he finds that angina sufferers are willing to put in the time if it gets rid of their pain. If the treatment is successful but angina eventually recurs, it can be repeated. Outcome varies—some patients obtain relief that lasts for years.

Note: While ECP is generally safe, doctors do not recommend it for people who have conditions such as phlebitis, peripheral artery disease or a leaky aortic valve, because it can lead to complications.

MORE EXTENSIVE USE OF ECP IN THE FUTURE?

Health insurers generally cover ECP for angina but only after standard medical and surgical care fails to control it. Dr. Conti notes that treatment may be beneficial earlier, for example as a complement to medical management before surgery proves necessary. Since this has not been demonstrated in trials, it's not typically covered by insurance. Data also suggests that ECP may benefit people with heart failure, but again further study is needed. If new research continues to demonstrate expanded benefits, however, treatment—and coverage for treatment—is likely to be extended as well.

Infection Protection for Cardiac Implant Patients

Bruce Wilkoff, MD, is director of Cardiac Pacing and Tachyarrhythmia Devices at the Cleveland Clinic and a professor of medicine at Cleveland Clinic Lerner College of Medicine at Case Western Reserve University in Ohio. He is also the president of the Heart Rhythm Society. HRSonline.org

Individuals with cardiac implantable electronic devices (CIEDs), such as pacemakers and cardioverter defibrillators, are at increased risk of infection. Sadly, 18% of patients with CIED infections do not survive for a year. For those who live, treatment can be economically devastating, with an average cost of more than $146,000.

Most CIED-related infections are caused by *Staphylococcus aureus* or *Staphylococcus epidermidis* bacteria. Infection can get started if, at the time of surgery, bacteria contaminate the surface of the device, the patient's skin or the area in the chest beneath the skin where the surgeon creates a "pocket" to hold the CIED. The surgeon's scrupulous attention to proper sterile techniques can greatly reduce but not completely eliminate this risk. Sometimes an infection develops soon after surgery, but in other cases it becomes apparent only after a year or more has passed.

Compared with the infection risk after an initial implantation, the risk is four to six times greater when a patient has another surgery to replace a device (for instance, because its battery is depleted, a component has stopped working or the patient requires a device with additional features).

Reason: Reopening the pocket where the device was placed may allow a colony of bacteria that the body had previously "walled off" to overwhelm the immune system's defenses. Since a CIED typically lasts about four to eight years, a patient is quite likely to need such repeat surgery.

Warning signs: There is no one symptom that appears in all cases of infection. *But see your doctor quickly if any of the following occur…*

- **You run a fever of 101 degrees or higher.**
- **There is swelling, redness or pain at the site where the device was implanted.**
- **The skin covering the device becomes dimpled or oozes.**
- **The device appears to be shifting position.**

Be especially vigilant about watching for such signs if you have diabetes or compromised kidney function. Either of these conditions can increase your susceptibility to CIED-related infection.

If you do get a CIED infection: Both the device and all of its leads (wires that deliver energy from the CIED to the heart muscle) need to be removed and replaced.

Reason: Staph bacteria can bind to a sticky substance called fibronectin that circulates in the blood and clings to the surface of implanted devices. Once this biofilm of persistent bacterial bugs takes hold, it is very antibiotic-resistant and almost impossible to get rid of without removing the device.

Before and after the surgery, for a period that can range from several days to several weeks, you receive antibiotics through an IV. You may be given a temporary pacemaker or an external defibrillator during this time. When the infection is gone, your doctor will schedule another surgery to implant a new CIED, often before you go home.

To reduce your risk for a subsequent infection: It is best to use an experienced cardiologist who does a high volume of device implantation and device change procedures. Ask the doctor and/or hospital whether they report the number of CIED procedures they do on a website or in a booklet—the larger the number, the better the outcomes tend to be. Also, patients sometimes ask to have the CIED implanted underneath a muscle so that it's less visible. But since this makes it more difficult to remove if an infection does develop, it's important to discuss the pros and cons with your doctor before opting for such placement. And, of course, follow your doctor's advice on minimizing CIED infection risk after surgery.

The Diet That Cures Heart Disease

Caldwell B. Esselstyn, Jr., MD, surgeon, clinician and researcher at the Cleveland Clinic for more than 35 years. He is author of *Prevent and Reverse Heart Disease: The Revolutionary, Scientifically Proven, Nutrition-Based Cure.* DrEsselstyn.com

In the mid-1980s, 17 people with severe heart disease had just about given up hope. They had undergone every available treatment, including drugs and surgery—all had failed. The group had experienced 49 cardiovascular events, including four heart attacks, three strokes, 15 cases of increased angina and seven bypass surgeries. Five of the patients were expected to die within a year.

Twelve years later, every one of the 17 was alive. They had had no cardiovascular events. The progression of their heart disease had been stopped—and, in many cases, reversed. Their angina went away—for some, within three weeks. In fact, they became virtually heart-attack proof. And there are hundreds of other patients with heart disease who have achieved the same remarkable results. *What you need to know...*

HOW THE DAMAGE IS DONE

Every year, more than half a million Americans die of coronary artery disease (CAD). Three times that number suffer heart attacks. In total, half of American men and one-third of women will have some form of heart disease during their lifetimes.

Heart disease develops in the endothelium, the lining of the arteries. There, endothelial cells manufacture a compound called nitric oxide that accomplishes four tasks crucial for healthy circulation...

- **Keeps blood smoothly flowing,** rather than becoming sticky and clotted.
- **Allows arteries to widen when the heart needs more blood,** such as when you run up a flight of stairs.
- **Stops muscle cells in arteries from growing into plaque**—the fatty gunk that blocks blood vessels.
- **Decreases inflammation in the plaque—** the process that can trigger a rupture in the cap or surface of a plaque, starting the clot-forming, artery-clogging cascade that causes a heart attack.

The type and amount of fat in the typical Western diet—from animal products, dairy foods and concentrated oils—assaults endothelial cells, cutting their production of nitric oxide.

Study: A researcher at University of Maryland School of Medicine fed a 900-calorie fast-food breakfast containing 50 grams of fat (mostly from sausages and hash browns) to a group of students and then measured their endothelial function. For six hours, the students had severely compromised endothelial function and decreased nitric oxide production. Another group of students ate a 900-calorie, no-fat breakfast—and had no significant change in endothelial function.

If a single meal can do that kind of damage, imagine the damage done by three fatty meals a day, seven days a week, 52 weeks a year.

PLANT-BASED NUTRITION

You can prevent, stop or reverse heart disease with a plant-based diet. *Here's what you can't eat—and what you can...*

- **What you cannot eat...**
  - No meat, poultry, fish or eggs. You will get plenty of protein from plant-based sources.
  - No dairy products. That means no butter, cheese, cream, ice cream, yogurt or milk—even skim milk, which, though lower in fat, still contains animal protein.
  - No oil of any kind—not a drop. That includes all oils, even virgin olive oil and canola.

What you may not know: At least 14% of olive oil is saturated fat—every bit as aggressive in promoting heart disease as the saturated fat in roast beef. A diet that includes oils—including monounsaturated oils from olive oil and canola oil—may slow the progression of heart disease, but it will not stop or reverse the disease.

  - Generally, no nuts or avocados. If you are eating a plant-based diet to prevent heart disease, you can have moderate amounts of nuts and avocados as long as your total cholesterol remains below 150 milligrams per deciliter (mg/dL). If you have heart disease and want to stop or reverse it, you should not eat these foods.

- **What you can eat...**
  - All vegetables.
  - Legumes—beans, peas, lentils.
  - Whole grains and products that are made from them, such as bread and pasta—as long as they do not contain added fats. Do not eat refined grains, which have been stripped of much of their fiber and nutrients. Avoid white rice and "enriched" flour products, which are found in many pastas, breads, bagels and baked goods.

- Fruits—but heart patients should limit consumption to three pieces a day and avoid drinking pure fruit juices. Too much fruit rapidly raises blood sugar, triggering a surge of insulin from the pancreas—which stimulates the liver to manufacture more cholesterol.
- Certain beverages, including water, seltzer water, oat milk, hazelnut milk, almond milk, no-fat soy milk, coffee and tea. Alcohol is fine in moderation (no more than two servings a day for men and one for women).

- **Supplements**

For maximum health, take five supplements daily...

- Multivitamin/mineral supplement.
- Vitamin B-12—1,000 micrograms (mcg).
- Calcium—1,000 milligrams (mg) (1,200 mg if you're over 60).
- Vitamin D-3—1,000 international units (IU).
- Flaxseed meal (ground flaxseed)—one tablespoon for the omega-3 fatty acids it provides. Sprinkle it on cereal.

THE CHOLESTEROL CONNECTION

If you eat the typical, high-fat Western diet, even if you also take a cholesterol-lowering statin drug, you will not protect yourself from heart disease—because the fat in the diet will damage the endothelium cells that produce nitric oxide.

In a study in *The New England Journal of Medicine*, patients took huge doses of statin drugs to lower total cholesterol below 150 but didn't change their diets—and 25% experienced a new cardiovascular event or died within the next 30 months.

Recommended: Eat a plant-based diet, and ask your doctor if you should also take a cholesterol-lowering medication. Strive to maintain a total cholesterol of less than 150 and LDL ("bad" cholesterol) below 85.

MODERATION DOESN'T WORK

The most common objection physicians have to this diet is that their patients will not follow it. But many patients with heart disease who find out that they have a choice—between invasive surgery and nutritional changes that will stop and reverse the disease—willingly adopt the diet.

Why not eat a less demanding diet, such as the low-fat diet recommended by the American Heart Association or the Mediterranean Diet?

Surprising: Research shows that people who maintain a so-called low-fat diet of 29% of calories from fat have the same rate of heart attacks and strokes as people who don't.

Natural Therapies for Atrial Fibrillation

Mark A. Stengler, NMD, naturopathic doctor and founder of the Stengler Center for Integrative Medicine in Encinitas, California. He is author or coauthor of numerous books, including *The Natural Physician's Healing Therapies* and *Bottom Line's Prescription for Natural Cures*, and author of the newsletter *Health Revelations*. MarkStengler.com

With atrial fibrillation, the heart's two upper chambers (the atria) do not fully contract, so blood isn't pumped out completely. This causes heart palpitations, light-headedness, chest pain and weakness. Such symptoms call for immediate medical attention, since atrial fibrillation raises the risk of blood clots and stroke. Drugs such as *digoxin* (Lanoxin), *propranolol* (Inderal) and *diltiazem* (Cardizem) help to slow the heart rate but may cause fatigue and dizziness.

Natural therapies that improve conduction of electrical currents in heart cells may allow you to decrease your medication dosages, thereby reducing the drugs' side effects. Take fish oil supplements at 1,000 mg of combined eicosapentaenoic acid (EPA) and docosahexaenoic acid (DHA) twice daily. If you use blood thinners, such as aspirin or *warfarin* (Coumadin), ask your doctor before taking fish oil. Also take the amino acid derivative L-carnitine (1,000 mg twice daily)...coenzyme Q10 (200 mg to 300 mg daily)...and magnesium (250 mg twice daily).

Which Exercises Are Best For Heart and Lung Disease?

John P. Porcari, PhD, program director of the Clinical Exercise Physiology (CEP) program at the University of Wisconsin–La Crosse.

Everyone agrees that exercise is good for you. The goal for most people should be at least 150 minutes of moderate aerobic activity a week, plus strength training two days a week, according to the Centers for Disease Control and Prevention.

But what if you have a chronic condition, such as heart disease or COPD, that makes exercise difficult—or raises your concern about injury?

While exercise is helpful for most chronic health problems, some activities are likely to be easier, more beneficial and less risky than others.* *Best workouts for the following chronic conditions that can cause chest pain...*

CARDIOVASCULAR DISEASE

A key benefit of exercise is reduced heart attack risk. But if you have already had a heart attack or undergone bypass surgery...or have symptoms, such as chest pain (angina), that signal established heart disease, you may worry that physical exertion is too risky.

For the vast majority of people with heart disease, it's not—if it's supervised. This usually involves initial and periodic testing to establish safe levels of exercise and monitoring of heart rate and blood pressure for some sessions. Once you're cleared, you can do most sessions on your own.

When performed at the proper intensity, standard aerobic activities are usually suitable. This means you can most likely walk, jog, use a stationary bike or treadmill (or even participate in aerobic dance) as long as you do it at a moderate level that doesn't raise your heart rate too high. Talk to your doctor about the heart rate you should strive for.

Once you have that number, you may want to wear a heart rate monitor—several models are widely available for under $100.

Another option: Use the "Talk Test." If you can talk while exercising, this will indicate with 95% accuracy that your heart rate is in a safe range.

If you have hypertension: Higher-intensity exercise may trigger potentially dangerous spikes in your blood pressure—talk to your doctor about appropriate heart rate goals, and remember to breathe (do not hold your breath) and stay away from heavier weights when doing strength training.

Important: Be sure to ask your doctor to reevaluate your target heart rate if you change blood pressure medication—some drugs, such as beta-blockers, will affect your heart rate.

LUNG DISEASE

Asthma, one of the most common lung diseases in the US, generally does not interfere with exercise unless you are performing an activity that's especially strenuous, such as running, which can trigger an attack ("exercise-induced asthma").

With exercise-induced asthma, the triggers vary from person to person. For example, working out in the cold is generally to be avoided (but a face mask or scarf may warm air sufficiently). Very vigorous exercise, such as squash or mountain biking, can cause difficulties for some people with asthma, who may do better alternating brief periods of intense and slower-paced activity (as used in interval training). Know your own triggers.

Swimming is also a good choice —the high humidity helps prevent drying of the airways, which can trigger an asthma attack.

If you use an inhaler such as albuterol to treat an asthma attack: Ask your doctor about taking a dose immediately before you exercise to help prevent an attack, and always carry your inhaler with you throughout the activity.

If you have chronic obstructive pulmonary disease (COPD): Exercise doesn't improve lung function, but it does build muscle endurance and improve one's tolerance for the shortness of breath that often accompa-

*Always talk to your doctor before starting a new exercise program. If you have a chronic illness, it may be useful to consult a physical therapist for advice on exercise dos and don'ts for your particular situation.

nies COPD (a condition that typically includes chronic bronchitis and/or emphysema).

Aerobic exercises that work the lower body (like walking or stationary cycling) are good, but the Schwinn Airdyne or NuStep provides a lower- and upper-body workout with the option of stopping the upper-body workout if breathing becomes more difficult.

Devil's Grip: The Mysterious Infectious Pain

Richard O'Brien, MD, associate professor of emergency medicine at The Commonwealth Medical College of Pennsylvania in Scranton.

When I caught a glimpse of Clara, a local college basketball coach in her mid-30s, clutching her chest as she was wheeled from triage to a cardiac bed in the emergency department, I was quite surprised. I knew that she was a serious athlete herself, which, along with her age, put her at low risk for heart problems. Her chart also showed that she had no risk factors for vascular or lung disease and hadn't suffered any recent injuries.

Clara's story began to unfold. She explained that over the previous four days she had gradually developed a low-grade fever, chills and body aches. Then, suddenly, that morning, she had been stricken with severe, sharp spells of pain on the right side of her chest. Pain episodes occurred every hour or so and lasted about 30 minutes. When I asked Clara to take a deep breath, it was very uncomfortable for her, and the painful area of her chest was extraordinarily tender to touch.

All these clues made me worry that Clara might have a pulmonary embolism (a potentially deadly blood clot in the lungs). An aneurysm in a major blood vessel, or even a case of pneumonia with unusual signs and symptoms, were also possibilities, though less likely. To see whether Clara had one of these very dangerous conditions, I ordered a "stat" CT scan of her chest. I was pleased but puzzled when her chest CT and the blood work that had just been analyzed were entirely normal.

Just as Clara had described, her chest pain continued to come and go every hour or so. To see if there was anything in her medical history that might give us more clues, I contacted Clara's family doctor as well as a cardiologist. Clara's family doctor admitted her to the cardiac unit and mentioned that the case sounded like the "Devil's Grip," a rather antiquated but entirely legitimate medical term for a rare condition that causes intense chest pain.

As it turns out, Clara's doctor was right. After 48 hours, she had fully recovered. We also got back positive results for Clara on a serum antibody test to Coxsackie B, the virus that causes pleurodynia (also known as the "Devil's Grip"). This viral infection of the muscles of the chest wall and often the upper abdomen causes excruciating pain that comes and goes in spasms for two to six days, then generally vanishes. Coxsackie B can be easily spread from one person to another—for example, by kissing, by sharing eating utensils or a drinking straw or by eating food that's been contaminated with the virus. Usually, a person's immune system does a good job of disarming the virus so the infection causes only a mild, flulike illness, but some people, like Clara, aren't so lucky.

Lesson learned: In rare cases, severe chest pain is due to a relatively benign illness, rather than a deadly cardiac, pulmonary, vascular or abdominal condition. Still, chest pain should always be immediately evaluated—no matter what your age or how healthy you think you are.

Hope for Pulmonary Hypertension

James Calvin, MD, professor of medicine, director, section of cardiology, department of internal medicine, Rush University Medical Center, Chicago.

Sometimes it is not technology or a new medication that makes the greatest difference in medical care but something far simpler. A new approach to treating pulmonary hypertension—a particularly dangerous type of high blood pressure that affects the arteries leading from the heart to the lungs—puts top specialists together as a "team" to work collaboratively with patients, with the goal of delivering a far better quality of care.

While specialists have always discussed their patients with one another, this approach takes the concept much further. Teamwork is built into every aspect of a patient's care to comprehensively address the many different causes of this complex disease. With this approach the doctors' combined specialized training and clinical experience leads to more accurate diagnoses and more successful treatment.

Patients can even schedule appointments with several different specialists on the same day in the same office, and the doctors can conveniently consult with one another.

HARD TO DIAGNOSE

Pulmonary hypertension is not uncommon, and doctors are well aware of its signs and causes, but it can nonetheless be tricky to diagnose because its symptoms mimic those of so many other heart and lung diseases.

This condition develops in people whose hearts have had to pump especially hard to push blood through increasingly stiff and narrow arteries. It has many causes, including heart, lung and liver problems...living at altitudes higher than 8,000 feet...and heredity in some cases can contribute, too. When the body must expend intense effort to bring blood through the lungs to the left side of the heart the eventual result is weakening of the heart muscle on the right side leading to heart failure or other potentially fatal complications. Shortness of breath is usually the first warning sign of pulmonary hypertension, but other common symptoms include fatigue...dizziness...fainting...chest pain...leg and ankle swelling...palpitations (fast heartbeat)...and bluish lips and skin.

How pulmonary hypertension is diagnosed: An echocardiogram, a form of ultrasound that enables your doctor to get a good look at your heart and pulmonary arteries, is usually the first step toward diagnosis. If "problems" are found, the next step is right heart catheterization, to measure how well blood moves through and to look for blockages or other abnormalities. Doctors often order other tests to obtain additional information on the extent of the patient's problem, possibly a chest X-ray, CT scan, MRI and/or pulmonary function assessment (a measure of how well the lungs take in and release air).

LIFE WITH PULMONARY HYPERTENSION

While treatment is complex, inroads have been made. A variety of medications may be used, and together, they can allow many patients to continue to live their lives fairly normally. *These may include...*

- **Vasodilators.** These drugs—including *epoprostenol* (Flolan) and *iloprost* (Ventavis)—widen blood vessels and reduce scarring in them. Patients used to have to come to the hospital or a doctor's office for intravenous (IV) administration of this therapy, but now new drugs can be taken orally by patients at home.
- **Endothelin Receptor Agonists.** ERAs—such as *bosentan* (Tracleer) or *ambrisentan* (Letairis)—block endothelin, a substance in blood vessel walls that causes them to narrow.
- **Calcium channel blockers.** Though these were once the first line of treatment, they work only 5% of the time.
- **Other drugs.** Your physician may also prescribe an anticoagulant such as *warfarin* (Coumadin)...a diuretic to prevent fluid accumulation...*sildenafil* (Revatio) to relax smooth muscle in pulmonary arteries...digoxin to help the heart pump blood...and/or oxygen to help you breathe.
- **Surgical treatments.** If drugs alone cannot control your condition, options include open-heart surgery to create an opening between the right and left chambers of the heart and relieve pressure on the right side...and, in very severe cases, a lung or heart-lung transplant (in patients with a diseased lung).

PUT YOURSELF ON THE TEAM

When you have pulmonary hypertension, it's vital to control any other underlying conditions (for example, religiously take your blood pressure medications).

For the best quality of life, keep your focus on making sensible, healthful daily lifestyle choices...

- **Get lots of rest.** Listen to your body. When you are tired, take a nap.
- **Follow a healthy diet.** In particular, avoid salt—which can increase swelling in your legs. Eat more whole foods and fewer salt-laden processed products.
- **Stay active.** Ask your doctor what level of exercise is safe for you.
- **Don't smoke.** Smoking severely damages your arteries, heart and lungs.
- **Avoid stress.** Improve your quality of life by meditating or practicing yoga or tai chi.
- **Eliminate saunas and hot baths.** These can cause your blood pressure to drop dangerously low.
- **Avoid high altitudes (including air travel).** Low oxygen levels worsen symptoms such as shortness of breath.

Pulmonary Embolism: Better Blood Clot Detection

Paul D. Stein, MD, professor of medicine, department of internal medicine, Wayne State University School of Medicine, Detroit.

Background: Computed tomography (CT) scans of the chest are used to detect pulmonary embolism, a potentially fatal blood clot in a lung artery.

Recent finding: In a study of 824 people, researchers evaluated the accuracy of chest CT scans alone or when combined with leg CT scans.

Result: Chest CT scans alone detected suspected clots in 83% of patients, while combined chest and leg scans detected clots in 90%.

Reason: CT scans of legs, where pulmonary embolisms usually originate, improve detection of pulmonary embolism.

If your doctor suspects a pulmonary embolism: Ask him/her if a leg CT scan should be done in addition to a chest CT scan.

What's That Spot on Your Lung?

Andrew J. Kaufman, MD, expert in advanced minimally invasive thoracic surgery and thoracic surgical oncology.

Imagine for a moment that your doctor has told you to get a routine chest X-ray or CT scan because you are having chest pain... are about to have shoulder surgery...or may have cracked a rib.

Then your doctor calls to say that the test unexpectedly detected a "spot" on your lung. Your first thought is, It might be lung cancer!...but take a deep breath.

Here are the steps you need to take to preserve your health and your sanity...

STEP 1: **Don't panic.** Most lung spots (dense areas within the lung that appear as white, shadowy areas on imaging tests) are not cancer. In fact, when doctors screen high-risk patients (people over age 55 who have smoked roughly 30 "pack years"—a pack year is defined as smoking one pack of cigarettes a day for a year) specifically for lung cancer, only about 1% to 2% of nodules that are detected on CT scans are cancerous.

When the spot is found incidentally—that is, during an imaging test that wasn't given because cancer was suspected—the risk is even lower.

Many conditions that don't have anything to do with cancer can cause a spot on the lung. *These include...*

- **Infection from tuberculosis,** pneumonia, bronchitis or other illness involving the lungs. (For more on infectious diseases and pain, see chapter 12, "Infectious Diseases.")
- **Inflammation from an autoimmune disease**—rheumatoid arthritis, for example, is a common cause of inflammatory lung nodules (see chapter 3, "Autoimmune and Related Diseases," for more information).
- **Scarring from pulmonary fibrosis or other lung disease.**
- **Environmental irritants,** such as asbestos, coal dust or silicone.

• **Environmental infection,** such as histoplasmosis, caused by fungus spores in bird or bat droppings. People can be exposed while demolishing old buildings, for example, or by spending time in bat-filled caves.

STEP 2: **Talk about your history.** If you've been told that you have a spot on your lung, make an appointment with the doctor who knows you best to review your medical history...take stock of your lung cancer risk...and decide your next steps.

First, your doctor, often in consultation with a radiologist, will want to compare the latest chest X-ray or CT scan with any previous imaging tests of your chest. It is possible that the spot has been there for years but wasn't previously identified. If the spot was present and hasn't grown for many years, the chance that it is malignant is low.

Next, discuss your recent health and personal risk factors for lung cancer with your doctor. Have you had a cough, the flu or a severe cold? Do you have an autoimmune disease? Have you had any risky environmental exposures? These all have the potential to cause lung spots.

If you have a history of another malignancy somewhere in your body, your doctor will want to rule out a metastasis to the lungs.

Of course, smoking history is very significant. Smokers have a higher risk for lung cancer...former smokers have a lower risk than active smokers...and nonsmokers have the lowest risk. For everyone, however, the risk for lung cancer increases with age.

Important: For reasons no one understands, the incidence of lung cancer is rising among never-smokers, especially women. Therefore, people who have never smoked should not assume that they can't have lung cancer. Any lung spot should be evaluated by an expert even if you don't have serious risk factors for lung cancer.

STEP 3: **Get follow-up testing.** If your nodule was found incidentally, you'll need focused follow-up imaging. For most people, the best option is a low-dose CT (LDCT) scan without IV contrast. This test gives a clear view of the nodule with minimal radiation.

The dose of radiation used in an LDCT is about the same as that used in a standard mammogram. The LDCT will let doctors see the size and qualities of the nodule.

For example...*

• **Small nodules**—spots that are less than one-fifth of an inch (5 mm) are very low risk but should be followed with surveillance in most cases. For example, such nodules should usually be monitored for two years at set time intervals to reveal if there is any growth in the nodule. A stable nodule without growth for two years is safely considered benign.

• **Larger nodules**—spots that are about one-third of an inch (8 mm) or greater demand a thorough workup. This may include a positron emission tomography (PET) scan, which involves an injection of radioactive tracers that light up to indicate areas that may be cancerous and would require a biopsy for confirmation, or a needle or surgical biopsy if the person's risk factors are high and the radiographic appearance warrants a tissue diagnosis.

• **Spiky nodules**—or those with an irregular surface—are generally more concerning than smooth nodules.

• **Solid and part-solid nodules**—meaning they have a solid density measurement throughout the entire spot or some solid component—are typically more concerning than nonsolid nodules.

• **More is usually better.** If your doctor says that you have multiple nodules (that is, more than one), the nodules are less likely to be cancer.

Because surveillance is the most practical way to determine whether a spot is dangerous, it's important to get expert recommendations. That's why decisions regarding surveillance are usually made by a multidisciplinary team that includes pulmonary doctors, thoracic surgeons and radiologists.

*The sizes and characteristics of nodules that require follow-up (as well as the schedule for such testing) may vary depending on the medical facility where you are receiving care. Many medical centers use the Fleischner Guidelines for Pulmonary Nodules, FleischnerSociety.org.

Even if a nodule is deemed benign, depending on your personal medical history, your doctor may recommend a yearly follow-up scan.

For example, if a person has a close relative with cancer (a first-degree relative such as a parent or sibling) or a history of heavy smoking, he/she will likely need an annual screening to check for new nodules that may develop and possibly become cancerous.

Important: You should not settle for an X-ray as a follow-up. An LDCT provides greater detail.

Among current or former heavy smokers, LDCT has been shown to reduce the risk for lung cancer deaths due to early detection. In the National Lung Screening Trial, more than 53,000 men and women (ages 55 to 74) who were current or former heavy smokers were randomly assigned to receive annual screenings with either LDCT or standard chest X-ray for three consecutive years. The LDCT group had 20% fewer lung cancer deaths than the X-ray group.

STEP 4: **Get a closer look.** If follow-up scans show that a nodule is getting larger and/or changing in appearance, your physician will need to take a biopsy to determine whether it's malignant.

If the nodule is easy to reach—for example, in the airway—a biopsy may be done with a very thin lighted instrument that is threaded through the mouth or nose and down the throat to snip off a piece of the nodule.

A needle biopsy may be preferred if the nodule is in the peripheral lung or near the chest wall.

A surgical biopsy that involves making an incision to remove a tissue sample may be needed if the approaches described above fail to make an adequate diagnosis or if the likelihood of cancer is considered high.

If lung cancer is diagnosed, then it is crucial to make a prompt appointment with a thoracic surgeon and/or oncologist to begin treatment.

Acid Reflux Can Cause Alarming Chest Pain

Julia Liu, MD, assistant professor, division of gastroenterology, University of Alberta Hospital, Edmonton, Canada.

In a study of 31 emergency room patients (median age 46) who complained of chest pain, 57% had acid levels in the esophagus high enough to indicate gastroesophageal reflux disease (GERD). Heartburn is the most common symptom of GERD, but the disorder also can cause chest pain, hoarseness and chronic cough with or without heartburn.

If you have any of these symptoms: Ask your doctor if GERD is a possible cause.

Caution: If you suffer severe chest pain that does not go away within five minutes, seek immediate medical care to rule out a heart-related cause.

The Hidden Cause of Chest Pain: It Could Be Your Esophagus

Richard Sheinbaum, MD, gastroenterologist and partner of Gastroenterology/Hepatology Associates in Stamford, Connecticut. He is an assistant clinical professor of medicine at Columbia University College of Physicians and Surgeons in New York City.

Heartburn is the most commonly recognized ailment associated with a malfunctioning esophagus, but there are some less well-known disorders involving this tube extending from your mouth to your stomach that can cause symptoms ranging from painful swallowing to unexplained chest pain. *What you need to know...*

WHAT GOES WRONG

The purpose of the esophagus is to deliver foods and liquids to the stomach. But it's not merely a hollow pipe, and it doesn't depend on gravity—that's why you can swallow when standing on your head.

How it works: When you swallow, waves of muscular contractions, known as peristalsis, ripple down the esophagus, propelling foods and liquids to the stomach. A muscular ring at the bottom of the esophagus, the lower esophageal sphincter (LES), briefly opens to allow foods to pass, then squeezes shut until the next swallow.

Gastroesophageal reflux disease (GERD)—most commonly characterized by chronic heartburn and/or sometimes chest pain—is caused by transient relaxation of the lower esophageal sphincter, which allows stomach contents to backwash into the esophagus.

The LES may also act up in patients with esophageal motility disorders—for example, it may fail to open at the right time or stay open when it shouldn't. Esophageal motility disorders often involve more frequent episodes of reflux than simple GERD. In other cases, the muscular contractions may be insufficient to propel food downward. Or the contractions may occur chaotically instead of sequentially, which prevents food or liquid from reaching the stomach.

Patients with these disorders typically experience difficulty passing food down the esophagus or chest pain from excess muscular contraction ("squeezing" tightness) and/or the upward splashes of stomach acid. Patients with such pain must first be checked for heart problems because the pain can be identical to the pain of angina or a heart attack.

Note: Motility disorders, though uncomfortable, generally aren't dangerous.

Exception: Achalasia (see below) is associated with infection and a small increased risk for esophageal cancer. *Main esophageal motility disorders…*

ACHALASIA

Achalasia is most common in middle-aged or older adults.

What happens: Over a period of years, patients experience a loss of function of the cells that control relaxation and tightening of the esophageal wall and sphincter. This might be due to a viral infection or an autoimmune disorder—the underlying cause of loss of cell function is still unknown.

As more and more cells lose function, the LES loses the ability to relax completely and peristaltic contractions become weak and chaotic, and foods and liquids are unable to easily pass through the esophagus into the stomach.

Result: This material accumulates in the esophagus, causing potentially deadly complications.

Patients may have difficulty swallowing, chest pain and/or regurgitation during/after meals. The main risk is that someone will regurgitate during sleep and aspirate some of the esophageal contents into the lungs, which can be fatal.

Diagnosis: Esophageal manometry, in which a tube is guided into the stomach, then slowly withdrawn, detects pressure changes and measures the peristaltic waves and lower esophageal sphincter pressure. Also, endoscopy, in which a viewing tube is inserted into the esophagus, is used to look for characteristic changes in the esophagus. Some patients will be given a special type of X-ray (barium swallow) to see how readily substances pass through the esophageal opening.

Main treatment: For some patients with mild-to-moderate achalasia, medications that relax the LES will be helpful. These medications include nitrates, such as nitroglycerin, and calcium channel blockers, such as *nifedipine* (Procardia, Adalat).

Note: Achalasia is usually progressive. Medication will give only temporary relief. *Other treatment options…*

- ***Botulinum toxin* (Botox),** injected into the LES, relaxes the muscle and allows foods/liquids to pass through. It brings relief in about 70% to 80% of patients. The injections have to be repeated once or twice a year. Botox poses little risk if administered by a qualified gastroenterologist.

- **Pneumatic dilatation,** in which a balloon is placed inside the LES and then inflated, stretches the muscle fibers and allows normal passage through the sphincter. It works in about two-thirds of patients, but many will need to repeat the procedure in a few years if symptoms reappear. The procedure is safe, but there's a small risk for perforation damage to the esophagus that requires immediate surgery to repair.

• **Heller myotomy,** in which a surgeon makes a small incision in the outer muscle layers of the LES. This procedure prevents the muscle from closing as tightly. Up to 90% of patients who have the procedure will experience long-lasting relief. Unfortunately, many also experience postsurgical heartburn because the LES relaxes too much and allows the upward passage of stomach acid.

DIFFUSE ESOPHAGEAL SPASM

With this condition, patients don't have the coordinated peristaltic waves that push food down the esophagus into the stomach. Instead, the esophagus contracts and relaxes with variable strength, but in a chaotic fashion. Patients are able to swallow, but it's often painful, and they also may experience severe chest pain from overly forceful contractions.

What happens: The spasms are thought to be caused by heartburn.

Diagnosis: Esophageal manometry is typically used to detect these chaotic pressure changes. The test also measures peristaltic waves.

Treatment: A proton pump inhibitor (PPI), such as *omeprazole* (Prilosec) or *lansoprazole* (Prevacid), can help prevent the reflux of stomach acid and may be used indefinitely for relief. Research has linked long-term use of PPIs to side effects such as increased fracture risk and calcium and magnesium depletion, so ask your doctor to monitor you closely. Patients also can be treated with nitrates or a calcium channel blocker if the discomfort is not caused by acid reflux.

NUTCRACKER ESOPHAGUS

The swallowing contractions are properly coordinated but too powerful with this condition. The main symptom is chest pain—some patients will also have difficulty swallowing. The causes are unknown, although patients who are overweight tend to have worse symptoms.

Diagnosis: Esophageal manometry to measure pressure.

Treatment: Most patients are treated with calcium channel blockers or nitrate medications. Therapy with Botox can be difficult because the excess pressure occurs throughout the length of the esophagus, a large area to treat with injections. A trial of PPI also can be effective.

SCLERODERMA

This autoimmune disease damages smooth-muscle tissue in the esophagus (and elsewhere in the body), reducing elasticity. Its effect is the opposite of that caused by achalasia. The LES is too relaxed rather than too tight. Most patients have severe acid reflux because the esophagus lacks the peristaltic activity to push the acid out.

Diagnosis: Blood tests will show the presence of antinuclear antibodies, the hallmark of autoimmune disease. Endoscopy will show inflammation of the lower esophagus.

Treatment: There isn't a cure for scleroderma. The main approach for patients with esophageal discomfort is to take a PPI drug to reduce acid reflux/heartburn.

Getting the Right Diagnosis: Do You Have GERD?

Anil Minocha, MD, professor of medicine at Louisiana State University and staff gastroenterologist at Overton Brooks VA Medical Center, both in Shreveport. He is the author of *How to Stop Heartburn*.

Nearly everyone suffers from heartburn from time to time, but frequent episodes (two or more times weekly) can signal a condition that must be taken seriously. Chronic heartburn, also known as gastroesophageal reflux disease (GERD), can lead to internal bleeding and scarring—even a deadly form of cancer.

A primary care doctor or gastroenterologist usually diagnoses GERD on the basis of heartburn-like symptoms. In some cases, the doctor will perform endoscopy, in which a thin, flexible, fiber-optic tube is passed through the throat to examine the esophagus and upper part of the stomach.

Ask your doctor about: An esophageal acidity test. With this procedure, a tiny device is placed in the esophagus to monitor levels of acidity for 24 hours (very high levels usually indicate GERD). This test typically is used when a patient has not responded to treatment or has atypical symptoms (such as chronic cough or hoarseness).

THE SURGICAL OPTION

Surgery usually is an option if drug treatment and alternative approaches have failed (see the following article).

In the standard procedure, called fundoplication, part of the upper stomach is wrapped around the LES to strengthen it. This operation can be performed with tiny incisions (laparoscopically), rather than by opening the chest.

Drug-Free Help for Chronic Heartburn

Kristina Conner, ND, assistant professor at National University of Health Sciences in Lombard, Illinois. She specializes in natural family medicine for women and children, naturopathic endocrinology and gastroenterology.

Jacob Teitelbaum, MD, board-certified internist and nationally known expert in the fields of chronic fatigue syndrome, fibromyalgia, sleep and pain. Based in Kailua-Kona, Hawaii, he is author of numerous books, including *The Fatigue and Fibromyalgia Solution*, *Pain-Free 1-2-3* and *Real Cause, Real Cure*. Vitality101.com

To break down food, the stomach produces about one quart of hydrochloric acid daily. At the base of the esophagus is the lower esophageal sphincter (LES), a band of muscle that opens to let swallowed food into the stomach, then shuts again. When the LES fails to close properly, stomach acid backs up into the esophagus and damages the esophageal lining. This is what happens with GERD. *What helps...*

ESOPHAGUS-SOOTHING SUPPLEMENTS

Taken alone or in combination for two to four months, the dietary supplements below promote esophageal healing. For dosages and guidelines on which supplements are most appropriate for you, consult a naturopathic physician. *Options...*

- **For quick heartburn relief,** try bicarbonate of soda (baking soda). One-half teaspoon of alkaline bicarbonate of soda (baking soda) in four ounces of water can quickly neutralize stomach acid and relieve the pain. Over-the-counter antacids with alkalinizing minerals (calcium combined with magnesium, such as Rolaids) also work—as little as one-quarter tablet can squelch the pain of heartburn. But there is some evidence that long-term use of calcium is associated with increased risk for heart attacks in women.
- **Calcium citrate powder mixed with water** helps tighten the LES and improves the esophagus's ability to push acid back into the stomach.
- **Deglycyrrhized licorice tablets** promote production of mucus that protects esophageal cells.
- **Marshmallow root lozenges** contain mucilage, a gelatinous substance that coats the gastrointestinal tract, soothes inflammation and heals cells lining the esophagus and stomach.
- **Slippery elm herbal tea** also provides mucilage. Drink it hot, not iced. Warm beverages are easier to absorb than cold drinks, which can tax gastrointestinal function.
- **Vitamin B complex,** including thiamine (B-1), pantothenic acid (B-5) and choline, promotes proper smooth-muscle activity of the esophagus to keep food moving in the right direction.
- **Take mastic gum.** This gum (resin) from an evergreen tree is a wonderful remedy for heartburn and indigestion. Take mastic gum in supplement form.
- **Digestive enzymes.** One of the primary reasons for indigestion in the US is lack of enzymes in food, which have been removed during processing.

Recommended product: The enzyme-containing supplement Complete GEST from Enzymatic Therapy. Take two capsules with every meal to digest food properly.

Caution: Some people find that digestive enzymes irritate the stomach. If this happens, start with GS-Similase—it's the gentler enzyme product. If it causes irritation, don't use it. Instead, use the DGL licorice and mastic gum remedies (see above) until your stomach feels better, usually in a month or two—and then start taking digestive enzymes. The enzymes are used long-term to support healthy digestion.

ANTI-GERD DIET

Foods that can exacerbate GERD by relaxing the LES muscle and/or increasing acidity generally are those that are spicy or high in fat or sugar. Some people find that symptoms are triggered by certain other foods, such as alcohol, carbonated beverages, citrus fruits and juices, chocolate, coffee, mint, onions and tomatoes. Contrary to the popular idea that dairy foods ease GERD, they actually can worsen symptoms. You do not necessarily need to give up all these foods forever, but you will feel better if you avoid them long enough to let your body recover.

What to do: Eliminate all potential troublemakers from your diet for two to four weeks, then reintroduce them one at a time. If eating a particular food brings on symptoms within a day, avoid it for another three to six months, then try it again. If GERD symptoms return, it is best to avoid this food henceforth. If no symptoms develop after the three- to six-month hiatus, you may be able to eat this food occasionally. But keep portions moderate.

Safe to eat: Foods unlikely to exacerbate GERD include those that are high in fiber, complex carbohydrates and/or minerals. Good choices include most fruits and vegetables (except those identified above as potential heartburn triggers)...lean meats and skinless poultry...and whole grains.

Eat slowly and chew carefully, giving your mouth—a key part of your digestive system—and stomach plenty of time to work. Don't overfill your stomach. Avoid eating while watching TV, driving, standing up or doing anything that takes attention away from your food and encourages you to rush or overeat.

Celebrate your food: Put out placemats, cloth napkins, even candles...as you eat, notice each food's taste, texture and aroma. You'll enjoy your food more and eat less—a double benefit.

While eating, also try to sip warm liquid rather than cold. Cold drinks slow and even can stop digestion. Drink warm liquids during meals to aid digestion.

CHAPTER 7

Emotional Hurt

How to Deal with a Tough Diagnosis

"You have cancer." "It's Alzheimer's." "The diagnosis is Parkinson's Disease." No one is ever truly prepared to find out that he or she has a chronic and/or life-threatening disease.

But it happens all the time. So even if this information doesn't apply to you right now, bookmark this article, because you never know when you—or a close friend or family member—might need it.

A serious diagnosis usually leads to a flood of emotions. In fact, some patients say that the mental aspect of dealing with a disease (coming to terms with it) can be even more challenging than the physical part (whether it's managing pain, fatigue, memory loss or other symptoms).

So we spoke with an expert about how to handle what goes on in your head when your body breaks down.

OVERCOMING DENIAL

Most people experience disbelief when they first learn that they have a serious health condition. They may be confident, intellectually, that the diagnosis is correct…and yet somehow, it just doesn't seem real. "The healthier you feel at the time of diagnosis, the more you may be in denial," said Walter Baile, MD, a professor in the departments of behavioral sciences and psychiatry at the University of Texas MD Anderson Cancer Center in Houston who counsels doctors on how to communicate delicately with patients who have cancer. If you truly doubt your doctor and need extra confirmation about your diagnosis, get a second opinion, he recommended. But beyond that, the best thing that you can do is give yourself some time for the diagnosis to sink in—as it will. "This could take anywhere from moments to days," he said.

Walter Baile, MD, professor of behavioral science and psychiatry, The University of Texas MD Anderson Cancer Center, Houston.

GETTING PAST YOUR FEARS

Once the disbelief has worn off, you may feel fearful and/or anxious. A lot of times, people are frightened and worried because they feel lost and out of control—they don't know what's going to happen next, said Dr. Baile. So the best way to reduce any panic or fright is by learning everything you can about your disorder or disease. Read any pamphlets your doctor gives you...check out books from the library on the topic...and search for information on legitimate medical websites, such as MedlinePlus.gov, the site for the National Institutes of Health. The more you know about your condition and what's ahead, the fewer surprises there will be and the more you will feel in control, said Dr. Baile.

STAYING POSITIVE

At this point, patients often become demoralized and can even feel grief. "Even though nobody has died, you can still experience a sense of loss," said Dr. Baile. After all, a serious illness can cause you to lose not only your health but also your job and/or financial stability—and you may worry about how it might negatively affect relationships with your loved ones and friends. At this stage, it's usually helpful to speak with a trained mental health counselor, such as a social worker, psychologist or psychiatrist, he said, because a counselor can help you manage stress and maintain optimism.

LETTING OTHERS IN

As you start to develop a more positive state of mind, follow this last piece of advice.

You might feel embarrassed at first to tell relatives and friends about your diagnosis, but keeping it hidden from the outside world may only make you feel lonely. "Remember that there is nothing to feel ashamed of, and the effect of holding feelings in is much more damaging than getting them on the table," said Dr. Baile. "You can't deal with your emotions when they're all locked inside." Plus, when more people are aware of your diagnosis, more people can help you cope with it.

If you're too tired of telling people the story of your diagnosis or if you're too busy going to medical appointments to share the news, appoint a close friend or family member to spread the word for you, he recommended. Or you could tell people via a single mass e-mail or Facebook status update or by using a website such as CaringBridge.org.

And join a support group full of people who have your condition—either a group that meets in person, an online group or both, said Dr. Baile. You can find one by talking to your doctor or by entering the phrase "support group" and then the name of your condition into any Web search engine. If talking with an entire group feels overwhelming, some hospitals have patient-to-patient programs that can match you one-on-one with someone who has (or had) your condition, so ask your doctor about that.

PTSD: A Hidden Danger After a Serious Illness

Robert London, MD, practicing physician/psychiatrist for more than three decades on the professorial staff of NYU School of Medicine in New York City. Dr. London also developed the short-term psychotherapy unit at the NYU Langone Medical Center and ran this program for 20 years. DrRobertLondon.com

Survivors of a traumatic medical situation—for example, a stay in the intensive care unit (ICU) or treatment for a heart attack or cancer—are at increased risk for post-traumatic stress disorder (PTSD).

Surprising fact: PTSD can strike weeks—or even years—after an illness. Symptoms may include nightmares, flashbacks, irritability and feeling detached (depersonalization) and emotionally numb. Ignoring PTSD after a serious medical situation carries its own risks. Without treatment, symptoms worsen, impacting the sufferer's social, family and work relationships.

HOW TO FIGHT PTSD

Anyone who suffers PTSD after a serious illness—or wants to help prevent it—can benefit from one or more of the following...*

*These therapies are generally covered by health insurance. Check with your insurer.

• **Cognitive behavioral therapy** typically involves weekly visits with a therapist for several months during which sufferers learn to reprocess the traumatic events by gaining a new perspective on the past trauma and improving skills to cope with the distressing thoughts that arise from it.

• **Prolonged exposure therapy** involves the patient revisiting the specific trauma in a safe environment through guided imagery until it's no longer distressing.

To find a psychologist or psychiatrist trained in these therapies, consult the Association for Behavioral and Cognitive Therapies, ABCT.org.

• **Hypnosis** helps people reprocess traumatic memories first by using relaxation strategies and then a series of visual images to slowly reintroduce the trauma. This is usually coupled with pleasant visualizations that reduce the anxiety of the traumatic memory. Patients generally require four to 16 sessions. To find a qualified hypnotherapist near you, consult the American Society of Clinical Hypnosis, ASCH.net.

Other therapies to consider...

• **EMDR.** With eye movement desensitization and reprocessing (EMDR), the therapist asks the patient to perform certain eye movements, such as following the therapist's finger from side to side, while the patient talks about the trauma. The exercise is then repeated, this time focusing on positive memories to help the brain reprocess the trauma so that the emotional distress is decreased. EMDR usually requires four to 12 sessions and has been approved as a PTSD treatment by the US Department of Defense. To find an EMDR-trained practitioner, consult the EMDR International Association, EMDRIA.org.

• **Medications.** Antidepressants known as selective serotonin reuptake inhibitors (SSRIs), which work by raising the level of the mood-boosting chemical serotonin in the brain, have been shown to help with PTSD, especially if depression is present. *Sertraline* (Zoloft) and *paroxetine* (Paxil) are two SSRIs that have been approved by the FDA specifically for PTSD.

• **Support groups.** Most PTSD sufferers find it helpful to join a support group of other people who have had similar experiences. Family members may also find comfort from support groups aimed at those caring for someone with PTSD. To find a support group near you, check the psychology/psychiatry department at your local hospital.

SPECIFIC STEPS THAT HELP

In addition to the steps above, the following strategies help prevent or treat PTSD in patients after...

• **An ICU stay.** Even though most ICU patients receive lifesaving care, ICUs are high-intensity settings with constant noise and bright lights, which can further traumatize an already vulnerable, perhaps disoriented patient. One-quarter of those admitted to a hospital ICU have symptoms of PTSD after their stays.

To prevent PTSD in ICU patients: Unlike most PTSD survivors, who have flashbacks about actual events, ICU patients often suffer flashbacks about delusions or hallucinations that occurred during their stays—a relatively common problem among these patients.

What helps...

• ICU diaries, in which nurses and family members record what's happening daily while the patient is hospitalized, are one way to reduce the risk for PTSD. After discharge, the patients are given the diary to review with a nurse or family member whenever the patient feels anxious. This process helps establish what actually occurred during the patient's stay rather than focusing on the frightening details of their misperceptions.

• Music therapy, which relaxes and distracts seriously ill patients during the hospital stay, helps reduce the likelihood of lasting psychological trauma. If permitted, a patient could listen to favorite music through headphones.

• **Heart attack.** Around 12% of heart attack sufferers develop PTSD, and those who do are more likely to experience a second heart attack. Some heart attack survivors may go into a state of anxiety or panic whenever they feel shortness of breath, fearing that another heart attack is on the way. This often creates a vicious circle of symptoms and worry.

To prevent heart-related PTSD: Heart patients should seek counseling to learn calming strategies such as relaxation techniques. Heart patients who have a lot of support from their families and friends—especially so that the patient can ask for help when needed—are also less likely to develop PTSD. Having this type of readily available assistance appears to reduce the feelings of vulnerability and helplessness, which so often occur in heart attack survivors.

• **Cancer.** PTSD can follow treatment for any type of cancer. As with other conditions, the more intense or frightening the situation, the higher the chance for PTSD.

To prevent cancer-related PTSD: For some patients, learning all the specifics of their disease from their doctors can help reduce anxiety, while others prefer to know as little as possible. In either case, talk to your doctor about your risk for recurrence and steps you can take to monitor for any early signs that the cancer may be returning.

As with other serious illnesses, family support is crucial in helping cancer patients readjust psychologically after treatment.

It Can Be Hard When Things Don't Happen

Nancy K. Schlossberg, EdD, professor emerita, department of counseling and personnel services, College of Education at University of Maryland, College Park. She is author of nine books, including *Too Young to Be Old*. TransitionsThroughLife.com

Coping with life transitions can be difficult for anyone. We expect big changes to affect us emotionally, whether positively or negatively. When we face an event such as starting or losing a job, retiring, moving, getting married (or remarried) or losing a loved one, our friends and family typically rally around to provide emotional support.

But when something we planned or counted on doesn't happen, we may not recognize the emotional impact—even though the adjustment may be just as challenging. That makes these nonevents especially hard for us to cope with.

WHAT ARE NONEVENTS?

Nonevents are changes you expected to happen but that do not occur as you had hoped.

Examples: You worked hard to receive a promotion that didn't come...you planned to retire at a certain age, but you do not have enough money to stop working...you were looking forward to becoming a grandparent, but your children choose not to have children of their own. There are many more expected things that just don't happen.

These disappointed expectations can affect your life in profound ways. You may feel a deep sense of failure or loss. Your identity and assumptions about your place in the world may be challenged. You may question your competence and worth.

Example #1: **A man who always wanted to be a commercial pilot joined the navy and was trained to fly.** When he left the military, he was crushed that he couldn't get a job with a major airline. He became a lawyer and no longer felt comfortable calling himself a pilot, but he deeply missed that identity. He felt envious of his friends who were working in areas that they felt passionate about.

Example #2: **A 60-year-old woman expressed dismay that she never became the poet she expected to be.** She had received poetry awards when she graduated from college, but after that, nothing happened. She was unable to get her work published and eventually gave up. She kept thinking about what might have been.

DIFFERENT TYPES

My colleagues and I at University of Maryland interviewed more than 100 people of all ages about how nonevents changed their lives. We identified several different categories of nonevents. Some nonevents are personal—they stem from our own choices, abilities and limitations.

Example: A woman always expected to lose the weight she gained decades earlier when she was pregnant. At age 60 and after many unsuccessful diets, she concluded that she would never have the slim figure she longed for.

Other nonevents are ripples, resulting from life choices made by the people around us.

Example: Not becoming a grandparent because your children don't have children.

There is a third category we investigated as well—it's not technically a nonevent but an event that turns out to be delayed, though it feels like a nonevent for many years to the person experiencing it.

Example: A woman who finally accepts that she will never marry and lives with her nonevent for decades. Then she meets someone at age 70 and marries for the first time, turning her nonevent into an event.

Because nonevents often are invisible to others, the people who experience them are likely to suffer alone. Those around them may not realize that support is needed. No one throws you a party for the book that did not get published or brings you chicken soup to comfort you about the grandchild you never had. This lack of support can prolong unhappiness and make it difficult to move on. But you can move on and become happier if you know how to help yourself with nonevents.

RECOVERING FROM NONEVENTS

My colleagues and I have found that people who recover successfully from nonevents follow these three steps...

1. Acknowledge the loss. Nonevents can be harder to spot than event-related transitions because they tend to be more gradual—the cherished goal or dream recedes further and further away. It is important to acknowledge what is bothering you and why you are feeling dismayed. You need to label the loss as a nonevent and tell the people close to you what you are experiencing.

Example: A former professor who ran a government agency was shaken when he learned that two of his former students had surpassed his professional achievements. Instead of being satisfied about the contribution he had made to the next generation, he felt envious and diminished. Only after admitting his disappointment in his own academic accomplishments was he able to refocus and begin taking pride in his former students' success.

Helpful: Tell the story of your lost dream to people you trust. Choose people who can listen empathetically and won't try to minimize your disappointment or try to talk you out of your feelings. If family and friends don't have this ability, talk to a therapist or clergyperson.

2. Grieve. Separating from a dream takes time, and the pain of disappointment may come and go in cycles. Find ways to express your grief.

Examples: Write in a daily journal...cry if you have the urge...seek spiritual solace in a house of worship or with a meditation group.

3. Refocus. This is the time to let go of old expectations and look at your nonevent differently. You need to begin to think of possible new ways you might live your life and identify new goals and dreams.

Developing rituals or rites of passage is a way to help people separate from the past and move to a new place.

Example: A young woman who had given up hope of marrying sent an announcement to her friends and family members saying that she was moving into a beautiful new apartment and that she had registered for housewarming gifts at Macy's.

Shifting focus is necessary as we shape new goals by identifying a new dream, a new vision, a new self.

Example: The lawyer who had wanted to become a commercial pilot began to see himself as someone with a satisfying hobby—he bought a small plane that he used to visit family and go on business trips. He realized that flying was essential to his well-being and that he could fly for fun instead of as a career. This outlet freed him to find enjoyment in his law career.

Because life does not follow a preordained script, it is important to have backup plans. All of us will have scripts for our lives that are interrupted and do not go according to plan. We cannot count on life just following a neat, arranged, linear script.

Don't Let Grief Endanger Your Health

Phyllis Kosminsky, PhD, clinical social worker specializing in grief, loss and trauma at the Darien, Connecticut–based Center for Hope/Family Centers, a nonprofit organization that offers services to people coping with a life-threatening illness or the loss of a loved one. She also is in private practice in Pleasantville, New York, and Norwalk, Connecticut. She is the author of *Getting Back to Life When Grief Won't Heal.*

When someone close to you dies, it's natural to grieve. The ache may never go away entirely, but you gradually accept that your loved one is gone, and you find a new way for life to feel normal.

But for up to 15% of bereaved people, intense grief can linger for years or even decades. This so-called complicated grief is powerful enough to disrupt the bereaved person's ability to work, get along with others and/or to find much pleasure in anything. Although elements of depression are present, complicated grief also is marked by chronic and persistent yearning and longing for the deceased...and an inability to accept the loss.

Especially in older adults, complicated grief can go undetected by doctors and family members—or even the sufferers themselves. Regardless of age, the condition can contribute to chronic depression, drug and alcohol abuse and certain infectious diseases (by weakening the immune system). In people who have heart disease, the emotional stress created by complicated grief can worsen their condition.

HURT BUT HEALING

A person who is grieving is bound to experience feelings of sadness, emptiness, loss—and often anger. Physical symptoms are also common. You lack energy and feel fatigued. You may have trouble sleeping—or do nothing but sleep. You find it hard to concentrate and may even wonder about the meaning of life. Some people lose their appetites, while others eat uncontrollably. Headaches, digestive problems, and other aches and pains often occur.

These grief responses may actually serve a purpose. The psychological pain and physical symptoms force you to slow down, giving your mind and body the opportunity to heal.

Important: There's no fixed timetable for grieving. No one can say "you should be over it" in three months, six months or even a year. As long as the general trend is toward feeling better, it's normal to have ups and downs.

GRIEF CAN BE COMPLICATED

If painful feelings last for more than a few months—and don't seem to be getting better—something may have gone wrong with the grieving process.

Red flags: Thoughts of the lost person constantly intrude throughout the day...or you're simply unable to speak about your loss...or normal life seems impossible, and you feel you can't survive without the person.

Complicated grief is more likely to occur if your relationship with the person you lost was characterized by...

- **Dependence.** We all depend on those we love. But such dependence is excessive when you can't let yourself acknowledge that the person you need so badly is dead and no longer there for you.
- **Ambivalence.** Virtually all relationships have some degree of ambivalence. For example, it's common to love a parent for his/her strength and reliability, but resent that person's tendency toward harsh judgment. Even in the most loving of marriages, anger comes up from time to time. Recognizing our negative feelings toward the deceased person can trigger guilt, so we instinctively push away those thoughts. However, the negative thoughts invariably find their way back into our consciousness, until we acknowledge them.

Regardless of the nature of the relationship, a sudden or otherwise traumatic death can complicate the task of grieving. You relive the moment—or keep trying to push it out of your mind. Problems also arise when death follows an extended illness, triggering both grief and guilt-inducing relief that the person is no longer suffering—and perhaps that you no longer have to take care of him.

ALLOWING YOURSELF TO GRIEVE

Grieving involves experiencing your full range of emotions, including anger, resentment and relief as well as sadness. Some of these feelings may be hard to bear, especially if you have no one with whom to share them. Most people find it helpful to have the emotional support of others.

What to do...

- **Don't isolate yourself.** Spend time with compassionate, understanding friends and family members who are willing to listen, and tell them how you feel.

If you need to talk to more than these people are willing to listen, consider joining a grief support group. Meeting regularly with people who share a similar loss gives you the opportunity to express your feelings. Local hospitals, hospices and mental-health facilities can help you find a support group.

Online support groups can be helpful if you live in a remote area, prefer not to deal with others face-to-face or lack transportation. To find an online support group, go to the Internet community GriefNet, GriefNet.org.

- **Be active.** For many people, doing is better than simply talking. Volunteer work can be especially healing—helping others diverts you from your own sadness and is a powerful way to help yourself.

Physical exercise also is a potent mood-lifter and a general aid to mental health. Anything that gets your body moving is a step in the right direction.

- **Take time to grieve.** Particularly if you have a busy schedule, spend five to 10 minutes a day in a quiet, private place where you feel safe and comfortable experiencing your grief. Focus on your feelings and on thoughts about the deceased. This way, if your grief intrudes during the day, you can remind yourself that you will have a chance to grieve at some point later.

WHEN TO GET HELP

If your own efforts to deal with grief aren't enough, a professional can help you find where and why you're stuck.

Consider therapy or counseling if you're showing signs of depression—you can't work, can't sleep, can't eat, can't get interested in anything or can't deal with other people. Ask your physician to direct you to a therapist or counselor with experience in dealing with grief. Or you can find a list of "thanatologists"—grief specialists—from the Association for Death Education and Counseling, 612-337-1808, ADEC.org.

You also may want to consult your doctor about short-term use of medication to help you function in your day-to-day activities.

How to Love Life Again After Losing a Spouse

Becky Aikman, New York–based journalist and author of *Saturday Night Widows: The Adventures of Six Friends Remaking Their Lives*, the memoir of a group that Aikman founded to help herself and five other widows focus on happiness rather than grief. BeckyAikman.com

Becky Aikman was in her 40s when she lost her husband to cancer. She formed a group with five other widows.

Their goal: To learn to live again after the worst thing that ever happened to them.

In the process, they found that some of the traditional thinking about loss and recovery wasn't helpful.

Here, advice for rebuilding your life—when you feel ready to do so—in the months or years after the death of your husband or wife...

AVOID COMMON TRAPS

Beware the missteps that can stand in the way of remaking your life.

- **Don't put off rebuilding because you haven't yet experienced the stages of grief.** In the late 1960s, psychiatrist Elisabeth Kübler-Ross popularized the idea that the grieving process has five predictable stages—denial, anger, bargaining, depression and acceptance. These "five stages of grief" have become so ingrained in our culture that some widows and widowers believe they can't be truly ready to move on with their lives if they haven't yet passed through each of them. In fact, these stages were never intended to apply to grieving spouses but only to those who were dying themselves.

People who lose a spouse often experience waves of emotion separated by periods of feeling relatively normal. Over time, the waves become less extreme and less frequent until the widow or widower feels ready to reengage with humanity.

• **Be wary of support groups.** These groups are supposed to help widows and widowers cope with their grief by talking about it with others. Trouble is, spending time with other grieving people and focusing your attention on your grief can make you sadder.

Give one of these groups a try if you think talking about your grief might help. But if you discover that it isn't for you, don't feel that your recovery depends on your continued attendance.

• **Make decisions based on what you want your life to look like in the future, not on maintaining the life you had before.** It can be very difficult to give up the plans we made with our late partners, but those plans might no longer be appropriate for us.

Example: Some widows hang onto the family home, even though they no longer need the space, and then feel isolated living in communities full of families. Many who move into smaller homes closer to other singles are glad they did.

FRIENDS

It might make sense to alter whom you socialize with or how you arrange to spend time with them...

• **Be proactive about making plans with friends.** You can't just sit at home waiting for friends to call with things for you to do. Your friends might go out of their way to extend invitations in the months immediately after your spouse passes away, but those invitations are likely to eventually dry up as your friends return to their normal patterns and forget that you're sitting home alone. It's up to you to contact them to make plans. Do this days or weeks in advance, when possible, to reduce the odds that they already will have made plans.

• **Construct a new circle of single friends.** If you and your late spouse were like most married couples, you probably socialized mainly with other married couples. You might start to feel like a fifth wheel if couples remain your only friends. If other members of your circle have also lost their spouses, make a particular effort to socialize with them. If you don't have unattached friends, ask your friends if they have other friends who have lost their partners or are otherwise unmarried and suggest that they be invited to get-togethers, too.

• **Get over any guilt about new romantic relationships.** Widows and widowers often worry that seeing someone new implies that their departed spouse wasn't really the love of their life. This isn't true—researchers have found that it's people who were very deeply in love with their departed spouses who are most likely to find love again.

ACTIVITIES

Certain pursuits are particularly worthwhile when you're trying to recover from the loss of a spouse.

• **Seek new experiences.** Explore new hobbies. Visit new places. Take classes in subjects you know little about.

Examples: I attended the opera, took architecture tours and joined a group of friends on a spa trip, all things I don't normally do.

Doing new things isn't just enjoyable—it also helps widows and widowers gain confidence in their ability to face new challenges. That can be very empowering for people worried that they might not have it in them to remake their lives after decades of marriage and routine.

• **Cook well for yourself.** Losing a spouse can mean losing the person who cooked for you...or losing the person for whom you cooked. Either way, the result often is a dramatic decline in the quality of the surviving spouse's meals. (When the survivor is the cook, he/she often concludes that it isn't worth preparing elaborate meals that no one else will eat.)

Dining out can be challenging, too. Many newly widowed people find it uncomfortable and boring to eat alone in restaurants.

But if you stop eating well after the loss of a spouse, you deny yourself an important source of pleasure when you need it most.

Your health might suffer, too, if you resort to junk food.

What to do: Make cooking good food a priority, even if you're the only one who will eat it. If your late spouse was the cook in the family, enroll in cooking classes. Not only can these classes teach you to cook well for yourself, but you also might meet new friends.

• **Travel with tour groups.** Travel is an excellent way to have new and enjoyable experiences, but many people find it awkward to travel alone, and not having someone to share travel experiences with can detract from the fun.

If you travel with a tour group, you'll have people with whom you can share the adventure. You might even form lasting friendships with other members of the group.

Helpful: Before signing up for a trip, call the tour operator to confirm that a significant number of the members of the group are single. It can be uncomfortable to be the only one traveling alone in a group.

Don't Live with Loneliness

Take action against loneliness, which is detrimental to both mental and physical health. Make small talk with strangers—simply chatting in person, not online, boosts well-being. Have as much face-to-face contact with friends and family as possible—use video conferencing if distance or health issues make that impossible. Use social media such as Facebook to create your own social networks, such as a book club where you share personal reactions with other readers. Invite neighbors over for coffee, and help them with small chores when you can. Try throwing a dinner party—eating together is a long-established method of connecting with people. Creative group endeavors, from crafts nights to choral singing, also can improve connection with others.

Roundup of experts on preventing loneliness, reported in *Psychology Today.*

Hidden Harms of Long-Ago Trauma: It's Never Too Late To Get Help

Vincent J. Felitti, MD, clinical professor of medicine at University of California, San Diego. Dr. Felitti is co-principal investigator of the Adverse Childhood Experiences (ACE) Study, one of the largest investigations of childhood abuse and neglect and later-life health and well-being.

If you've ever suffered physical, sexual or emotional abuse, you might think that psychological scars are the only long-lasting damage. But that couldn't be further from the truth.

A lingering threat: Volumes of scientific evidence show that these negative experiences also increase risk for chronic disease and early death...even when the incidents occurred several years earlier.

LANDMARK INVESTIGATION

The Adverse Childhood Experiences (ACE) Study, a massive collaborative research project cosponsored by the Centers for Disease Control and Prevention, looked at the backgrounds of 17,000 adults, beginning in 1995 at Kaiser Permanente in San Diego. With more than 20 years of follow-up, the study offers crucial insights into the physical effects of abuse and mistreatment.

In the original research, two-thirds of the study's middle-class participants reported at least one incident of childhood trauma or neglect. More specifically, 28% reported physical abuse...and 21% said they were abused sexually. More than one in five people reported three or more categories of adverse childhood experiences, or ACEs. (To determine your own ACE score, see next page.)

THE HEALTH RISKS ARE REAL

The ACE Study determined that the more of these experiences a person has suffered, the higher his/her risk is for a range of mental and physical health conditions.

For example, compared with participants who did not experience any abuses or mistreatment, those who reported four categories of adverse childhood experiences were twice as likely to be diagnosed with lung cancer and/or depression as adults. They also had a fourfold increase in chronic lung disease, such as chronic obstructive pulmonary disease (COPD), and a sevenfold increase in alcoholism. A person with six or more categories of ACEs had their life expectancy shortened by nearly 20 years.

WHY PHYSICAL HEALTH SUFFERS

It's easy to imagine how trauma would affect a person's mental health. But why would it also impact physical health? *Long-term research has identified such factors as...*

• **Coping mechanisms.** Trauma victims are more likely to use self-soothing habits, such as smoking, drinking, overeating and drug abuse, which are helpful in the short term but are known risk factors in the long term for many chronic health problems.

• **Complex brain-mediated effects.** Chronic stress due to ACEs can distort the function of brain networks, resulting in immune system suppression, which in turn can lead to a variety of diseases. In addition, it causes the release of pro-inflammatory chemicals that are responsible for additional diseases such as heart disease, pulmonary fibrosis, etc.

WHAT HELPS MOST

If you experienced trauma as a child, it is never too late to get help to reverse or at least moderate the negative physical and/or emotional effects of ACEs. *The strategies below, which tend to yield positive results more quickly than psychotherapy and/or antidepressants, are likely to also be helpful for those who experienced trauma as an adult...*

• **Tell a trusted person.** People who have experienced childhood trauma often carry the secret into adulthood. Victims of abuse feel shame and assume that they did something wrong to deserve the abuse. By simply telling someone, and having that person continue to accept you, the shame dissipates.

• **Try eye movement desensitization and reprocessing (EMDR).** The American Psychiatric Association recognizes this therapy as an effective treatment for trauma. Studies have found that trauma victims no longer had signs of post-traumatic stress disorder after as few as three 90-minute EMDR sessions.

How it works: During EMDR, a clinician asks the patient to hold a traumatic memory in mind while the therapist moves one or two fingers from side to side, or diagonally, in front of the patient's eyes. This guides the eyes to move as they do during the rapid eye movement (REM) sleep phase, during which the most active dreaming occurs. Dreaming can help process trauma and move it to long-term memory, enabling the patient to feel as if it is now resolved and only in the past.

The therapist repeats the process multiple times as needed, until the distress related to the targeted memory is gone and a positive belief replaces it. For example, a rape victim shifts from feeling horror and self-disgust to feeling empowered—*I survived it and I am strong.*

To find an EMDR clinician near you, visit the website of the EMDR Institute at EMDR.com. Check with your health insurer to see if your policy covers the treatment.

• **Consider clinical hypnosis.** This method helps patients identify past events or experiences that are causing problems. With hypnotherapy, a trained practitioner uses imagery and presents ideas or suggestions during a state of concentrated attention that helps bring about desired changes in thinking.

To find a certified hypnosis professional in your area, visit the website of the American Society of Clinical Hypnosis at ASCH.net. Check with your health insurer to see if clinical hypnosis is covered.

HOW TRAUMATIC WAS YOUR CHILDHOOD?

For each of the following questions, give yourself one point for every "yes" answer. *During your first 18 years of life...*

1. Did a parent or other adult in the household often swear at you, insult you, put you down or humiliate you? Or act in a way that made you afraid that you might be physically hurt?

2. Did a parent or other adult in the household often push, grab, slap or throw something at you? Or ever hit you so hard that you had marks or were injured?

3. Did an adult or person at least five years older than you ever touch or fondle

you or have you touch his/her body in a sexual way? Or try to or actually have oral, anal or vaginal sex with you?

4. Did you often feel that no one in your family loved you or thought you were important or special? Or that your family didn't look out for one another, feel close to one another or support one another?

5. Did you often feel that you didn't have enough to eat, had to wear dirty clothes and had no one to protect you? Or that your parents were too drunk or high to take care of you or take you to the doctor if you needed it?

6. Were your parents ever separated or divorced?

7. Was your mother or stepmother often pushed, grabbed or slapped? Or did she often have something thrown at her? Or was she sometimes or often kicked, bitten, hit with a fist or hit with something hard? Or ever repeatedly hit for at least a few minutes or threatened with a gun or knife?

8. Did you live with anyone who was a problem drinker or an alcoholic or who used street drugs?

9. Was a household member depressed or mentally ill, or did a household member attempt suicide?

10. Did a household member go to prison?

Takeaway: If you score a four or higher, tell your doctor about your history of abuse and follow the recommendations in the main article. If these steps don't help, consult a trained therapist.

Let Go of Toxic Memories

Thomas H. Crook III, PhD, CEO of Cognitive Research Corporation and a psychologist in private practice in St. Petersburg, Florida. He is author of numerous books, including *The Memory Advantage.* CogRes.com

---

Good or bad, happy or sad, our memories are a huge part of who we are. They can help us repeat our successes, motivate us to learn from our mistakes and provide the framework for our sense of ourselves as individuals.

But when painful or counterproductive memories echo over and over in our heads, they drain our mental energy and lessen our joy.

Self-defense: Learn how toxic memories form—then develop skills to defuse their power.

ORIGINS OF MEMORIES

Much of the way we see ourselves is rooted in childhood experiences, and the memories of those early events can be intense. Not every unpleasant childhood experience becomes a toxic memory, however. In fact, similar situations can create similar memories—yet produce very different effects.

Example: Two women remember feeling humiliated in first grade for being unable to read. Whenever the first woman thinks of this, she also reminds herself of how she excelled at math. For her, this early memory is tied to feelings of success. But when the second woman recalls her six-year-old self, she views those first failures with reading as the start of every struggle she has ever faced and every challenge she has ever avoided. For her, this unhappy memory is toxic.

Not all toxic memories are rooted in childhood. They can form at any time, especially during emotional upheaval.

For instance: The memory of losing his job turns toxic if a man feels enraged whenever he thinks of it. The memory of a bitter divorce becomes toxic if a woman is too afraid ever to date again.

An exceptionally traumatic event, such as being a victim of a violent crime, understandably can cause extreme fear, anger and sadness. But the memory turns especially toxic if a woman blames herself—believing, for instance, "I was sexually assaulted because I danced too provocatively"—rather than rightfully blaming the assailant.

HOW MEMORIES CAN HURT

If poisonous memories repeatedly invade our thoughts, reinforcing negative feelings about ourselves or others, we may have...

• **Diminished pleasure in life, as even happy occasions are overshadowed by images from the past.**

Example: At her daughter's wedding, a woman obsesses about how aloof her own mother was. Such thoughts increase a person's risk for depression and/or anxiety disorders.

• **Low self-esteem and missed opportunities for growth.**

Example: Having always been picked last for teams in gym class, a woman habitually labels herself as clumsy—and refuses to exercise or to socialize with friends on the golf course.

• **Inability to respond appropriately to new situations.**

Example: Continued resentment over having been laid off may negatively affect a woman's manner and the impression she makes on job interviews.

• **Chronically elevated levels of stress hormones.** These have damaging effects on blood pressure, blood sugar, digestion and immunity, increasing risk for heart disease, diabetes and gastric disorders.

BREAKING THE HABIT

A toxic memory turned constant companion is as much a bad habit as a bad memory—and like any bad habit, it can be broken. *Steps...*

1. Select a favorite positive memory. You can choose an event that specifically contradicts your toxic memory (for instance, the day you learned to ski despite being a "hopeless klutz")...or choose a completely unrelated experience, such as your first date with your husband.

2. Write down as many details as you can recall. Where did you go? What did you wear? Did you dance to a certain song or see a stunning sunset? How did that first kiss feel? Tap into all your senses.

3. Practice conjuring up this happy memory. Let this personal "movie" play inside your head during relaxed moments. Soon you'll be able to recall it vividly at will, even when stressed or depressed.

4. Mentally hit an "eject" button whenever a toxic memory pops into your head, replacing it with thoughts of the happy memory.

FULFILLING EMOTIONAL NEEDS

If the technique above isn't working, your toxic memory may be more than a bad habit—it may be fulfilling some unmet need. Ask yourself, "How am I benefiting by holding onto this painful memory?" This insight will help you explore more productive ways to meet that need, thus diminishing the power of the toxic memory. *Consider...*

• **Does thinking of yourself as unlucky let you avoid taking responsibility for your life?** On a sheet of paper, make two columns, labeled "good luck" and "bad luck," then list examples from your own life of each type of experience. You will see that your whole life hasn't been a series of misfortunes. Next, identify the role played by your own efforts—rather than good luck—in creating each positive experience...and give yourself due credit.

• **Is there a certain pleasure for you in resenting other people for past unpleasantness?** (Be honest with yourself!) Develop a habit of doing small favors that make people respond to you in a positive way. Smile at everyone you pass on the sidewalk, yield to other drivers trying to enter your lane, say a sincere "thank you" to a surly cashier. A conscious and voluntary decision to be of service to others can help you overcome old resentments, relegate toxic memories to the past and find pleasure in the here and now.

If you feel traumatized: After an extremely traumatic experience, it is normal to fixate on the event for a time. However, if you are seriously disturbed by recurrent memories of the trauma months or even years later, you may have post-traumatic stress disorder (PTSD). Symptoms include nightmares or obsessive mental reenactments of the event... frequent fear or anger...trouble concentrating...feelings of guilt, hopelessness or emotional numbness.

Defusing traumatic memories may require the help of a mental-health professional.

Recommended: Cognitive-behavioral therapy (CBT), which focuses on changing harmful thought patterns rather than on lengthy exploration of past experiences.

Referrals: National Association of Cognitive-Behavioral Therapists, NACBT.org. With CBT, even seriously toxic memories can become more manageable—and you can move on with your life.

Overcoming the Pain of Sexual Abuse Memories

Wendy Maltz, LCSW, DST, psychotherapist, lecturer and sex therapist based in Eugene, Oregon, who has written six books on sexuality including *The Sexual Healing Journey: A Guide for Survivors of Sexual Abuse.* HealthySex.com

A recent social movement, in which women (and some men) bravely come forth to tell their stories of sexual harassment, abuse and violence, has felled the careers of some of the most powerful men in business, politics, media and entertainment—even as it empowers the abused to stand up for their rights.

For many people, however, these stories, while inspiring, can trigger very painful memories—even bring new ones to light that you may have suppressed. To learn how to deal with these, we spoke with Wendy Maltz, LCSW, DST, a psychotherapist, lecturer and sex therapist. (*Note*: These recommendations apply to anyone—including men—who has been a victim of sexual abuse.)

The truth is, there are many paths to healing. *Here is how to find the ones that are a good fit for you...*

- **Honor your experiences.** Don't minimize your experiences or compare them with someone else's experiences that seem even worse. Each event of sexual harassment, abuse or violence—from catcalls to crude remarks to groping and beyond—is an invasion of your privacy and an attempt to diminish your dignity that can make you feel vulnerable, violated and humiliated. The appropriate response to yourself in each experience is compassion and understanding.

- **Don't overshare on social media.** The #MeToo hashtag allows anyone to make a valuable public statement without getting into the details of what happened. But sharing specifics or naming names is riskier because what goes online stays there forever, and you can't control how others might respond to your story or use it against you in the future. If your goal is to push the problem of sexual abuse out into the sunshine by saying more than "me, too" and you're willing to face potential personal consequences of that, then sharing specifics of your #MeToo experience is an option you can be proud of. But I think it's counterproductive to expect that you'll find healing on social media.

- **Use your memories to heal.** It's upsetting to remember the painful past, but the resurfacing of old memories provides an opportunity for deeper healing. It's a chance to recognize how strong you are. Even if you feel you haven't fully resolved what happened, focus on the extent to which you withstood the incident and moved forward in spite of it.

- **Talk to someone you know who is sympathetic.** Not everyone wants to share his/her story—it's OK to stay silent forever or until you feel ready to talk—but if you do, decide how much you want to disclose and to whom. Disclosure can help dispel feelings of isolation and shame. It can feel freeing to finally receive the validation and comfort you deserve. Choose someone carefully—whether a spouse, friend, relative, clergy member or family doctor—who you know understands the prevalence and significance of sexual violence. Such a person is most likely to provide helpful support.

One way to gauge whether someone is a good person to talk to: Begin by bringing up sexual abuse in general or via a news story. Pay attention to how the person responds. Does he express sympathy with abuse victims or, instead, challenge or doubt their stories? Then you might talk in general about your own experience without going into specifics

("This kind of thing happened to me, too") and feel out the response before saying more. Remember that once you share details, you can't take them back. That's why it's wiser to reveal small amounts of general information at first and then more only if it feels important and right to do so. Keep in mind that friends, family members and others are not therapists and may have difficulty hearing specifics and explicit information. You don't need to share a lot to receive some understanding and caring from people you know.

- **Find strength in numbers.** If confiding in one person isn't for you or if you feel you could benefit from joining with others in an active healing process, there are a number of support groups for survivors of sexual abuse or violence. Find local groups and resources on RAINN—the Rape, Abuse & Incest National Network (RAINN.org/statistics/victims-sexual-violence—just type in your zip code).

- **Read helpful books or listen to podcasts.** Reading about or listening to other survivors' stories can show you there's a light at the end of the tunnel. If you find the details too upsetting, you can skim over those parts to get to the recommendations. Some books to try include *The Courage to Heal* and my book *The Sexual Healing Journey*. Sometimes just listening to others' stories is therapeutic. Safe Space Radio features conversations on sex abuse and related topics.

- **Seek counseling.** I'm not a fan of digging up the past for no reason. But if the abuse you suffered in the past is affecting your mental and physical health or harming your ability to be intimate—or if you want to understand better how it has influenced your life—find a therapist. Sex abuse recovery therapists can help you undo negative thinking patterns and develop skills for self-care, self-compassion and speaking up for yourself. Ask your doctor or a rape crisis center for therapists who have worked with sex abuse survivors. It's also OK to make trial appointments with two or three therapists and see which one is the best fit.

SHOULD I CONFRONT THE ABUSER?

Counseling can be particularly helpful if the person who abused or harassed you has resurfaced or somehow still is a part of your life. A therapist can help you work out whether you want to call out this person's behavior. There's no single right answer—unless you believe that someone else, especially a child, is in danger. Then it's your responsibility to do whatever is necessary, including calling the police, to avert future abuse.

Choosing to confront an abuser depends on your emotional strength, what you want to accomplish and who else is involved, including other potential victims, and how cooperative and safe they are. The best scenario is to confront the person with the guidance and presence of a trained professional. When therapists facilitate such conversations, they can help you prepare well and move the discussion along to a resolution. But if that's not possible, it may be appropriate to enlist a supportive friend to be there. Remember, confrontations are not always necessary or advised.

As an alternative, you may decide to confront your abuser through a letter or a phone call or by e-mail. These, too, are best accomplished with a therapist's guidance. Focus on the power of asserting your truth, rather than making the success of the interaction whether you receive a specific response.

Figure out beforehand how you'll handle your abuser's reaction. Many offenders will deny the extent of the abuse, minimize it or blame the survivor in some way. And all of that can be really upsetting, so you want to be emotionally prepared and supported.

HEALING OUR CULTURE

Finally, it's important to realize that sexual violence is a cultural problem. I challenge anyone to turn on the TV and not find a program on some channel where a woman has been or is about to be sexually intimidated in some form. Sexual aggression against women is a common feature in popular pornography, as well. It's become entertainment, and we've become desensitized to it.

We can't keep role-modeling negative behaviors and expect change or expect the victims to mop up the mess. Instead, we must change our behavior in terms of what we tolerate in the media and as bystanders. When something that is meant "as a joke" is demeaning, say so. When you see abuse, call it out—if necessary, to the authorities.

Reclaiming Your Life After Trauma

Judy Kuriansky, PhD, clinical psychologist and sex therapist on the adjunct faculty of Teachers College, Columbia University, in New York City. She is the author of five books, including *The Complete Idiot's Guide to a Healthy Relationship.* DrJudy.com

You come home to find your house burglarized...your daughter has a serious car accident...you're laid off from a job you need and love...a friend loses her battle with cancer...or seemingly out of the blue, your husband demands a divorce. Such shocking and traumatic events wreak havoc with your emotions, leaving you struggling to pick up the pieces of your life. Nothing can make that task easy, but there are ways to make the challenge less daunting. *Here's what can help you cope after a trauma...*

• **Expect a myriad of reactions.** A disaster in your personal life inevitably triggers a range of reactions on many levels—emotional (panic, rage, desperation)...cognitive (confusion, indecision, obsessive thoughts)...physical (palpitations, breathlessness, insomnia, aches)...and spiritual (questioning your faith or the meaning of life). Simply knowing that these experiences are normal can buffer their impact a bit.

• **Call yourself a survivor.** When you catch yourself thinking of yourself as a victim, try substituting the word survivor—you'll feel less helpless and more empowered.

• **Remember how you coped with past traumas.** Even if the current crisis is more severe than any difficulty you faced before, the coping techniques you used successfully in the past can be invaluable to you now. Do whatever makes you feel better—burn off anger in a fast-paced Zumba class, ease tension with a soothing bubble bath, find solace in the meditative repetition of weeding a garden. The stress that accompanies a crisis increases your risk for illness, so safeguard your health by eating well and getting to bed early. In talking with others, strive for balance—neither isolating yourself completely from friends and family nor obsessively repeating every detail of the trauma to anyone who's near. Reveal your feelings at your own pace, choosing trustworthy confidants who listen empathically and help you process your experience and emotions.

• **Stay in the present.** There's no point in beating yourself up for a past event that you could not have foreseen or prevented ("If only I had told Aunt Trudy not to live in tornado country")...nor does it help to catastrophize about the future ("What if I never find another job and wind up on the streets?").

Better: Resume your normal daily activities to the extent possible...and take what comfort you can in small pleasures of the present moment. If you were to blame—for instance, you fell asleep at the wheel and caused an accident—you'll no doubt feel remorseful about what's past and must make whatever reparations you can, but try to focus mostly on learning lessons so you can prevent similar events in the future.

• **Consider professional help.** It is normal for a sense of loss to linger for a long time or to resurface on occasion (commonly on an anniversary). But it's best to see a counselor with expertise in bereavement or crisis counseling if you find it impossible to function...if extreme distress persists for more than a month...if people who know you well express concern about your behavior, appearance or well-being...or if you're tempted to "self-medicate" the pain away with excessive alcohol, pills or food or unsafe sexual activities. Get referrals from your doctor...or check online search engines for local grief therapists or counselors who treat post-traumatic stress disorder, then check out their credentials.

• **Let the crisis serve as a catalyst for change.** Trauma provides an opportunity for reevaluating priorities. Decide what's truly important to you and take new directions accordingly—for instance, by finally pursuing your dream career, devoting more time to cherished relationships or embarking on a spiritual journey that will enrich the rest of your life.

Using Video Games to Overcome Emotional Pain

Jayne Gackenbach, PhD, department of psychology, Grant MacEwan University, Edmonton, Alberta, Canada.

Critics regularly blame video games for everything from contributing to a slothful youth culture to encouraging aggressive behavior—but now some scientists are telling a different story, citing a litany of health benefits such as stress reduction, improved mood, pain management, lower heart rate, faster reaction time and better problem-solving abilities. And a recent Oxford University study suggests that games similar to the old classic Tetris, an engrossing game in which a player quickly stacks and organizes colorful blocks as they cascade down the screen, can actually help prevent and treat post-traumatic stress disorder (PTSD).

GAME ON—TETRIS VS. PTSD

Disturbing flashbacks, intensely vivid mental images of a past traumatic experience, are a common symptom of PTSD that can develop after experiences such as accidents, abuse, sexual molestation or military combat. Earlier research suggests that there is a six-hour window in which victims "consolidate" memories following a traumatic event. At Oxford, researchers theorized that distracting the brain during this period could act as a "cognitive vaccine" against flashbacks.

To test their hypothesis, the investigators asked 40 male volunteers (average age 23) to watch a 12-minute video. It graphically depicted a road accident that resulted in injury and death. The video was followed by a 30-minute unstructured break with no distractions provided except, for half the participants, 10 minutes of playing Tetris. Both groups were monitored for flashbacks over the following week—those who had played Tetris reported experiencing significantly fewer than those who had not played.

The Oxford researchers concluded that distracting the brain with a Tetris-like game after a traumatic event helps prevent the mental integration of traumatic images and reduces the intensity and frequency of unwanted, involuntary flashbacks.

YOU'RE IN CONTROL

Playing this type of video game may provide enough cognitive engagement to divert the brain from the normal "rev up" of the autonomic nervous system—the fight-or-flight response. It also puts the player into a mental state that combines concentration and relaxation. And people feel helpless in stressful or traumatic situations, whereas the opposite is true when you play a video game—you can take control, a feeling that can be particularly beneficial in countering the effects of PTSD.

Hopefully nobody reading this suffers an event traumatic enough that they'd need to try to erase the anguish with a video game. And

Panic Attacks Increase Risk for Heart Attack and Stroke

Panic attacks are characterized by sudden fear and anxiety, sweating, shortness of breath, choking sensation, chills and chest pain.

Recent finding: Older women who had one or more panic attacks in the past six months had four times more risk for a heart attack within the next six months than women who had no panic attacks... and three times more risk for stroke.

Self-defense: If you are having panic attacks, see your doctor.

Jordan Smoller, MD, ScD, associate professor of psychiatry, Harvard Medical School, and director of the psychiatric genetics program in mood and anxiety disorders, Massachusetts General Hospital, both in Boston, and leader of a study of 3,369 women, published in *Archives of General Psychiatry*.

it's safe to say that no health expert would advise playing these games for extended periods of time...but there may be some very practical ways these findings can be put to use in everyday life. For instance, if you suffer from chronic pain, this may be a way to distract yourself from what hurts and allow your brain to stop the continuous feedback loop that chronic pain can create.

Another idea: A short round of the absorbing video game Angry Birds (or another one) may be a helpful timeout during a stressful period. As with all medical therapies, it seems that the wise use of video games is starting to fall into place right where logic would put it—the right amount, at the right time, and not more.

Take Charge of Your Anger To Protect Your Health

W. Robert Nay, PhD, clinical psychologist and clinical associate professor of psychiatry at Georgetown University School of Medicine in Washington, DC. The author of *Taking Charge of Anger*, he is in private practice in McLean, Virginia, and Annapolis, Maryland, and trains professionals in anger management. WRobertNay.com

All you have to do is pick up a newspaper or go online to read a story about the many ways that poorly managed anger ruins lives—in schools, offices, relationships and more. Every week, I treat patients who simply "can't" control their anger. These are usually good, caring people, but their inability to handle their intense feelings of anger hurts their relationships, their ability to work effectively—and their health.

What anger does to your body and effective ways to defuse it...

YOUR BODY ON ANGER

In small doses, anger can be a helpful emotion—it signals to you and others that important needs are not being met. Perhaps you've been lied to by a loved one or feel overburdened by demands from the family.

If you can learn to manage your irate feelings, you can use them as energy to solve problems. For instance, if you see a neighbor illegally burning leaves, instead of starting an argument, you can remain calm and educate him/her about safer ways to dispose of his trash.

However, if you're not able to effectively manage anger, it can blaze out of control. When this happens, you feel threatened, and the primitive fight-or-flight response kicks in to prepare your body mentally and physically for survival. Without conscious thought, adrenaline is released, shoulders tense, the heart beats faster and blood rushes to the face, all of which can have a negative impact on your health.

Anger can contribute to...

- **Heart attack and stroke.** Anger increases your heart rate and blood pressure, raising the risk of developing coronary heart disease (or suffering further complications if you already have it). Because of the fight-or-flight response, your red blood cells become more "sticky" (to increase clotting ability in case you are injured), while your liver releases more fats into your blood (for muscles to burn)—both of which increase odds of a cardiac event.

- **Stomach problems.** When you're fuming, blood from your stomach and gastrointestinal (GI) system is diverted to your brain and muscles, which can contribute to stomach upset, acid reflux, nausea, changes in bowel and urination frequency and irritable bowel syndrome (IBS).

- **Muscle tension.** Your muscles tighten in a state of anger—they become poised to help you "fight" or "flee" from the situation. The shoulders, neck, forehead and jaw are all typical hot spots. As anger continues, soreness or musculoskeletal pain may occur.

- **Breathing issues.** When you're feeling outraged, respiration speeds up in an effort to deliver blood to the brain and muscles, resulting in shallow breathing and sensations of chest heaviness and throat constriction.

Also, blood vessels in the face, hands and elsewhere constrict during anger. Your face and neck might feel flushed or warm ("hot under the collar") or may even look bright red.

ANGER MANAGEMENT

If you experience any of these effects, anger is likely impacting your health in a negative way. Besides the symptoms mentioned above, you may notice that you are constantly on edge and have trouble relaxing. You also could have little energy, and the simplest activity might seem overwhelming.

But, if you're aware of your anger being triggered, you can effectively manage it to help prevent harmful automatic responses from happening and harming your health.

The following techniques will build your self-awareness and help you better manage your anger by promoting deep relaxation. Do them when you first notice signs of anger in your body. The first step for each technique is to sit down, lean back and let the chair support your back.

- **Deep breathing.** Relax your stomach muscles and breathe in through your nose, allowing your lungs to completely fill with air and expand into the abdominal area. Exhale very slowly through your pursed lips, as if you were letting air out of a small valve. As you exhale, silently count backward from 10 to one, which helps distract you from thoughts of anger. Doing this can help you feel calm and secure. Many people are so used to shallow chest breathing that this may feel odd at first. It becomes more natural with practice. About 15 minutes before bedtime, practice deep breathing for three to five minutes, so you can use it as needed. It also helps promote deep sleep.

- **Progressive muscle relaxation.*** Starting with your fists, begin tensing specific muscle groups (in the forearms, shoulders and legs, for example) for 10 to 15 seconds each. Tense each group until it's quivering. Take a small breath toward the end of the tensing period, then release your breath and the tension. Repeat, then move on to the next muscle group.

*If you have a muscle disorder or chronic pain, check with your doctor before starting this technique as it could worsen these conditions.

Muscle relaxation helps make you aware of when your muscles are tensing and gives you a simple way to relax them. Do this exercise for at least 15 minutes once each day for the first two weeks. Then use when needed.

Time to get help? If you have extreme fight-or-flight symptoms, are getting angry more often or if others are complaining about your temper, seek professional help. Visit the American Psychological Association at Locator.APA.org to find an anger-management expert.

3 SMART WAYS TO DEFUSE ANGER

- **Sit down!** Your brain interprets a seated or reclining position as safe and relaxing, interrupting the flow of anger-enhancing adrenaline. The next time you're in an argument, get yourself (and the other person) to sit down. Say something like, "Let's sit and discuss this." If you're already sitting down when angered, try leaning back and relaxing your muscles.

- **Never go to bed angry.** Research proves that the old saying is right! A recent study found that hitting the sack after having negative emotions appears to reinforce them. Try to resolve disagreements before saying good night.

- **Become an observer.** The next time your blood boils, step back and view the situation from a distance. Evaluate how angry you are on a scale of 0 to 100. Then project what may happen if you don't lower that figure by using some of the techniques here. This will help you remain calm.

The Healing Power of Forgiveness

Ellis Cose, contributing editor to *Newsweek* and *Weekend Edition* commentator for National Public Radio. He is author of several books, most recently, *Bone to Pick: Of Forgiveness, Reconciliation, Reparation and Revenge.*

Recent studies about forgiveness have proven what major religions advocate—showing your antagonists compassion and letting go of the desire for revenge can improve your psychological and physical health.

Example: In a study of 71 people conducted at Hope College in Michigan, researchers found that forgiveness lowered risk of heart problems. Participants were asked to recall hurtful memories about friends, lovers, parents and siblings. Their heart rates and blood pressure tested significantly lower after they had forgiven the people who had hurt them.

Even once we know the benefits, many of us find it hard to forgive. It's easier and seems more satisfying to strike back—or to fantasize about it—than to turn the other cheek. Can forgiveness really improve our lives? How can we learn to forgive?

We spoke to renowned journalist and commentator Ellis Cose. During his distinguished career, he has interviewed victims of some of the worst atrocities of our time—survivors of the Holocaust and African genocides...adults molested by priests in childhood...parents of children murdered by people now on death row...and families of those killed in the September 11 terrorist attacks. Cose was amazed at how many of these ordinary human beings found the capacity and willingness to forgive—and were better off for it.

• How do I forgive when it seems impossible?

There are basically three steps...

Step 1: **Get some perspective on your pain and anger.** People who were able to get on with their lives refused to see themselves as victims. If your spouse cheats on you and leaves, you aren't an unlovable dupe—you're a devoted person who was stronger than your spouse.

Step 2: **Attempt to empathize with the person who hurt you.** Think about what he/she was feeling at the time of the transgression, and understand the pressures and factors that made him commit harmful acts. This doesn't mean that the acts were justified. It means that you have put yourself in the transgressor's shoes. This is the crux of forgiving and perhaps the hardest part.

Rejection Causes Physical Pain

Heartbreak causes physical pain as well as emotional pain.

Recent finding: The same brain regions associated with bodily pain become active when a person feels rejected by someone he/she loves.

Ethan Kross, PhD, assistant professor, department of psychology, University of Michigan, Ann Arbor, and leader of a study published in *Proceedings of the National Academy of Sciences of the United States of America.*

Step 3: **Stop thinking of forgiveness in absolute terms.** Many people fantasize that their compassion will inspire gratitude from the person who hurt them, followed by a reconciliation and a state of peace and comfort. What you often get is partial relief—a release of your most intense anger—that allows you to move on.

• Doesn't forgiving let people off the hook when they should be held accountable for their actions?

Finding a genuine way to respond with compassion may seem like letting abusers get away with their actions, but it actually benefits you more than the person you forgive. Victims told me that forgiveness was a psychological tool to heal their own wounds so that they could lead happier, more positive lives.

Think about how much energy it costs you to hold on to past incidents, feeling resentful over actions and remarks made years ago. By admitting that you can't change the past and renouncing the hold your anger has on you, you become stronger and more effective.

For example, Nelson Mandela spent 26 years in prison in South Africa, confined to a small cell with a bucket for a toilet and daily hard labor in a limestone quarry. When he was freed at age 72, he felt bitter toward his captors but was determined to not let it ruin the rest of his life. "Resentment," he said, "is like drinking poison and waiting for it to kill your enemy."

• To forgive, don't I need an apology from the person who hurt me?

It's easier to feel compassion if the perpetrator acknowledges what he/she has done and expresses regret—but victims told me that making forgiveness contingent upon an apology gives control of your emotions to someone who wasn't worthy in the first place. The result is that you cling to your anger and perpetuate your victimization.

• Is revenge ever helpful?

For superficial injustices, a small revenge can help healing. For instance, a coworker purposely embarrassed me. Later that day, I said I was driving home. The coworker said he was going that way, but I didn't offer him a ride. He knew that he was being snubbed and it was a warning to treat me respectfully.

However, the greater the injustice you suffer, the more vital a role forgiveness plays in your future well-being. I interviewed many parents whose children had been murdered. They often became obsessed with the killer's trial, hounded the district attorney's office for a capital murder charge and witnessed the execution years later—but vengeance offered only short-term relief. It was swallowed up by grief and rage at the realization that their loved one still wasn't coming back. Only forgiving let them move on with their lives.

• Are certain injustices so horrifying that they cannot be forgiven?

Each person must answer that for himself, but let me address it this way. The Holocaust survivor and Nazi hunter Simon Wiesenthal told the story of being imprisoned in a German concentration camp during World War II. He listened to the deathbed confession of a 22-year-old German soldier who had asked to confess to a Jewish prisoner. The Nazi said that he had herded Jews in the Ukraine into a building, tossed grenades into it and shot those who tried to run. The soldier wanted a Jew to forgive him. Wiesenthal opted not to respond, silently rejecting the plea for absolution.

When the war was over, Wiesenthal paid a visit to the mother of the Nazi soldier. Tempted as he was to tell the mother about the murders, he could not shatter her illusions about her dead son. He merely told her that he had been asked to convey greetings from her son and sat silently as she called her son a "good boy."

• What if I just can't forgive? Is there something positive I can do to feel better?

People who struggle with forgiveness sometimes engage in "constructive revenge." They take aggressive action aimed not directly at their abuser but at a larger goal that fights the kind of thing the person has done. This transforms their suffering into something nobler.

Example: I spent some time with Azim Khamisa, an investment consultant in La Jolla, California. A decade ago, his son Tariq, a 20-year-old student at San Diego State University, was jumped by a gang while delivering pizzas. A 14-year-old named Tony Hicks shot Tariq in the heart. Hicks pled guilty to first-degree murder. He was sentenced as an adult to 25 years to life.

The sentence brought Azim Khamisa no relief. What did save him was starting a foundation in his son's name that holds forums at schools to teach kids about the consequences of violence. His perspective on his son's death began to change, and that mitigated his rage.

Khamisa was able to develop a relationship with Hicks's grandfather, who also had been devastated by the murder. The two men forged an alliance and now make appearances together promoting nonviolence.

Tap Away Fears And Phobias

Shoshana Garfield, PhD, psychologist, registered trauma specialist and neurolinguistic programming master practitioner in practice in Uplands, Wales. UnlimitedEmotionalFreedom.com

Is it possible to "tap away" fearful images and obsessions? There is an emotional-healing terapy that does just that. Called Thought Field Therapy (TFT), the technique is designed to help people permanently free themselves from phobias (strong, irrational fears of things that pose little or no actual danger), such as fear of spiders or of public speaking...and even from post-traumatic stress disorder (PTSD), an anxiety disorder that can develop after a terrifying event in which grave harm occurred or was threatened. No medications are used, so there are no side effects. TFT falls within the field of energy psychology (similar to Emotional Freedom Technique, or EFT, see page 507 for more information). TFT involves thinking about the feared object or event while tapping specific points on the face and body and humming, counting or moving the eyes.

TFT has roots in acupuncture, in that you tap on points that correspond to energy meridians. This helps unblock the body's energy system, which can become overwhelmed by fear. TFT also simultaneously provides sensory data to the right brain (the emotional side) and left brain (the logical side). This stimulates activity of both brain hemispheres and of the corpus callosum that connects them...deactivates signals associated with fear-triggered hyperarousal of the limbic system...and "rewires" cognitive function, releasing distress.

Evidence: In a 2010 study, PTSD patients treated with TFT showed dramatic decreases in nightmares, flashbacks, concentration problems, jumpiness, aggression and isolation. Other studies have demonstrated TFT's effectiveness in reducing depression...and in patients with anxiety disorder, EEG scans showed that abnormal brain wave patterns associated with anxiety normalized after TFT treatment.

One case study included a woman who had a lifelong fear of water. After more than a year of ineffective conventional treatment, she was instructed to tap a spot under each eye while looking at a swimming pool. After a few minutes of tapping, she said that she no longer felt any fear, then ran to the pool and splashed water on her face—something she could not do previously.

TRYING TFT FOR YOURSELF

For best results, work with a psychologist trained in TFT who can provide testimonials from other patients with phobias similar to yours.

Try Horseback Riding

Giddyup! Therapeutic horseback riding could help military veterans with PTSD.

Report: Vets who participated in a riding program had 87% declines in PTSD scores after just six weeks.

University of Missouri College of Veterinary Medicine.

Referrals: Association for Comprehensive Energy Psychology (visit EnergyPsych.org and click on "Find a Practitioner")...or Association for the Advancement of Meridian Energy Techniques (visit AAMET.org)...or Dr. Roger Callahan (RogerCallahan.com). Results might be seen after just one treatment for a simple phobia or might take nine months or longer for PTSD. Are you skeptical? That's OK—because TFT can be quite effective even if you don't believe in it.

For simple fears that are not deeply interwoven with complex traumas, you may find relief on your own with the tapping sequence below. Practice it several times until you know the steps...then do the sequence whenever you anticipate or encounter the feared object or event. (Use common sense, of course—for instance, by tapping before you get behind the wheel, rather than while you are driving.) The routine takes just a few minutes and, though it may seem complicated at first, it soon becomes second nature.

Demo: YouTube.com/watch?v=ntWUsL5hZJ0.

Step 1: **Focus attention on the thing you fear.** For instance, visualize a spider or imagine driving through a construction zone.

Important: Keep thinking about the object of your fear throughout your TFT session.

Step 2: **Rate your fear level on a scale of zero to 10.** Zero would indicate no distress whatsoever and 10 would be the worst it could possibly be. Remember this number.

Step 3: **Tap.** Use the tips of the index and middle fingers of either hand to tap firmly (but not hard enough to hurt) five to 10 times, at a moderately fast pace. First tap four inches below either armpit (women: the center of the band on your bra)...then tap one inch below the center of either eye.

Step 4: **Perform the nine-step "gamut sequence."** Make a loose fist with your nondominant hand and locate what TFT practitioners call the gamut spot on the back of that hand, in the hollow an inch below the knuckles of the ring and little fingers. Start tapping this gamut spot with the index and middle fingers of your dominant hand.

Continuing tapping, giving five to 10 taps for each of the following actions.

Gamut sequence: Open eyes wide...close eyes...open eyes and (keeping head still) look down and to the left...look down and to the right...roll eyes around counterclockwise... roll eyes around clockwise...hum a few bars of any song (activating the right brain)...count aloud from one to five (activating the left brain)...hum again. When finished, repeat the gamut sequence a second time.

Step 5: **Rate your fear again, from zero to 10.** If your score has dropped to zero, terrific! If it has not, repeat all the TFT steps one or more times, continuing to visualize the object of your phobia. Then, again rate your fear level—which may now be much lower.

CHAPTER 8

Exercise Injury and Pain Prevention

4 Dangerous Fitness Myths—Half-Truths Can Turn Your Exercise Regimen Into an Injury Trap

Don't believe everything you hear when you are trying to get in shape or stay in shape. There are plenty of myths and half-truths.

Among the most dangerous fitness myths to avoid...

***FITNESS MYTH #1:* A little pain means you're getting maximum benefit from your workout.** Despite the popular cliché "no pain, no gain," you should never feel prolonged, stabbing or sharp pain during a workout or continue to exercise when something hurts.

The risk: Pain means damage. It could be a warning sign that you have overstressed or overstretched a muscle, tendon or ligament. It also can indicate joint damage. People who continue to exercise when they hurt risk more serious injuries, such as torn muscles or tendinitis (inflammation of a tendon).

Exception: A little soreness after exercise means that you have had a good workout. When you exercise hard, the muscles develop microscopic tears that lead to rebuilding of tissue and an increase in strength. If you are very sore, however, you have overworked your muscles.

Warning: Don't believe the myth that you can exercise longer and harder if you take an anti-inflammatory pain reliever, such as *ibuprofen* (Motrin), before going to the gym. Taking a preworkout anti-inflammatory may reduce muscle performance and prevent you from feeling an injury while working out.

Important: If you have arthritis or another painful condition that requires daily treat-

Wayne Westcott, PhD, director of the Exercise Science Program, Quincy College, Massachusetts. He is the author or coauthor of several fitness books, including *Get Stronger, Feel Younger.*

ment with aspirin, ibuprofen or another anti-inflammatory medication, ask your doctor if it's safe to take the drug prior to workouts. The combination of exercise and anti-inflammatories might increase the risk for damage to the gastrointestinal lining, according to recent research.

***FITNESS MYTH #2:* You should stretch before exercising.** Trainers used to advise everyone to stretch before lifting weights, going for a run, etc. Do not do it.

The risk: Tendons and ligaments take longer to warm up than muscles. People who stretch when they're "cold" are more likely to suffer from muscle and tendon strains and other injuries than those who begin their workouts with a progressive warm-up. Static stretches, in which you stretch a muscle to a point of tension and hold the stretch for a certain period of time, can be particularly harmful before a workout.

Recent finding: New research also has shown that people who do static stretches before working out can't exercise as long and may have reduced muscle strength.

Exception: You can start a workout with dynamic stretches, slow movements that mimic the exercise patterns you're about to do. Before taking a run, for example, you could do some fast walking and slow jogging. This type of stretching is safe and prepares the muscles for exercise.

Also: Stretch after vigorous activity. That's when muscles and tendons have the best blood flow and elasticity, and you're less likely to get injured. *Good postworkout stretches...*

- **Figure Four.** Sit on the floor with both legs out in front of you. Bend your left leg, placing the sole of your left foot against your right inner thigh. With your right hand, reach for your right ankle and hold for 30 seconds. Perform twice on each side to stretch your hamstrings and calves.
- **Letter T.** Lie faceup on the floor with your arms in a T-position. Slowly cross your left leg over your body, allowing your torso to rotate so that your left foot is near your right hand. Keep your leg as straight as possible. Hold for 20 seconds. Perform twice on each side to stretch your hips and lower back.

***FITNESS MYTH #3:* Do not rest during workouts.** You have probably heard that the best strength-training workouts involve nonstop action, with no rest (or very little rest) between exercises.

The risk: Failing to rest will cause muscle fatigue and poor form, a common cause of injuries. Also, you won't fully train the muscles because they need time to recover.

When you're working the same muscles, you need to rest 30 to 90 seconds between sets.

Example: Do eight to 12 biceps curls... take a 30- to 90-second break...then curl the weight again.

Exception: With circuit training, you move quickly from one exercise to the next. You might do a biceps exercise, then a leg exercise, then return to the biceps. Even though you're constantly moving (and getting a good cardiovascular workout), you're allowing one group of muscles to rest while you work a different part of the body.

***FITNESS MYTH #4:* High-heat exercise works the muscles more.** Some people believe that high-temperature workouts—including "hot" yoga, spinning and others in which the room temperature may be 90°F or even hotter—make the muscles more limber and improve the body's ability to remove toxins.

I do not recommend it. For the average person, exercising in high temperatures will reduce their performance because the body has to work harder to fend off the heat.

The risk: It forces the heart to do double-duty—not only to bring oxygen to the muscles and remove wastes that accumulate during exercise, but also to pump more blood to the skin to dissipate the extra heat. If you're tempted to try high-heat workouts, ask your doctor first.

More from Dr. Westcott...

Save Your Back

"Core"-strengthening exercises help prevent low-back pain by strengthening abdominal and back muscles. However, one of the most popular of these workouts, which involves lying on your back and simultaneously raising both legs in the air, causes a pronounced arch in the low back that can trigger—or worsen—low-back pain.

Better: Bicycle maneuver. Lie with your lower back pressed against the floor, your hands clasped behind your head and your knees bent. Simultaneously lift your head and shoulders off the floor. Bring your left knee to your right elbow, while straightening your right leg. Using a bicycle-pedaling motion, alternate sides. Extend your legs as far as you comfortably can without arching your back.

Typical number of reps: 10 to 15 times on each leg with slow and controlled movements.

How to Exercise When You're Sore

Does exercising when muscles are sore ease the discomfort—or increase the risk for injury?

After intense exercise, muscles are sore because your workout caused small tears in the tissues. Exercising strenuously again the next day (or even the day after that, if you are still sore) delays healing and perpetuates soreness. It also slightly elevates the risk for injury because your muscles won't be at peak strength.

Better: When you are sore, stick to light cardio exercise (walking, low-resistance stationary cycling) for the next day or two. This promotes blood flow, facilitating delivery of nutrients to muscles and speeding healing.

Wayne Westcott, PhD, director of the Exercise Science Program, Quincy College, Massachusetts. He is the author or coauthor of 24 fitness books, including *Get Stronger, Feel Younger.*

Don't Give Up on the Treadmill...Be Safe

Rebecca Shannonhouse, editor, *Bottom Line Health*, with Wayne L. Westcott, PhD, director of the Exercise Science Program, Quincy College, Massachusetts.

It's true that treadmill workouts can be riskier than many other types of exercise. You might strain a muscle on an exercise bike or lose your grip when lifting weights, but at least you control the motion. A treadmill, once you turn it on, just keeps going.

"We insist that people on treadmills wear shut-off safety straps, which shut down the machine if they start drifting too far backward or stumble," says Wayne L. Westcott, PhD, director of the Exercise Science Program at Quincy College in Massachusetts.

But the treadmill is also effective. A study in *The Journal of the American Medical Association* found that it was better at improving heart-lung fitness than other equipment, such as a stair-stepper, stationary bike or rowing machine.

What's the solution? Fatal accidents involving treadmills are rare—30 deaths were reported from 2003 to 2012. The risk from not using a treadmill (or getting some form of exercise) is much greater. Just be sure to learn the machine's safety features, read the instructions—and check with your doctor before starting an exercise program (to assess, for example, your heart health and balance).

More Treadmill Safety...

Barry A. Franklin, PhD, director of preventive cardiology/cardiac rehabilitation at William Beaumont Hospital in Royal Oak, Michigan. He is coauthor of *One Heart, Two Feet.* CreativeWalking.com

Treadmills are generally a safe way to exercise, but accidental falls can happen. *To stay safe...*

- **Always straddle the treadmill before turning it on,** and don't assume it will always start at a slow, comfortable speed.

- **Always warm up and cool down before and after the aerobic phase of your workout.** Never suddenly stop the treadmill.

• **Skip the ankle weights.** You've probably seen people at the gym wearing ankle weights while walking on the treadmill. It's safer to avoid. They can strain the lower extremities, increasing your risk for orthopedic or musculoskeletal problems.

Better approach: Try walking with a backpack carrying a comfortable amount of weight. You'll burn more calories than you would if you were walking without one. A snug fit will keep the weight close to your spine and hips—which may help you avoid balance problems and improve your bone density.

Safe Workouts for Women

Wayne Westcott, PhD, director of the Exercise Science Program, Quincy College, Massachusetts. He is the author or coauthor of several fitness books, including *Get Stronger, Feel Younger.*

Exercise machines can provide excellent workouts. But unfortunately, a woman may wind up with injuries if she uses a machine improperly—or if the machine is not suitable for a person her size.

Benefits: Cardiovascular exercise helps you control or lose weight...reduces blood pressure and cholesterol...and boosts energy and mood.*

Do a cardio workout for 30 minutes or more at least three times a week. Begin with a five-minute warm-up, working up to your target speed...and end with a five-minute cooldown, gradually slowing your pace. For the 20 minutes in between, work hard enough to give your heart a workout, but not so hard that you risk overtaxing it.

To gauge effort: If you can talk normally, work harder...if you barely have the breath to get a word out, ease up. Interval workouts—alternating every few minutes between bursts of intense activity and periods of lighter activity—burn more calories than a single sustained pace.

RECOMMENDED: TREADMILL

You walk or run on a flat or inclined surface as the treadmill records your time, mileage, heart rate and/or calories burned. A preset program can automatically generate varying speeds and inclines.

Especially beneficial for: Women with or at risk for osteoporosis (brittle bone disease). Walking is a weight-bearing exercise that increases bone density...and the treadmill's shock-absorbing platform is easier on joints than pavement.

To use: Start by setting the speed at two miles per hour, then slowly increase your pace. Move naturally, keeping your head up and staying in the center of the belt.

Safety alert: Holding the handrails while walking rapidly or running forces your body into an unnatural posture, increasing the risk for muscle strain—so once you have your balance, let go. Use a safety key with a cord that clips to your clothing and connects to the emergency "off" switch so that the treadmill belt will immediately stop moving if you fall.

RECOMMENDED: STATIONARY BICYCLE

An upright bike looks and feels like a regular road bike. With a recumbent bike, the rider sits on a wide saddle, leaning against a backrest, legs out in front. Both types give an equally good cardio workout.

Especially beneficial for: Women with balance problems, because there is no risk of falling...and overweight women, because it supports the body and allows adjustable levels of external resistance rather than working against the user's own body weight. A recumbent bike is most comfortable for people with back problems or limited mobility.

To use: Every few minutes, alternate "sprints" of fast, low-resistance pedaling..."climbs" of slow, high-resistance pedaling...and recovery intervals of moderately paced, medium-resistance pedaling. To work shin muscles, use pedal straps or toe clips so that you can pull up as well as push down while pedaling.

*Check with your doctor before beginning any exercise program, especially if you are pregnant, are new to exercise, have recently recovered from an injury or have a chronic disease.

Safety alert: Improper seat height can lead to knee injuries. When one pedal is pushed all the way down, your knee should be slightly bent—never fully extended. If the seat adjusts forward and aft, position it so that knees align with your ankles rather than extending beyond your toes. If you have narrow hips and the distance between the pedals seems too wide, see if a different brand of bike feels more comfortable. To reduce back and shoulder strain on an upright bike, raise the handlebars.

USE WITH CAUTION: STAIR-STEPPER

This machine provides a challenging workout because you work against your own body weight and your center of gravity moves up and down with every step.

Problem: Users may lean heavily on the handrails to keep their balance and to take weight off the legs. This increases the risk for injury to the wrists...and misaligns the spine, which can strain the back.

Solution: To avoid falls, keep only your fingertips on the rails, using a light touch...maintain a moderate pace that does not challenge your balance. Do not set the height of the rise too high (as if taking stairs two at a time)—the stepping motion should feel natural. For good posture, keep shoulders and hips aligned and imagine trying to touch the top of your head to the ceiling.

Note: The stair-stepper may not be appropriate if you are overweight or new to exercise and feel discouraged by the difficulty of the workout...have problems with your joints...or have any trouble with balance.

USE WITH CAUTION: ELLIPTICAL TRAINER

This low-impact machine combines the leg motions of stair climbing with cross-country skiing to work the lower body. Some styles include movable arm poles, adding an upper-body component.

Problem: For short-legged women, the elliptical can force a longer-than-normal stride that may strain the knees, hips and/or lower back.

Solution: The goal is to move smoothly with good posture. If your movement feels awkward or jerky, decrease the stride setting (try 16 inches). If this does not help, avoid the elliptical trainer.

RECOMMENDED: STRENGTH-TRAINING

Next, add strength-training machines, which build muscle...fortify tendons and ligaments... increase bone density...improve posture... boost mood...and raise metabolic rate so that you burn more fat.

Best: Do a strength-training workout two to three times per week, leaving at least one day between workouts so that muscles can recover. Start with a gentle warm-up of three to five minutes, doing an activity that involves the whole body, such as jumping jacks. Then use the machines for a total of 20 to 30 minutes.

Machine styles and weight increments vary depending on the manufacturer. If the machines in your gym do not have the same increments as the starting weight guidelines below, ask a trainer if it is possible to modify the options. *On each machine...*

- **Perform one to three sets of eight to 12 repetitions,** resting for one minute between sets.
- **If you can't complete eight repetitions using the starting guidelines, reduce the weight.** When it becomes easy to complete one set of 12 reps, try two sets, then three. When it becomes easy to do three sets, increase the weight.
- **Control the motion at all times.** Count slowly to two as you raise the weight...count to four as you lower the weight.
- **Exhale as you raise the weight...inhale as you lower the weight.** This helps keep blood pressure down.

Finish workouts with a three-minute walk to cool down. Then do three minutes of gentle stretching to maintain flexibility, holding each stretch for 15 to 30 seconds.

New research: Stretching promotes additional gains in strength.

Address each major muscle group to keep muscles in balance—otherwise the weaker muscles could be prone to injury. *A complete workout typically includes…*

• **Lat pull-down.**

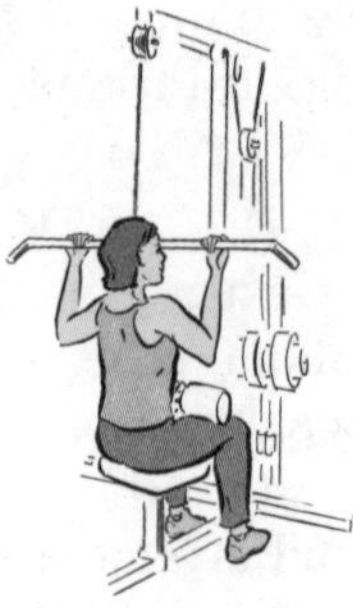

Muscles worked: The latissimus dorsi (upper back) and biceps—muscles used in daily life for lifting and carrying (for example, grocery bags).

To use: Sit tall, facing the machine, with thighs tucked beneath the pads to stabilize your lower body. Reach up, palms facing you and slightly farther than shoulder-width apart, and grasp the bar hanging overhead. Squeeze shoulder blades together as you pull the bar down a few inches in front of your face…stop at chin level…then raise the bar to starting position. Start with 35 pounds if you're in your 40s…32.5 pounds in your 50s…30 pounds in your 60s…27.5 pounds in your 70s…25 pounds in your 80s and beyond.

Safety alert: Never pull the bar behind your head. This can injure the neck and shoulders. It is safe to grasp the bar with palms facing away—but muscles get a better workout when palms face you.

• **Shoulder press.**

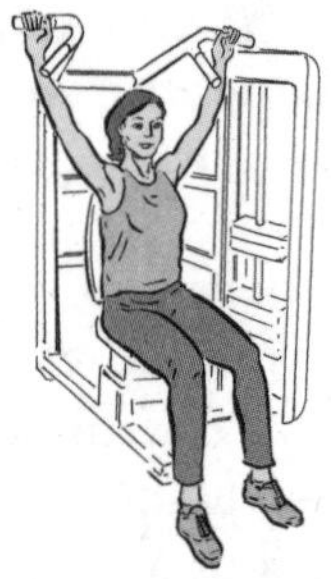

Muscles worked: Shoulders, triceps (back of the arms) and base of the neck—used when placing items on a high shelf.

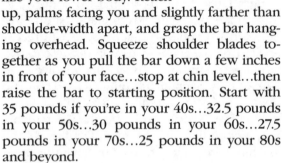

To use: Sit erect, hips and shoulder blades pressed against the backrest. With hands at shoulder height, palms facing forward and arms bent, grasp the outer set of handles and push up until arms are nearly straight…then lower to starting position. Start with 30 pounds if you're in your 40s…27.5 pounds in your 50s…25 pounds in your 60s…22.5 pounds in your 70s…20 pounds in your 80s and beyond.

Safety alert: If you have shoulder problems, such as with your rotator cuff, use the inner handles, palms facing each other—this is easier.

• **Chest press.**

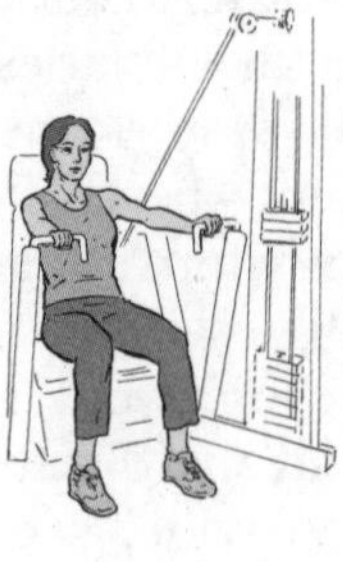

Muscles worked: Pectorals (front of the chest) and triceps—used for pushing a lawn mower or wheelchair.

To use: Sit erect with arms bent, hands at chest height, palms facing forward. Grasp handles and press forward, elbows pointing to the sides (not down), until arms are nearly straight…then bend elbows and return to starting position. Start with 35 pounds if you're in your 40s…32.5 pounds in your 50s…30 pounds in your 60s…27.5 pounds in your 70s…25 pounds in your 80s and beyond.

Safety alert: Do not lean forward—keep head up and entire back pressed against the backrest to avoid neck and low-back strain.

• **Biceps curl.**

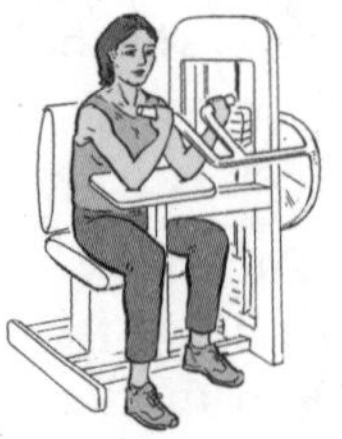

Muscles worked: Biceps and forearms—needed for lifting and carrying.

To use: Sit with arms out in front, elbows resting on the padded platform. Palms facing you, grasp handles and bend elbows to bring hands toward your chest…then straighten arms to return to starting position. Start with 30 pounds if you're in your 40s…27.5 pounds in your 50s…25 pounds in your 60s…22.5 pounds in your 70s…20 pounds in your 80s and beyond.

Safety alert: Elbows are prone to hyperextension—so to prevent joint injury when lowering the bar, stop when elbows are still slightly bent. If your lower back arches, reduce the weight to prevent back strain.

• **Leg press.**

Muscles worked: Quadriceps and hamstrings (fronts and backs of thighs), inner thighs and buttocks—vital for walking and climbing stairs.

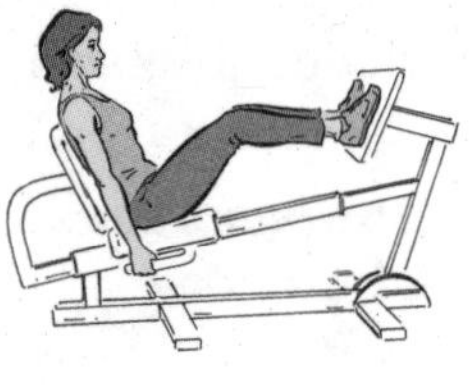

To use: Sit and recline against the backrest, legs raised in front of you, knees at a 90-degree angle, feet flat and hip-width apart on the movable platform. Slowly straighten legs until knees are almost straight, pressing with heels to push platform away...then bend knees to return to starting position. Start with 85 pounds if you're in your 40s...80 pounds in your 50s...75 pounds in your 60s...70 pounds in your 70s...65 pounds in your 80s and beyond.

Safety alert: To protect knees, do not straighten legs completely...keep thighs parallel to align knees.

- **Ab crunch machine.**

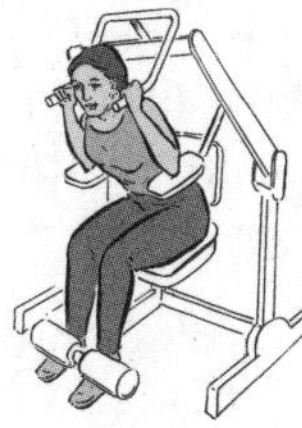

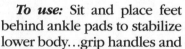

Muscles worked: Abdominals—which help maintain posture and combat belly bulge.

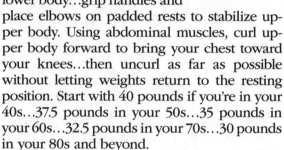

To use: Sit and place feet behind ankle pads to stabilize lower body...grip handles and place elbows on padded rests to stabilize upper body. Using abdominal muscles, curl upper body forward to bring your chest toward your knees...then uncurl as far as possible without letting weights return to the resting position. Start with 40 pounds if you're in your 40s...37.5 pounds in your 50s...35 pounds in your 60s...32.5 pounds in your 70s...30 pounds in your 80s and beyond.

Safety alert: Keep head and spine aligned to prevent neck injury.

Illustrations by Chris Andrews/Getty Images.

How to Run Injury Free

Danny Dreyer creator of ChiRunning and ChiWalking, forms of moving that blend the subtle inner focuses of Tai Chi with running and walking. He is author of *ChiRunning: A Revolutionary Approach to Effortless, Injury-free Running* and *ChiWalking: Fitness Walking for Lifelong Health and Energy.*

Many people love to run, but hate how much it can hurt afterward. ChiRunning offers a solution. It blends the internal power of tai chi with the aerobic benefits of running. ChiRunning is a technique that emphasizes proper form, core strength and relaxation, enabling you to run efficiently, safely and injury free, moving with grace and fluidity.

TAI CHI + RUNNING = CHIRUNNING

The ChiRunning technique was developed by running coach and ultramarathoner Danny Dreyer as a solution to his own vexing knee pain, which flared up during runs and left him feeling achy and exhausted afterward. He incorporated the practice of tai chi into his running and was thrilled to discover that he not only could run without pain, but that his runs left him feeling renewed and energized.

Tai chi is an ancient Chinese martial arts practice that uses the power of your mind to harness chi ("energy") from the body's center (the core muscle group, which includes lower back and abdominal muscles). According to the principles of tai chi, any type of movement, such as running or walking, can draw its strength from the core muscles, not from the legs and arms. Tai chi helps the flow of chi by teaching the practitioner to maintain a body that is well-aligned, yet relaxed.

GRAVITY PROPELS YOU

Focusing on core muscles for ChiRunning lets runners overcome the two major forces that typically work against them—the force of gravity and the force of the road coming at them. It's a natural way to run. Leaning forward reduces, and in fact nearly eliminates, the braking motion of your feet as they hit the ground.

Imagine that your spine is strong—the source of great power—and your arms and legs are loose and light. By maintaining strong posture and relaxing the rest of your body while you run, more energy can flow from your core throughout your body. Since you aren't using the legs for propulsion, ChiRunning can reduce or eliminate most of the overuse injuries associated with running, including shin splints, hamstring injury, and hip and knee problems, and it reduces pounding so there are no impact (joint) injuries. Moreover, because your body is not overworked or pounded from the run, recovery time is much quicker, leaving you feeling more energized after your run.

THE CHIRUNNING TECHNIQUE

The first step to ChiRunning is learning how to hold a tall, elongated posture while you run, allowing your structural alignment to support your body weight, not your legs. Stabilize your posture by "leveling" your pelvis (consciously lift up the front) while you run. To know how this feels, stand up tall and place your hand on your lower abdomen with your thumb in your belly button and your fingers resting across your lower abdomen. Now, shorten the distance between your thumb and fingers by pulling up on your pubic bone.

Once you have this posture working for you, fall slightly forward, keeping your posture line straight. Picture your spine as a straight arrow that begins at your ankles and ends at the top of your head.

Holding both the posture and slight forward tilt, begin to run. Bend your knees. Lean forward at the ankles, rather than at the waist, to avoid putting unwanted pressure on your back and knees. Keep your hips, shoulders and ankles in a straight line.

Let gravity work with momentum to propel you. Proper ChiRunning form involves a balancing act. You're not leaning too far forward or too far back—just allow gravity to pull you along. With each step, as your heels lift off the ground, your legs will swing to the rear and your feet will plant underneath you, rather than in front of you.

Relax your arms, legs and everything else. Use your core muscles to maintain your structure and hold your torso straight. Envision your core muscles bringing the rest of your body, including your joints, muscles, arms and legs, along for the ride. Always keep your shoulders low and relaxed.

Quiet your mind. Concentrate on leaning forward, using your core to move you, bringing your focus back to this whenever you begin to strain or your thoughts to wander. This helps maintain proper form.

Breathe. Even, relaxed breathing will give you power and help you stay relaxed throughout your run.

CHIWALKING WORKS TOO

You can also try ChiWalking, by the way. The technique for this integrates tai chi and the proper biomechanics of walking—good posture, loose joints, engaging core muscles and relaxing the arms and legs. When you try ChiWalking, slow it down, be mindful and relaxed, and try to perfect your stride. ChiRunning and ChiWalking are similar to other mindful practices such as yoga and Pilates, in which the focus is on technique, not on short-term goals such as running faster, going farther or losing weight. The pleasant side effect may be that you will get in shape and lose unwanted weight.

For more information about ChiRunning and ChiWalking, visit ChiRunning.com.

How to Prevent Shin Splints

Wayne Westcott, PhD, director of the Exercise Science Program, Quincy College, Massachusetts. He is the author or coauthor of 24 fitness books, including *Get Stronger, Feel Younger.*

"Shin splints" is a general term for muscle pain along the shins, usually caused by a muscle imbalance—strong calf muscles and weaker shin muscles. *Solution...*

- **Thread a 24-inch–long shoestring through the center hole in a two- to five-pound weight plate.** Tie the ends together so you have one big loop with the weight on it (like a key on a key ring). Sit on a countertop with your knees bent and feet dangling about 12 inches above the floor.

- **Wrap the loop of string several times around the toe box of one sneaker so the weight dangles below your toes.** Let your toes point down...then flex your foot to bring your toes up as high as you can. Point again, then flex while angling your foot slightly to lead with your little toe. On your third repetition, lead with your big toe. Do 15 reps, then switch sides. Work up to three sets every other day.

Are You Hurting Your Knees?

Wayne Westcott, PhD, director of the Exercise Science Program, Quincy College, Massachusetts. He is the author or coauthor of 24 fitness books, including *Get Stronger, Feel Younger.*

If jogging up a flight of stairs is part of your workout, are you hurting your knees?

Maybe, but you can modify your routine to reduce your chance of knee (and hip, lower back and muscular) injuries. Your best bet is to jog up the stairs, then walk back down.

Here's why: When you're running, the fraction of time your feet are in contact with the ground and supporting your weight decreases. Add the impact of bouncing, and the average "landing force" absorbed by your ankles, knees and hips is about three times your body weight. (Walking reduces the landing force absorption by about half.) Jogging up those stairs reduces this force because your foot does not drop as far as it would on level ground. Jogging down the stairs increases the landing force because your foot has to fall farther. Walking, of course, is a lower-impact exercise and less risky.

The Truth About Sit-Ups

Vik Khanna, PA, MHS, physician assistant, exercise coach and health-care consultant in Chesterfield, Missouri. He is the conditioning coach for the Missouri Karate Association and coauthor of *Ten Commandments of Faith and Fitness: A Practical Guide for Health and Wellness.* ExercisewithVik.com

There are few exercises as quintessential as the sit-up. Virtually all of us did them in gym classes when we were growing up. Many people still regularly perform sit-ups in an effort to strengthen the muscles of the core (abdomen, sides and lower back). But conventional sit-ups may cause more harm than good.

Recent development: In a report in *The United States Army Medical Department Journal*, more than half the injuries caused by the army's standard fitness test were linked to sit-ups. Various branches of the US Armed Forces are now evaluating the use of sit-ups. So what does that mean for people who need core conditioning in their fitness regimens? *Here's the latest thinking...*

TOO HARD ON THE SPINE

Sit-ups not only target mainly the rectus abdominis, the wall of abdominal muscles that bridges the area between the rib cage and the hips but also make excessive use of the hip flexors to raise the torso up toward the knees. The side oblique muscles and lower back, which are crucial for everyday activities, are left out.

But suppose that you are moving a heavy piece of furniture. Strong abdominals will help, but so will strength and stability in the back, sides and legs—areas that are not helped by sit-ups. You'll move better—with more balance and power and less risk for injury—when you exercise all the core muscles as an integrated unit.

A real downside: The most common way people do sit-ups leads them to curl their upper body into a "C shape" as they rise from the floor, which puts tremendous stress on the spinal column. This increases risk for disk herniation, back or nerve pain and muscle strain in the lower back.

A BETTER CORE WORKOUT

Based on my research and work as a conditioning coach for athletes, I believe the following exercises are superior to sit-ups because multiple muscle groups are worked together. In general, a healthy adult can do these exercises three or more times a week.

- **Forearm plank.** Known in yoga as the dolphin plank, it is a whole-body exercise that works the core as well as the shoulder girdle, buttocks and legs. A straight-arm plank puts more emphasis on the triceps (muscles on the back of the upper arm) and the shoulders, while the forearm plank also works the core and hips. The forearm plank is a better choice for people with

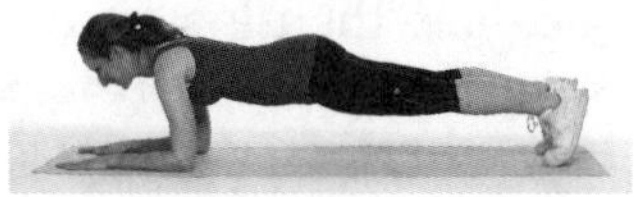

limited shoulder stability or arm strength or who have carpal tunnel syndrome or other wrist problems.

What to do: Once you're in position (imagine the upper position of a push-up, except that your forearms are on the floor and your upper arms are perpendicular to the floor), focus on keeping your body and head in one straight line looking at a spot on the floor just in front of your hands.

Tighten your abdominal muscles—this will help you hold the position and keep your back straight. It's harder than it looks, especially as the seconds pass and you realize how thoroughly you must engage your muscles from your toes to your shoulders to keep from collapsing to the floor. Keep your jaw relaxed, and breathe deeply throughout the exercise.

I try to hold the position for two or more minutes. For beginners, 10 to 15 seconds is about the limit. If you can hold the position with good form for 30 to 60 seconds, you are probably strong enough to try some variations. *For example...*

While holding the plank, lift one leg a few inches off the floor...flex the foot toward your knee or point the toes backward. Hold for a few seconds. Repeat with the other leg.

• **Side plank.** This variation of the forearm plank is challenging because you support your weight on just one arm, using the oblique muscles in your sides, the deep transverse abdominal muscles and many muscles in the hips, low back and thighs.

What to do: Lie on your right side while resting on your forearm. Contract your abdominal, side and hip muscles, and raise your hips off the floor until your body is in a straight line. Hold the position for at least 30 seconds, then lower yourself back down and switch sides. Alternate sides until you have done three on each side.

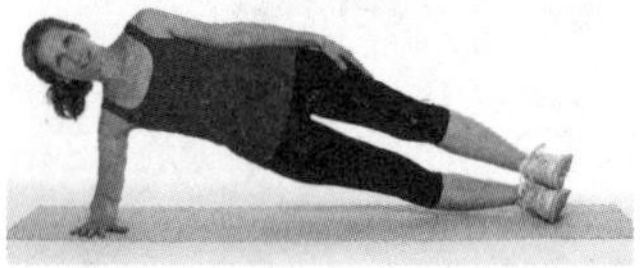

• **The McGill curl-up.** Developed by the spine researcher Stuart McGill, this movement is an abdominal crunch with a surprisingly small range of motion that works multiple core muscles. In this exercise, you barely come off the floor, and you never force your spinal column into that hazardous "C" shape.

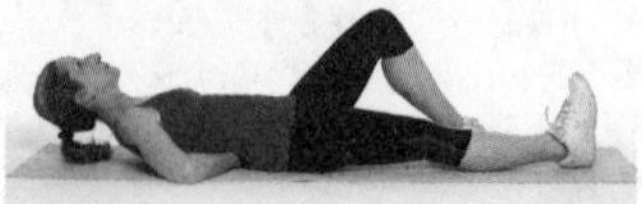

What to do: Lie on your back, with one foot planted flat on the floor and the other leg straight out. Place one hand on top of the other under the arch in your lower back. This preserves the natural curve and reduces spine pressure.

Keeping your neck in a neutral position, contract your abdominal and oblique muscles so that your upper body just comes up off the floor. You may feel your shoulder blades lose contact with the ground, but your back should remain straight, while your hands support the curve in your lower back. Hold the position for a few seconds, then lower back down. Do three to five reps with your left leg bent and then three to five with the right leg bent. Try to work up to three to five reps held for about 10 seconds each on each side.

Also: Don't tuck your chin into your chest during the rising motion, and don't curl your back or round your shoulders. Keep your upper body in a straight line by activating only the abdominal and oblique muscles. This keeps your spinal column in a safe and supported position, reducing the risk for muscle strain and spinal disk damage.

Bananas to Exercise Pain!

Eating bananas lessens aches and pains from exercise. Bicyclists had reduced inflammation during recovery if they ate bananas during rides instead of consuming sports drinks or water. They had less evidence of an enzyme that causes pain and inflammation, which usually is treated with drugs such as ibuprofen. It may be that antioxidants and other nutrients from bananas are all the body needs to perform better and recover faster.

David C. Nieman, DrPH, professor of health and exercise science at Appalachian State University, Kannapolis, North Carolina.

Workout Fatigue

Wayne Westcott, PhD, director of the Exercise Science Program, Quincy College, Massachusetts. He is the author or coauthor of 24 fitness books, including *Get Stronger, Feel Younger.*

Fatigue can be a factor in injuries among athletes...both amateur and professional alike.

If you participate in a high-impact activity, such as basketball, considerable stress is placed on your feet, ankles, Achilles tendons, knees, hips, the low back and muscles in the buttocks and legs. While running is a much more controlled aerobic exercise, it too stresses the same body parts, which could increase the risk for musculoskeletal injuries, especially in those who exercise frequently.

If you sense tightness, weakness or pain in any of these areas, substitute non–weight bearing endurance exercises, such as cycling, rowing or swimming, for your run or high-impact activity.

Supplements for Sore Muscles After Exercise

JoAnn Yanez, ND, naturopathic physician and medical consultant in Sioux Falls, South Dakota, and a past board member of the Council on Naturopathic Medical Education and the New York Association of Naturopathic Physicians. DrYanez.com

A sore muscle is an injured muscle. When you push a muscle past its capacity, its cell membranes rupture...substances from within the cells pour into the bloodstream, triggering an inflammatory response... and inflammation causes pain.

If you are always very sore after exercise—too sore to do normal daily activities—you may be pushing yourself too hard or working out incorrectly. If that is the case, a better approach than taking supplements is to reduce the intensity and/or duration of your workouts and ask a professional trainer to review your technique. Also, always stretch and rehydrate immediately after exercising.

That said, if you are prone to occasional soreness—for instance, after an especially challenging day of bicycling or a new exercise class that works your muscles in unaccustomed ways—supplements may provide some relief.

Important: Ask your naturopathic physician whether any or all of the following supplements are appropriate for you and discuss whether the typical dosages should be modified. *To use as needed for post-workout muscle soreness, consider...*

- **Turmeric,** a spice whose active ingredient, curcumin, has powerful anti-inflammatory effects. Studies suggest that turmeric eases other inflammation-related discomforts, such as arthritis, morning stiffness and minor sprains—so although there isn't much research on whether turmeric relieves acute muscle soreness, it makes sense that it might...and anecdotally people say that it helps.

Typical dosage: 400 mg of curcumin three times daily (as used in arthritis studies).

- **Fish oil,** another anti-inflammatory.

Typical dosage: 2,000 mg daily.

- **Vitamin C,** an antioxidant that helps tissues heal.

Typical dosage: 1,000 mg daily.

Even more effective: A combination product, such as Emergen-C (original formula), EmergenC.com, that replenishes vitamin C as well as the electrolytes and B vitamins lost during exercise.

A Fruit That Gives Muscle Aches the Boot

Encarna Aguayo, PhD, associate professor, department of food engineering, Universidad Politécnica de Cartagena, Spain. Her study was published in *Journal of Agricultural and Food Chemistry.*

Muscle soreness is the big downside of working out.

Ginger Eases Muscle Pain and Inflammation Caused by Exercise

In a recent finding, exercisers who consumed two grams (about one teaspoon) of raw or heated ginger had 23% to 25% less pain after exercise than those who did not consume ginger. Volunteers consumed the ginger daily for eight days prior to exercising and three days afterward.

Recommendation: Add fresh ginger to your diet for faster workout recovery.

Christopher D. Black, PhD, assistant professor, department of kinesiology, Georgia College and State University, Milledgeville, and leader of a study published in *The Journal of Pain.*

Good news: When athletes drank 16 ounces of watermelon juice an hour before exercise, they had less muscle soreness than when they did not drink it.

Theory: Watermelon contains L-citrulline, an amino acid that boosts blood flow and oxygen in muscles, reducing pain.

To ease sore muscles: Try eating some watermelon (or drinking the juice if you have a juicer).

No More Heartburn After a Workout

William D. Chey, MD, professor of internal medicine, University of Michigan, Ann Arbor, quoted in *Shape.*

Prevent heartburn after a workout by avoiding fatty and greasy foods before working out...and waiting a few hours after eating to exercise.

Also: Sip water slowly during and after your workout to avoid filling your stomach with water and air.

If you still get heartburn: Try taking an over-the-counter medicine, such as Pepcid or Zantac, 30 minutes before your workout...or talk to your doctor.

CHAPTER 9

Foot, Gout and Leg Pain

Oh, My Aching Foot! Help For Common Causes of Foot and Leg Pain

The average person walks the equivalent of four times around the world in his/her lifetime. No wonder foot problems plague more than three-quarters of US adults! The good news is that we can take steps on our own to relieve the pain. *Here are the most common symptoms and problems—and what you can do...*

ACHILLES TENDONITIS

Symptoms: Pain above the heel or in the back of the leg.

Even though the tendon in the back of the heel is the strongest and largest in the body, it's still among the most vulnerable—and when it hurts, it can hurt a lot.

Inflammation of the tendon, known as Achilles tendonitis, usually is due to overuse. The tendon gets weaker and susceptible to injuries with age. If you overwork the tendon—say, by spending a few hours on the dance floor or the basketball court—the fibers can develop small tears and get inflamed. It typically takes at least three months for it to heal completely. In the meantime, don't engage in high-impact exercises such as running, and switch to low-impact activities such as biking or swimming. *Also...*

- **Start with ice.** Ice is one of the best ways to reduce inflammation and help the tendon heal. When you first feel pain at the back of the heel, apply an ice pack for up to 20 minutes. Keep applying ice throughout the day—and keep the heel elevated as much as possible for a few days. You can further reduce inflammation by taking aspirin or ibuprofen.

Johanna S. Youner, DPM, podiatrist and cosmetic foot surgeon in New York City. She is a spokesperson for the American Podiatric Medical Association and a delegate of the New York State Podiatric Medical Association. HealthyFeetNY.net

• **Supplements also can help heal a painful Achilles tendon.**

I recommend choosing one from each of the following categories: Vitamin C, glucosamine or chondroitin sulfate to help build ligaments...fish oil, boswellia extract, devil's claw or quercetin to decrease inflammation...and the enzymes pancreatin, papain, bromelain or trypsin to relieve pain. Check with your doctor, since they could interact with medications. Follow label directions.

• **Try heel lifts.** These are thin wedges that slip into your shoes. Raising the heel as little as one-eighth of an inch reduces stress and helps the tendon heal quicker. Use lifts in both shoes so that your body is balanced. I like Spenco Rx Heel Cushions and AliMed Heel Lifts. Both are available online and in pharmacies and some stores.

Important: If you can't stand up on your toes even for a second, there's a good chance that the tendon has ruptured (completely torn). Surgery is the only treatment for a ruptured Achilles tendon.

MORTON'S NEUROMA

Symptoms: Feels as if a pebble is in your shoe...pain in the ball of the foot.

Morton's neuroma is a thickened nerve in the ball of your foot. It typically causes sharp pain or burning that gets worse when you walk. The abnormal growth of nerve tissue is the body's response to irritation—usually from shoes that are too tight or from wearing high heels. Anything that puts repetitive pressure on the toes, including activities such as jogging, can cause Morton's neuroma.

• **Wear wider shoes.** Giving the toes more room to move reduces pressure and causes the neuroma to shrink back to normal, possibly within a month or two.

• **Stretch your toes.** The nerve may be trapped under a ligament in the foot. Stretches will lengthen the ligament and open up space over the nerve. A few times a day, use your fingers to bend your toes up and down. Stretch them as far as you comfortably can, and repeat the stretches about a dozen times.

PLANTAR FASCIITIS

Symptoms: Stabbing pain in the heel of the foot.

A thick band of tissue (the plantar fascia) runs across the bottom of the foot. It connects the heel bone to the toes and creates the arch. Small tears in the tissue can cause burning/stabbing pain, particularly in the morning.

Important: Get a second opinion if your doctor recommends surgery. About 90% of cases heal with conservative care within a year.

• **Apply ice.** Hold an ice pack over the painful area for 15 or 20 minutes, three or four times a day.

• **Replace your shoe insoles.** The Powerstep brand of insoles support and cushion the plantar fascia and help it heal more quickly. You can buy insoles at pharmacies, sporting-goods stores and online for $15 to $60. In many cases, they work as well as prescription products (which can cost $550).

• **Use a tennis ball or rolling pin to gently roll along the bottom of your foot (while sitting).**

• **Take aspirin or ibuprofen to reduce pain and inflammation.**

• **Replace worn-out athletic shoes.** They stop cushioning your feet after about 500 miles of use.

• **See your doctor if the pain isn't gone within three months.** He/she might recommend a steroid injection. Used judiciously, steroid injections can help heal a chronically inflamed area quickly. Three steroid injections per area are the maximum for one year—more than that in a year can weaken tissue.

SHIN SPLINTS

Symptoms: Pain that runs along the bone on the front of your lower leg.

Shin splints are caused by inflammation that affects muscles and the underlying bone. They usually are caused by activities that involve sudden stops and starts, such as aerobics, jogging, tennis and basketball. They also occur in people who walk a lot in hard-soled shoes.

• **Use ice to reduce inflammation.** It's the most effective treatment for bone and ligament trauma. When you are in pain, ice the area of the leg—10 minutes on and 10 minutes off, as needed.

• **Try arch supports.** They slip into your shoes and support the bottom of the foot. They reduce stress on the lower leg and will help shin splints heal more quickly. I like the brands Powerstep (see above) and Superfeet.

• **Talk to your doctor about bone stimulation.** If the pain of a shin splint lasts more than a few months, you may have a stress fracture at the tibia. Your doctor might recommend a bone stimulator, a prescription device that uses ultrasound or electrical currents to stimulate new bone growth. Bone stimulators are worn daily for a minimum of three hours per day for 90 to 180 days.

BUNIONS

Symptoms: Bump and pain at the base of the big toe.

A bunion is a bony hump that forms on the outside of the foot, where the big toe emerges from the foot. Take it seriously, even if it doesn't hurt. It means that your big toe is pushing in the wrong direction. It can lead to joint damage, as well as a misalignment of the other toes.

Some people are born with a tendency to develop bunions. More often, they are caused by narrow, ill-fitting shoes (particularly high heels) that press the toes into odd positions.

• **Wear sensible shoes.** "Sensible" means that the shoes are wide enough to allow your toes to move. Avoid shoes with sharply pointed toes or heels higher than two inches.

• **Do foot exercises to relieve symptoms and increase flexibility.** Point and flex your toes, or massage the bottom of your foot with a golf ball.

• **See a doctor if the bunion is painful or getting larger.** It will get worse unless you take care of it. The treatment might be as simple as a custom-made shoe insert that will reduce pressure on the affected joint. Surgery (bunionectomy) is recommended only if the bunion is persistently painful and doesn't get better with other treatments.

Fix Your Feet for Under $75

Johanna S. Youner, DPM, podiatric surgeon in private practice and attending physician at New York–Presbyterian/Lower Manhattan Hospital, both in New York City. Dr. Youner is a board-certified foot surgeon and a Fellow of the American College of Foot and Ankle Surgeons. HealthyFeetNY.com

For less than $75, you can choose a handful of excellent over-the-counter (OTC) products that will relieve foot pain and keep your toenails and the skin on your feet healthy—without seeing a doctor.

Caution: If your foot pain is daily or doesn't improve with the products mentioned in this article, see a podiatrist for advice.

FOR BETTER SUPPORT

Well-made, foam-padded insoles that go inside your shoes work like shock absorbers, alleviating pressure and stress on the foot. Insoles help restore balance, increase stability and reduce pain—not just in your feet but also in your knees, hips and back.

Important: If an insole does not feel comfortable in the shoe, then it's not right for you—these are not devices that you "break in." *Before you buy expensive, custom-fit orthotics, consider trying these OTC insoles...*

• **Superfeet insoles are available in a variety of styles for men's and women's shoes.** For example, Superfeet Delux Dress-fit ($29.95, Zappos.com) are slim enough to slip inside any women's shoe, but they work best in flats or shoes with heels up to one-and-a-half inches. Superfeet Premium Blue insoles ($44.95, Zappos.com), available for men and women, are designed for cleated athletic footwear and most types of casual and dress shoes.

• **Powerstep ProTech Full Length Orthotics** ($30 to $40, Amazon.com), also available for men and women, are especially helpful for pain in your arch or heel due, for example, to plantar fasciitis. If you have this condition, which causes inflammation of the tissue along the bottom of the feet, you'll likely benefit a lot by using these insoles.

Important: Insoles can be transferred from shoe to shoe (depending on the size of each one) but should be replaced yearly or more often if they no longer relieve pain.

TO FIGHT DRY SKIN AND CALLUSES

To prevent dry skin and calluses on your feet, you need a moisturizing cream that contains a keratolytic (descaling) agent to strip away the layers of dead skin so the moisturizer can do its work. *To restore your feet's skin, try one of the following products with keratolytic agents...*

- **Gehwol Med Callus Cream** ($16.99 for 2.6 ounces, Amazon.com).
- **Kerasal One Step Exfoliating Moisturizer Foot Therapy** ($10.99 for one ounce, CVS.com).

Apply the cream after your shower, when the skin is softened a bit. Twelve to 24 hours later, rub the area gently with a pumice sponge, which is less damaging to use than a pumice stone. Be very gentle if you have cracks in your feet, especially if you've lost some of the feeling in your feet (due to neuropathy, for example). If you're using one of the moisturizing products and it stops working, switch to the other.

FOR FUNGAL INFECTIONS

These common infections—often due to athlete's foot, which can be contracted by walking barefoot in a public shower, for example—cause thickened, disfigured toenails that sometimes curl inward.

You'll need a doctor's prescription for antifungal cream, such as Ertaczo or Naftin...or maybe even oral medication, such as terbinafine (Lamisil). *To speed the recovery process and help prevent recurrences, try this nail cream...*

- **Kerasal Fungal Nail Renewal Treatment** ($27.49 for 0.33 ounce, CVS.com) contains acids and other ingredients that soften the nail, reduce its thickness and improve its appearance, usually within two weeks of nightly use.

S-T-R-E-T-C-H To Stop Heel Pain

John Furia, MD, sports medicine physician with Sun Orthopaedics and Sports Medicine, in Lewisburg, Pennsylvania, author of *Collegiate Fitness: A Guide to Healthy Living*.

Paul Langer, DPM, clinical faculty member of the University of Minnesota, podiatrist at Minnesota Orthopedic Specialists in Minnesota and author of *Great Feet for Life: Footcare and Footwear for Healthy Aging*.

Heel pain—usually caused by plantar fasciitis—is one of the most common problems seen by podiatrists, accounting for an estimated 15 to 30% of all visits.

What happens: The long ligament on the bottom of the foot—the plantar fascia—tugs and pulls at the tissue in the heel, separating it at the bone and inflaming the area.

There are many risk factors for plantar fasciitis, including aging; overweight; high-impact recreational activities, such as running or basketball; standing on your feet all day and frequently wearing non-supportive footwear, such as flip-flops.

But no matter the cause, there's an easy way to fix the problem. *S-t-r-e-t-c-h...*

THE PAIN-RELIEVING STRETCH

Here are instructions for a pain-relieving stretch. Perform the stretch in a seated position.

1. Cross your affected foot over the knee of your other leg.

2. Grasp the toes of your painful foot and bend your toes back toward your shin.

3. Place your thumb along the plantar fascia and rub it to stretch it.

4. The fascia should feel like a tight band along the bottom of your foot when stretched.

5. Hold the stretch for 10 seconds. Repeat it 10 to 20 times.

Best: Do the stretch first thing in the morning, before getting out of bed. You can also do it after any long periods of sitting.

Important: If there's a sharp pain in your heel when you get up, you should have stretched before standing.

MORE WAYS TO STOP THE PAIN

There are several other ways to help clear up an acute bout of plantar fasciitis and prevent recurrences of the problem. *They include...*

- **Don't go barefoot or in slippers around the house.**
- **Ice the affected foot with a 12- or 16-ounce frozen water bottle, setting it on the floor and rolling the foot over it for 15 to 20 minutes, several times a day.**

No More Foot Blisters

Joan Wilen and Lydia Wilen are folk-remedy experts based in New York City who have spent decades collecting "cures from the cupboard." They are authors of *Bottom Line's Treasury of Home Remedies & Natural Cures.*

To prevent blisters, generously apply any type of stick antiperspirant or deodorant to the bottom of your feet before you go jogging or hiking. The antiperspirant should prevent the friction that causes blisters. You can also use other types of lubricants to prevent blisters, such as petroleum jelly (available at drugstores) and BodyGlide (available at sporting-goods stores or online at Bodyglide.com).

High Heels: Pain Maker

Mark G. Mandato, DPM, attending podiatrist, Kings County Hospital Center, Brooklyn.

High heels force the pelvis to tilt, changing your center of gravity. To compensate, your low back arches, placing a strain on back muscles. High heels also cause prolonged contraction of the Achilles tendon, creating calf pain. *Before and after wearing heels...*

- **Stretch your back.** Sit in a chair, feet on the floor. Chin tucked, slowly curl your torso forward, bringing forehead toward knees and reaching hands toward toes...hold 10 seconds...slowly return to starting position. Repeat 10 times.
- **Stretch your calves.** Stand 18 inches away from a wall, hands pressed against the wall at shoulder level. Bending your left knee slightly, step your right foot back 12 to 18 inches. Press right heel into the floor...lean forward until you feel a stretch in the right calf...hold 10 seconds...return to starting position. Repeat five times with each leg.

Best: Limit time spent in high heels.

Promising New Treatment for Painful Heels

Luca M. Sconfienza, MD, radiologist at Policlinico San Donato in Milan, Italy, and lead author of a study of 44 people, presented at a meeting of the Radiological Society of North America.

If you dread getting out of bed because it hurts to put weight on your heel (particularly in the morning or after standing for a long time), chances are that you have plantar fasciitis—persistent, painful inflammation of a large ligament on the bottom of the foot. Usually it is treated with rest, exercises, splints and arch supports...steroid injections...a series of shockwave treatments (often uncomfortable)...or surgery.

Encouraging: A recent study investigated a new single-treatment therapy. Under ultrasound guidance, after injecting local anesthesia, researchers repeatedly punctured affected areas with a needle, creating a bit of bleeding (which hastens healing by increasing blood flow to the area)...then injected an anti-inflammatory steroid.

Results: 95% of study participants were symptom-free within three weeks and remained so throughout the four- to six-month follow-up period.

Best: If you have severe plantar fasciitis that has not responded to noninvasive therapies, talk to your podiatrist about this technique, called dry-needling with steroid injection.

More research is needed before it could become standard protocol—but results are promising.

Pain in Your Big Toe? You May Have Gout

Robert T. Keenan, MD, MPH, rheumatologist and assistant professor of medicine in the division of rheumatology at Duke University School of Medicine and medical director of the Infusion Center at Duke University Medical Center, both in Durham, North Carolina.

Approximately six million Americans suffer from gout, the most common form of inflammatory arthritis. Although gout is most often associated with pain, it is now thought that the condition also increases risk for hypertension and cardiovascular disease.

AGONIZING ATTACKS

Gout often strikes at the base of the big toe, causing pain that increases for eight to 12 hours and subsides within three to 10 days without treatment. Other joints can also be affected. The attacks are intermittent and unpredictable. They may occur every few weeks or months, once or twice a year or every few years. But without treatment, the attacks generally increase in duration as well as frequency.

The risks: Untreated gout can cause permanent joint damage. Some patients progress from recurrent gout to tophaceous gout, a severe form in which lumps of urate crystals form in and around joints or even under the skin. Gout increases the risk for kidney stones, and patients who don't achieve good control of their elevated uric acid levels are more likely to develop cardiovascular disease than those without gout.

EASY TO DIAGNOSE

Patients who are suspected of having gout are usually advised to have a blood test to measure uric acid. However, some asymptomatic patients have high levels of uric acid, while those in the midst of an attack may have apparently normal levels (3 mg/dL to 7 mg/dL). Typically, the uric acid level peaks around two weeks after an acute attack.

Joint aspiration is the best test for gout, especially in its early stages. Your doctor will insert a needle into the inflamed joint (lidocaine and numbing sprays minimize the pain of the needle) and withdraw fluid, which is then examined under a microscope. The presence of urate crystals means that you have gout, regardless of the uric acid concentrations in your blood.

Ultrasound is now used by some doctors to diagnose gout. It's painless and completely noninvasive. It's good for detecting gout (which may not be evident with a physical exam), but harder to diagnose in the early stages without joint aspiration.

BEST TREATMENTS

Treating gout is a two-step process. Depending on the severity of the attack, various medications can be used to reduce pain and inflammation.

Examples: Nonsteroidal anti-inflammatory drugs, such as *ibuprofen* (Motrin)...*colchicine* (Colcrys), the oldest medication used for treating gout...and corticosteroids, which serve as fast-acting anti-inflammatories.

To reduce uric acid, medications such as the following are taken one to two weeks after a gout attack (using these drugs during a gout attack can worsen symptoms)...

- ***Febuxostat* (Uloric)** is the first new oral drug for gout in 40 years. Taken daily, it can reduce uric acid to an optimal level within a few weeks. Most people with gout need to continue taking this drug indefinitely, but in rare cases it can be discontinued after about a year without subsequent flare-ups.
- ***Allopurinol* (Zyloprim, Aloprim),** like febuxostat, reduces uric acid concentrations. It's much less expensive than febuxostat ($40 versus $185 for 30 tablets), and it works well for most patients. It usually takes at least six to eight weeks to see a reduction in uric acid levels and may take subsequent dose increases to reduce uric acid to an appropriate level. An older gout drug, allopurinol is more likely to cause kidney problems than febuxostat.

DASH Away from Gout

The DASH diet (Dietary Approaches to Stop Hypertension)—developed to lower blood pressure—can reduce uric acid levels enough to prevent gout flare-ups. The diet is rich in whole grains, fruits, vegetables and low-fat dairy...and low in salt, red meat, sweets and saturated fats. It sometimes can work as well as antigout medication.

Stephen P. Juraschek, MD, PhD, research and clinical fellow, The Johns Hopkins University School of Medicine, Baltimore.

- ***Probenecid*** **(Benemid, Probalan)** increases the excretion of uric acid by the kidneys. Most patients who take it can achieve reductions in uric acid levels within two weeks. Potential side effects include kidney stones, gastrointestinal upset and rash. Probenecid can't be taken by patients with kidney disease.
- ***Pegloticase*** **(Krystexxa)** has just been approved by the FDA for the treatment of refractory gout, which can't be managed with other approaches. It's given by intravenous infusion once every two weeks. Side effects may include nausea, confusion and vomiting.

LIFESTYLE APPROACHES

People with gout were traditionally advised to avoid foods high in purines (such as anchovies and organ meats), which are metabolized to form uric acid. Research shows that this approach reduces uric acid levels only minimally, but in combination with drug therapy, exercise and weight loss, may help to prevent attacks. *Other strategies...*

- **Consume low-fat dairy.** Research shows that a high intake of low-fat milk and low-fat yogurt reduced the risk for gout by 50%. The benefit was mainly seen in those who consumed two or more eight-ounce glasses of skim milk daily—milk proteins reduce uric acid levels.
- **Avoid beer and liquor.** Both can raise uric acid and precipitate gout attacks. Beer contains the greatest amount of purines. Wine is thought to have antioxidant compounds that may mitigate the effects that alcohol has on gout.
- **Eliminate high-fructose corn syrup (HFCS).** This sweetener, commonly used in snacks, soft drinks and other processed foods, raises uric acid.

To minimize intake of HFCS: Eat whole, natural foods such as fresh vegetables, fruits and grains.

- **Get enough vitamin C.** Consuming at least 500 mg of vitamin C daily can reduce uric acid, but it may take large doses (at least 1,500 mg daily) to significantly reduce levels. Use caution, however, because high-dose vitamin C may cause upset stomach, diarrhea and kidney stones.

Best option: Dietary sources such as strawberries (one cup fresh contains 98 mg of vitamin C).

- **Eat cherries.** A 2010 study showed that one tablespoon of cherry juice concentrate (the equivalent of 45 to 60 cherries) twice a day cut gout attacks by more than 50%.

What Is Turf Toe?—Common Problem, Simple Solution

Johanna S. Youner, DPM, podiatrist, cosmetic foot surgeon and attending podiatric physician at New York Downtown Hospital in New York City. HealthyFeetNY.net

Anyone who has had "turf toe" knows how debilitating it can be. And it doesn't just sideline athletes. Anyone can get it.

EXCRUCIATING PAIN

Turf toe, as the name suggests, tends to occur in athletes who play on artificial grass. The turf grips the bottoms of their flexible athletic shoes. This is good for traction, but it also can "trap" the foot when players move at high speeds and sharp angles, forcing the big toe to bend sharply upward.

Off the playing field, this type of injury is simply called a sprain. Anything that forces the toe joint to hyperextend, or bend too far upward, can stretch or tear ligaments and sometimes damage the joint itself.

Among nonathletes, this usually occurs in the first or second joints of the big toe. It's often due to footwear. Shoes that are very soft don't provide enough support to prevent excessive joint movement.

Age plays a role, too. After about age 50, the ligaments have stretched, and there is less fat padding the bottom of the feet.

WHAT GOES WRONG

When you're walking or running, the big toe is the last part of the foot to leave the ground. On "push-off," up to eight times your weight is transferred to the first joint of the big toe, and the toe easily can be forced beyond its normal range of motion.

Result: The ligaments stretch and may tear slightly or—if the sprain is severe—completely rupture.

FASTER HEALING

You don't have to see a doctor right away if you think you have a mild or moderate sprain. Take care of it yourself (see below) for a week to 10 days. If it seems to be getting better—there's a daily decrease in pain and swelling—it probably will heal on its own.

Your doctor usually can diagnose a sprain just by asking about the history of the injury and seeing where and when it hurts. Imaging tests such as X-rays or MRIs are needed only if your doctor thinks the sprain is severe and that there might be bone damage.

For faster healing...

- **Take an anti-inflammatory,** such as *ibuprofen* (Advil) or *naproxen sodium* (Aleve), following the directions on the label. It will decrease inflammation, helping to heal the injury. It also will reduce pain.
- **Rest.** Sprains heal slowly because the connective tissues have a limited blood supply. It can take weeks or even months for the damaged tissues to repair. Resting the joint is critical—keep your weight off the foot as much as possible. You may want to use crutches or at least elevate the foot on a pillow whenever you're sitting down. Elevating the foot decreases swelling and thus promotes healing.

Also important: Frequently ice the area on the first day after the injury. This reduces inflammation. You can use a cold pack, available in pharmacies, or wrap ice cubes in a small towel and hold them on the joint for 15 to 20 minutes at a time. Ice as frequently as you want as long as the area warms in between and there is normal sensation.

- **Splint the toe with a buddy splint.** Loosely tape the big toe to the toe next to it. This will keep it more stable and accelerate healing. Put a strip of gauze under the tape to prevent chafing.

Helpful: You can buy a stiff-bottomed shoe, known as a postoperative shoe, in a pharmacy. It will keep the toe from flexing.

Cost: About $20.

- **Exercise the toe.** When the pain and swelling are gone, exercise the toe to strengthen muscles and restore its normal range of motion.

Examples: While sitting, use the toe to trace an imaginary alphabet...or put a towel on the floor, and repeatedly pick it up with your toes.

SHOES FOR PREVENTION

Nonathletes who injure the big toe usually can blame their shoes. In New York City, I often see women rushing around in ballet flats. They're comfortable and lightweight but offer no support—and no protection from concrete sidewalks and curbs.

Similarly, women who wear high heels are putting a lot of unnecessary pressure on the big toe—they're forcing it to hyperextend. It's fine to wear heels on special occasions but risky when you're doing a lot of walking.

In general, women should wear firm shoes with relatively low heels. Men do better with firm but lightweight shoes, such as those made by Rockport, rather than with stiff dress shoes.

Also helpful: You can add protection to any shoe by using an over-the-counter neoprene insert. They're inexpensive and add support and cushioning.

Shoes for Hammertoe

Johanna Youner, DPM, podiatric surgeon in private practice in New York City. HealthyFeetNY.net

Are there any fashionable women's shoe options that would be comfortable for hammertoes and subsequent leg pain?

There are actually many choices. You need a shoe with maximum support, so look for a more rigid shoe with a sturdy heel and cushioned footbed to help support your feet. A high toe box (vertical room at the front of the shoe) protects hammertoes from additional friction.

The best shoe for hammertoes is a tie-up oxford, since the foot does not have to work to keep it on. Other trendy styles that give good support are low-height "flatforms" (flats on a platform)...and booties (a cross between boots and shoes).

Expect to pay at least $75 for a good pair of shoes. Look for shoes that have the seal of acceptance from the American Podiatric Medical Association, which means they have been found to promote good foot health. Good brands (for women and men) include Clarks, Ecco, Rockport, ASICS and Vionic.

No More Foot and Leg Pain: Exercise Your Foot Core

Patrick O. McKeon, PhD, certified athletic trainer and assistant professor in the department of exercise and sport sciences at Ithaca College in Ithaca, New York.

Just about every workout these days includes "core" exercises that strengthen muscles in the abdomen and lower back. That's because you need a strong core for balance, posture and everyday movements.

But there's another core muscle group that you probably haven't thought about. New research suggests that a strong foot core might be the key to avoiding painful plantar fasciitis, shin splints, Achilles tendinitis, bursitis and other common foot and leg problems.

Latest development: Research now suggests that strengthening the intrinsic muscles by walking barefoot* and doing certain simple foot exercises (see below) can help prevent and treat the common foot and leg problems mentioned earlier.

THE CASE AGAINST SHOES

Shoes protect your feet from rough surfaces and harmful organisms and keep your toes warm. But they do not contribute to foot strength.

Millions of people worldwide go shoeless most of the time—and have stronger feet because of it. A study published in the podiatry journal *The Foot* found that modern-day Zulus, who often go barefoot, have the healthiest feet, while shoe-wearing Europeans have the unhealthiest feet.

EXERCISING YOUR FOOT CORE

In addition to walking barefoot whenever you can, exercise that is performed barefoot, such as yoga and Pilates, will also strengthen your feet. But for a simple and effective foot core workout, try the following exercises.

Important: Before you begin the exercises, sit down with one foot flat on the ground. Roll your ankle out to lift the ball of your foot off the ground. Then roll your foot the other way to lift your little toe off the ground. Keep doing this until you can sense where the midpoint is between these two extremes. This point is the subtalar neutral, the optimal position for the foot to be in to adapt to the demands placed on it. Repeat with the other foot.

- **"Short foot" exercise.**

What to do: Sit in a chair with your bare feet flat on the floor. Engage the intrinsic muscles by sliding your big toes back toward the heels, but without curling the toes. (You're temporarily making your feet shorter—hence the name of the exercise.) Hold the stretch for about six seconds. Do this eight to 10 times, rest for about a minute, then repeat the cycle two more times. Do the sequence at least a few times a day on each foot.

*Do not walk barefoot if you have diabetic neuropathy.

Note: It can be difficult to get the hang of this exercise because we're not used to engaging these muscles. You'll know you're doing it right when the foot arches rise.

Once you've mastered this movement, you can work the muscles harder by doing this exercise while standing...or by standing on one foot. Studies have shown that people who do this exercise have improvements in balance as well as arch height within four weeks.

- **Quarter roll exercise.**

What to do: Place a quarter under the ball of each foot, just behind the big toes. While standing, rise up slightly on your toes. Try to roll your feet so that your weight is directly over the quarters (or as close as you can get). Hold the position for five to 10 seconds, rest for about a minute and repeat eight to 10 times. Do the sequence at least a few times a day.

As your muscles get stronger, you can increase the difficulty of the exercise by raising your heels higher or by rising up on one foot at a time.

Sore Feet? Four Feel-Better Yoga Poses

Roger Cole, PhD, internationally recognized, certified Iyengar yoga teacher who trained at the Iyengar Yoga Institutes in San Francisco and Pune, India. RogerColeYoga.com

---

Our poor feet pay the price—in the form of pain, inflammation and misalignments—for our habit of wearing high-heeled, pointy-toed, stylish-but-not-sensible shoes. Despite the daily wear-and-tear from our favorite shoes, certain yoga postures can help feet feel and function better.

The greatest thing yoga can do for foot health is to help restore normal "foot posture." That means equal weight on the inner and outer foot...arches lifted...toes spread apart evenly...and usually feet pointing straight ahead. The four poses below can help you achieve this correct foot posture.

Why "foot yoga" works: The following three standing poses challenge your ability to keep weight equally distributed on the "four corners" of the foot—the ball of the big toe, ball of the little toe, inner heel and outer heel. Each pose makes the weight distribution uneven in one way or another. So the act of bringing the feet back to neutral strengthens certain muscles and stretches others, while also training your nervous system to "find center" with your feet. The fourth pose is a kneeling posture. It stretches the top of the foot while temporarily taking tension off the inflammation-prone plantar fascia (a band of tissue that runs the length of the sole).

Check with your doctor before beginning, as not all yoga poses are appropriate for all people.

Suggestion: Start by holding the standing poses for five to 15 seconds per side, working your way up to 30 seconds per side...start by holding the kneeling pose for 10 to 30 seconds, gradually increasing to one minute. For best results, practice daily.

The basic instructions below will get you started. Be sure to incorporate foot-focus how-tos. For more detailed instructions and photos of each pose, go to the *Yoga Journal* demo links listed with each pose. *Poses to try...*

- **Vrksasana (Tree pose).** Stand on right foot, right knee straight. Bend left knee and place sole of left foot on inner right thigh, so toes point down and left knee points out to side. Raise arms straight overhead and hold pose. Repeat on other side.

Foot focus: Concentrate on keeping weight evenly distributed among all four corners of the supporting foot. This strengthens the calf and shin muscles that balance the foot and stretches the plantar fascia.

Demo: YogaJournal.com/poses/496.

- **Utthita Parsvakonasana (Extended side angle pose).** Stand with feet spread about three-and-a-half feet apart, right toes turned a little to the left and left toes facing sideways at a 90-degree angle. Bend left knee until knee is directly above ankle. Lean to left side by bending at left hip, placing left forearm on thigh or placing left hand on floor. Extend right arm diagonally overhead. Keeping torso facing forward (not turned toward floor), hold pose. Repeat on other side.

Foot focus: Press outer edge of back foot down into floor before you start going into the pose…keep it there throughout. Also, as you bend front leg, do not allow weight to shift to inner edge of that foot—keep knee aligned over ankle.

Demo: YogaJournal.com/poses/749.

• **Virabhadrasana 1 (Warrior 1 pose).** Stand with left foot about three-and-a-half feet in front of right foot, toes facing forward. Now turn right foot outward so toes are on a 30-degree angle. Bend left knee, bit by bit, directly toward left foot. Keep hips facing forward. Raise arms straight overhead and hold pose. Repeat on other side.

Foot focus: Before bending front knee, press outer corner of back heel firmly into floor. Keeping that part of heel down, slowly begin to bend front knee. When outer corner of back heel begins to lift, press it firmly back into floor and don't bend front knee any further—you have gone as far as you should. This pose strengthens key muscles that lift the arch of the foot, while also stretching some of the muscles whose tightness can flatten the arch.

Demo: YogaJournal.com/poses/1708.

• **Virasana (Hero pose).** Kneel with tops of feet on floor. Keep knees close to each another but not touching…spread feet apart slightly wider than hip width. Place a prop (such as a yoga block or thick book) on floor between ankles, then lower pelvis so hips are supported by the prop.

Foot focus: Keep thighs parallel and feet pointing backward in line with shins. If the stretch at the top of the ankles is too intense, support the ankles by draping them over a rolled blanket.

Demo: YogaJournal.com/poses/490.

Easy Cure for Leg Cramps at Night

Barbara Bergin, MD, orthopedic surgeon, Texas Orthopedics, Sports & Rehabilitation Associates, Austin.

If you're occasionally plagued by leg cramps (and you know that they're the harmless kind), a possible solution is in your sock drawer.

Here's what you do: Take out a pair of socks, and put them on your feet!

Here's why it works: Cold feet constrict blood vessels, which slows down blood circulation in your legs, including to the muscles in your legs. Keeping your feet warm in the evening, including during the two or three hours before you go to bed, restores better circulation to your feet and legs. So if you usually kick off your shoes and socks at the end of the day and pad around the house barefoot, don some cozy slippers instead! And wear socks to bed.

For extra-toasty toes: You also can tuck a hot water bottle under the covers at the foot of the bed. Or take a bath before bed—and spike the tub with Epsom salts to increase the muscle-relaxing effects.

Natural Help for Vein Pain

Mark A. Stengler, NMD, naturopathic doctor and founder of the Stengler Center for Integrative Medicine in Encinitas, California. He is author or coauthor of numerous books, including *The Natural Physician's Healing Therapies* and *Bottom Line's Prescription for Natural Cures*, and author of the newsletter *Health Revelations*. MarkStengler.com

Carolee, a 61-year-old patient of mine, began experiencing severe pain in her lower right leg. Because the results of her ultrasound were normal, I diagnosed Carolee as having chronic venous insufficiency—poor blood flow through the veins of the legs. At the time she had severe pain, there was stress on her circulatory system because she was somewhat overweight and had recently taken a long flight (which can impede blood flow).

Even though her ultrasound was normal, I was concerned about blood clots. I recommended natto-kinase, a protein-digesting enzyme capsule that improves circulation through blood vessels and breaks down clot-forming proteins. I also asked her to start taking an herbal formula containing horse chestnut extract (made from seeds of the horse chestnut tree)...butcher's broom root extract (a shrub of the lily family)...and gotu kola leaf extract (a perennial plant native to India, China, Australia and parts of South Africa). Horse chestnut and butcher's broom improve the function of vein valves, so that they prevent the backflow of venous blood. Gotu kola strengthens vein walls, so that they don't distend and pool blood. Carolee had access to a whirlpool tub, so I recommended that four times each day she alternate sitting on the side with her legs in the whirlpool for two minutes and putting her legs in the nearby pool's cooler water for 30 seconds. Alternating hot and cold and the massaging action of the whirlpool improves circulation. Exercise and elevation are recommended for people who don't have access to whirlpools.

Carolee reported great improvement within one week and had no remaining symptoms one month later. She continues to take the supplements to prevent the problem from recurring.

Bilberry for Varicose Veins

Jamey Wallace, ND, naturopathic physician and chief medical officer at Bastyr Center for Natural Health in Seattle.

Bilberry can help improve circulation. This antioxidant-rich fruit is tasty in jams and pies—and useful as a natural remedy.

Typical dose: If you have a circulatory problem, such as varicose veins, atherosclerosis or venous insufficiency, take an 80-mg capsule, once or twice a day. For diabetic retinopathy, take 160 mg, twice a day.

Caution: Be sure to speak to your doctor before trying bilberry if you use blood-thinning drugs (this herb may increase bleeding risk) or take diabetes medication (bilberry may lower blood sugar).

Natural Treatments for Peripheral Artery Disease

Catherine Ulbricht, PharmD, cofounder of the Somerville, Massachusetts–based Natural Standard Research Collaboration, which collects data on natural therapies, and senior attending pharmacist at Massachusetts General Hospital in Boston. She is also the author of *Natural Standard Herbal Pharmacotherapy.*

You are walking or climbing up a set of stairs, and suddenly you notice a dull, cramping pain in your leg. Before you write off the pain as simply a sign of overexertion or just a normal part of growing older, consider this: You may have intermittent claudication, the most common symptom of peripheral artery disease (PAD).

PAD, also known as peripheral vascular disease, is a condition in which arteries and veins in your limbs, usually in the legs and feet, are blocked or narrowed by fatty deposits that reduce blood flow.

Intermittent claudication, leg discomfort (typically in the calf) that occurs during exertion or exercise and is relieved by rest, usually is the first symptom of PAD. But other possible symptoms may include leg sores that won't heal (chronic venous ulcers)...varicose veins (chronic venous insufficiency)...paleness (pallor) or discoloration (a blue tint) of the legs...or cold legs.

Why is "a little leg trouble" so significant?

If it's due to PAD, you have got a red flag that other arteries, including those in the heart and brain, may also be blocked. In fact, people with PAD have a two- to sixfold increased risk for heart attack or stroke.

An estimated eight million to 12 million Americans—including up to one in five people age 60 or older—are believed to have PAD. While many individuals who have PAD experience the symptoms described earlier, some have no symptoms at all.

Those at greatest risk: Anyone who smokes or has elevated cholesterol, high blood pressure or diabetes is at increased risk for PAD.

What you need to know…

BETTER TREATMENT RESULTS

The standard treatment for PAD typically includes lifestyle changes (such as quitting smoking, getting regular exercise and eating a healthful diet). Medical treatment may include medication, such as one of the two drugs approved by the FDA for PAD—*pentoxifylline* (Trental) and *cilostazol* (Pletal)—and, in severe cases, surgery.

For even better results: Strong scientific evidence now indicates that several natural therapies—used in conjunction with these treatments—may help slow the progression of PAD and improve a variety of symptoms more effectively than standard treatment alone can.

Important: Before trying any of the following therapies, talk to your doctor to determine which might work best for you, what the most effective dose is for you and what side effects and drug interactions may occur.

Do not take more than one of the following therapies at the same time—this will increase bleeding risk.

Among the most effective natural therapies for PAD…

- **Ginkgo biloba.** A standardized extract from the leaf of the ginkgo biloba tree, which is commonly taken to improve memory, is one of the top-selling herbs in the US. But the strongest scientific evidence for ginkgo biloba may well be in the treatment of PAD.

Scientific evidence: Numerous studies currently show that ginkgo biloba extract can decrease leg pain that occurs with exercise or at rest. The daily doses used in the studies ranged from 80 mg to 320 mg.

Warning: Because it thins the blood and may increase risk for bleeding, ginkgo biloba should be used with caution if you also take a blood thinner, such as warfarin (Coumadin) or aspirin. In addition, ginkgo biloba should not be taken within two weeks of undergoing surgery.

- **Grape seed extract.** Grapes, including the fruit, leaves and seeds, have been used medicinally since the time of the ancient Greeks. Grape seed extract is rich in oligomeric proanthocyanidins, antioxidants that integrative practitioners in Europe use to treat varicose veins, chronic leg ulcers and other symptoms of PAD.

Scientific evidence: In several recent studies, grape seed extract was found to reduce the symptoms of poor circulation in leg veins, which can include nighttime cramps, swelling, heaviness, itching, tingling, burning, numbness and nerve pain.

Caution: Don't use this supplement if you're allergic to grapes. It should be used with caution if you take a blood thinner.

- **Hesperidin.** This flavonoid is found in unripe citrus fruits, such as oranges, grapefruits, lemons and tangerines.

Scientific evidence: Research now shows that hesperidin may strengthen veins and tiny blood vessels called capillaries, easing the symptoms of venous insufficiency. Hesperidin also has been shown to reduce leg symptoms such as pain, cramps, heaviness and neuropathy (burning, tingling and numbness). Some hesperidin products also contain *diosmin* (Daflon), a prescription medication that is used to treat venous disease…vitamin C…or the herb butcher's broom—all of which strengthen the effects of hesperidin.

Caution: Many drugs can react with hesperidin. If you take a diabetes medication, antihypertensive, blood thinner, muscle relaxant, antacid or antinausea medication, be sure to use this supplement cautiously and promptly alert your doctor if you experience any new symptoms after starting to use hesperidin.

- **Horse chestnut seed extract.** The seeds, leaves, bark and flowers of this tree, which is native to Europe, have been used for centuries in herbal medicine.

Scientific evidence: Several studies now indicate that horse chestnut seed extract may be helpful for venous insufficiency, decreasing leg pain, fatigue, itchiness and swelling.

Caution: Horse chestnut may lower blood sugar and interfere with diabetes medication.

- **L-carnitine.** Also known as acetyl-L-carnitine, this amino acid may improve circulation and help with PAD symptoms.

New finding: Taking L-carnitine in addition to the PAD medication cilostazol increased walking distance in people with intermittent claudication up to 46% more than taking cilostazol alone, reported researchers from the University of Colorado School of Medicine in a recent issue of *Vascular Medicine*.

- **Inositol nicotinate.** This is a form of niacin (vitamin B-3) that is less likely to create the typical "flushing" (redness and heat) that is produced by high doses of niacin.

Several studies show that it is helpful in treating PAD. It is commonly used in the UK to treat intermittent claudication.

- **Policosanol.** This is a natural cholesterol-lowering compound made primarily from the wax of cane sugar. Comparative studies show that policosanol treats intermittent claudication as effectively as the prescription blood thinner *ticlopidine* (Ticlid) and more effectively than the cholesterol-lowering statin *lovastatin* (Mevacor).

OTHER THERAPIES

You may read or hear that acupuncture, biofeedback, chelation therapy, garlic, omega-3 fatty acids and vitamin E can help with PAD.

However: The effectiveness of these particular therapies is uncertain at this time. For this reason, it is best to forgo these approaches until more scientific evidence becomes available.

Both Arm Exercises and Walking Help Painful Peripheral Artery Disease

Diane J. Treat-Jacobson, PhD, RN, assistant professor of nursing, University of Minnesota School of Nursing, Minneapolis.

Arm exercises as well as walking may help PAD. In patients with PAD, blood flow to arteries, particularly in the legs, is blocked by fatty deposits, causing pain and cramping in the legs while walking. People with PAD are at high risk for heart attack or stroke.

Recent research: Thirty-five PAD patients were assigned to either a no-exercise control group or to groups that performed aerobic arm exercises (using a device with bicycle-like pedals cranked by hand), treadmill walking or a combination of the two activities. All exercisers worked out for one hour, three times a week for 12 weeks in a supervised setting.

Result: After three months, people in all three exercise groups, but not in the control group, could walk about one-and-a-half blocks farther without pain and up to three blocks farther after they had rested.

Theory: Aerobic arm exercises, which are an especially good option for PAD patients who have trouble walking, are believed to have a systemic effect that improves overall cardiovascular function and fitness.

If you have PAD: Ask your doctor whether walking and/or doing aerobic arm exercises for one hour at least three times a week could help you.

Stretch If You Have PAD

Neel P. Chokshi, MD, MBA, medical director, Cardiology and Fitness Program, University of Pennsylvania, Philadelphia. Study presented at the American Heart Association's Arteriosclerosis, Thrombosis and Vascular Biology/Peripheral Vascular Disease 2017 Scientific Sessions.

In a small study from Florida State University College of Medicine in Tallahassee, patients with peripheral artery disease who stretched their calf muscles for 30 minutes a day, five days a week for a month improved both blood flow to their calves and their walking ability. They were able to walk farther during a timed period (six minutes)...and they were able to walk for a longer distance without needing to stop and rest because of discomfort.

A physical therapist can show you how to stretch effectively to relieve your PAD—and recommend for how long and how often you should do it.

The Diabetes Complication That Kills More People Than Most Cancers

James M. Horton, MD, chair of the Standards and Practice Guidelines Committee of the Infectious Diseases Society of America. IDsociety.org

A foot or leg amputation is one of the most dreaded complications of diabetes. In the US, more than 65,000 such amputations occur each year.

But the tragedy does not stop there. According to recent research, about half of all people who have a foot amputation die within five years of the surgery—a worse mortality rate than most cancers. That's partly because diabetic patients who have amputations often have poorer glycemic control and more complications such as kidney disease. Amputation also can lead to increased pressure on the remaining limb and the possibility of new ulcers and infections.

What you need to know...

HOW FOOT INFECTIONS START

Diabetes can lead to foot infections in two main ways—peripheral neuropathy (nerve damage that can cause loss of sensation in the feet)...and ischemia (inadequate blood flow).

Small wounds can lead to big trouble. About 25% of people with diabetes will develop a foot ulcer—ranging from mild to severe—at some point in their lives. Any ulcer, blister, cut or irritation has the potential to become infected. If the infection becomes too severe to treat effectively with antibiotics, amputation of a foot or leg may be the only way to prevent the infection from spreading throughout the body and save the person's life.

A FAST-MOVING DANGER

Sores on the foot can progress rapidly. While some foot sores remain unchanged for months, it is possible for an irritation to lead to an open wound (ulcer), infection and amputation in as little as a few days. That is why experts recommend that people with diabetes seek medical care promptly for any open sore on the feet or any new area of redness or irritation that could possibly lead to an open wound.

Important: Fully half of diabetic foot ulcers are infected and require immediate medical treatment and sometimes hospitalization.

Don't try to diagnose yourself—diagnosis requires a trained medical expert. An ulcer that appears very small on the surface could have actually spread underneath the skin, so you very well could be seeing just a small portion of the infection.

WHAT YOUR DOCTOR WILL DO

The first step is to identify the bacteria causing the infection. To do this, physicians collect specimens from deep inside the wound. Once the bacteria have been identified, the proper antibiotics can be prescribed.

Physicians also need to know the magnitude of the infection—for example, whether there is bone infection, abscesses or other internal problems. Therefore, all diabetes patients who

Watch Your Feet

Charcot foot (a condition in which bones in the foot weaken and break) is common in people with diabetes and/or peripheral neuropathy. They may have a loss of feeling in the feet due to nerve damage and are sometimes unaware that they have Charcot foot until it causes severe deformities.

If you have diabetes and/or peripheral neuropathy: See a podiatrist or orthopedic surgeon to be monitored for Charcot foot, which can be treated with surgery and/or specialized footwear. Warning signs include sudden swelling or pain of the foot and/or leg.

Valerie L. Schade, DPM, FACFAS, podiatric surgeon, Tacoma, Washington.

have new foot infections should have X-rays. If more detailed imaging is needed, an MRI or a bone scan may be ordered.

The doctor will then classify the wound and infection as mild, moderate or severe and create a treatment plan.

HOW TO GET THE BEST TREATMENT

Each person's wound is unique, so there are no cookie-cutter treatment plans. *However, most treatment plans should include...*

- **A diabetic foot-care team.** For moderate or severe infections, a team of experts should coordinate treatment. This will be done for you—by the hospital or your primary care physician. The number of specialists on the team depends on the patient's specific needs but may include experts in podiatry and vascular surgery. In rural or smaller communities, this may be done via online communication with experts from larger hospitals (telemedicine).

- **Antibiotic treatment.** Milder infections usually involve a single bacterium. Antibiotics will typically be needed for about one week. With more severe infections, multiple bacteria are likely involved, so you will require multiple antibiotics, and treatment will need to continue for a longer period—sometimes four weeks or more if bone is affected.

If the infection is severe...or even moderate but complicated by, say, poor blood circulation, hospitalization may be required for a few days to a few weeks, depending on the course of the recovery.

- **Wound care.** Many patients who have foot infections receive antibiotic therapy only, which is often insufficient. Proper wound care is also necessary. In addition to frequent wound cleansing and dressing changes, this may include surgical removal of dead tissue (debridement)...and the use of specially designed shoes or shoe inserts—provided by a podiatrist—to redistribute pressure off the wound (off-loading).

- **Surgery.** Surgery doesn't always mean amputation. It is sometimes used not only to remove dead or damaged tissue or bone but also to improve blood flow to the foot.

If an infection fails to improve: The first question physicians know to ask is: "Is the patient complying with wound care instructions?" Too many patients lose a leg because they don't take their antibiotics as prescribed or care for the injury as prescribed.

Never forget: Following your doctors' specific orders could literally mean the difference between having one leg or two.

FOOT CARE IS CRITICAL IF YOU HAVE DIABETES

To protect yourself from foot injuries...

- **Never walk barefoot, even around the house.**

- **Don't wear sandals**—the straps can irritate the side of the foot.

- **Wear thick socks with soft leather shoes.** Leather is a good choice because it "breathes," molds to the feet and does not retain moisture. Laced-up shoes with cushioned soles provide the most support.

In addition, pharmacies carry special "diabetic socks" that protect and cushion your feet without cutting off circulation at the ankle. These socks usually have no seams that could chafe. They also wick moisture away from feet, which reduces risk for infection and foot ulcers.

- **See a podiatrist.** This physician can advise you on the proper care of common foot problems, such as blisters, corns and ingrown toenails. A podiatrist can also help you find appropriate footwear—even if you have foot deformities. Ask your primary care physician or endocrinologist for a recommendation, or consult the American Podiatric Medical Association, APMA.org.

Also: Inspect your feet every day. Otherwise, you may miss a developing infection. Look for areas of redness, blisters or open sores, particularly in the areas most prone to injury—the bottoms and bony inner and outer edges of the feet.

A Foot Problem That Gets Misdiagnosed

Mitchell Yass, DPT, a Florida–based physical therapist and creator of the Yass Method for treating chronic pain. He is the author of *Overpower Pain: The Strength Training Program That Stops Pain Without Drugs or Surgery.* MitchellYass.com

If you're age 50 or older, overweight and have recently experienced pain, tingling or numbness in one or both feet, you fit the classic profile of a person with diabetic neuropathy.

This condition occurs when diabetes leads to nerve damage, which most often affects the feet. Sometimes DN hurts, while other times it creates an inability to feel pain, heat or cold. This loss of sensation is serious, because a sore or ulcer can go unnoticed, become infected and sometimes lead to a foot or leg amputation—so your doctor diagnoses you with DN.

Here's the kicker: You may not have DN—or diabetes. Even though people who are overweight are at much greater risk for type 2 diabetes, you may not have the disease.

WHAT ELSE COULD IT BE?

If your doctor has diagnosed you with DN, make sure that your blood tests (such as a fasting blood glucose test) confirm that you actually have diabetes. If you are not diabetic but your physician insists it's DN, it's time to find a new doctor. But if you don't have DN, then what's causing your foot problems?

UNRAVELING THE CLUES

Based on my experience treating hundreds of patients with foot pain who were misdiagnosed with DN, I recommend special exercises.

To ensure that you're doing the most effective exercises, it's crucial to isolate where you're experiencing pain or numbness in your foot—is it all over...on top...or on the bottom? *What the location may mean...**

If your entire foot is affected—it could be sciatica. This condition, characterized by shooting pain that travels down one or both legs, can occur when the piriformis muscle in the buttocks compresses the sciatic nerve, which runs down the leg before branching off in the foot. The result can be gluteal pain, as well as pain, numbness or a "pins and needles" feeling in the foot. Sciatica often occurs when the gluteus medius muscle above the hip joint is weak, leading the piriformis muscle to compensate.**

Self-test for a weak gluteus medius muscle: Look at yourself in a mirror while standing casually. Does one hip naturally sit higher than the other? A higher hip indicates that the lower back muscle on that side is overworked and shortened, pulling the hip higher. This points to sciatica—not DN—as the cause of your foot discomfort.

To strengthen the muscles of the weaker hip, do these two exercises...

- **Hip abduction.** Lie on your side, with your bottom leg bent at the knee and your top leg (the weaker one) extended in a straight line. Rotate the foot of your extended leg slightly so that your toes point down and your heel is the first to rise. Raise your top leg several inches keeping it parallel with the floor, then lower it, keeping movements controlled.

Perform two to three sets of 10 repetitions, two or three times a week. If doing 10 repetitions is easy, add a weighted ankle cuff (available online). Begin with a one-pound weight and increase weight when the exercise becomes too easy. Do the exercise on your weak leg only.

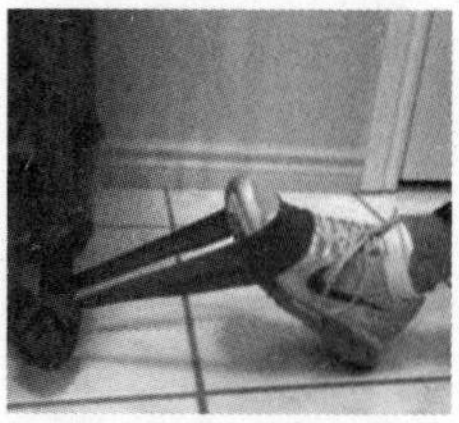

- **Dorsiflexion.** Slip one end of an elastic resistance band around a sturdy table leg. While wearing sneakers, sit on the floor facing the table. Extend your weak leg, bend your knee and slip the other end of the resistance band over your instep. Point and flex, keeping the heel stationary and movements slow and controlled. Perform two to three sets of 10 repetitions, two or three times a week, on your weak leg only.

*If your foot pain, regardless of location, isn't eliminated by these exercises in four weeks, see a neurologist.

**If sciatica causes severe pain or you have trouble controlling your bowels or bladder, see a doctor right away,

If just the top of the foot is affected—you may have a pinched peroneal nerve. This happens more frequently in people with strained hip muscles. Symptoms are similar to those of weak gluteal muscles. Unlike sciatica, however, there's no gluteal pain, and the altered foot sensation is on the top of the foot only—not all over. To strengthen hip muscles, perform the two exercises above, plus this exercise...

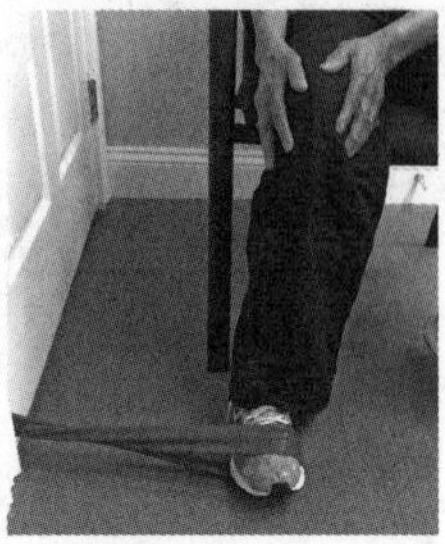

• **Inversion.** Knot a resistance band on one end, and place the knotted end behind a closed door. Sit in a chair, parallel to the door. Loop the other end of the resistance band around your instep. Angle your toes slightly to the outside of the heel, then stretch the band until toes are in line with the heel. Perform two to three sets of 10 repetitions, two or three times a week, on your weak leg only, using slow and controlled motions.

If pain is in the sole of your foot—you may have a collapsed arch.

What can happen: If the gluteus medius or the muscles that support the arch are weak, your arch may flatten. When this occurs, the sole of your mid-foot will be flat on the floor when you stand or walk, compressing nerves in the bottom of the foot. This triggers tingling and/or numbness in the sole.

Self-test for a collapsed arch: Wet the sole of your foot, shake off any excess water, then step on a brown paper bag. If the arch side of your footprint is filled in, you may have a collapsed arch.

To alleviate pain, do all three of the exercises above.

CHAPTER 10

Hands and Arms Pain

Do You Have Aching or Numb Hands?

Hands are vulnerable to mechanical difficulties because of their intricate networks of bones, nerves, muscles, ligaments and tendons—all of which are located in the narrow, relatively unprotected areas of the wrist, palm and fingers.

Each year, about 17% of Americans over age 55 report having hand pain. But if you count the full range of potential symptoms—including numbness, tingling, burning sensations and "frozen" fingers—the number of hand problems is much higher. *Common hand disorders...*

ARTHRITIS

Although arthritis can occur in any hand joint, one of the most frequently affected locations is at the base of the thumb, where the thumb bones connect to the trapezium bone in the wrist. This very flexible joint is in constant use and takes the most stress of any hand joint—the thumb is used anytime we need to hold an object.

Symptoms: Mild or severe pain, usually at the base of the hand between the thumb and the wrist.

First treatment step: Use a brace that surrounds the thumb and connects to the hand. This reduces stress on the joint and may decrease the painful joint inflammation associated with arthritis. Such braces are available at drugstores. Your doctor also may recommend prescription anti-inflammatory medications or over-the-counter (OTC) painkillers, such as *ibuprofen* (Advil) or buffered aspirin (to prevent gastrointestinal upset). If two or three weeks of bracing quiets the pain, this treatment can be repeated as needed.

Terry R. Light, MD, Dr. William M. Scholl Professor and chairman of the department of orthopedic surgery and rehabilitation, Loyola University, Chicago, Stritch School of Medicine in Maywood, Illinois, and author of more than 50 medical journal articles.

If symptoms continue or worsen: Pain can be relieved with injections of cortisone, a powerful anti-inflammatory, into the arthritic joint at the base of the thumb. Although frequent cortisone injections can cause thinning of joint cartilage and weakening of joint ligaments, injections can be given for as long as they work. That's because cartilage is already destroyed by the arthritis, so the injections do more good than harm.

If all else fails: Surgery offers a permanent solution.* The most popular involves removing the affected joint by taking out the trapezium wrist bone, which is about the size of a sugar cube. Once this bone is removed, the thumb can be anchored and cushioned by a piece of tendon taken from the forearm.

Within a year after surgery, most patients report good pain relief and enough range of motion to allow normal daily activities. Common risks associated with this surgery include sensory nerve damage, scar tenderness and persistent pain.

CARPAL TUNNEL SYNDROME

The median nerve runs from the neck, arm and forearm to the hand, passing a "tunnel" formed by the bones of the wrist and a thick band of tissue called the transverse carpal ligament. Anything that narrows the tunnel, such as a fracture or swelling of the surrounding tissue, can pinch the nerve, causing carpal tunnel syndrome (CTS).

No one knows what causes CTS. Now experts even question the common assumption that it is due to repetitive strain, which can occur during typing or using machinery. CTS is more common in people with diabetes, rheumatoid arthritis and thyroid disease—perhaps because these conditions are often linked to inflammation.

Symptoms: Numbness in the fingers nearest your thumb, especially at night. You also may experience tingling, burning, or mild or severe pain in the fingers.

First treatment step: Use a custom-made wrist brace (available from hand therapists) or a store-bought brace at night. Both relieve nerve pressure. If symptoms improve within six weeks, no other treatment is needed.

If symptoms continue or worsen: An injection of cortisone can eliminate pain and numbness for about three months. Because cortisone can harm soft tissue, additional injections are rarely given.

If all else fails: A surgeon can cut the transverse carpal ligament, making room for the nerve, which reduces pain and improves strength and sensation. Full recovery usually takes about three months.

This surgery is successful in about 90% of cases, and it carries a low risk for complications, such as nerve damage.

TRIGGER FINGER

Each finger has one or two tendons that slide through a tunnel formed by a series of fibrous bands. The tendons normally glide smoothly as you flex your fingers. If the band at the base of the finger narrows or the tendons thicken or swell, the tendons may catch or become stuck. The cause of trigger finger is unknown, but it is more common in people with diabetes and rheumatoid arthritis.

Symptoms: Mild pain or tenderness in the palm at the base of one or more fingers. There may be a popping or clicking sensation while opening and closing the hand.

First treatment step: Rest the affected finger—using a brace to limit its use. Cut back on hand-related activities for two to four weeks.

If symptoms continue or worsen: Cortisone injections into the band at the base of the finger can relieve inflammation. Up to three injections (over a lifetime) may be given.

If all else fails: A surgeon can make a small incision at the base of the finger and cut the fibrous band, freeing the tendon. Normal activity can be resumed within two weeks. Nerve injury, though rare, is a possible complication of this surgery.

DUPUYTREN'S CONTRACTURE

This disorder causes abnormal tissue growth in the palm and the fingers, eventually causing the fingers to flex or curl. It is seen mainly

*To find a hand surgeon in your area, contact the American Society for Surgery of the Hand (847-384-8300, ASSH.org).

in men of Northern European ancestry, but its causes are unknown.

Symptoms: The first sign is usually a small lump or nodule in the palm. Later, patients are unable to completely straighten the fingers.

First treatment step: This disorder is not dangerous, and it may take years before hand function is affected. Diagnosis is based on a physical exam.

If symptoms continue or worsen: In some cases, cortisone injections may be given if the nodule becomes painful.

If the contracture is keeping you from doing things you love, a surgeon can remove the abnormal tissue. The success rate for the surgery depends on the extent of the disorder, and risks can include nerve damage, blood vessel damage, skin healing problems and infection.

Surgery-Free Help for Trigger Finger

Mitchell Yass, DPT, a Florida–based physical therapist and creator of the Yass Method for treating chronic pain. He is the author of *Overpower Pain: The Strength Training Program That Stops Pain Without Drugs or Surgery* and *The Pain Cure Rx: The Yass Method for Diagnosing and Resolving Chronic Pain* and host of the PBS special *The Pain Prescription*. MitchellYass.com

Trigger finger is the result of the person flexing or bending the finger, but the problem usually stems from the elbow, not the finger joint. The tendons performing the act are the finger tendons on the palm side of the hand. When the finger flexors shorten, the finger extensors (the muscles on the opposite side of the hand) must lengthen. These muscle/tendon mechanisms originate at the elbow and end at the last joint near the tip of the finger.

If these muscles strain, they tend to shorten. If they shorten enough, they lose their ability to lengthen over all the joints—including the wrist and finger joints, so that when a finger is bent enough, these muscles can get stuck. So the inability to straighten the finger after it has been bent is not a result of some effect on the finger flexor muscle. It is the fact that the length of the finger extensor has been so altered that it can no longer perform its function of straightening the finger.

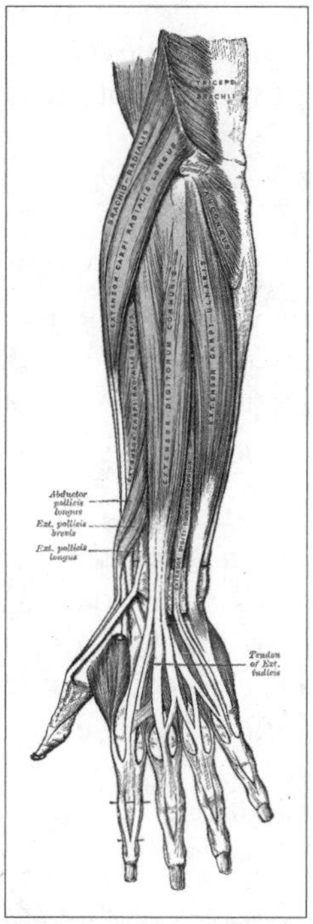

The muscles that need to be strengthened are the finger extensors, wrist extensors and then two muscles in the shoulder and shoulder blade region that support the arm and any objects that are held. A simply stretch of the wrist and finger extensors can be used in the short term to return the finger extensors to their optimal length to allow them to function properly and end the trigger finger. Here is the full routine.

Perform these exercises three times a week. For each exercise, do three sets of 10 repetitions with a one-minute break between sets. Continually increase the resistance until the muscles are strong enough to perform your functional activities without strain or other symptoms.

FINGER EXTENSION

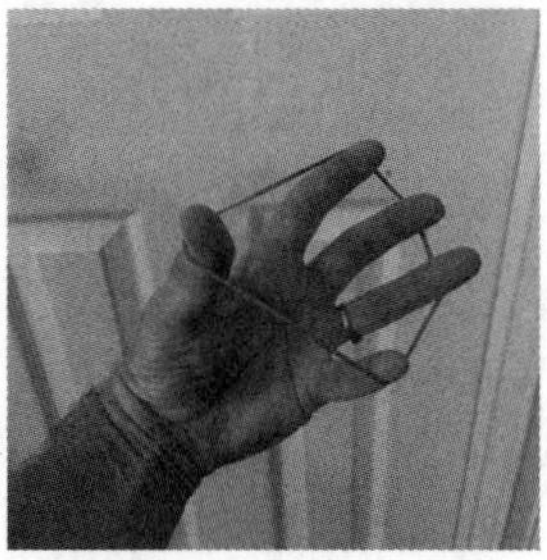

START

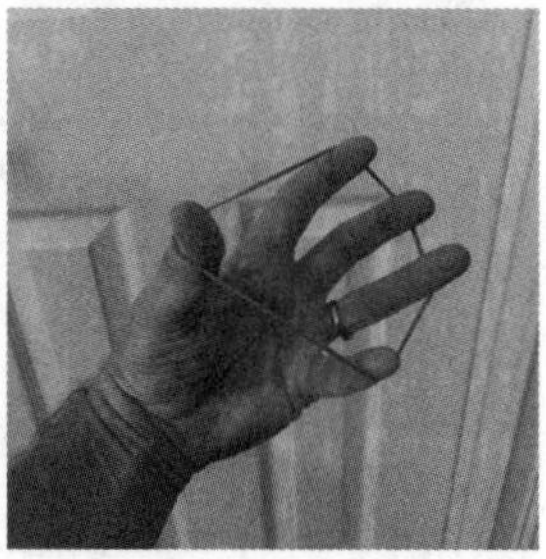

FINISH

Place a rubber band around your hand so the band is touching the finger tips at the level of the farthest joint. Open the fingers as far as you can, then return to the start position. Try to emphasize the use of the affected finger as much as possible.

WRIST EXTENSION

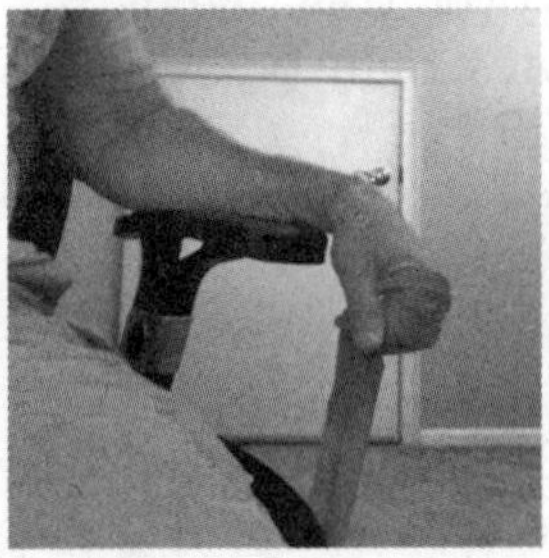

START

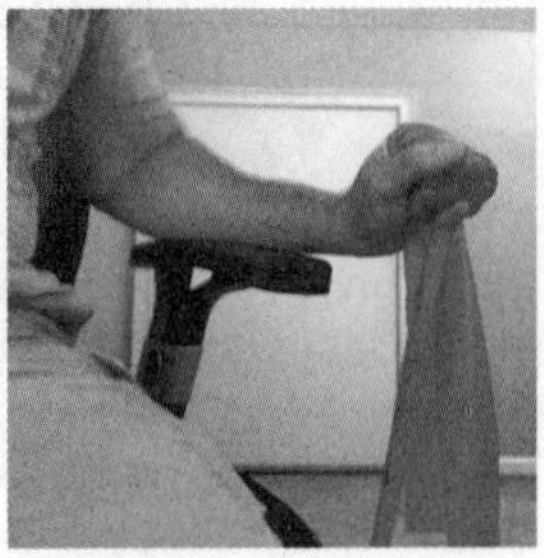

FINISH

Attach a resistance band to the leg of a chair. Wrap the other end around the hand until resistance is obtained at the start position. Start with the wrist pointing down as much as possible. Then raise the wrist as high as possible while keeping the forearm on the arm of the chair. Return to the start position.

LAT PULLDOWN

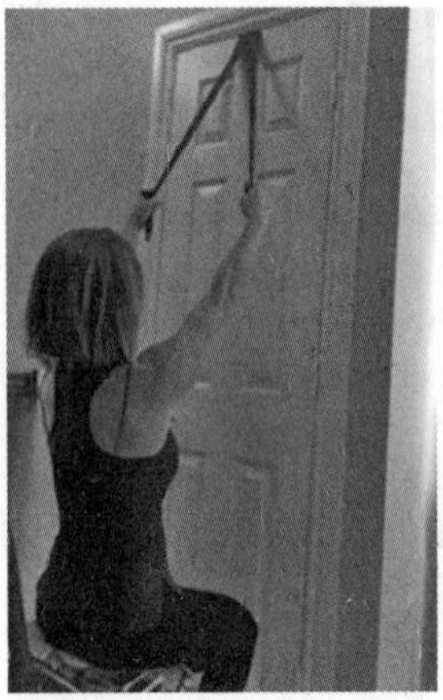

START

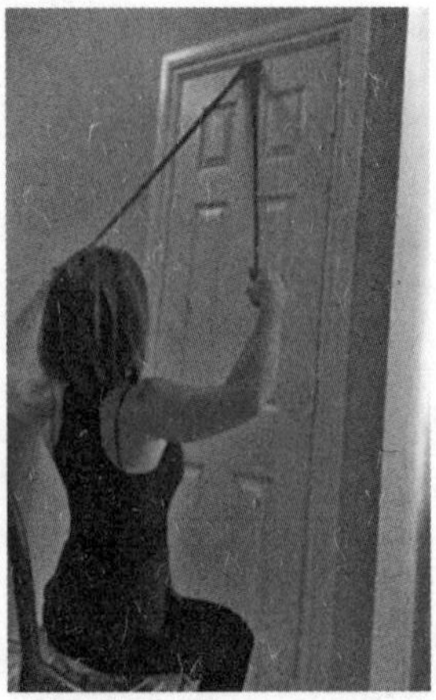

FINISH

Tie a knot in the center of a fitness band and secure behind the top of a closed door. Sit in a chair facing the door. Leaning back with an angle at the hip of about 30 degrees, reach up for the elastic band so that the start position begins with the arms nearly straight and the elbows just unlocked. Pull down, keeping your arms wide and bringing the elbows just below shoulder height and slightly behind the line of the shoulders. At this point, you should feel the shoulder blades squeeze together (the elbows will barely reach behind the line of the shoulders if performing this exercise correctly). Then return to the start position. If the elbows start to drop so they are lower than the shoulders, you are using the incorrect muscles to perform the exercise.

LOWER TRAP EXERCISE

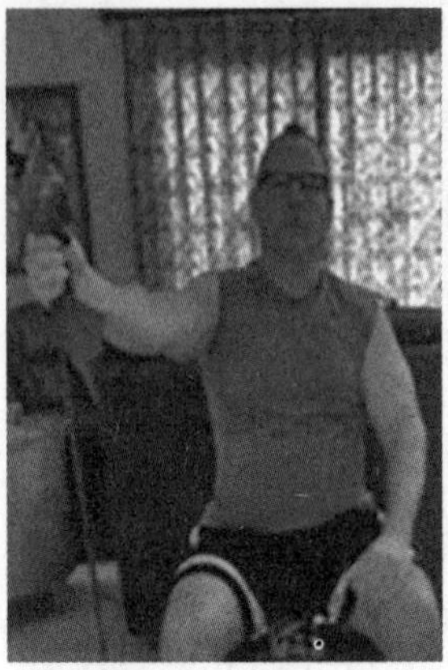

START

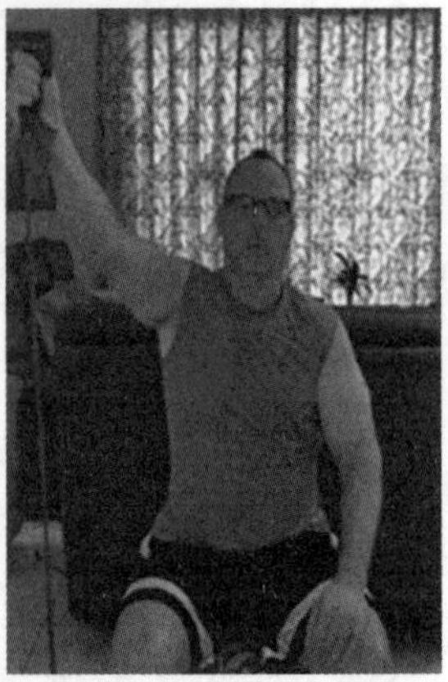

FINISH

This exercise is critical to achieving complete functional capacity of the shoulder. To perform this exercise, sit in a sturdy chair and lean back slightly—about 10 degrees. This will prevent the resistance from pulling you forward. Start with your arm halfway between pointing straight forward and pointing straight to the side, with your hand at shoulder height and your elbow just unlocked. Begin to raise the resistance until the arm reaches about 130 to 140 degrees (about the height of the ear). Then return to the start position at shoulder height. Make sure you are sitting and are supported with a chair back if possible. You want to be leaning back about 10 degrees to prevent the resistance from pulling you forward.

WRIST AND FINGER EXTENSOR STRETCH

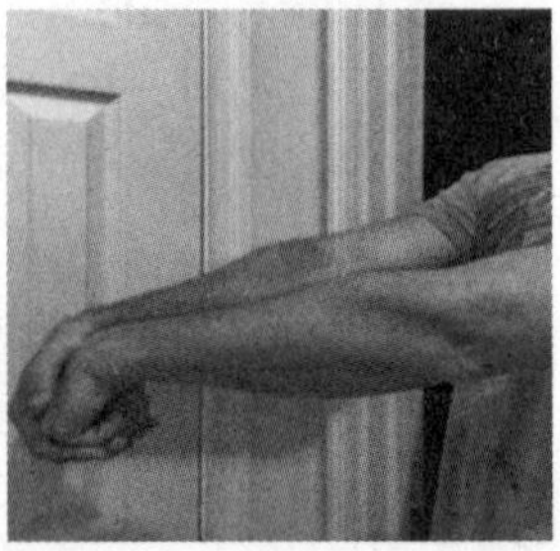

Wrap the fingers of the unaffected hand around the affected hand. Try to bend the wrist down while trying to close the fingers into a fist. Make sure that the elbow of the arm being stretched is maintained in a straight position. This allows the wrist and finger extensors to be lengthened optimally. Hold the stretch for 20 seconds. Pause, and repeat the stretch.

This stretch can be performed as often as you choose during the course of the day every day to maximize the length of the wrist and finger extensors.

Keep Your Hands Young and Strong—7 Simple Exercises Reduce Pain and Stiffness

Anjum Lone, OTR/L, CHT, occupational and certified hand therapist and chief of the department of occupational therapy at Phelps Memorial Hospital Center in Sleepy Hollow, New York.

If you have been diagnosed with arthritis, it's wise to protect your hands right away. Approximately 40% of arthritis patients must eventually restrict their daily activities because of joint pain or stiffness—and the hands often get the worst of it.

Both osteoarthritis (known as "wear-and-tear" arthritis) and rheumatoid arthritis (an autoimmune disease) can damage cartilage and sometimes the bones themselves. (For natural remedies to help ease rheumatoid arthritis, click here.)

What's missing from the typical arthritis prescription: Unfortunately, most patients with either type of arthritis do not recognize the importance of simple daily hand exercises, which can improve joint lubrication...increase your range of motion and hand strength...and maintain or restore function. These exercises also are helpful for people who have a hand injury or who heavily use their hands.

SAVE YOUR HANDS WITH EXERCISE

Most hand and wrist exercises can be done at home without equipment. But don't exercise during flare-ups, particularly if you have rheumatoid arthritis. Patients who ignore the pain and overuse their hands and wrists are more likely to suffer long-term damage, including joint deformity.

Important: Warm the joints before doing these exercises—this helps prevent microtears that can occur when stretching cold tissue. Simply run warm water over your hands in the sink for a few minutes right before the exercises. Or you can warm them with a heating pad.

Before doing the hand exercises here, it also helps to use the fingers of the other hand to rub and knead the area you'll be exercising. This self-massage improves circulation to the area and reduces swelling.

If you have osteoarthritis or rheumatoid arthritis, do the following exercises five times on each hand—and work up to 10 times, if possible. The entire sequence should take no more than five minutes. Perform the sequence two to three times a day.*

1. Tendon glides.

Purpose: Keeps the tendons functioning well to help move all the finger joints through their full range of motion.

What to do: Rest your elbow on a table with your forearm and hand raised (fingertips pointed to the ceiling). Bend the fingers at the middle joint (form a hook with your fingers), and hold this position for a moment. Then bend the fingers into a fist, hiding your nails. Don't clench—just fold your fingers gently while keeping the wrist in a "neutral" position. Now make a modified fist with your nails showing. Next, raise your fingers so that they are bent at a 90-degree angle and your thumb is resting against your index finger (your hand will look similar to a bird's beak). Hold each position for three seconds.

2. Thumb active range of motion.

Purpose: Improves your ability to move your thumb in all directions. Do the movements gently so that you don't feel any pain.

What to do: Rest your elbow on a table with your forearm and hand in the air. Touch the tip of the thumb to the tip of each finger (or get as close as you can). Then, flex the tip of your thumb toward the palm. Hold each of these positions for three seconds.

3. Web-space massage.

*For more exercises, see an occupational therapist. To find one, consult the American Occupational Therapy Association. AOTA.org

Purpose: Using one hand to massage the other hand strengthens muscles in the "active" hand while increasing circulation in the "passive" hand.

What to do: Clasp your left hand with your right hand as if you are shaking hands. With firm but gentle pressure, use the length of your left thumb to massage the web (space between the thumb and the index finger) next to your right thumb. Then, reverse the position and massage the web next to your left thumb. Massage each web for 30 seconds.

4. Wrist active range of motion.

Purpose: To maintain proper positioning of the wrist, which helps keep the fingers in correct alignment.

What to do: Rest your right forearm on a table with your wrist hanging off the edge and your palm pointing downward—you'll be moving only your wrist. Then place your left hand on top of your right forearm to keep it stable. With the fingers on your right hand held together gently, raise the wrist as high as it will comfortably go. Hold for three seconds.

Next, make a fist and raise it so the knuckles point upward. Now, lower the fist toward the floor. Hold each position for three seconds.

5. Digit extension.

Purpose: Strengthens the muscles that pull the fingers straight—the movement prevents chronic contractions that can lead to joint deformity.

What to do: Warm up by placing the palms and fingers of both hands together and pressing the hands gently for five seconds. Then place your palms flat on a table. One at a time, raise each finger. Then lift all the fingers on one hand simultaneously while keeping your palm flat on the table. Hold each movement for five seconds.

6. Wrist flexion/extension.

Purpose: Stretches and promotes muscle length in the forearm. Forearm muscles move the wrist and fingers. Flexion (bending your wrist so that your palm approaches the forearm) and extension (bending your wrist in the opposite direction) help maintain wrist strength and range of motion.

What to do: Hold your right hand in the air, palm down. Bend the wrist upward so that the tips of your fingers are pointed toward the ceiling. Place your left hand against the fingers (on the palm side) and gently push so that the back of your right hand moves toward the top of your right forearm. Hold for 15 seconds. Switch hands and repeat.

Now, bend your right wrist downward so that the fingers are pointed at the floor. Place your left hand against the back of your right hand and gently push so your palm moves toward the bottom of the forearm. Hold 15 seconds. Switch and repeat.

7. Finger-walking exercises.

Purpose: Strengthens fingers in the opposite direction of a deformity. This exercise is particularly helpful for rheumatoid arthritis patients.

What to do: Put one hand on a flat surface. Lift the index finger up and move it toward the thumb, then place the finger down. Next, lift the middle finger and move it toward the index finger. Lift the ring finger and move it toward the middle finger. Finally, lift the little finger and move it toward the ring finger. Repeat on your other hand.

When Fingers Don't Work Right

Lawrence C. Hurst, MD, professor and chair of the department of orthopedics and chief of the division of hand surgery at Stony Brook University in Stony Brook, New York. He is author of numerous studies on hand disorders and led research on the new nonsurgical treatment for Dupuytren's disease.

Finger problems can make it hard to cook, carry groceries, use a computer or do any number of everyday activities...and they frequently involve significant pain and even deformity.

Good news: Most conditions that affect the fingers are treatable. Nonsurgical approaches are tried first. If these fail, surgery usually succeeds. Depending on the disorder, recovery from surgery takes several weeks to several months and may include physical therapy.

The sooner a finger problem is treated, the better the outcome is likely to be—so see your doctor if you have any of the symptoms below. If your doctor advises, visit a hand specialist.

Referrals: American Association for Hand Surgery, HandSurgery.org.

What you need to know if your...

- **Finger straightens with a snap or click.** This is trigger finger, in which the affected finger gets stuck in the bent position, then releases suddenly when pushed straight. Pain and stiffness are common...middle and ring fingers are most often affected.

How it develops: Finger flexion (bending) depends on flexor tendons that run from the forearm to each finger. A tubelike sheath surrounds the tendons. If a tendon or sheath becomes inflamed due to injury, overuse or the effects of diabetes or rheumatoid arthritis, a nodule (bump) forms and traps the tendon when the finger is bent. (For an exercise cure, see page 239.)

Your doctor may have you take an over-the-counter nonsteroidal anti-inflammatory drug (NSAID), such as *ibuprofen* (Advil) or *naproxen* (Aleve), for two to four weeks. For persistent inflammation, cortisone injections often help.

If surgery is necessary: Through a small incision in the palm, the surgeon cuts open the entrance to the sheath to enlarge it so that the tendon can move without getting stuck.

- **Finger curls toward the palm.** This progressive condition, Dupuytren's (duh-pwee-tranz) disease, can affect just one finger —usually the ring or little finger—or several fingers. It develops when connective-tissue ligaments beneath the skin thicken into nodules, then form cords of scarlike tissue that extend into the fingers. The cords then shorten, causing fingers to contract like claws. Risk for Dupuytren's is elevated if a parent or grandparent had it...if you have diabetes, seizures or thyroid problems...or if you are or were a smoker or heavy drinker.

New treatment: Surgery used to be the only option—but with a new technique, the cords are injected with *collagenase clostridium histolyticum* (Xiaflex), which dissolves the scar tissue. The next day, the surgeon breaks the weakened cords with manual manipulation (local anesthesia may be used), restoring finger movement. The FDA approved Xiaflex in February 2010.

A treatment used in Europe (though less common in the US) is needle aponeurotomy. After injecting local anesthesia, the surgeon repeatedly punctures the cord with a needle to weaken it, then breaks it down by manual manipulation.

Surgery for Dupuytren's can be complicated because the surgeon must remove the tissue causing the contracture, but it usually is successful.

Note: After Xiaflex or surgery for Dupuytren's, the condition recurs in about 10% to 15% of cases. After needle aponeurotomy, recurrence rate is higher.

- **Top joint droops.** With mallet finger, the tip of the finger bends forward and won't straighten. Typically it happens after the fingertip gets jammed into something, damaging the extensor tendon near the base of the fingernail.

For treatment, the finger is splinted around the clock for about six weeks...then over the next six weeks, the splint is worn only at night. Surgery generally is done only if the initial injury also caused a bone fracture or joint misalignment that requires surgical repair.

- **Wrist swells and hurts on the thumb side.** With de Quervain's tenosynovitis, the sheath around the tendons on the thumb side of the wrist becomes inflamed, inhibiting the tendons' movement. This causes swelling at the base of the thumb...intense pain in the thumb and forearm...and difficulty grasping, pinching or turning your wrist.

The disorder typically arises due to repetitive overuse of or injury to the thumb or wrist. It is most common after age 50—but it often afflicts new mothers, whose tendons and sheaths swelled during pregnancy.

Nonsurgical treatment includes immobilizing the thumb with a splint for four to six weeks and taking anti-inflammatories. Cortisone may be injected into the sheath. In severe cases, surgery opens the tight, inflamed sheath, reducing pressure and allowing tendons to glide smoothly.

• **Fingers feel tingly, numb and weak.** With carpal tunnel syndrome, the thumb, index and middle fingers are most often affected...sharp pain may travel from the wrist through the arm.

What happens: The carpal tunnel (a channel in the wrist) is composed of bone and a fibrous band called the transverse carpal ligament. The median nerve, which controls sensation in all fingers except the little finger and part of the ring finger, runs through the tunnel, as do flexor tendons and their lining tissues. When lining tissues get inflamed or the ligament thickens, it creates pressure on the median nerve. Carpal tunnel syndrome is linked to repetitive movements...some evidence suggests a possible link to hypothyroidism, rheumatoid arthritis, diabetes, excess weight, pregnancy and menopause.

In the early stages, wrist splinting at night plus oral anti-inflammatories or cortisone injections bring relief. Once symptoms ease, your doctor may suggest stretching and strengthening exercises to help prevent recurrences. Some patients report improvement from acupuncture or chiropractic care, though there are no large-scale scientific studies backing these.

The most common surgical technique, open release surgery, involves making an inch-long incision in the wrist or palm and dividing the transverse carpal ligament to enlarge the carpal tunnel. Endoscopic release surgery, which may minimize scarring but has a higher risk for nerve injury, uses a mini camera and other instruments inserted via one or two small incisions.

• **Little and ring fingers feel numb.** This is ulnar nerve entrapment. It occurs when the ulnar nerve, which runs through the arm and controls the little finger and part of the ring finger, gets compressed at the elbow due to injury or swelling. If untreated, muscles in the affected fingers may atrophy and sensation may be lost.

You need to wear a splint that keeps the elbow straight at night...avoid putting pressure on the elbow...and take anti-inflammatories. Your doctor may demonstrate arm exercises that ease pressure on the nerve. If necessary, a surgeon can free the entrapped nerve by moving it to a different position within the elbow...or by widening the tunnel at the elbow through which the nerve passes.

Finger-Joint Replacement

Scott W. Wolfe, MD, director of the hand surgical fellowship program and attending orthopedic surgeon at the Hospital for Special Surgery in New York City. He is a professor of orthopedic surgery at Weill Medical College of Cornell University, also in New York City.

If you have finger pain that's so severe that medication and hand exercises don't provide adequate relief, joint replacement may be the next step. Until recently, the traditional surgical procedure, joint fusion, controlled the pain associated with arthritic or injured fingers but severely limited their flexibility.

Now: Specialized hand surgeons are able to replace damaged finger joints with a technique that is similar to hip- or knee-replacement surgery. Called joint replacement, or arthroplasty, the procedure not only relieves pain due to osteoarthritis and rheumatoid arthritis, but also provides enough flexibility so that you can use a tennis racket, golf club or garden tools.

What you need to know about this breakthrough procedure...

ARE YOU A CANDIDATE?

Finger-joint replacements are far less common than knee or hip replacement—in part because the intricate bone structure and miniature size of the finger joints make the procedure more challenging for surgeons to perform. But this procedure has now advanced to the point that individuals who have not received adequate relief from other medical treatments should think about having finger-joint replacement, particularly if they have an active lifestyle.

The decision to get a finger joint replaced is primarily based on one's level of disability—how much pain you continue to experience after trying other medical treatments and the degree to which your activities are limited.

The finger joints most often replaced are the proximal interphalangeal (PIP) joint (second joint from the fingertip) and the metacarpophalangeal (MCP) joint (knuckle joint).

Any type of joint replacement is major surgery, but finger-joint replacement is relatively safe. For example, the risk for infection is relatively low—in part because the hand has an excellent blood supply, which helps prevent bacteria from entering the site of the wound. Nerves can be damaged during the procedure, which can lead to numbness and a loss of sensation, but this is a rare occurrence.

GETTING A FINGER-JOINT REPLACEMENT

If you are interested in getting a finger-joint replacement, it's important to consult an experienced hand surgeon who performs dozens of these surgeries a year. Often, surgeons at university teaching hospitals have experience with less common procedures such as these.*

The procedure takes about an hour to perform on each joint that is being replaced. Some patients receive more than one finger-joint replacement—and, in some cases, during a single operation.

The operation does not require an inpatient hospital stay or general anesthesia. Instead, a nerve block is used to numb the arm—which allows for a quicker recovery—and patients can go home the same day.

During the procedure, the surgeon makes a small incision on the finger and removes the damaged finger joint. An artificial joint, which in many respects resembles a miniature total knee replacement, is inserted and then cemented into place.

New development: Previously, surgeons accessed damaged finger joints through the back of the hand, which delayed recovery because tendons and soft tissue were often damaged during the procedure. A less invasive approach involves accessing the finger from the palm side, which limits damage to the soft tissues and tendons.

The most commonly used material for artificial finger joints is silicone. There are no long-term studies indicating how long these artificial joints will last. However, implant fractures commonly occur after seven to 10 years.

The finger-joint replacements made of pyrolytic carbon, a type of material often used for mechanical heart valves, are the newest artificial joints available. Initially, the results were favorable when these joints were used for joint damage caused by arthritis or injury, but some recent studies have demonstrated less-favorable outcomes with these prostheses, and they are still being evaluated.

Yet another option is a two-part implant coated with a cobalt chrome surface—the same materials used in many knee and hip replacements. This provides a high degree of durability and flexibility.

WHAT TO EXPECT AFTER SURGERY

Some patients begin rehabilitation one to two days after surgery, but others may need more time to heal. A removable splint is worn for four to five weeks after the procedure to keep the joint stable and help soft tissues heal and become stronger.

It is important to meet with a physical therapist twice weekly for six to eight weeks. During this time, patients learn strengthening exercises and methods to protect their new joints against excess stress. If the artificial joint loosens or gets infected, it may have to be removed and replaced with a fused joint that does not bend.

Within about eight to 10 weeks after finger-joint replacement, patients regain about two-thirds of their finger's normal range of motion, on average. By that point, patients are able to resume their usual activities—even golf, tennis or gardening, for example. However, recovering patients continue to tape the finger with the new joint to an adjacent finger for additional support whenever they're performing these types of activities, which require a grip and release motion.

For travelers: The devices used in finger-joint replacement are unlikely to set off scanners at airports (or in courtrooms). But just in

*To find a hand surgeon near you, consult the American Society for Surgery of the Hand. ASSH.org.

case, most doctors provide their patients with an X-ray and/or a report indicating that they have had a finger joint replaced.

You Can Have Strong, Pain-Free Hands

Mary Formby, OT, CHT, certified hand therapist at the Curtis National Hand Center at MedStar Union Memorial Hospital in Baltimore. She has practiced hand rehabilitation medicine for more than 25 years and was a contributor to the textbook *Hand and Upper Extremity Rehabilitation*. CurtisHand.com

It's hard to imagine how indispensable your hands are until arthritis limits your ability to use them as you once did. The simplest things, such as turning a doorknob, using a key or opening a jar of pickles, can be intensely painful—or even impossible.

Fortunately, hand exercises can help improve strength and flexibility. Just be sure to do them in moderation—and stop when it hurts!

What most people don't realize: You can make hand exercises more fun by adding a ball, putty and other simple tools to your workouts. You can also do these exercises while you watch TV, so the program can entertain you even if the workout doesn't.

WHO NEEDS TO EXERCISE?

Osteoarthritis ("wear-and-tear" arthritis) and rheumatoid arthritis (an autoimmune disease) can strike any joint in the body, but when the hands are affected, our day-to-day tasks become difficult.

Examples: An inability to grasp small objects (such as dropped coins or earrings)…or lift or carry more than 10 pounds (such as grocery store purchases). The carpometacarpal (CMC) joint in the thumb is often one of the affected joints, particularly in older women. Stiffness and pain of the CMC joint makes any kind of gripping difficult.

Self-test: Hold up your hand with the palm facing you. Can you touch the tip of your thumb to each fingertip…and bring the thumb to the base of the little finger? Also, can you make a fist and touch each fingertip to your palm? If you can't—or if you struggle with any of the activities described above—you might benefit from hand exercises.

HOW TO START

In conventional workouts, people are often advised to do many repetitions for each exercise. This might not be advisable for people with hand pain. High-repetition exercises can strain tendons and cause overuse injuries.

Muscles work and become stronger during both isometric (holding) exercises and repetitive movements, but holding exercises are less stressful to arthritic joints.

Important: The exercises in this article are helpful for a variety of hand symptoms and conditions, but anyone with significant hand limitations should work with an occupational or a physical therapist, preferably with the additional credential of certified hand therapist (CHT). You can find a CHT in your area by going to HTCC.org and clicking on "Find a CHT."

What you will need: For the exercises described below, you will need the following items—a hand therapy ball…a small piece of sponge (about the size of a golf ball) or a cotton ball…a rubber band…and hand therapy putty. Sets that include soft, medium and firm balls or putty are available online for about $12 each. Start with soft!

Stretch first: Before using any resistance, start with a few stretches to maximize your flexibility.

Examples: Stretch your thumb gently away from the side of your hand, then toward the bottom of your little finger…make a full fist…then spread your fingers all the way apart. Repeat on the other hand. Do these stretches a few times each.

READY, SET…GO!

Do each exercise below for 10 seconds (extend the time to 20, then 30 seconds as your hands get stronger). Relax your hands for a few seconds, then repeat. Continue this cycle for a total of about one minute for each exercise on each hand. You can increase the time gradually to up to three minutes. If you can, do each exercise daily.

- **Ball squeezes.** This exercise can increase overall hand strength, but don't overdo it. Squeezing the ball too often—or too hard—can lead to "trigger finger" (stenosing tenosynovitis), in which a finger gets stuck in a bent position. Stop the exercise if it's painful!

What to do: Hold a ball in your palm... squeeze it with your thumb and fingers...then relax. If your hands are weak or painful, be sure to start with a soft ball. As you improve, you can progress to a harder ball or even a tennis ball. Let your hand be your guide for timing the progression.

- **Scissor squeeze.** This exercise strengthens muscles between the fingers (known as intrinsic muscles). It can help to improve grip strength and is unlikely to cause overuse injuries.

What to do: Simply squeeze a piece of sponge or a cotton ball between two fingers. Hold the item between the index and middle finger, then between the middle and ring finger, then between the ring and small finger. Try to keep the little joints of your fingers straight as you do this.

- **Thumb roll.** This simple exercise can increase thumb mobility and improve your ability to grip things.

What to do: Place a ball in the palm of your hand. Using just your thumb, roll the ball from side to side...and in a circular motion.

- **Finger flicks.** The finger muscles are small, so this easy movement does strengthen them.

What to do: Place a ball on a table in front of your loosely closed fist. Flick the ball away from you with the back of each fingertip (by straightening the fingers), and repeat with your other hand. If you're doing it with a partner, he/she can flick it right back. Stop before you get tired. If you are alone, catch the ball with your other hand.

- **Finger spread.** This exercise improves finger range of motion, which helps with holding large objects, etc.

What to do: With your hand held in front of you, place a rubber band around your thumb and all your fingertips. Spread your fingers out to stretch the rubber band...hold...relax... then repeat.

- **Squeeze, roll, spread and pinch.** This exercise combines flexion, extension and "pinch" movements.

What to do: Mold the putty into a ball. Then roll out the putty with your palm into a cylinder. Next shape the putty into a circle on a table. Place your fingertips inside the circle and stretch it out with your thumb/fingers. You can lift the putty off the table to spread your fingers.

Now mold the putty into a ball again and pinch it using a "three-point pinch"—that is, use the tips of your thumb, index and middle fingers. People with hand arthritis should try to limit their use of a "lateral pinch," in which they pinch with the thumb against the side of the index finger (as though holding a key). This type of pinch pattern can irritate the thumb's CMC joint. When possible, use a three-point pinch—it helps to protect the CMC joint.

Got Wrist Pain That Won't Go Away?

Randall W. Culp, MD, orthopedic surgeon at The Philadelphia Hand Center and a professor of orthopedic surgery at the Jefferson Medical College of Thomas Jefferson University, both in Philadelphia. Handcenters.com

Millions of Americans have had hip, knee or shoulder replacements to relieve pain and improve their mobility.

Now: A similar procedure can be done on the wrist, a joint that used to be considered too complex to remove and replace.

With wrist replacement, or arthroplasty, patients can achieve pain relief while retaining more mobility than was possible with earlier procedures.

What you need to know...

A NEW APPROACH

Approximately 27 million American adults suffer from osteoarthritis—a condition that frequently affects the wrist. Millions more have rheumatoid arthritis or osteoporosis, conditions that also can lead to permanent damage to the wrist and other joints.

Until recently, the main surgical treatment for arthritic and damaged wrists was fusion, in which wrist bones are permanently fused to prevent the bones from rubbing together and causing pain. Fusion is very effective at easing pain but, depending on the procedure, allows for little or no joint movement.

Unlike the hip and knee joints, which have only two bones each, the wrists have eight bones—10 if you count those in the forearm. The challenge for manufacturers was to design an artificial joint that gave patients a wide range of movement but also was durable enough to justify the risks and discomfort of surgery.

WHO SHOULD CONSIDER A WRIST REPLACEMENT?

Wrist replacement is a good choice for people whose persistent pain and stiffness interferes with their daily activities, and who have not been helped by medical treatments such as rest, splinting, stretching exercises and/or the use of anti-inflammatory medications.

Important: There isn't enough data to predict how long the new wrist replacements will last. We think they'll last 10 to 15 years—but no one knows for sure.

Because of this, I advise patients—particularly those who are younger and have decades of life ahead of them—to wait as long as they possibly can before having surgery. When a wrist replacement wears out, pain results and a new artificial wrist joint or fusion will be required.

Cost is also a factor. A total wrist replacement costs significantly more than wrist fusion. For this reason, patients with limited or no insurance might decide that the lower cost of a fusion procedure justifies having less wrist mobility.

Exception: If you've already had one wrist fused and need treatment for the other wrist, I always recommend joint replacement. You need at least one mobile wrist for many of the activities of daily living, such as brushing your teeth, buttoning a shirt, etc.

GETTING A WRIST REPLACEMENT

If you're considering a wrist replacement, look for an orthopedic hand surgeon with experience in wrist replacements.*

Wrist replacement is typically a 45-minute outpatient surgery that doesn't require general anesthesia—a nerve block is used to numb the arm.

The surgeon makes a two- to three-inch incision on the back of the wrist and removes the arthritic/damaged joint. The artificial joint, made of plastic and steel, is then inserted. There is a separate component that attaches to the radius, one of the bones in the forearm.

New development: We've found that many younger patients do just as well when they have a hemiarthroplasty, which involves replacing only half of the joint.

Hemiarthroplasty is a less extensive procedure that leaves more of the carpal bones in the wrist in place. This is important because an implant on the carpal bones is more likely to loosen and become unattached from those bones than other parts of the joint.

Unlike hip and knee replacements, arthroplasty usually doesn't use bone cement. The prosthesis has a roughened surface that allows the body's natural bone to grow into and anchor the steel parts, a process known as porous in-growth. It's stronger and more stable than cement.

Long-term complications (after 10 to 15 years), including joint loosening or damage to the components, occur in 2% to 3% of arthroplasty cases. A revision replacement or fusion is required to treat the pain that occurs in these patients.

Postsurgical infection is possible but is no more likely with wrist replacement than with other surgical procedures.

WHAT TO EXPECT AFTER SURGERY

Patients regain, on average, about half of their normal wrist motion, usually within three to four months of wrist-replacement surgery. This range of motion, accompanied by a roughly equal level of fine control, is typically enough to do just about anything you want, including activities such as gardening, golf and

*To find a hand surgeon near you, visit the American Society for Surgery of the Hand at ASSH.org.

tennis. In some cases, patients may regain up to 75% of their normal wrist motion following wrist replacement.

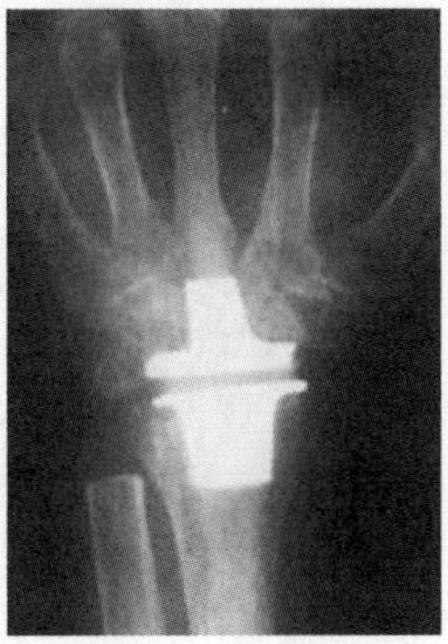

X-ray of a rheumatoid arthritis patient's wrist after wrist replacement.

However, as a precaution, I advise my patients who have undergone wrist replacement not to lift anything heavier than about 10 pounds for the rest of their lives to avoid loosening the joint.

For four weeks following wrist-replacement surgery, a splint or cast is worn to keep the joint stable while it heals.

After that, patients meet regularly with a physical therapist—usually twice weekly for about two to four months—to perform stretching and strengthening exercises.

Caution: Unlike hip and knee replacements, the smaller devices used in wrist replacement may not set off scanners at airports—but we've had reports that they will set off scanners used in other settings, such as in courtrooms. Ask your doctor for a card that explains that you've had the procedure.

Also important: Bacteria can readily proliferate on foreign material in the body, including artificial joints. A lingering infection, even if you don't have symptoms, can loosen the implant.

Be sure to mention to your dentist and all of your doctors that you have an artificial joint. You may be advised to take antibiotics for a few days prior to dental and medical procedures to help avoid infection.

Mystery Wrist Pain Solved

Richard Berger, MD, PhD, hand specialist, department of orthopedic surgery, Mayo Clinic College of Medicine, Rochester, Minnesota.

Imagine suffering, possibly for years, with a chronic pain in your wrist that puzzles every doctor you consult. You have MRIs, which look normal. The pain strikes almost every time you lift or twist your forearm, keeping you from enjoying the things you like to do, and sometimes making it difficult to perform your job. Your wrist is stable, but nothing seems to help the pain. This problem perplexed orthopedist and hand specialist Richard Berger, MD, PhD, of the Mayo Clinic in Rochester, Minnesota, many times over the years, as patients complained about a persistent pain just beneath the palm and on the pinky side of the wrist. When Dr. Berger pressed on the spot, patients would wince, both because it was exactly the site of their pain and because pressing on it hurt terribly.

Dr. Berger described the "aha" insight that helped him solve this puzzle. It occurred when he was looking arthroscopically into a patient's wrist joint while pressing the painful spot externally. Suddenly he realized that he was not looking at the surface of the whole UT (ulnotriquetral) ligament, which runs through this part of the wrist. Instead he saw that the ligament had, in fact, split open lengthwise, though it appeared normal on the surface. This explained why these injured wrists remained stable—the ligament is not torn across, as generally happens with ligament injuries so it continues to hold the bones in place—and is why most MRIs show nothing unusual. This particular form of injury had not previously been identified, so there was no way to treat it. Fortunately, the cure for this painful problem is relatively simple—doctors stitch the ligament together arthroscopically, and patients then spend six weeks in a cast. Dr. Berger said that more than 90% of those on whom he has performed this procedure get relief from their pain.

THE ROOT OF THE INJURY

What causes this type of injury? It can result from a twisting action in sports such as tennis or basketball, when the arm turns in one direction and is impacted by something coming at it from the other. But about half the time there is no obvious precipitating event. Pain that starts as a minor annoyance eventually becomes more and more unbearable. The diagnosis is remarkably simple—if pressing on the wrist in that specific spot creates a sharp pain, it is a sure indicator of the injury.

Information about the split UT ligament and its treatment is just beginning to get out among orthopedic surgeons, says Dr Berger. Consequently, if you suspect it may apply to you, seek a consultation at a large, cutting-edge orthopedic facility that will more likely have some experience with this.

That Shooting Pain in Your Arm Could Be Carpal Tunnel Syndrome

Scott Zashin, MD, certified rheumatologist in private practice, ScottZashinMD.com, and clinical associate professor of medicine at University of Texas Southwestern Medical School in Dallas.

You are driving the car or talking on the phone—and feel aching, tingling, numbness or burning in your thumb, index and middle fingers. You wake up during the night with pain shooting up your arm or down into your palm and fingers. You drop things because of a sudden weakness in your hand or wrist. You may suffer from carpal tunnel syndrome (CTS).

Most people think that CTS is caused only by repetitive hand or wrist movements, including those made by typists, carpenters, people who handle vibrating machinery, such as power tools, or supermarket checkout counter workers. But doctors now know that this painful ailment can have a variety of unexpected causes, which can make diagnosis tricky. About one million Americans are diagnosed annually with the condition.

CTS occurs when the median nerve, which runs down the forearm into the hand, becomes irritated. At the point where it passes through the wrist, this nerve is surrounded by a protective tunnel of bone and ligaments. If this area becomes inflamed or swollen, pressure on the nerve can cause the symptoms mentioned above.

Good news: Once CTS is diagnosed, pain-free hand function can usually be restored through a combination of rest and anti-inflammatory medication. And if that doesn't work, a simple operation probably will.

THE MANY CAUSES OF CTS

Doctors now believe that CTS results from a combination of factors. Jobs or activities involving repetitive hand or wrist movements can help bring it on. But so can sleeping with your wrists bent inward 90 degrees or more (which decreases the size of the carpal tunnel passage). CTS also can result from medical conditions, including rheumatoid arthritis, hypothyroidism (low thyroid activity) and diabetes. Menopause and fluid retention from pregnancy may also give rise to symptoms.

CTS tends to run in families—most likely due to inherited wrist structure. Women are three times as likely as men to develop CTS, probably because their carpal tunnel passages tend to be smaller.

DIAGNOSING CTS

Many primary care doctors diagnose and treat CTS—so first ask your own doctor if he/she can handle your case. If not, your doctor can refer you to either a rheumatologist, neurologist or hand surgeon, all of whom treat CTS. (CTS is considered a neurological condition because it is brought about by impingement of the nerve by the bone and connective tissue.)

Most physicians begin by taking a complete medical history of the patient, which is im-

Help for Carpal Tunnel

Wearing a wrist splint, especially at night, helps decrease tendon swelling and eases the symptoms of carpal tunnel for many people. In some cases, a corticosteroid injection into the carpal tunnel may also provide relief.

Terry R. Light, MD, professor of orthopaedic surgery and rehabilitation, Loyola University Stritch School of Medicine, Maywood, Illinois.

portant since this can determine if the condition is caused by an underlying ailment, such as arthritis or diabetes, or a different kind of nerve impingement. If the patient complains of achiness, tingling, burning or numbness in one hand or pain extending out from one wrist, CTS is strongly suspected—particularly if pain occurs at night, a common symptom. Signs that it is not CTS include symptoms that occur in both hands, which may indicate rheumatoid arthritis or hypothyroidism. In this case, an evaluation for rheumatoid arthritis and thyroid blood test are in order. (Persistent numbness or tingling in the hands can also be a sign of nerve damage due to long-standing diabetes.)

Or, it could be damage to a different nerve, especially if the pinky or non-thumb side of the ring finger is involved (since that is a sign of cubital tunnel syndrome, in which the ulnar nerve, which runs from the collarbone through the inside of the elbow and forearm to the pinky, is entrapped).

Diagnostic tests usually include a physical exam to determine the location of the pain—these may consist of testing the feeling and strength in the fingers and hand…tapping the underside of the wrist…or placing the backs of both hands together. The physician also will want to rule out the possibility of other muscle or nerve disorders, including muscular dystrophy, peripheral neuropathy or nerve lesions (any nerve injury). To do this, he will perform a nerve conduction study, in which a computerized system measures the amount of electricity that is being conducted along the nerve, something a physical exam can't pick up. An underlying nerve disorder will show a reduction in nerve transmission different from that of a compression injury like carpal tunnel syndrome.

Another type of test is an electromyogram, in which small needles are used to measure electrical activity in the muscles of the hand and wrist. If these tests are inconclusive, you may be referred to a neurologist for a complete neuroelectrical exam. Nerve testing is not always accurate and depends on the expertise of the doctor performing the test.

TREATING CTS

When CTS is caused by another condition, such as diabetes or arthritis, treating the condition may alleviate CTS. Treatment might also involve taking pressure off the affected area by resting it, stopping any activities that may contribute to the symptoms and placing the wrist in a splint to hold it in a neutral position, maximizing the space inside the carpal tunnel.

A nonsteroidal anti-inflammatory drug (NSAID), such as *ibuprofen* (Advil, Motrin) or *naproxen* (Aleve, Naprosyn), is typically prescribed as well. (Consult your doctor about how much is safe for you to take.)

Applying a cold pack to the affected area may also help temporarily relieve symptoms. If pain persists, your doctor may suggest injecting the steroid cortisone into the wrist to further reduce inflammation. Alternative treatments, such as acupuncture, have not been clinically proven to be effective.

With these treatments, most people begin feeling better within a week. However, in severe cases, CTS may continue to interfere with daily activities…or pain and numbness may persist for six months or more. A carpal tunnel release operation by a hand surgeon or neurosurgeon may then be required. In this procedure, which is currently performed on about 577,000 Americans annually, the ligament pressing on the median nerve is cut. The procedure may be done laparoscopically, a minimally invasive procedure in which a thin tube containing a camera is inserted through a small incision in the wrist, or it may be done through an open incision at the base of the palm. Both surgeries are performed under local anesthesia, and the patient goes home the same day. Full recovery generally takes six to 12 weeks and may include physical therapy. While a small number of patients report some lingering pain, numbness or weakness, 70% of patients are satisfied with the results of their surgery.

PREVENTING A RECURRENCE

If CTS is caused by an underlying condition, such as diabetes, it's important to keep that condition under control. Some people also need to avoid or modify activities that may have contributed to the symptoms in order to help prevent a recurrence. This may include giving up or cutting back on certain hobbies and activities that put stress on your wrists and hands...and evaluating your position when you use a computer at a desk.

Example: Make sure that your chair and desk are at the right height. Your chair should be adjusted so that your feet are flat on the floor and your elbows are at or above keyboard height when your arms hang naturally. Some people with CTS are helped by a keyboard wrist support that maintains a neutral position for the wrists.

Easy Exercises Relieve Carpal Tunnel

Kelly Jo Wantz, certified hand therapist, Kernan Orthopaedics and Rehabilitation Hospital, Baltimore.

It won't kill you—but when you have carpal tunnel syndrome, the numbness, tingling and/or throbbing pain in your wrist and hand can seriously degrade your life. It can be difficult to work...to pursue sports and hobbies...even to just relax. And common treatments can be frustrating or even risky.

Wearing a wrist guard every night and at least part of the day can be uncomfortable, and the guard can interfere with daily activities, such as typing on a computer. Surgery, another treatment for the condition, helps relieve symptoms but, as with any surgery, has risks, including nerve damage, infection, scarring and loss of wrist function.

Fortunately, you can ease the pain of carpal tunnel syndrome with a few simple stretches, according to Kelly Jo Wantz, a certified hand therapist at the Kernan Orthopaedics and Rehabilitation Hospital in Baltimore. *She told us how to do them...*

WHAT NOT TO DO

First, Wantz explained one reason why we may get carpal tunnel syndrome—and why it hurts so much! The trouble zone, she said, is just below the center of the wrist, a narrow tunnel through which the median nerve and nine tendons connect from the forearm to the hand and fingers. One potential cause is a constant repetitive motion (such as typing, gardening, chopping food and handling tools), which eventually can cause the median nerve and tendons to swell. That makes the tunnel squeeze the nerve and tendons, which causes the discomfort.

Many people assume that exercises to strengthen the wrist will relieve carpal tunnel, Wantz said—in fact, it's the opposite. She explained that squeezing a rubber ball and lifting small weights actually add to the problem by increasing inflammation in the tendons and median nerve.

As an alternative strategy, Wantz and many other therapists get good results from certain specific, light hand stretches. These are safe for almost everyone, but of course, check with your own doctor before trying them.

SOOTHING STRETCHES

Wantz recommends a multipart exercise called tendon gliding, which is designed to ease pressure on the tendons and, therefore, ease pain in the carpal tunnel. You can do this sequence sitting or standing. Do it five times to complete one "set," and do three sets scattered throughout the day every day.

Home position: Hold your arm down straight at your side and, bending your elbow, raise your forearm so your hand is at shoulder height, palm facing out. Spread your thumb from your fingers, but hold your four fingers together, as if indicating "halt!" Hold that position for three seconds. You will return your hand to this "home position" after each of the following exercises.

Claw position: From the home position, curl the middle and upper fingers (the parts of your fingers above your middle knuckles) to their natural touch points on the top of the palm. Hold this position for three seconds and then return to the home position.

Full-fist position: Curl your fingers into a complete, tight fist, keeping your thumb at the side of your index finger. Hold for three seconds, then return to home.

Table-top position: Bend your fingers (not your thumb) only from the lowest knuckles so that the fingers are perpendicular to your palm, creating a "table-top" position. Hold for three seconds, then return to home.

Flat position: Bend the middle and lowest knuckle joints until the tips of your fingers lie flat against the base of your palm. Hold for three seconds, then return to home.

Of course, if these stretches ever cause you any pain, stop doing them and consult with your doctor.

Got Pain in Your Elbow?

Sabrina M. Strickland, MD, orthopedic surgeon and specialist in sports medicine at the Hospital for Special Surgery and assistant professor at Weill Cornell Medical College, both in New York City. She is also chief of orthopedics at the Bronx Veterans Affairs Medical Center in Bronx, New York.

Virtually all adults suffer a bone or joint (orthopedic) injury at some point in their lives. Often complicated by damage to nearby muscles or ligaments, orthopedic complaints, such as tennis elbow, can severely limit movement and sometimes cause excruciating pain.

Although surgery is available to correct most orthopedic injuries, about 80% of cases can be treated with appropriate home care, such as rest, anti-inflammatory drugs and applications of ice and/or heat.

Best treatments for the most common orthopedic complaint, tennis elbow...

About 90% of patients who get tennis elbow (lateral epicondylitis) do not play tennis. The condition is caused by overuse of the extensor tendon, which runs from the wrist to the elbow. People who flex the wrist repeatedly—from prolonged hammering or painting, for example, or from poor tennis form—are at greatest risk.

Symptoms: Pain that radiates from the elbow to the forearm and/or wrist...pain when bending the wrist...or tenderness on the outside of the elbow.

Texting Can Be Dangerous to Your Hands, Arms and More...

Carpal tunnel... Texting and tapping damage nerves in your hands and arms. Overuse of your cell phone, tablet or gaming device may result in carpal tunnel syndrome (damage to the median nerve in the hand). A recent study found that 45.5% of those who used these devices five or more hours daily suffered pain, tingling and potential damage to the hand and wrist due to the repetitive and often awkward finger and wrist movements required. But even less intensive use may lead to musculoskeletal discomfort in different regions, such as the neck and shoulders. It's worse for those who use multiple devices or operate their phone with just one hand.

Peter White, PhD, department of health technology and informatics, The Hong Kong Polytechnic University, Kowloon.

Thumb pain... Handheld electronics may cause thumb pain. Typing on iPads and cell phones can cause painful swelling of the thumb.

Self-defense: When typing, use a pencil eraser or a plug-in keyboard that has larger buttons. Take breaks from typing, and rest arms on a cushion for support while typing.

Alan Hedge, director, Human Factors and Ergonomics Research Group, Cornell University, Ithaca, New York.

Medical experts used to think that tennis elbow was mainly due to inflammation.

Finding: The real problem is a condition in the cells of the tendon, known as tendinosis, in which wear and tear is thought to cause degeneration of the tendon. Experimental treatments, such as injecting platelet-rich plasma, are meant to promote tissue repair rather than fight inflammation.

Main treatment: About 90% of people with tennis elbow recover with rest and the use of ice. Also, patients should use a counterforce brace, which limits stress on the proximal part of the tendon (near the elbow). Avoid painful activities for two weeks, then gradually resume them with use of the brace.

Helpful: An exercise that lengthens the muscle and accelerates healing.

What to do: While keeping the wrist straight, hold a hammer in the hand of the affected arm. With the palm facing down, slowly bend the wrist downward. At the bottom of the movement, switch the hammer to the other hand to avoid lifting the weight with your bad arm. Repeat eight to 10 times, a few times a day.

Surgical option: Fewer than 10% of patients with tennis elbow will require surgery. The goal is to remove dead tissue from the area to encourage the formation of new blood vessels and healthy tissue.

Patients typically are able to resume most activities in four to six weeks, and to resume tennis and other sports in four to six months. In rare cases, nerve and/or ligament damage may occur.

Cupping Eases Pain

Andreas Michalsen, MD, professor of medicine, Charité Medical University, Berlin, Germany, and leader of a study of 52 people.

Among carpal tunnel patients, those who underwent cupping on the neck and shoulders reported significantly more improvement than those treated with heating pads.

Theory: Cupping stimulates blood and lymph flow, improving nerve function.

Referrals to practitioners: American Association of Acupuncture and Oriental Medicine, 866-455-7999, AAAOMonline.org.

Hope for Sore Arms: Platelet Treatment May Be Easy Fix For Tendon Pain

Allan Mishra, MD, orthopedic surgeon at Menlo Medical Clinicat Stanford University Medical Center, Menlo Park, California. ApexPRP.com

Tennis elbow is an especially stubborn condition and an extremely painful one. For the most part, tennis elbow goes away after a few months (with or without treatment), but for some people the problem recurs and can become chronic. Treatment has traditionally consisted of rest, non-steroidal anti-inflammatory drugs (NSAIDs) such as Advil or Motrin, wearing a brace, and physical therapy—with corticosteroid injections as a last non-surgical resort. If all else fails, patients can have surgery to repair the damaged tendon, though surgery is not always successful. Tennis elbow can now be successfully treated with platelet-rich plasma, a component of a patient's own blood.

WHAT PLATELET TREATMENT IS

This remarkably simple approach may someday become the treatment of choice. Platelet-rich plasma has been used to augment bone grafting during oral and maxillofacial surgery. A recent study involved 20 patients with severe tennis elbow, none of whom had improved with extensive and prolonged non-surgical treatment. These patients had suffered from tennis elbow for about 15 months and judged their pain as "severe" (a mean score of 82 on a scale of 100 as maximum pain).

For the study, blood was taken from each of the patients, 15 who later were injected with platelets derived from their own blood donation, which was spun in the lab to isolate platelets. The platelet-rich plasma contained a concentration of their own platelets suspended in plasma. The remaining five received an anesthetic injection. To encourage absorption of the platelets, each tendon was injected six times with a total of one-half teaspoon of protein-rich plasma directly at that site, allowing the platelets to seep in. The entire procedure takes about half an hour. Afterward, patients were required to rest through the following day and then to start a stretching program. Two weeks later, they started a program to strengthen the arm. All patients were tested at four and eight weeks and again at six months. At eight weeks after the initial injection, the patients treated with the platelet preparation reported a 60% reduction in their pain compared with a 16% reduction in the control group. This reduction was statistically significant. Improvement continued in the platelet group. When these patients were evaluated at six months, they had approximately 81% less pain. Two years later, most of these patients reported complete satisfaction, all having returned to normal daily activities, with 94% once again active in work or sports.

WHY DOES IT WORK?

There are two possible reasons why this treatment works. First, the platelets are rich in growth factors that help trigger the healing process. The platelets do not, however, contain enough of these factors to boost or speed healing as quickly as platelet-rich plasma, but theories include that the process works because the growth factors signal the need to bring new repair to the area. A few days following the platelet injection, some patients reported that the surrounding area became warm and swollen, which means that the body may have circulated bone-marrow derived stem cells there...facilitating on-going repair. Adding credibility to that theory, these patients did not experience any worsening of their symptoms. Since this procedure uses their own blood, rejection is not an issue and there have been no serious side effects reported. Nevertheles, the procedure is still experimental and in limited use, so discuss with your doctor current availability.

Making Injections Less Painful

Lindsay Uman, PhD, clinical psychologist at the IWK Health Centre in Halifax, Nova Scotia.

Fear of needles is not unique to childhood—it's estimated that 21% of Americans are terrified of them. For many people, needle fear leads to health problems as they avoid routine blood tests and vaccinations, and for those with diabetes or another chronic condition requiring regular injections, needle anxiety can turn into a nightmare.

Less Ouch!

Research now confirms that your mother was right. Watching an injection does make pain more intense. What's a good way to reduce the pain? Look away!

Pain.

THE WORST THINGS TO SAY

Not surprisingly, techniques to ease needle fear in adults are similar to those for children.

Here's the funny thing: Studies show that most well-meaning nurses, doctors and phlebotomists actually have a habit of saying just the wrong thing to nervous patients. Their intentions are the best, but the results are not.

Their first mistake? The very human impulse to be reassuring. If someone keeps saying there is nothing to worry about, the message generally received is that there is something you really do need to worry about.

The second-worst mistake? Criticizing patients' fear by telling them to "Get a grip," "Get over it" or "Don't be a baby"—belittling messages that would make anyone feel worse.

The third kind of phrase often heard but best not uttered? A "pre-apology," such as saying "Sorry about this," as the elastic strap is wound tightly around the arm. This only brings more fear and distress.

WHAT DOES HELP

If you have ever felt weak or silly because you couldn't talk yourself out of the fear of needles, give yourself a break—as with most fears, this one isn't rational, so you can't expect rational talk (from yourself or anyone else) to help. *Instead, you can try the following...*

- **Distraction.** This is number one in effectiveness and can include anything from blowing bubbles for young children to putting on headphones and playing music for adults. Chatting about the weather or the latest news...even making up stories about people around you and saying them aloud if you enjoy being creative...talking about anything but the needle will be helpful.

• **Relaxation techniques.** These can help, especially when practiced shortly before the procedure—calm breathing, positive imagery, a few minutes of meditation, whatever relaxes a nervous patient is the way to go. Not only do techniques for relaxing the mind ease fear—they also reduce muscle tension that could otherwise make shots more painful.

• **Skin-numbing creams.** A product called EMLA, available by prescription, combines the anesthetics lidocaine and prilocaine and will numb the area, but for best results, you need to apply the cream 30 to 60 minutes in advance. For some people, using the cream provides a calming psychological effect that comes just from knowing that the physical pain will be reduced.

If your fear of needles continues to be a problem, consider talking with a cognitive behavioral therapist or any psychologist trained in anxiety-reducing techniques—these professionals likely can help you. Ask your doctor or local hospital for a referral. For some people, it takes only a few sessions for a patient to put needle fear into the past.

Should You Ease the Pain of a Shot...or Not?

Sergei Frenzel, ND, MD, naturopathic doctor in private practice, Milford, Connecticut.

Is it OK to take an over-the-counter pain reliever to minimize the discomfort of a vaccination shot?

Not really—and here's why. The purpose of vaccination is to create an immune reaction...and that includes inflammation. Pain is a natural consequence of inflammation. If you try to reduce the pain and inflammation, whether with a pain-relieving drug or with ice, it may decrease the effectiveness of the vaccination, research suggests. For instance, in a study published in *The Lancet,* babies who received *acetaminophen* (Tylenol) after their injections produced significantly fewer antibodies against the diseases for which they had been vaccinated than babies who were not given the pain reliever. It makes sense that this same effect might apply to adults.

Think of it this way—pain actually is a good sign that your body is reacting to the vaccine the way you want it to. The discomfort should go away within about 10 hours. If it has been more than a day and your arm is still very sore, alert the doctor who prescribed the injection. You may need to be evaluated to make sure there are no other forces at play.

CHAPTER 11

Headaches

Headaches That Stump Doctors and How to Finally Get Relief

When you are in the throes of a headache, you do not care what is causing the pain. You just want relief. But not all headaches or migraines respond to the same treatment—and the wrong approach can keep you locked in your misery or even worsen the pain.

Should you take a migraine pill or a powerful pain reliever? Or would it be better to lie down in a cool, dark room or even go for a run? The answer depends on what is really causing your headache.

The problem is, there are more than 300 different causes of headaches, and just over half of people who have severe headaches are properly diagnosed.

What makes a difference: The more you know about symptoms associated with different types of headaches, the better equipped you'll be to help your doctor pinpoint the underlying cause of your pain. Unusual symptoms, which often occur with headaches, are easily misinterpreted.

THE HEADACHE MYSTERY

Surprisingly, these common types of headaches can be difficult for some doctors to diagnose. *For example...*

- **Migraine with aura.** The main symptom is throbbing or pounding head pain that occurs during or shortly after an aura (visual disturbances such as blurred vision...white, black or colored dots...flashing light...or blind spots). Nausea and, less frequently, vomiting may also occur. Severe migraines may develop without an aura, too.

Alan M. Rapoport, MD, clinical professor of neurology at The David Geffen School of Medicine at the University of California in Los Angeles and president of the International Headache Society.

Symptoms that can be misdiagnosed: Numbness or tingling or even weakness on one side of the face or body and/or speech difficulties—all of which may be misdiagnosed as stroke—and increased sensitivity to touch (called allodynia) can be symptoms of migraine with aura. So can dizziness, a runny nose or tearing eyes.

Important: Most "sinus" headaches are really migraines.

Best treatment: Most individuals diagnosed with migraine are aware of lifestyle changes that can help—this includes avoiding triggers such as caffeine, certain odors and the artificial sweetener aspartame...eating a healthful diet...and exercising regularly. Most important, do not miss or delay meals—this commonly triggers migraines.

Medication also may be needed but should be taken promptly for the best results. For example, if a triptan migraine drug, such as *sumatriptan* (Imitrex), or similar medication is prescribed, be sure to take it within the first 60 minutes of the migraine (the sooner, the better).

Supplements, including vitamin B-2, magnesium and coenzyme Q10, may be taken daily as a preventive. They may help by increasing energy in the nerve cells.

- **Episodic cluster headache.** Unlike most headaches, cluster headaches strike more men than women, with excruciating and sudden daily headaches one to three times per day, always on one side of the head, in or around an eye. The headaches can last from 15 minutes to three hours and often persist for one to three months, about once a year.

While a migraine sufferer's pain may improve when relaxing in a cool, dark room, a cluster headache patient may get some relief from walking or even running.

Symptoms that can be misdiagnosed: Doctors may misdiagnose cluster headaches as sinusitis or a tooth problem because the pain extends to the sinuses, upper teeth, back of the head or even the neck.

Best treatment: To treat cluster headaches, steroid pills may be taken daily for a week or two. An injection of sumatriptan may be given for each headache. Nasal spray triptans such as *zolmitriptan* (Zomig) also may be tried, and breathing pure oxygen via a mask may help. If cluster headaches persist, the calcium channel blocker *verapamil* (Verelan) is usually prescribed. If these therapies fail, patients may need a nerve block—an injection of anesthetics and steroids in the occipital nerve, which immediately numbs the pain. A tiny electrical device also can be implanted to stimulate the nerve.

- **Episodic tension-type headache.** Most adults get these headaches occasionally. They cause squeezing or pressing (nonthrobbing) pain, often on both sides of the head. Stress is the usual trigger. Muscles in the back of the neck and scalp tighten, which may cause headache pain.

Symptoms that can be misdiagnosed: Some tension-type headaches are so severe that they are misdiagnosed as migraines, and patients are prescribed migraine medication that is not always helpful.

Best treatment: Most people with tension-type headaches get some relief from over-the-counter drugs, such as aspirin, *naproxen* (Aleve) or *acetaminophen* (Tylenol). There are two other effective but underused treatments—removing yourself from the stressful situation and getting any kind of aerobic exercise.

GETTING THE HELP YOU NEED

To properly diagnose your headaches, your physician should review your medical history and your family's medical history, conduct a physical examination and rule out other possible causes of head pain, such as an aneurysm or a congenital malformation. Be sure that you thoroughly describe your symptoms to your doctor.

What helps most: Keeping a headache diary, either in a notebook or on a computer or tablet, is crucial to getting the right diagnosis. This diary should include such information as the time of day your headaches occur...the specific location and type of pain (for example, throbbing, pressing or piercing)...other symptoms (such as nausea, light sensitivity or dizziness)...food you ate before the headache...and activities before the headache developed. There are several headache diary templates available online, such as MigraineTrust.org/living-with-migraine/coping-managing/keeping-a-migraine-diary.

If you don't get relief after working with your physician for a few months, consider consulting a headache specialist or neurologist. Board-certified headache specialists are the best qualified to treat headaches. To find one near you, consult ProMyHealth.org.

Is It a Migraine, Low Blood Sugar, a Seizure... Or a Stroke?

Edward Jauch, MD, professor and director, division of emergency medicine, professor, department of neurosciences, comprehensive stroke program, and director, acute stroke trials, Medical University of South Carolina, Charleston.

They're called stroke mimics. The symptoms are similar to a stroke—slurred speech, a weakness on one side of your body and confusion—but what you're experiencing is actually low blood sugar, a migraine or another condition. If you know you have diabetes, suffer from migraines, have a seizure disorder or other conditions, you may be tempted to ignore possible stroke symptoms.

That's a big mistake.

Reason: When you're having a stroke, minutes—even seconds—count. Getting emergency treatment with blood clot–dissolving medications—typically tissue plasminogen activator (tPA)—or other therapies can mean the difference between life and death and can dramatically affect recovery. To learn more about stroke mimics, we spoke with Edward Jauch, MD, director of the division of emergency medicine at the Medical University of South Carolina.

MIMIC #1: **Low Blood Sugar (Hypoglycemia).** When blood sugar dips too low, a common problem for people who take medication for diabetes, the symptoms mimic a stroke—confusion, feeling dizzy or light-headed, slurred speech and/or muscle weakness.

Clues that it may be hypoglycemia, not stroke: Symptoms may build up slowly, rather than occur suddenly, as they do with a stroke. If you do a finger prick and discover your blood sugar is low, and if symptoms resolve after eating a glucose tablet or drinking a half cup of fruit juice, it's likely not a stroke.

But if you have any doubts, call 911. Be sure to tell the EMS professionals that the patient is a diabetic so they can rule out hypoglycemia with a finger-prick test—and maybe save a trip to the ER. It's actually standard practice to test everyone's glucose right away, whether or not they have diabetes, but it's not always followed, says Dr. Jauch.

MIMIC #2: **Hemiplegic Migraine.** You may remember when the newscaster Serene Branson frighteningly lost her speech during a live broadcast, and everyone thought she had had a stroke. Well, it turned out to be a hemiplegic migraine. This type of migraine can cause loss of speech, weakness and other strokelike symptoms.

Clues that it may be a migraine, not a stroke...

- **You know you get migraines,** the pain is familiar, and an aura precedes the symptoms.
- **The headache comes on gradually,** over several minutes or longer, intensifies to a peak and tends to be throbbing or a dull ache.
- **You have known triggers such as stress,** caffeine, foods, weather changes, etc.
- **You have visual disturbances such as seeing flashing lights or wavy lines.**

Signs that it may be a stroke, not a migraine...

- **You're older than 50, and you've never had a migraine.** Migraines don't tend to develop after age 50.
- **The headache comes on suddenly and is the worst headache of your life.**
- **You have visual disturbances that involve loss of part of your visual field**—you may bump into things because you don't see them, for example.

As always, when in doubt, call 911. It's particularly important for people who get migraines frequently to pay attention to possible stroke symptoms. "There's a small increased risk for stroke in people who have migraines, but we are still researching if treatment of a migraine reduces stroke risk," says Dr. Jauch.

MIMIC #3: **A Seizure.** Some seizures leave people with neurological symptoms such as difficulty speaking or a weakness in one or more limbs often on one side of the body, known as Todd's paralysis. "When you have a seizure, your brain turns off, just like when you shut down a computer," Dr. Jauch explains. "When you turn the computer back on, it takes a while to boot up. Your brain, too, may take some time to get back to normal."

Clues that it may be a seizure…

- **The patient has a history of seizures, a bite mark on the side of the tongue**—or confusion that gradually improves.
- **Typically symptoms subside with time… from a few minutes to a few hours.**

Clues that it may be a stroke: If there is confusion, it is persistent and doesn't improve.

If you're concerned that it's a stroke, time isn't on your side. EMS guidelines state that the ER team should consider stroke if someone has a seizure and has symptoms of neurological deficits, such as weakness, numbness or language issues, particularly if the patient doesn't have a history of seizures. Sometimes, seizures are symptoms of a stroke.

MIMIC #4: **Bell's Palsy.** Bell's palsy causes facial drooping, but it's not because of a stroke. It's typically caused by a viral infection such as shingles or the flu or Lyme disease that leads to an inflammation or infection in the facial nerve (called the seventh cranial nerve). It can also cause your eyelid to droop, drooling, dryness of the eye or mouth or excessive tearing in one eye. Though this is easy for the pros to diagnose, patients often confuse it with a stroke.

Clues that it may be Bell's palsy…

- **It typically causes significant facial distortion including the forehead.** Facial symptoms are your only symptoms.

Clues that it may be a stroke…

- **You're older than 60,** when Bell's palsy becomes less common.
- **You have other stroke symptoms,** not just facial droop.

Not sure? You know what to do—call 911.

MIMIC #5: **A Brain Tumor.** Brain tumors can also cause symptoms that mimic stroke, such as headache, confusion, nausea, weakness and disturbance in the way you walk.

Clues that it's a brain tumor rather than a stroke: Symptoms are headaches that are worse in the morning, when coughing, exercising or changing position.

Both are serious ailments, of course, so these symptoms, whatever the cause, require immediate attention. For any of these unexplained symptoms, you would likely be given a CT scan, which would pick up the tumor versus signs of a stroke.

WHAT HAPPENS IF I THINK IT'S A STROKE AND IT'S NOT?

Stroke mimics confuse even health-care professionals. In one study, about 20% of the time when neurologists thought patients were having a stroke, the cause was a different condition. The result can be getting a CT scan and treatment when it's not needed, with all the anxiety that entails. But the risk for harm is much lower than having a stroke and not getting it promptly treated.

Here's what you can do: Help health-care professionals by giving them the right information. Let them know if the symptoms came on suddenly (common in strokes) or more gradually (uncommon), and let them know when the symptoms began or when the person was last known to be normal. If the patient has diabetes or is subject to frequent migraines

Pure Oxygen for Cluster Headaches

Pure oxygen may relieve cluster headaches. Delivered with a face mask, 100% oxygen may relieve a painful cluster headache in 15 to 30 minutes. Oxygen treatment, when available, is inexpensive and better than drugs such as triptans, which have side effects. But oxygen does not prevent cluster headaches—it only stops them once they start—and it has no effect on other forms of headache such as migraines.

Mayo Clinic Health Letter.

or has a seizure disorder, tell the EMS professionals right away. Also let them know if the person takes any form of regular medications. It'll help them sort things out quicker.

HOW TO SPEED UP STROKE TREATMENT

Everyone should know the classic signs of a stroke, made easy to remember with the acronym FAST...

- **Face drooping.** One side of the face may droop or become numb. Ask the person to smile, and check to see if the smile is uneven.
- **Arm weakness.** One arm only may be weak or numb. Ask the person to raise both arms, and check to see if one arm drifts downward.
- **Speech problems.** Speech may be slurred, or the person may have trouble speaking or being understood. Ask the person to repeat a simple sentence, such as "The sun is shining."
- **Time,** as in, act quickly! If you think you or someone you're with is having a stroke, call 911 immediately. If you use the ambulance, you will get to the hospital faster, you see a doctor faster, you get a CT scan faster, you're more likely to get tPA, and you're more likely to get it faster. After calling 911, check the time so that the first responders know when symptoms started. When the ambulance arrives—and again when you get to the ER—say the word "stroke" if you think that's what you or the patient is having. Don't just say, "My arm is numb" or "I'm dizzy." The sooner someone says, "I think I'm having a stroke," the sooner health-care providers can start the proven system called the "Stroke Chain of Survival."

Aimovig Gets FDA Nod as a Migraine Preventive Drug

The news release "FDA Approves Novel Preventive Treatment for Migraine," May 17, 2018.

As every migraine sufferer knows all too well, when that granddaddy of all headaches strikes, you can be laid up for days with throbbing head pain, nausea and/or vomiting and sensitivity to light and sound.

A new way to stop it: The FDA has approved a new once-monthly injectable drug, *erenumab-aooe* (Aimovig), that helps reduce the number of days that migraineurs are affected by these debilitating headaches.

Even though medical experts still have not determined exactly what causes migraines, they have recently discovered that the levels of a molecule called calcitonin gene-related peptide (CGRP) rise in brain cells during migraine pain. Aimovig is the first drug that works by blocking the activity of CGRP.

Scientific evidence: To test the new treatment, three clinical trials, including 955 patients with different types of migraine, were conducted. Two of the trials enrolled people with episodic migraine (four to 14 headache days per month). Patients in the first study who used Aimovig over a six-month period reported one to two fewer monthly migraine days, on average, than those who received a placebo. Patients in the second study, which

What Is a Migraine?

A migraine headache is a cascade of electrical, chemical and inflammation-related blood vessel changes that occur in the brain, typically in distinct stages, but they can overlap...

- **Prodrome.** The warning stage. You may feel "off," irritable or moody...have amplified senses, such as a heightened sense of smell...and crave certain foods, such as sweets.
- **Aura.** Usually occurring five to 60 minutes before an attack, it involves visual disturbances such as flashing lights, zigzag lines or blind spots.
- **Headache.** Pain, mild to severe, often described as intense pounding or pressure, usually on one side of the head.
- **Postdrome.** The recovery period. You may feel fatigued over the next few hours or days.

Morris Levin, MD, chief of the Division of Headache Medicine and director of the Headache Center at UCSF Medical Center in San Francisco.

lasted three months, reported an average of one fewer migraine day per month than those in the placebo group. Put another way, that's 24 to 48 fewer hours per month without headache pain.

The third study enrolled patients with chronic migraine (15 or more headache days per month for three or more months). Over a three-month period, the Aimovig users reported an average of two-and-one-half fewer monthly migraine days than those who used a placebo. That's 60 fewer hours per month without headache pain.

Eric Bastings, MD, deputy director of the Division of Neurology Products in the FDA's Center for Drug Evaluation and Research, called the medication a "novel option" to help minimize the suffering caused by migraines. "We need new treatments for this painful and often debilitating condition."

Migraines are most commonly treated with over-the-counter (OTC) and prescription-strength pain relievers...a class of medications known as triptans...antinausea drugs...and, in some cases, injections of the well-known wrinkle treatment Botox, which was FDA-approved for chronic migraines in 2010. The effectiveness of these medications varies depending on the patient.

The Aimovig injection can be self-administered. The most common side effects reported by patients in the clinical trials were constipation, along with pain, redness, itching, tenderness or bruising at the injection site.

Important: Be sure to check with your insurer about coverage for Aimovig. Due to its high cost, insurers may require migraine patients to try other less expensive generic drugs before approving coverage for Aimovig.

Also: Check with your doctor and pharmacist about potential side effects and interactions with other medicines.

Nondrug approaches can also help to control migraine symptoms. Read the following articles for natural relief.

Women: How to Relieve Migraine Pain

Alan M. Rapoport, MD, clinical professor of neurology at the David Geffen School of Medicine, University of California, Los Angeles. Founder and director emeritus of The New England Center for Headache in Stamford, Connecticut, he has coauthored nine books on headache, including *Conquering Daily Headache.*

Three times as many women as men suffer from migraine. The culprit may be women's fluctuating levels of the hormone estrogen.

There are about 36 million migraineurs in the US, including 18% of all female teens and adults. Many remain undiagnosed or undertreated—even though migraine can cause unbearable pain.

Good news: There is a lot you can do to halt or alleviate migraine headaches and perhaps even prevent them altogether.

WHAT IS MIGRAINE?

Research suggests that migraine involves an electrical phenomenon in the cortex of the brain...dysfunction in the brain stem... inflammation around and dilation of blood vessels in membranes that cover the brain...increases of the brain chemical calcitonin gene-related peptide (CGRP)...and/or decreases in the brain chemical serotonin.

A migraine attack causes severe throbbing pain, often on one side of the head or behind one eye...nausea and vomiting...and/or sensitivity to light, sound and smells. Movement can intensify pain.

About half of all migraine headaches are preceded by several hours by a prodrome (early warning), consisting of irritability, depression, fatigue, yawning, food cravings and/or increased or decreased urination. Up to one-third of migraine attacks are immediately preceded by a 20-to-30-minute visual aura—colored dots, zigzag lines, flashing lights or blind spots in the visual field—sometimes accompanied by speech problems and tingling or weakness on one side of the body. (If you have no history of aura but suddenly develop any of these symptoms, seek medical help—it could be a stroke.)

If not effectively treated, migraine attacks last, on average, 12 to 48 hours. They typically occur one to three times per month—often around the time of a woman's period—but can occur almost daily.

If your migraine attacks are not responding to whatever treatment you currently use, see your doctor. If he/she cannot help, ask to be referred to a neurologist or headache specialist for an exam, blood tests and/or imaging tests (such as a CT or MRI scan) of the brain. This should lead to an accurate diagnosis and the most effective treatment possible.

NONDRUG PREVENTION STRATEGIES

To reduce migraine frequency...

• **Avoid triggers.** Keep a headache log to identify substances and situations that bring on your migraine attacks. Common triggers include alcohol, chocolate, cured meats and aged cheeses...caffeine (or caffeine withdrawal)...stress...high altitude...bright sun and flickering lights.

• **Stick to a schedule.** Going too long without eating can bring on a migraine attack, as can getting too little or too much sleep. Eat four or five small, low-sugar meals daily, spread evenly throughout the day...maintain consistent bedtimes and waking times.

• **Reduce stress.** Get moderate exercise daily...make time for activities you enjoy...use relaxation techniques, such as meditation and deep breathing. Try biofeedback—during a session, you wear sensors on your head and/or hands...and a monitor provides visual and auditory feedback on muscle activity and hand temperature, so you know when you're succeeding in relaxing.

• **Try nutritional supplements.** Some evidence suggests that supplementation helps prevent migraine. With your doctor's approval, try one or any combination of the following—magnesium salts at 400 mg daily...vitamin B-2 (riboflavin) at 400 mg daily...the herb butterbur at 50 mg three times daily (for purity, I recommend the Petadolex brand)...coenzyme Q10 (CoQ10) at 300 mg daily...and one hour before bedtime, the hormone melatonin at 3 mg nightly.

• **Consider complementary therapies.** Although I have seen little proof of effectiveness in literature, many people say they get migraine relief from acupuncture, massage or physical therapy...a dental appliance that minimizes nighttime jaw clenching (see page 269)...and/or cervical spine manipulation by a chiropractor. I tell my patients that they can use any therapies they find helpful (though I advise against sudden chiropractic manipulation of the neck for patients over age 35).

MEDICATIONS FOR MIGRAINE

When an attack begins, you have less than 90 minutes in which to halt it with drugs—so take medication as soon as you sense an impending attack. Limit use to two days per week—overuse can cause rebound headaches. To ease the pain until medication takes effect, apply cold compresses. *Medications to try...*

• **Nonprescription pain relievers.** Some migraineurs respond to over-the-counter (OTC) products. Taking them as directed on the label and with lots of water, use trial and error to see if any of these work for you—aspirin, *ibuprofen* (Advil), *naproxen* (Aleve)...or *acetaminophen*, either alone (Tylenol) or combined with caffeine (Excedrin Migraine).

• **Prescription drugs.** If OTC drugs don't work, you may need something stronger. *Your doctor will use trial and error to discover which of the following works best for you...*

• A triptan. Fast-acting oral triptans include *sumatriptan* (Imitrex), *zolmitriptan* (Zomig), *rizatriptan* (Maxalt), *almotriptan* (Axert) and eletriptan (Relpax). Two other triptans—*naratriptan* (Amerge) and *frovatriptan* (Frova)—take longer to work but last longer. Side effects of all triptans include tiredness, dizziness and a warm sensation.

Some triptans can be given by nasal spray or injection. These bypass the digestive system, making them more appropriate than oral drugs for migraine patients who suffer from nausea and vomiting.

• *Dihydroergotamine* (DHE) nasal spray (Migranal) or injections (DHE 45). DHE should not be taken within 24 hours of using a triptan.

Caution: Because triptans and DHE constrict blood vessels, they should not be used if you have vascular or heart disease, high blood pressure or a history of stroke...and should be used only under medical supervision if you have cardiac risk factors, such as smoking, obesity, high cholesterol, diabetes or a family history of early heart disease.

- **Daily preventive medication.** Consider this if you have more than three attacks monthly or severe attacks that do not respond to triptans or DHE. Options include cardiac medications called beta-blockers, such as *propranolol* (Inderal) or *timolol* (Blocadren)...or the antiseizure drugs *divalproex* (Depakote) or *topiramate* (Topamax). A doctor must monitor use.

- **Monthly preventive medication.** For menstrual migraine, for three days before your period, take OTC naproxen at one tablet three times daily...or long-acting prescription frovatriptan twice daily.

Alternative: Ask your gynecologist about using an estrogen patch (Estraderm) for three to five days before your period.

Good news: After menopause, migraine attacks usually diminish.

BOTOX FOR MIGRAINE

When other treatments fail, some doctors offer injections of prescription *Botulinim toxin* (Botox). This use of Botox is "off label"—meaning it is legal but the drug has not been FDA-approved for this purpose. Since the therapy is considered experimental, insurance generally does not cover it. If a clinical trial, now in its final stage, shows Botox to be effective against migraine, it may earn FDA approval within a few years.

Some evidence suggests that multiple Botox injections in the head and/or neck can reduce the severity and frequency of migraine attacks for three to four months by decreasing the release of certain chemicals from nerve endings. Cost varies widely, from $700 to $2,000 or more.

Sex Can Ease Migraine Pain

James R. Couch, MD, PhD, professor and former chair of neurology, University of Oklahoma Health Sciences Center, Oklahoma City, and leader of a study of 82 women with migraines, published in *Headache: The Journal of Head and Face Pain.*

Women who have sex when they feel a migraine coming on experience less head and neck pain, fatigue and moodiness. Nearly one-third of women who had sex at the start of a migraine reported reduced symptoms...and for 12%, sex stopped the migraine completely.

Possible reason: Sex and orgasm boost levels of the pleasure hormone serotonin—which is known to be low in migraine sufferers.

Subtle Signals Hold Clues to Prevent Migraines

Peter Goadsby, MD, PhD, researcher, director, Headache Center, University of California, San Francisco. His study was published in *Neurology.*

Many migraine patients experience a common pool of symptoms during the premonitory phase—several hours to several days before a migraine headache actually begins. Some of these warning signals actually have nothing to do with head pain. That can mean neck discomfort, unusual tiredness, yawning, changes in appetite, excessive urinating or thirst, craving something sweet or savory, or mood changes, such as feeling unusually cranky or anxious. In fact, it's all pretty primitive symptomatology from a brain perspective. And it's there if you know what to look for!

In our study, 97 migraine sufferers recorded their nonheadache symptoms on electronic diaries for three months and noted when migraines struck. Patients were able to correctly predict the onset of full-blown headaches from premonitory symptoms in 72% of diary entries. The most common of these symptoms were fatigue (experienced by 72%), difficulty concentrating (51%) and stiff neck (50%).

Links to Migraine Headaches

Chewing gum... Gum-chewing teens may be giving themselves migraines by stressing the TMJ joint, a common cause of headaches.

A recent study showed that headaches disappeared entirely in 19 of 30 teens who gave up chewing gum for a month.

Tel Aviv University.

Lightbulbs... Energy-saving lightbulbs might trigger migraines and epileptic seizures. Fluorescent low-energy lightbulbs have a high rate of "flicker" that normally is not noticeable. But the British Migraine Action Association says that the flicker may trigger migraine headaches, and the organization Epilepsy Action reports that the bulbs apparently have triggered seizures in a small number of epilepsy sufferers. If you or any family member suffers from these conditions, consult your doctor before installing such bulbs.

Karen Manning, spokesperson, Migraine Action Association, Great Oakley, Northamptonshire, England. Migraine.org.uk

Child abuse... When researchers studied 1,348 migraine sufferers, 58% reported emotional, physical or sexual abuse in childhood—a substantially higher percentage than in the general population.

Theory: Excessive childhood stress may permanently change the brain's response to stress, contributing to migraines.

If you have migraines: Inform your doctor of any adverse childhood events. This will help him/her identify strategies, such as cognitive behavioral therapy, to reduce stress that may trigger migraines.

Gretchen E. Tietjen, MD, professor and chair, neurology department, University of Toledo College of Medicine, Ohio.

Lightning... Chronic headache sufferers had a 31% higher risk for headaches when lightning struck within 25 miles of their homes—and migraine sufferers had a 28% higher risk for migraines.

Reason: Possibly related to lightning's electromagnetic waves.

Study of 90 people led by researchers at University of Cincinnati College of Medicine, published in *Cephalalgia*.

Anxiety... Generalized anxiety disorder (persistent and excessive worry) is three times more likely to occur among migraine sufferers than those who don't get migraines, according to a study of more than 21,000 adults.

Interesting detail: Men with migraines were twice as likely to have anxiety disorder as women with migraines—possibly because men are less likely to take migraine medication and may have less emotional support.

Esme Fuller-Thomson, PhD, Sandra Rotman chair in social work, University of Toronto, Ontario, Canada.

Yawning, which occurred in about one-quarter of the headache sufferers, was a whopping 96% predictive of migraines.

Premonitory symptoms reported in the study: Feeling tired or weary, dizziness, lots of energy or hyperactivity, excessive yawning, face paler than usual, stiff neck, light sensitivity, noise sensitivity, blurred vision, sensitive skin, constipation, frequent urination, nausea/vomiting, unusual hunger or food cravings, excessive thirst, feeling intolerant or irritable, feeling unusually emotional, difficulty with thinking, difficulty with reading or writing, difficulty with speech, difficulty with concentration.

So what's different in all of this from the more familiar symptoms of migraine—known as the aura stage, which includes seeing flashing lights or wavy lines? For one thing, the warning signs tend to show up a lot earlier—in some cases, three days before the headache pain. Even more interesting is how the chicken-and-egg question is being turned on its head with this research. Until now, doctors and patients have focused on identifying behaviors that they assume play a role in triggering migraine—eating chocolate, for example. With the recent research, it seems that the urge to eat chocolate actually could mean that the attack has already started, with the sign being a craving for sweets.

Current research is concentrating on using functional imaging of the brain to reveal which regions are involved in migraines and how they interplay with symptoms.

Already, however, the latest findings give migraine sufferers something new to try. Every migraine sufferer knows that interrupting the pain early can cut the headache short. Now, by taking medicines such as naproxen or ibuprofen at the first sign of a premonitory symptom, they may be able to reduce or even prevent the pain.

Lifestyle adjustments may help as well. Avoiding a noisy party, bright lights or too much red wine, for instance, once you experience an early symptom could be a very wise move indeed.

Generally, if you recognize the symptoms, a good strategy is to pull back from typical triggers when you feel them. Try not to stay up late, not skip a meal, not push the envelope when the envelope is already pretty thin. Keeping a step ahead of triggering a migraine means practicing regularity in all things.

Precision-Tinted Lenses Help Prevent Migraines

Jie Huang, PhD, associate professor of radiology, Michigan State University, East Lansing.

Helen Irlen, MA, LMFT, learning disability specialist, Long Beach,California.

For many migraine sufferers, simply looking at certain visual patterns, such as stripes or polka dots, can trigger a severe headache. It can be especially problematic when the patterns involve flashes of light…such as when driving in a wooded area when the sun and the tree canopy create a pattern of light/shadow, light/shadow…or when sunlight is coming in through partially closed blinds…or even when exposed to almost imperceptibly flickering lights (including fluorescent bulbs).

Fortunately, many people who have regular migraines experience far fewer when they wear customized precision tinted lenses (PTLs), either as glasses or as contact lenses. (They are sometimes also called "precision ophthalmic tints" or "precision spectral filters.")

ARE PTLS RIGHT FOR YOU?

Here's what Helen Irlen, MA, LMFT, learning disability specialist who developed Irlen Spectral Filters (her version of PTLs), had to say…

Irlen Spectral Filters are tinted lenses that come in a variety of colors and can be used in both glasses and contact lenses—and you don't need a prescription from an ophthalmologist to buy them. They're one of only a few types of PTLs that are available in the US. (Another type is available from the University of Utah's John A. Moran Eye Center in Salt Lake City, Utah, at 801-581-2352, Healthcare.utah.edu/moran.)

Irlen PTLs are customized for each individual. When used in glasses, they look like tinted sunglasses from the outside, but when you wear them and look through them, they don't color what you see. Costs vary according to region. If you wear glasses, then you can use whatever frames you like and whatever lenses suit your vision (even progressive lenses)—one of Irlen's labs will tint them for you for about $75. Contact lenses can be tinted as well, and they do not change the color of your eyes (only the pupil area is tinted). For more information, visit Irlen.com.

Breakthrough Device For Migraine Pain

Morris Levin, MD, chief of the Division of Headache Medicine and director of the Headache Center at UCSF Medical Center in San Francisco. He is coauthor of *Understanding Your Migraines: A Guide for Patients and Families*. Dr. Levin is board-certified in neurology, pain medicine and headache medicine.

The FDA recently approved Cefaly, a noninvasive nerve stimulator that looks like a headband and is worn across the forehead. It delivers tiny, painless electrical pulses to the upper branch of the trigeminal nerve—the nerve responsible for sensations in your face and head. When inflamed, the trigeminal nerve overresponds to stimuli, possibly causing migraine pain.

Theory: Repeated pinging with electrical pulses might make the trigeminal nerve less sensitive to stimulation. In a recent Italian study, using Cefaly 20 minutes daily for four months reduced migraine frequency by more than 50%.

The device costs $349, plus $25 for three sets of electrodes (each set lasts about one month), and can be ordered online at Cefaly.us. It requires a prescription from your doctor and may not be covered by insurance. (Cefaly should not be used if you have a cardiac pacemaker, an implanted or wearable defibrillator, an implanted metallic or electronic device in your head or have pain of unknown origin.)

Supplements for Migraines

Mark A. Stengler, NMD, naturopathic doctor and founder of the Stengler Center for Integrative Medicine in Encinitas, California. He is author or coauthor of numerous books, including *The Natural Physician's Healing Therapies* and *Bottom Line's Prescription for Natural Cures*, and author of the newsletter *Health Revelations*. MarkStengler.com

Numerous studies confirm the benefits of the vitamin-like coenzyme Q10 (CoQ10)...riboflavin (vitamin B-2)...and the mineral magnesium to alleviate migraines. Taking just one of these three natural substances can decrease migraine severity and/or frequency by about half. In my experience, when patients regularly take all three, overall improvement can exceed 75%.

Theory: An abnormal lag in brain cells' energy production triggers the blood vessel dilation that leads to a migraine. These three nutrients support the mitochondria—structures in cells that convert oxygen and nutrients into chemical energy to power the cells' metabolic activities—helping them to work more effectively and thereby preventing migraines.

Daily prevention strategy: I suggest using all three of these substances if you get migraines once or more per month. Take them for four months. If you notice improvement, continue indefinitely. *Dosages and guidelines for people age 12 and up...*

- **CoQ10 at 100 mg three times daily.** Occasional side effects, such as mild heartburn or nausea, can be avoided by taking CoQ10 with meals. Swiss and Belgian researchers gave 42 patients a placebo or CoQ10 at 100 mg three times daily for three months. Migraine frequency fell by at least half in 47% of patients taking CoQ10, compared with 14% of the placebo group. CoQ10 users also had less nausea.

- **Riboflavin at 400 mg once daily.** B vitamins work best when in balance with one another, so take an additional B complex or multivitamin. In a Belgian study, 55 migraine patients took either a placebo or 400 mg of riboflavin daily. Frequency and duration of migraines decreased by at least half in 59% of riboflavin users, compared with 15% of placebo users. Research suggests that combining riboflavin with beta-blockers (cardiovascular drugs sometimes prescribed for migraines) may be more effective at preventing migraines than either therapy used alone.

- **Magnesium at 200 mg twice daily** (reduce dosage if you develop diarrhea). Least likely to cause loose stool is the magnesium glycinate form. Estimates show that 70% to 80% of the US population is deficient in magnesium. Oral magnesium supplementation may reduce the frequency and duration of migraines.

Possible reason: Upon exposure to a migraine trigger, excess calcium flows into brain cells, causing a sudden constriction of blood vessels...and magnesium supplementation combats this by normalizing the balance of minerals in the brain. In addition, intravenous (IV) magnesium can give fast relief from acute migraine symptoms.

A Holistic Approach to Chronic Headaches

Alexander Mauskop, MD, director of the New York Headache Center in New York City. He is the author of *What Your Doctor May Not Tell You About Migraines.* NYHeadache.com

All the natural therapies described earlier help prevent migraines, but you're likely to achieve even better results if you adopt a "holistic" approach that includes the following steps. These strategies also help guard against chronic tension headaches but are overlooked by many doctors. *My advice...*

• **Get regular aerobic exercise.** Exercise supplies more blood to the brain and boosts levels of feel-good hormones known as endorphins, which help fight migraines. Physical activity also helps release muscle tension that contributes to tension-type headaches.

Scientific evidence: In data collected from 43,770 Swedes, men and women who regularly worked out were less likely to have migraines and recurring headaches than those who did not exercise.

Helpful: Do some type of moderate-intensity aerobic activity for at least 30 minutes five times a week.

• **Use relaxation techniques.** A mind-body approach, such as progressive muscle relaxation (deliberately tensing then releasing muscles from toe to head)...guided imagery (in which you create calm, peaceful images in your mind)...or breathing exercises (a method of slow inhalation and exhalation), can ease muscle tension and relax blood vessels to help prevent migraines and tension headaches.

Also helpful: Biofeedback, which involves learning to control such involuntary functions as skin temperature, heart rate or muscle tension while sensors are attached to the body, helps prevent migraines and tension headaches. Biofeedback usually can be learned in about eight sessions and should be practiced daily by migraine and tension headache sufferers. To find a biofeedback practitioner near you, consult the Biofeedback Certification Institute of America (866-908-8713, BCIA.org).

Migraine Triggers

In susceptible individuals, certain foods and/or situations can bring on a migraine. To identify your triggers, keep a diary for four weeks, noting when your migraines occur and looking for patterns.

Common food culprits...

- **Alcohol,** especially red wine and beer
- **Caffeine**
- **Chocolate**
- **Cheese,** especially aged (Parmesan, Asiago)
- **Fermented foods** (miso, sauerkraut)
- **Monosodium glutamate** (a flavoring)
- **Nitrates** (a type of preservative)
- **Pickled foods** (dill pickles, olives, capers)
- **Shellfish**
- **Wheat**

Situational triggers...

- **Changes in weather, altitude, time zone**
- **Dehydration**
- **Fatigue, sleep problems**
- **Glaring lights**
- **Perfumes, powerful odors**
- **Stress**

Mark A. Stengler, NMD, naturopathic doctor and founder of the Stengler Center for Integrative Medicine in Encinitas, California. He is author or coauthor of numerous books, including *The Natural Physician's Healing Therapies* and *Bottom Line's Prescription for Natural Cures,* and author of the newsletter *Health Revelations.* MarkStengler.com

• **Try acupuncture.** There's good evidence that this centuries-old needling technique can reduce the severity and frequency of migraines and tension headaches.* It typically requires at least 10 sessions to see benefits. Ask your health insurer whether acupuncture is covered. If not, each session, typically an hour long, will cost $50 to $100, depending on your location.

If you feel that you are developing a migraine or tension headache: Perform a sim-

*To find an acupuncturist near you, go to the National Certification Commission for Acupuncture and Oriental Medicine website (NCCAOM.org) and click on "Find a Practitioner."

ple acupressure treatment on yourself to help relieve headache pain.

What to do: Place your right thumb on the webbing at the base of your left thumb and index finger, and your right index finger on the palm side of this point. Gently squeeze and massage this area, using small circular motions, for one to two minutes. Repeat on the right hand.

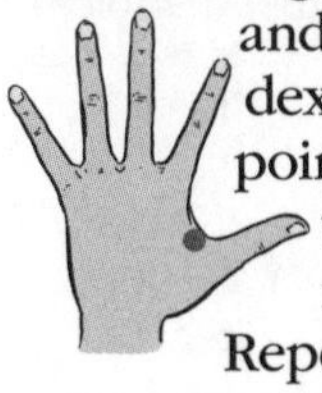

Illustration: Shawn Banner

Pepper to the Rescue!

Eliminate migraine pain with pepper. Capsaicin, an ingredient in cayenne pepper, cuts off neurotransmitters in the brain that cause headache pain.

Best: Dissolve one-quarter teaspoon of cayenne powder in four ounces of warm water. Dip a cotton swab into the solution, and apply the liquid inside your nostrils. It will burn—and by the time the burning stops, the headache pain will be reduced and sometimes gone altogether.

Eric Yarnell, ND, assistant professor, department of botanical medicine, Bastyr University, Kenmore, Washington.

Coffee Helps Migraines

Samantha Brody, ND, LAc, naturopathic doctor, licensed acupuncturist and owner of Evergreen Natural Health Center in Portland, Oregon. She has lectured extensively to lay and professional audiences across the country. DrSamantha.com

What if you could stop a migraine in its tracks? Many people can with a simple home remedy that's readily available.

Here's why: The pain of a migraine headache is usually caused by dilated, or widened, blood vessels, pressing against nerves.

Home remedy: Drinking coffee can constrict those blood vessels, relieving pain.

What to do: At the first sign of a headache, drink an eight-ounce cup of coffee (or about two cups of black tea). If the remedy is going to help, you should experience pain relief in about 20 minutes.

Coffee is most likely to work if you don't ordinarily drink it or consume other caffeine-containing beverages, such as tea or energy drinks.

For even greater relief: Try adding an ice pack to the back of your neck or head for a few minutes to further constrict dilated vessels.

Red flags: If you have insomnia, high blood pressure, anxiety or chronic fatigue—all of which coffee can worsen—this remedy probably isn't for you. Also, for some people, caffeine can trigger a migraine.

Electromagnetic Energy for Migraine Relief

Richard Lipton, MD, director, Montefiore Headache Center, New York City.

The FDA-approved Spring Transcranial Magnetic Stimulator (SpringTMS), a device that a migraine patient can hold on the back of his/her head, releases electromagnetic energy to the brain. In a recent study of 113 adults who have migraines with the sensory disturbance known as an aura, nearly 38% were free of pain within two hours after using the device—more than twice as many as those migraine sufferers who didn't use it.

How it works: Electromagnetic energy stimulates a part of the brain that can ease migraine pain. Side effects can include temporary dizziness.

Dental Device for Migraines

Michael Steinberg, DDS, dentist in private practice, New York City.

Migraine pain usually stems from the trigeminal nerve, which also is involved in jaw clenching. When worn through the night, the nociceptive trigeminal inhibition tension suppression system (NTI-TSS) dental mouthpiece reduces the intensity of clenching and frequency of migraines by 77%.

Cost: $450 and up. It may be covered by insurance, depending on your plan.

If You Get Migraines from Computer Use...

Alan Rapoport, MD, clinical professor of neurology, David Geffen School of Medicine at UCLA, Los Angeles.

Flickering lights, flashes of light, bright sun and light from some computer monitors can trigger migraines or worsen such headaches. This may be because the visual cortex, which allows us to see, becomes overexcited in migraine sufferers.

To disarm light triggers: Reduce the intensity of computer-screen illumination...avoid fluorescent lights (especially malfunctioning ones that flash) and lights that blink or flicker...tint contact lenses and/or glasses...wear hats with visors or sunglasses outdoors on bright days...and go to completely dark rooms when migraines strike.

If severe attacks persist, ask your doctor about taking a regimen of supplements that may help prevent migraines. This may include 200 milligrams (mg) of magnesium, 200 mg of vitamin B-2, 75 mg of butterbur, all twice daily...300 mg of CoQ10 once daily...and 3 mg of melatonin at night. Or ask about prescription drugs, such as the anticonvulsant *topiramate* (Topamax) or the antidepressant *amitriptyline* (Elavil)—both may help prevent migraines.

The Ayurvedic Approach to Headaches

Trupti Gokani, MD, is a board-certified neurologist and director of North Shore Headache & Wellness, an integrative clinic in Highland Park, Illinois. NorthShoreHeadache.com

According to the principles of Ayurvedic medicine, headache tendencies are to some extent preordained by your dosha, or mind-body type. But that doesn't mean you have to live with the pain. Just as your dosha determines the type and frequency of your headaches, it determines their antidotes, too. *Here's why...*

In Ayurveda, an ancient system of healing wisdom, the three basic doshas—vata, pitta and kapha—are said to be derived from the five elements of earth, air, water, fire and space. Your dosha shapes everything about you, from your physique to your personality to the particular maladies you're most vulnerable to.

To reduce the frequency of your headaches and minimize discomfort when they do arise, first, identify your predominant dosha...then follow the appropriate dosha-balancing strategies.

Note: Products mentioned below are sold in health-food stores and generally are safe, but it is best to work with an Ayurvedic practitioner who can ensure that they are right for you and suggest dosages.

The three doshas...

• **VATA.** Linked to the elements of air and space, people with this dosha tend to be energetic, lean and muscular. Vatas also are excitable, anxious and reactive...are prone to joint or muscle aches, constipation and/or gas (which can create stress that contributes to headaches)...and often feel cold.

Headache type: If you are a vata, you are vulnerable to tension headaches. The pain may be a throbbing in the back of your head or neck or it may feel like a constricting band around your head. Typically, headaches arise when you push yourself too hard, disrupt your schedule or repress your emotions. *What helps...*

• Sticking to a schedule is important for vatas. Get up and go to bed at the same time each day...have meals on a regular schedule, too.

• Eat plenty of warm, cooked foods that are high in fiber. To aid digestion, season foods with cinnamon, cumin, fennel and/or ginger.

• Drink warm or hot water throughout the day. Avoid cold drinks, which aggravate vata.

• Supplement with magnesium, which is calming. For patients with a vata imbalance, also consider the herbs jata mamsi and brahmi to promote relaxation...and triphala to help heal digestive distress.

• **PITTA.** Associated with fire and water, pitta is the dosha linked to metabolism and inflammation. Pitta people tend to be intense "type A" perfectionists...and often feel too warm even when others are cold.

Headache type: If you are a pitta, you are prone to migraines. Typically (but not always) the pain is in the eye area on the right side and is accompanied by nausea, light sensitivity and irritability. *What helps...*

• Cool down by eating more fresh fruits and salads...and season foods with cooling herbs, such as cilantro and turmeric. Avoid spicy foods and hot beverages, which worsen a pitta imbalance.

• After meals, drink one-quarter cup of aloe vera juice or chew a slice of turmeric root.

• Relax in the evening. Pitta women often keep going at full steam long past bedtime, then have trouble sleeping, thus increasing migraine risk. Try to go to bed by 10 pm.

• Lighten up. Noting that she herself falls into the pitta category, Dr. Gokani said, "We're the folks who need to relax, have some fun and allow life to flow a bit more, which may include allowing mistakes—our own and other people's—to just happen."

• **KAPHA.** Governed by the elements of earth and water, kapha is associated with stability and groundedness. Kaphas may suffer from congestion, fluid retention, body stiffness and lethargy.

Headache type: If you are a kapha, you are prone to sinus headaches, which affect the forehead and face and intensify when you bend down. *What helps...*

Try Feverfew

Feverfew has been used for centuries to prevent and relieve migraine. Studies show that it can reduce migraine frequency and severity.

Try: A total of 50 mg to 125 mg/day (tablet or capsule) divided into three doses. Feverfew thins blood—don't take it if you are on aspirin therapy or take a blood thinner such as *warfarin* (Coumadin). Also avoid it if you are allergic to ragweed. Other side effects include joint aches and gastrointestinal disturbances.

Morris Levin, MD, chief of the Division of Headache Medicine and director of the Headache Center at UCSF Medical Center in San Francisco. He is coauthor of *Understanding Your Migraines: A Guide for Patients and Families*. Dr. Levin is board-certified in neurology, pain medicine and headache medicine.

• Avoid antihistamines, which can impair your system's natural efforts to self-cleanse. Instead, to irrigate the sinuses and relieve the congestion that can lead to or exacerbate sinus headaches, use a neti pot daily (or less frequently if nasal passages become too dry). You can follow this with a treatment called nasya. It involves placing a few drops of medicated sesame oil in each nostril using a dropper or the tip of your pinky finger to help lubricate nasal passages, calm the mind and relieve headaches.

• Reduce your intake of dairy products and foods that contain gluten (a protein in wheat, rye and barley), since these are difficult to digest.

• Season foods with energizing hot spices, such as black pepper, cinnamon, cloves, ginger and mustard seed.

• Incorporate more movement in your day to stimulate your sluggish system.

Especially beneficial: Get up no later than 6 am and take a walk outdoors. Early-morning air is filled with the energy force prana, which can help keep you energized and headache-free all day.

Hypnotic Relaxation: Relieve Your Head Pain in Minutes

Yacov Ezra, MD, assistant head of neurology at Soroka University Medical Center and a lecturer at Ben-Gurion University, both in Be'er Sheva, Israel.

Taking a painkiller now and then may not be a problem if you have occasional tension headaches. But it's a different story if you frequently get that steady ache on both sides of your head—you probably know the feeling…it's a little like your head is being squeezed in a vise! With regular use, nonsteroidal anti-inflammatory drugs (NSAIDs) such as *ibuprofen* (Motrin) can lead to stomach problems and other side effects, while *acetaminophen* (Tylenol) can put the health of your liver at risk.

There is also the trap of getting "rebound" headaches—a common complication when a frequent headache sufferer overuses medication to fight the constant pain.

A missing link: In the quest to quell the pain of tension-type headaches, one crucial point often gets overlooked—up to 88% of these headaches are believed to be caused by stress. On top of that, nearly half of people suffering from chronic tension-type headaches also have depression or anxiety disorders, which painkillers don't treat.

Many doctors prescribe *amitriptyline* (Elavil), a tricyclic antidepressant, to boost mood and help regulate pain signals. This drug helps some people with tension-type headaches, but it, like other medication, has its share of bothersome side effects—dizziness, drowsiness and dry mouth, to name just a few. What's the answer?

RESEARCH UNCOVERS A BETTER SOLUTION

Researchers gave 98 people with frequent or chronic tension-type headaches the choice of using amitriptyline or trying "hypnotic-relaxation therapy"—a technique that induces a deeply relaxed, focused state. After up to a year of follow-up, 74% of patients in the hypnotic-relaxation group had a 50% reduction in headache frequency, compared with 58% of patients in the amitriptyline group.

Anyone can use hypnotic relaxation. People with tension headaches who try the technique are usually surprised by the simplicity of it. In fact, it takes just a few minutes to learn the progressive muscle relaxation and focused breathing exercises underlying the technique. *How to begin…**

- **Find a quiet, private space that's distraction free.** Turn off your cell phone.
- **Get comfortable on a chair or couch** (sitting or lying down).
- **Close your eyes and empty your mind of thoughts (as much as possible).** When intrusive thoughts return, simply acknowledge them and allow them to "drift away."
- **Breathe slowly and deeply, visualizing tension leaving your body with each exhale.** Imagine vitality entering your body with each inhale.
- **Progressively relax your body's major muscle groups,** beginning with your toes and then moving through the calves, thighs, hips, stomach, hands, arms, shoulders, neck, face and head. Stay in this relaxed state for a number of minutes, noticing the rising and falling of your chest. Now, imagine that you are at the top of a flight of 10 steps. Tell yourself that you are going to walk down the steps and count backward from 10 as you picture yourself descending each step. Feel yourself becoming more relaxed with each step.

How to create a hypnotic trance: Your next task is to self-induce a hypnotic trance using what is known as a "safe-place technique."

What to do: With your eyes closed and while breathing deeply, mentally take yourself to a place that feels calm and safe. This could be a quiet forest, a sunny beach or a serene mountaintop. What do you see, smell, hear and taste? How do you feel in this place? Engage all your senses. After a few minutes, begin repeating suggestions to yourself that

*If you have difficulty with this technique, consult a trained hypnotherapist who is also a medical doctor or psychologist.

reinforce a sense of well-being and lack of pain in your head.

These suggestions may include statements such as: The muscles in my head and neck are completely relaxed...my head is completely pain-free. The entire relaxation session takes only about 10 minutes. Ideally, headache sufferers should use hypnotic relaxation three times daily to guard against stressors that trigger tension-type headaches...it can also be used as soon as a headache starts to develop so the sufferer can quickly gain control over the pain. If pain medication is still needed, hypnotic relaxation will likely allow for a reduced dose.

Better Exercise for Migraine Sufferers

People who suffer from migraines often avoid exercise out of fear it will trigger or worsen a headache.

New finding: When 20 migraine patients exercised on stationary bicycles for 40 minutes three times weekly for three months, only one participant suffered an exercise-induced headache.

If you suffer from migraines: Ask your doctor whether cycling (on a stationary bike or outdoors) would be an appropriate type of exercise for you.

Jane Carlsson, PhD, professor of physiotherapy, Sahlgrenska Academy, University of Gothenburg, Sweden.

Reflexology Fix for Headaches

Bill Flocco, reflexology teacher and researcher, founder and director of the American Academy of Reflexology, based in Los Angeles and author of several books on reflexology.

Reflexology, which was developed by three medical professionals in the early 20th century, involves applying pressure to specific areas—known as "reflex points"—located on the feet, hands and ears.

Bonus: You can perform many basic forms of reflexology on yourself or a partner.*

For best results, work on all of the reflex points described here for at least five minutes twice a day, four or more times a week. Relief can be experienced within minutes, but it sometimes takes days or weeks of repeatedly working on the appropriate reflex areas to get results.

To fix a headache: Start with the hand corresponding to the side of your head where the pain is most noticeable. On the back of that hand, locate a point about an inch below the base knuckle of your index finger in the fleshy web between your index finger and thumb. Place the tip of the thumb of your other hand on this point and the tip of your index finger of the other hand on the palm side of this point, squeezing to find a spot that's slightly thicker and more tender than the surrounding area. While maintaining steady pressure, gently move the tip of your thumb in small circles over this spot. It usually takes about five minutes of work to alleviate a tension headache, and up to an hour to reduce or eliminate a migraine headache.

Caution: This point should not be worked on during the first trimester of pregnancy, as it could have an adverse effect on the fetus. Instead, work only on the related point on the ear, as described in the next column.

After you have completed the hand reflexology, locate the small, hard flap of cartilage at the top of your earlobe, then feel where this flap and the earlobe meet. With the tip of your thumb on the front of the ear and the tip of your index finger behind the ear, gently squeeze this point between your index finger and thumb, feeling for a spot that's slightly thicker and more tender than the surrounding area. Squeeze both ears at once, holding for five to 10 minutes, while resting your elbows on a table or desk.

*To find a certified reflexologist in your area, contact the American Reflexology Certification Board, 303-933-6921, ARCB.net.

Homeopathy for Headaches

Dana Ullman, MPH, director of Homeopathic Educational Services in Berkeley, California, and author of several books on homeopathy, including *Everybody's Guide to Homeopathic Medicines* and the regularly updated e-book *Homeopathic Family Medicine: Evidence-Based Nanopharmacology.* Homeopathic.com

Imagine taking a super-small amount of a substance that would cause your health problem if you took a normal quantity of it—and expecting that infinitesimal dose to heal you.

Well, that's exactly what happens when you take a homeopathic remedy.

HOW DOES HOMEOPATHY WORK?

Conventional medicine looks at symptoms as problems and tries to fix them with drugs or surgery. Homeopathy looks at symptoms as signs that the body-mind is attempting to defend and heal itself. (For example, the pain and redness of inflammation is a sign that the immune system is activating to heal the area.)

And homeopathy uses homeopathic medicines—repeatedly diluted preparations of herbs, minerals and other natural substances—to stimulate the vital force that is producing the symptom, so the symptom can complete itself, leading to full recovery.

MIGRAINE RELIEF

Researchers in Germany tracked 212 people who had suffered from migraine headaches for an average of 15 years—and had used homeopathy for the last two years. (Nine out of ten of the patients had used conventional medicine before turning to homeopathy.)

After two years of homeopathic treatment, the average severity of migraines had decreased by 70% (with 20% of patients "fully cured"). Overall, "migraine severity showed marked and long-standing improvement under homeopathic treatment," reported the researchers in *The Journal of Alternative and Complementary Medicine.*

And there was also a big improvement in "quality of life"—the ability to happily and energetically participate in everyday activities.

PICKING THE RIGHT MEDICINE

Start with a conventional homeopathic formula for headaches that combines several remedies, such as Hyland's Headache Homeopathic Formula or Headache Soothe from Native Remedies. Follow the dosage recommendations on the label.

If a homeopathic formula doesn't work, try experimenting with single remedies, such as Belladonna, Byronia, Nux Vomica, Pulsatilla, Gelsemium, Iris, Sanguinaria and Spigelia.

Homeopathic remedies are widely available in stores where supplements are sold and online.

Doses: Take the single remedy every two hours, until you start to feel better, using a potency as low as 6X or 6C and as high as 30X or 30C dose. (The "X" and "C" are indications of the potency of the remedy, with higher numbers being more potent.) After that, take the medicine only if your symptoms start to worsen again. If the symptoms aren't any better after two or three doses, try another one of the remedies.

For optimal results: If self-care doesn't work, consider seeing a professional homeopath. The homeopathic physician doesn't treat one disease or one system of the body—he or she treats the whole body-mind, and that's the best way to achieve better health.

Healthful Snack Can Fix Your Headache

Lydia Wilen and Joan Wilen, folk-remedy experts based in New York City. They are coauthors of many books, including *Bottom Line's Household Magic.*

Researchers tell us that almonds contain lots of salicylates, the pain-relieving ingredient in aspirin. Eating 15 raw almonds will do the work of one aspirin. While it may take a little longer for the headache to vanish, you won't run the risk of side effects. Almonds also have been shown to reduce cholesterol, build strong bones and teeth, and boost brain function, so if you eat almonds in moderation on a regular basis, the side effects you get are nothing but good. (Of course, if you have a nut or a salicylate allergy, don't try this at home—or anywhere!)

CHAPTER 12

Infectious Diseases

You're Never Too Old To Catch an STD

Painful urination or vaginal discharge may make you suspect a bladder or yeast infection—but those symptoms could instead signal a sexually transmitted disease (STD). Though people tend to associate STDs with adolescents and young adults, doctors report an alarming rise among older patients. *Reasons...*

- **Erectile dysfunction drugs allow older men to be more sexually active than before.** The more partners you have—and the more partners your partner has had—the greater your STD risk.
- **Condoms reduce the risk for catching some STDs**—but after menopause, when there is no need for contraception, couples are far less likely to use condoms.
- **As women age, the vaginal wall thins and lubrication diminishes, leaving tissues more prone to damage and infection during sex.**

PLAYING IT SAFE

The surest ways to avoid getting an STD are to abstain from sex, including oral sex, or to be in a long-term relationship in which you both are monogamous. *Otherwise...*

- **Before beginning a new relationship, you and your potential partner should both get tested for STDs.**
- **Have your male partner use latex condoms consistently.**
- **If you develop STD symptoms** (as described below), stop having sex and see your doctor promptly.
- **If an STD is diagnosed, abstain from sex** (including oral sex) until treatment is completed.

Kimberly Workowski, MD, associate professor of medicine at Emory University and chief of the guidelines unit in the epidemiology and surveillance branch of the Division of STD Prevention at the Centers for Disease Control and Prevention, both in Atlanta. CDC.gov/std

• **Your current partner must be tested and treated at the same time so he doesn't reinfect you.**

• **Notify anyone else with whom you had sex in the last six months**—he should get checked, too.

WHAT TO WATCH FOR

Some STDs can be cured with antibiotics. For other types there is no cure—so contagion control is essential. *Be on the lookout for...*

• **Chlamydia.** This bacterial infection of the genital tract is so widespread that testing is recommended for all sexually active women age 25 or under...and for women of any age who have a new sex partner or multiple partners.

Symptoms: Some women experience pain when urinating and/or an abnormal vaginal discharge...many others have no early symptoms. If infection spreads to the fallopian tubes, it can cause serious pelvic inflammation, intense pain and infertility. Men may have a penile discharge or pain when urinating.

Medical care: Diagnosis is based on a urine test or a cervical swab. Treatment is one dose of the antibiotic *azithromycin* (Zithromax) or a seven-day course of doxycycline.

• **Genital Herpes.** This viral disease stays in the body indefinitely, causing repeated outbreaks.

Symptoms: Women and men develop painful genital ulcers (blisters) that can take several weeks to heal...women may have difficulty emptying the bladder.

Medical care: Diagnosis is made with a viral culture. There is no cure, but outbreaks diminish in frequency and severity over time. An oral antiviral drug, such as *famciclovir* (Famvir) or *valacyclovir* (Valtrex), taken daily or at the start of an outbreak, minimizes symptoms.

Contagion control: To reduce the risk of catching or passing on herpes, always have your male partner use a latex condom—the virus can be transmitted even in the absence of active symptoms. Abstain from sex (oral sex, too) during outbreaks.

• **HIV (human immunodeficiency virus).** Everyone who is evaluated for an STD and all pregnant women should be screened for HIV infection. Some people with HIV infection develop acquired immunodeficiency syndrome (AIDS).

Symptoms: Signs may develop within weeks or may not appear for up to 10 years. Early symptoms are vague—fever, malaise, skin rash. Later symptoms include severe diarrhea, weight loss, chills and vulnerability to other infections and some cancers.

Medical care: Blood or saliva tests are used for diagnosis. With the Home Access HIV-1 Test System (about $44 at drugstores), blood is collected from a finger prick and mailed in for testing. Individualized drug combinations can significantly slow disease progression.

Contagion control: To minimize the risk of contracting or transmitting HIV, correct and consistent condom use is recommended.

• **HPV (human papillomavirus).** Certain HPV strains cause genital warts in women and men. HPV can lead to cervical cancer and other malignancies in women. HPV also is linked to some oral cancers in people infected through oral sex.

Symptoms: Warts appear as small flesh-colored growths—flat, raised or cauliflower-shaped—on or around the genitals. They may itch and may bleed with intercourse.

Medical care: Genital warts are diagnosed visually. Tests for HPV infection can be done along with a Pap test...or if Pap results are abnormal. Warts can be removed with topical medication, laser or other methods—but may recur.

Contagion control: Usually HPV goes away on its own.

Best: Get regular Pap tests (following the schedule recommended by your doctor), which can detect early cellular changes from HPV infection.

• **Trichomoniasis.** A protozoan parasite causes this. Women may develop vaginal symptoms from a recent sexual encounter...or from one that occurred years or even decades ago due to lingering infection in the glands surrounding the urethra.

Symptoms: Women develop frothy, smelly, greenish vaginal discharge...genital itching... and/or discomfort during intercourse and urination. Men may have a slight penile discharge or a burning sensation upon urination or ejaculation.

Medical care: Women are diagnosed with a lab test of vaginal secretions...men get a urine culture or urethral swab. Usually a single dose of the antibiotic *metronidazole* (Flagyl) or *tinidazole* (Tindamax) cures the infection.

You Have H. Pylori—Now What?

Andrew L. Rubman, ND, founder and director, Southbury Clinic for Traditional Medicines, Southbury, Connecticut. Southburyclinic.com

Eric Yarnell, ND, clinical supervisor at Bastyr University's Center for Natural Health, Seattle.

You've been bothered by chronic indigestion, perhaps leading your doctor to order an endoscopy so he/she could look down your esophagus and into your stomach with a camera, and, give you some tests. The finding? For many, it's that their digestive system is harboring the intestinal bacteria *H. pylori*...now what?

In 1982, when H. pylori was discovered to be at the root of stomach ulcers, the medical community celebrated, immediately deciding that the news meant ulcers could be cured by an intense course of antibiotics to kill off all those nasty bacteria. But now we know that a wise treatment path for people with H. pylori is not so straightforward. Yes, the bacteria are linked to a host of gastrointestinal (GI) problems, including ulcers and even gastric cancer. But many of us carry H. pylori around in our systems without ill effects, and doctors have found that eliminating it entirely is associated with other problems, including esophageal cancer.

FRIEND OR FOE?

Should we kill H. pylori every time we detect it? Probably not, says Eric Yarnell, ND, a clinical supervisor at Bastyr University's Center for Natural Health in Seattle. When he sees patients with H. pylori-related complaints, including inflammation, pain and other symptoms, his goal is to restore comfort by replenishing the stomach's natural defenses against the bacteria overgrowth that has thrown the system out of balance...but he aims for full elimination of the particular bacterium itself only in cases of recurrent illness or associated cancers.

SHOULD YOU FOLLOW DOCTORS' ORDERS?

Conventional medical treatment of H. pylori infection uses a 14-day course of an antibiotic (usually clarithromycin or amoxicillin) to remove H. pylori from the stomach...as well as the antimicrobial *metronidazole* (Flagyl)... and either a bismuth-salt preparation to blunt inflammation and soothe the tissue or (more likely) an antacid proton pump inhibitor (PPI), such as *esomeprazole* (Nexium), *omeprazole* (Prilosec) or *lansoprazole* (Prevacid). A combination of prescription drugs (*lansoprazole, amoxicillin* and *clarithromycin*) was recently approved (called Prevpac) for treatment. If this triple therapy fails to make your symptoms go away, your doctor will next try instead "quadruple therapy"—tetracycline, metronidazole, a PPI and the bismuth compound for an additional 14 days. Many doctors also will prescribe the PPIs even longer, up to an additional three weeks.

Andrew L. Rubman, ND, disagrees with this approach. He warns that these regimens bring significant side effects. If you take a PPI for longer than two weeks, you reduce your stomach's ability to produce adequate amounts of acid to digest food and also reduce its innate ability to protect you from dangerous pathogens. Antibiotics indiscriminately suppress many beneficial bacteria as well as the ones making you sick and as a result can lead to the emergence of antibiotic-resistant strains of H. pylori, paradoxically placing you at greater risk for digestive disorders.

A BETTER WAY: NATURAL THERAPIES

Rather than attempting to eradicate H. pylori, some doctors may seek to get it back in "balance" by first calming irritation and inflammation and then restoring proper stomach function, including adequate acid production to stabilize H. pylori and prevent its overgrowth.

This safe and natural approach may include...

- **Bismuth-based therapy.** Bismuth salts, originally believed to simply coat ulcers and physically block erosive stomach acid, now are known to directly attack and impair H. pylori.
- **Digestive enzymes.** Once irritation is resolved, hydrochloric acid (usually the supplement betaine hydrochloride) helps reestablish efficient acid production, which may have been interrupted by the infection but is necessary for normal digestion.
- **Manuka honey.** Evidence supporting the use of this New Zealand honey is largely anecdotal, but you may find that taking some before meals and before bed helps combat H. pylori. Discuss with your doctor how much to take if you want to try this therapy.
- **Mastic gum.** This natural resin from the sap of the mastic tree (*Pistacia lentiscus*), which grows mainly on the Greek island of Chios, inhibits H. pylori growth, according to a study in *The New England Journal of Medicine*. Capsules can be found at iHerb.com and in health-food stores.
- **Broccoli sprouts.** A small Japanese trial suggests that broccoli sprouts activate protective enzymes. Unlike mature heads, the sprouts contain high levels of sulforaphane, a potent natural weapon against H. pylori colonization. These can be eaten in salads or on sandwiches as a way to help keep H. pylori in check.
- **Bovine lactoferrin.** Studies show that this protein from cows (consumed as a powder added to shakes and smoothies) improves the effectiveness of other therapies against H. pylori. It can be purchased at iHerb.com and in some health-food stores.

Rather than eradicating H. pylori entirely, a better approach is to tame the bacteria so it can play a healthful, not harmful, role in your digestive system.

Seek immediate medical attention if you experience these symptoms: Vomit blood or what looks like coffee grounds...having bloody or tarry black stools...or experiencing sudden, severe and persistent abdominal pain.

Important: While you may not be able to eliminate exposure to H. pylori, people who maintain a healthy lifestyle—a diet of nutrient-rich whole foods, no smoking, regular exercise, alcohol in moderation only, etc.—are more likely to have robust immune systems and less likely to develop active infections or discomfort even if H. pylori is in their systems.

Update on Shingles: A New Vaccine and Better Self-Care

Lindsay C. Strowd, MD, assistant professor of dermatology at Wake Forest Baptist Health in Winston-Salem, North Carolina. Her research has appeared in *Journal of the American Academy of Dermatology*, *The American Journal of Dermatopathology* and other professional journals.

Shingles is one of those dreaded conditions that you may not think too much about—until it's your turn to endure the ravages of this painful viral infection.

Recent development: There's a new vaccine that provides better protection than the previous one. But despite all the attention it's getting, many people are still unaware of some key details.

Reality check: Because some people—vaccinated or not—still do develop shingles, you also need to know how to best treat the condition and use self-care measures to curb the suffering.

THE SHINGLES VACCINE

The first vaccine for adult shingles, Zostavax, was FDA approved in 2006. It was found to prevent shingles in about half of people who received the single shot.

What you may not realize: Shingles is much more than a skin rash. It's a viral infection that starts with a rash but usually doesn't stop there. The rash can be intensely painful and can lead to severe nerve pain that's potentially permanent. And in some cases, shingles can increase stroke risk.

Shingrix, the shingles vaccine that was FDA approved in late 2017, is about 97% effective against shingles during the first year. Its effectiveness wanes over time, but experts predict that it will continue to reduce infections by about 85% over four years. Research has shown that it's particularly effective in older adults, who face the highest risk for shingles.

What you may not realize: The new vaccine is also recommended for those who were previously vaccinated with Zostavax. Even if you've already received the older vaccine, the CDC recommends getting the new one.

Also important: Just because you've already had shingles, it doesn't mean you're off the hook—you can get shingles more than once. *Other key facts to know about the new vaccine...*

- **It requires two doses instead of one.** While the original shingles vaccine was given in a single dose, Shingrix requires two doses—given about two to six months apart.
- **It's pricey.** Shingrix is about $280 for both shots total, roughly the same cost as the single-shot original vaccine. Most insurance, including Medicare, is expected to cover the new vaccine, but you'll want to check before getting the shots.
- **There's some discomfort from the shot,** which involves mainly arm swelling and localized pain—this is typical with most injections. But about half of patients age 70 and older report more bothersome side effects, including widespread muscle pain, fatigue and/or headaches. Most side effects are temporary and last about 24 to 48 hours.
- **The vaccine's duration is uncertain.** Most vaccines lose their protection over time. The older shingles vaccine seems to lose some of its protection after about five or six years. Shingrix has not been used long enough to determine exactly how many years of protection it will give. And patients may need revaccination at some point after the original vaccination series.
- **Shingrix uses killed viruses, while Zostavax uses live viruses.** Those with impaired immune systems cannot receive live vaccines. If you have been told in the past that you cannot get the shingles vaccine due to an impaired immune system, ask your doctor about Shingrix.
- **Shingrix can be given starting at age 50,** while Zostavax was given to those age 60 and older.

My advice: Everyone age 50 or older and any adult with an impaired immune system should ask a doctor about getting the new vaccine.

IF YOU DO GET SHINGLES

If you get vaccinated but develop shingles anyway, the rash will typically be milder with less severe pain, and the illness will be shorter in duration. Plus, there will be less risk for serious complications such as permanent nerve damage.

Shingles typically starts with one to five days of shooting or burning pain, numbness, tingling, itching and/or skin sensitivity. Some people also have flulike symptoms—headache, chills and fever. The affected skin will then develop redness and small blisters filled with fluid. If you get these symptoms, see your doctor right away—early diagnosis and treatment can help shorten the course of the attack and improve symptoms.

If the pain is severe: Ask your doctor about *gabapentin* (Neurontin), an antiseizure drug that also relieves nerve pain. Topical lidocaine, available over-the-counter, can help with pain as well.

Complications: The shingles rash sometimes occurs on the face or near the eyes. In these cases, the virus can enter the optic nerve and cause vision loss. And in very rare cases, the shingles virus can infect the brain and cause inflammation of the brain (encephalitis).

Important: Seek immediate medical care if the rash is near your eye or on your nose or it continues spreading to other parts of your body.

Best self-care options...

- **Try a cool-water compress...or oatmeal/baking soda baths,** which can reduce itching and discomfort. For a compress, soak and wring out a soft washcloth with cool water and apply it to the rash for five to 10 minutes, several times per day. For baths, add colloidal oatmeal/baking soda to cool bathwater. Soak for 10 minutes once a day.

• **Coat the rash with a thick ointment such as petroleum jelly, Aquaphor or unscented A&D Ointment, then cover the area with a bandage.** Ointments are soothing, and the bandage will protect the area from the friction caused by clothing.

• **Wear loose, natural-fiber clothes (such as cotton).** They're more comfortable than polyester or other synthetic fabrics.

THE SHINGLES TRAP

About 90% of adults had chicken pox (varicella-zoster virus) early in life. Once you've been exposed to this virus, it retreats to the nervous system and lies dormant. The virus can reactivate later in life, usually after age 50, and cause shingles.

Sometimes shingles will be reactivated during periods of extreme stress on the body—for example, during a bad illness. People with weakened immune systems—the elderly...those with chronic diseases...and/or patients taking immune-suppressing medications for conditions such as rheumatoid arthritis or lupus or using chemotherapy drugs—are at greater risk of developing shingles.

The Fight Against Lingering Shingles Pain

Salim M. Hayek, MD, PhD, chief of the division of pain medicine at University Hospitals Case Medical Center and an associate professor at Case Western Reserve University School of Medicine, both in Cleveland. He is board-certified in pain medicine and anesthesiology.

Women have the unfortunate distinction of being more susceptible than men to the painful skin disease herpes zoster, otherwise known as shingles.

Surprising: Though shingles has long been considered a once-in-a-lifetime affliction, a recent Mayo Clinic study revealed that more than 5% of sufferers experienced a second bout within the follow-up period, which averaged eight years...and that recurrences were 60% more likely in women.

Shingles develops when the varicella-zoster virus—the same virus that causes chicken pox and then goes into hiding in nerve cells—becomes reactivated at a time when a person's immune function is reduced. Shingles risk rises with age as immunity gradually declines. The virus follows a nerve path that leads out from the spine, traveling around one side of the body and surfacing at nerve endings in the skin. The inflamed nerve becomes extremely painful and the affected skin (which reflects the location of that nerve path) erupts in clusters of fluid-filled blisters that take two to four weeks to crust over and heal.

Bad as shingles can be, an even scarier threat is a complication called postherpetic neuralgia (PHN) that develops in about 20% of shingles patients. PHN is characterized by intense nerve pain that lingers for months or years after the blisters themselves have healed. According to Salim M. Hayek, MD, PhD, chief of the division of pain medicine at University Hospitals Case Medical Center in Cleveland, the burning, stabbing sensations of PHN can be so severe that even the feeling of clothing or a breeze against the skin can be unbearable—and PHN sufferers often experience depression, isolation and concentration problems. *Self-defense...*

For prevention: Get vaccinated. The FDA recently lowered the approved age for receiving the shingles vaccine, Zostavax, from 60 to 50. The vaccine reduces shingles risk by an estimated 55% to 70%...and it reduces PHN risk by 67%. Vaccinated people who do develop shingles typically experience milder outbreaks and may be less vulnerable to recurrences than unvaccinated ones.

For a shingles outbreak: The first sign of shingles usually is a tingling, burning or itching sensation on the skin, most often on one side of the torso (though it can develop anywhere). This usually is followed within a few days by a red, blotchy rash that later blisters...some patients also have a headache and fever.

Important: If you have possible symptoms of shingles, see your physician immediately. If taken within 72 hours of the onset of the rash, a prescription antiviral drug such as *acyclovir* (Zovirax), *famciclovir* (Famvir) or *valacyclovir* (Valtrex) can lessen the severity of shingles and significantly reduce PHN risk.

For pain relief: If over-the-counter painkillers don't do the job, ask your doctor about taking prescription-strength ibuprofen, acetaminophen with codeine, *tramadol* (Ultram) or other pain medication.

For PHN: There is no cure (except, in some cases, time), but there are ways to manage the persistent pain of PHN. *These include...*

- **Mindfulness-based stress reduction.** A program developed at the University of Massachusetts Medical School combines yoga, meditation, support groups and individually tailored instruction to improve quality of life for PHN patients and other pain sufferers. Visit UMassMed.edu/cfm/mindfullness-based-programs for information, then check your local hospitals for similar programs.
- **Topical medications.** These inhibit damaged nerve cells in the skin from sending pain messages to the brain. The prescription skin patch Lidoderm, which contains lidocaine, is applied at home and worn for up to 12 hours per day. The prescription skin patch Qutenza, which contains capsaicin (the "hot" substance in chili peppers), is applied at the doctor's office in a one-hour procedure and replaced after three months. Nonprescription topical capsaicin products, such as the ointment Zostrix, may help—but patients should follow instructions carefully and some still may not be able to tolerate the burning sensation when capsaicin is first applied, Dr. Hayek said.
- **Oral medications.** Options include the neuropathic pain drug *pregabalin* (Lyrica)... the anticonvulsant *gabapentin* (Neurontin)... the SNRI antidepressant *duloxetine* (Cymbalta)...a tricyclic antidepressant, such as *amitriptyline* (Elavil)...and opioids, such as *oxycodone* (Oxycontin).

Topical and oral PHN medications can have potentially serious side effects, Dr. Hayek cautioned—so it is important to work closely with your physician when using such drugs to manage PHN pain.

Natural Rx for Shingles

Chris Meletis, ND, executive director, the Institute for Healthy Aging. He is author of several books including *Better Sex Naturally, Complete Guide to Safe Herbs* and *Instant Guide to Drug-Herb Interactions.*

In most people, shingles resolves itself by five or six very uncomfortable weeks...although, for a few patients, a painful and debilitating complication called postherpetic neuralgia (PHN) can linger for many more months and even years. In fact, the recent development of a vaccine for shingles was partly to shield people from the possibility of PHN. While the vaccination is now a reality and is available to people ages 60 and over, natural treatments can also ease the discomfort of shingles and possibly reduce the amount of time it normally takes to run its course, as well as develop PHN.

NATURAL RX FOR SHINGLES

The first recommendation for shingles patients is to take vitamin B-12. The reason, most importantly, is that B-12 has been shown to help prevent PHN. It also helps bolster energy levels and eases the discomfort of the outbreak. I often prescribes 1 mg of B-12 in the form of methylcobalamin twice a day, preferably under the tongue (sublingually). Continue this for the duration of the outbreak and for two to three months after the resolution of the rash and other symptoms.

Another useful vitamin for combating shingles is vitamin C. A potent antioxidant, vitamin C bolsters the immune system and helps patients cope with the stress of the disease. Some people find that vitamin C helps dry blisters as well and reduces pain to some degree and it may also hinder development of PHN. The dosage for many of my patients is 1,000 mg two to three times a day with meals. Vitamin C can cause diarrhea, in which case patients are directed to ease up slightly on

Homeopathy for Shingles

If you're looking for natural help, try one of the following remedies (all sold in health-food stores). If lesions have appeared on the face, take *Apis mellifica.* For shingles on the left side of your chest, use *Ranunculus bulbosus.* If lesions cause burning pain that eases with a warm compress, try *Arsenicum album.* Whichever remedy you use, take three 30C pellets twice a day for three days, dissolving pellets under your tongue. (Do not take within 30 minutes of meals.) If there's no improvement or you feel worse, discontinue use. For chronic or recurring shingles, see a homeopath.

Edward Shalts, MD, DHt (diplomate in homeotherapeutics), faculty member, Continuum Center for Health and Healing, Beth Israel Medical Center, New York City, and author of *Easy Homeopathy.*

dosage until they find the maximum level that is tolerated. If nerve pain does remain after the lesions have resolved, lipoic acid at a dose of 300 mg two to three times a day can be helpful.

One amino acid plays a particularly interesting role in shingles. L-lysine has been shown to be helpful in combating viruses, including another type of herpes virus called herpes simplex-1 that typically causes so-called fever blisters on the lips and herpes-simplex 2, which typically causes outbreaks of lesions on the genitalia. Use of L-lysine, however, must be prescribed and monitored carefully by a trained professional. L-lysine is contraindicated in pregnant women and those with elevated cholesterol or triglyceride levels.

TOPICAL RELIEF

Of course it is important to have topical balms and creams to soothe the itching and pain of the rash. There are several available that can be helpful. Lysine cream is one (but do not put on open sores) and lemon balm is another. After the sores heal, a variety of capsaicin-containing creams on the market may provide pain relief. Capsaicin, the substance that adds heat to hot peppers, is said to inhibit nerve cells from sending pain messages to the brain. Capsaicin creams come in a variety of strengths.

Whichever one you select, start small by using just a dab and apply four times a day. It will sting when you first put it on, but don't let that fool you. Stick with it since it will help. After applying, wash hands with soap and water to avoid irritation on other parts of your skin.

Finally, I remind all shingles patients that the body needs time to restore itself. You may not feel inclined to do much else as you battle shingles, so use the time to take it easy and get lots of rest.

Rhus Toxicodendron— A Soother for Shingles and More...

Mark A. Stengler, NMD, a naturopathic doctor and founder of the Stengler Center for Integrative Medicine in Encinitas, California. He is author or coauthor of numerous books, including *The Natural Physician's Healing Therapies* and *Bottom Line's Prescription for Natural Cures,* and author of the newsletter *Health Revelations.* MarkStengler.com

Rhus toxicodendron (pronounced roos tox-ih-ko-den-dron) is the homeopathic dilution of poison oak. We know this as a plant that causes a nasty, blistering rash. However, this homeopathic is one of the best skin remedies for relieving symptoms in people who have touched poison ivy. It is also effective in treating eczema, where the skin is very itchy and feels better after the application of very hot water.

I have also used this for people with shingles. The itching, burning pain of the shingles blisters can be relieved in a few days with rhus tox.

Dosage: The typical dosage for rhus tox is 30C potency taken two to three times daily for a day or two for conditions such as stiffness from overexertion. For long-term use for eczema or arthritis, I generally start with a lower dose such as 6C taken two to three times daily.

What are the side effects?: While rhus tox has few side effects, some people may experience skin irritation. People with chronic eczema or arthritis may experience a flare-up of their condition at the beginning of treatment. This is usually a sign that the remedy is working (known as a healing aggravation).

If you do have a flare-up and you begin taking the rhus tox less frequently, you'll probably notice that the flare-up subsides. Soon after, you'll probably notice an improvement in your condition.

If you are not sure whether you should use rhus tox, consult a homeopathic practitioner.

Recommendations for...

- **Flu.** Rhus tox is a good remedy for the type of flu that makes your joints and muscles stiff.

- **Herpes.** Cold sores on the mouth or face, or genital herpes outbreaks can be helped greatly with rhus tox.

- **Shingles.** This dormant chicken-pox virus erupts when the immune system is weakened. Many elderly people suffer from excruciating pain that is often not relieved with conventional medicines. Rhus tox has worked wonders in several cases I have treated.

- **Strains.** Rhus tox should be used when ligaments and tendons are strained. It helps speed up the recovery process. Athletes should have a supply of rhus tox available at all times.

- **Urticaria.** Urticaria is a fancy way of saying hives. For hive breakouts that do not require emergency treatment (such as when the throat closes), rhus tox helps to relieve the itching and works to heal the lesions more quickly. It is also effective for relieving itching caused by mosquito bites.

Natural Help for Ear Infections

Mark A. Stengler, NMD, licensed naturopathic medical doctor in private practice, Encinitas, California... adjunct associate clinical professor at the National College of Natural Medicine, Portland, Oregon...author of *The Natural Physician's Healing Therapies* and coauthor of *Prescription for Natural Cures* (both from Bottom Line Books).

The natural treatments below work well for most bacterial and viral ear infections. For mild pain, try eardrops alone. If pain is moderate to severe or does not ease after one or two applications of eardrops, use all three remedies. Therapies generally are safe for adults and children of all ages. Products are sold in health-food stores.

- **Garlic/mullein/St. John's wort eardrops relieve pain and have antibacterial and antiviral effects.** Hold the capped bottle under hot water until warm...then place three drops in the affected ear three to four times daily. Do not use if the eardrum is ruptured (indicated by pus in the ear).

Try: Eclectic Institute Ear Drops (800-332-4372, EclecticHerb.com).

- **Homeopathic chamomilla (from the chamomile plant) reduces pain and fever.**

Dosage: Two 30C potency pellets four times daily.

Dosage: Two 30C potency pellets four times daily.

- **Echinacea/goldenseal herbal formula strengthens the immune response.** Use as directed, typically four times daily. For children, choose an alcohol-free product.

Pain relief: Run one facecloth under hot water and another under cold water to make compresses. Hold the hot compress over the ear for two minutes, then switch to the cold compress for 30 seconds. Repeat twice. Do in the morning, midday and evening for two days to reduce congestion and draw healing immune cells to the area.

I consider antibiotics for an ear infection when a patient has pus in the middle ear (seen during an exam)...has a fever of 104°F or higher for more than 24 hours or any fever

Antibiotics for Ear Infections?

Antibiotics may not be necessary for most kids' ear infections. Eighty percent of children with ear infections get better on their own in about three days, according to a recent study. Antibiotics may cause side effects such as rash or diarrhea. And overuse of antibiotics may be responsible for the increase in stronger, drug-resistant bacteria.

Helpful: Ask your pediatrician to write a prescription for antibiotics to be filled only if your child gets worse or if the infection has not cleared up within two to three days. Give your child ibuprofen or acetaminophen to help relieve pain.

Tumaini Coker, MD, pediatrician, Mattel Children's Hospital, University of California, Los Angeles, and leader of a systematic review of 135 studies on acute ear infections, published in *The Journal of the American Medical Association.*

for more than 48 hours...has rapidly worsening symptoms...or does not respond to natural treatments within two days.

Don't Let the Flu Turn Into Pneumonia

William Schaffner, MD, an infectious disease specialist at Vanderbilt University Medical Center in Nashville and medical director of the National Foundation for Infectious Diseases. NFID.org

The flu lands hundreds of thousands of people in the hospital each year and kills tens of thousands. But flu that leads to pneumonia is even deadlier.

Startling statistic: Flu-plus-pneumonia ranks eighth in leading causes of death in the US.

THE FLU/PNEUMONIA COMBO

Every year, pneumonia affects more than one million Americans—and about 50,000 die. People most susceptible to pneumonia include the elderly, especially nursing home residents and individuals who have chronic health conditions such as heart or lung disease. The flu-to-pneumonia progression isn't the only cause of pneumonia, of course, but since the combo is so deadly—and often so preventable—it's worth special attention.

Here's what happens: You get the flu, a contagious respiratory illness caused by an influenza virus. You get the typical symptoms—sore throat, cough, body aches, fever, headaches and chills. But the flu also makes your lungs more susceptible to a bacterial infection caused by *Streptococcus pneumoniae*, the most common cause of pneumonia in adults.

When that happens, air sacs fill with pus and other liquid, making it harder for oxygen to reach the bloodstream and making it difficult to breathe. Death can come from organs that are starved of oxygen—or from a blood infection (sepsis).

Here's how to protect yourself...

STEP ONE: **Get a Flu Shot**

If you don't get the flu, you won't be at risk for that combination of flu virus/*S. pneumoniae* that is so dangerous to susceptible people. Getting a flu shot is the best way to protect yourself. It is recommended for everyone over the age of six months. While not 100% effective, it does offer substantial protection.

Why a flu shot is so important: A bad flu year means that pneumonia cases could potentially soar.

STEP TWO: **Make Sure You're Up-to-Date on Pneumonia Vaccination**

Effective vaccines exist against S. pneumoniae, which, as described earlier, causes the vast majority of pneumonia cases in adults. Everyone age 65 and older should be vaccinated—yet only about 50% of healthy adults in this age group are. Some adults need protection before they turn 65—smokers and anyone with a chronic health condition (heart or lung disease, diabetes, asthma, etc.). *For the best protection, you'll need two different vaccines, spaced out over a year or more...*

- **Start with a onetime-only dose of the pneumococcal conjugate vaccine called**

PCV13 (Prevnar 13), which protects against 13 types of pneumococcal bacteria.

- **One year later, get a dose of pneumococcal polysaccharide vaccine PPSV23 (Pneumovax),** which protects against 23 strains of pneumococcal bacteria. Prevnar 13 primes your immune system so that Pneumovax works better than it would if you took it by itself.
- **Based on your age and health,** your doctor may advise another dose of Pneumovax five years later.

***STEP THREE:* Watch Your Meds**

Certain health conditions and medications can affect your susceptibility to pneumonia...

- **Steroids and other immunosuppressive drugs can make you more susceptible to pneumonia.** These drugs interfere with the immune response, so your body can't fight off infection as easily.

Low-dose steroids, even taken long-term, may not increase pneumonia risk, but higher doses (such as 20 mg a day) can do so in as little as two weeks. If you need a high-dose steroid to control your condition, be especially vigilant during flu season—get vaccinated, wash your hands frequently, stay away from crowds, and call your doctor at the first sign of illness such as a sore throat.

- **Acid-suppressive medications,** such as proton pump inhibitors including *omeprazole* (Prilosec), as well as histamine-2 receptor antagonists including *ranitidine* (Zantac), inhibit the production of stomach acids. But these acids help keep harmful gut bacteria in check.

Less acid means more potential for harmful bacteria to colonize and eventually enter the lungs. Unless your doctor prescribes these on a long-term basis (a rare occurrence), use them only for short periods of time—no more than four weeks for heartburn/gastroesophageal reflux disease (GERD), for example.

- **Pneumonia occurs less often in adults who get routine dental checkups.** Routine dental visits can help decrease the overall amount of bacteria in your mouth, including those that can cause pneumonia in susceptible people.

Bonus: A healthy mouth reduces heart disease risk, too.

IF YOU DO GET THE FLU...

Since the flu shot doesn't always prevent infection, be on the lookout for symptoms including feeling feverish, chills, body aches, sore throat and fatigue. If you suspect that you have the flu, call your doctor. You may be a candidate for prescription antiviral medication such as *oseltamivir* (Tamiflu), which can shorten your illness duration and possibly decrease the odds of it progressing to pneumonia. But you need to take it within a day or two of the first symptoms for it to be effective.

PNEUMONIA AND YOUR HEART

Adults hospitalized with pneumonia have a heightened risk for cardiovascular problems including sudden heart attack, often with no warning signs.

What happens: Oxygen deprivation from a bout of pneumonia can starve cardiac muscle cells so that they function less well or even die off. One study found that within the first month of pneumonia diagnosis, the risk for stroke, heart attack or death due to heart disease grew by as much as fourfold...and remained elevated for years. Patients recovering from pneumonia also are predisposed to developing it again—another good reason to prevent it in the first place.

Lyme Ticks Are on the March ...and with New Diseases

Richard Horowitz, MD, medical director of the Hudson Valley Healing Arts Center, in Hyde Park, New York. He is the author of *How Can I Get Better? An Action Plan for Treating Resistant Lyme and Chronic Disease.*

Lyme disease* used to be thought of as a Northeastern problem.

Don't make that mistake. *Here's why...*

*If you've been treated for Lyme and your symptoms don't improve, you may want to see a Lyme-MSIDS specialist. To find such a doctor in your area, consult the Lyme Disease Association, LymeDisease-Association.org, or the International Lyme and Associated Diseases Society, ILADS.org.

• **Today, Lyme-infected deer ticks are found in most states**—covering nearly half of all US counties.

• **The epidemic continues to explode not only in the Northeast,** but also in north central states. In Wisconsin, Iowa and Minnesota, it's up by 250% since 1998, according to the Centers for Disease Control and Prevention (CDC).

• **Lyme ticks are now found on both coasts and in the South.**

• **They are spreading serious new diseases as well.** A single tick bite can transmit many disease-causing organisms. These so-called "coinfections" often persist even after a person takes antibiotics (the standard treatment for Lyme).

Yes, there are hot spots, but even in places like the Carolinas, Texas and Florida, there are reports of Lyme. In fact, an estimated 300,000 people are diagnosed with Lyme disease in the US each year, according to the CDC.

OTHER TICK-BORNE INFECTIONS

If you have Lyme-like symptoms that don't improve after a month of antibiotic treatment, ask your doctor to check for simultaneous infections. Even if you have tested negative for Lyme, you could still be infected with a similar organism that causes Lyme-like symptoms but isn't detectable with the standard tests for Lyme.

Tick-borne coinfections…

• **Babesiosis.** This parasitic infection is spreading rapidly in the US. Babesiosis has been reported across the country from the East Coast (New York) to the upper Midwest and West Coast (Washington State and California). It typically causes malaria-like symptoms—such as chills, sweating and fever—that occur intermittently, sometimes for years. It also can cause shortness of breath and an unexplained cough.

How it's diagnosed: Blood tests that check for the infecting organism (*Babesia*). It's important to test for different *Babesia* species—and do DNA and RNA testing if babesiosis is suspected, but the antibody titer is negative.

Typical treatment: I often rotate combinations of different antibiotics with antimalarial drugs and herbs.

Example: *Clindamycin* (Cleocin) combined with *atovaquone* (Mepron) and *azithromycin* (Zithromax) and/or *sulfamethoxazole/trimethoprim* (Septra) with the herbs artemisia and cryptolepis. I have found these regimens help reduce Babesia symptoms.

Also helpful: Curcumin, the yellow plant pigment in the spice turmeric. It reduces inflammation that may be caused by babesiosis as well as Lyme disease. If you want to try a curcumin supplement, follow label directions.

• **Ehrlichiosis/Anaplasmosis.** This is a bacterial infection that typically causes a high fever accompanied by severe headaches, muscle pain and fatigue. It's among the most common coinfections found in Lyme patients.

How it's diagnosed: Antibody blood tests help to diagnose ehrlichiosis/anaplasmosis, but a low white blood cell count, low platelet count and elevated liver enzymes are also signs that the infection is present.

Typical treatment: Doxycycline or other tetracycline antibiotics.

• **Bartonella.** Also known as cat scratch disease, this bacterial illness was once thought to be transmitted to people only from cat scratches or bites. It is now known that *Bartonella* also can be spread by ticks, fleas and biting flies.

A classic *Bartonella* infection usually causes a rash or papule (a small, red, raised bump on the skin), along with swelling of the lymph nodes, but patients who also have Lyme-MSIDS usually have more intense symptoms. For example, they may not have a rash but could experience seizures and severe nerve pain, burning, tingling or numbness as well as severe memory and concentration problems.

How it's diagnosed: Antibody blood tests as well as DNA and RNA testing.

Typical treatment: Doxycycline, combined with rifampin or other medications such as a quinolone antibiotic like Cipro.

ACT QUICKLY

The majority of patients with Lyme disease will recover completely—and quickly—when they take antibiotics within two to four weeks after a bite from an infected tick.

If you do not get better within a month after taking antibiotics, and the additional testing shows that you do not have a tick-borne coinfection, it's possible that blood tests missed the infection, you have one or more other tick-borne coinfections and/or you're still infected with the Lyme bacterium and need further treatment.

Helpful: Because inflammation can cause —or increase—the symptoms of Lyme and other tick-borne infections, *I often advise patients to take* small doses of *naltrexone* (ReVia). This prescription medication, which is also used for alcohol/opiate dependency, reduces inflammation and helps regulate an overstimulated immune system.

Naltrexone can be combined with over-the-counter anti-inflammatory supplements, including the antioxidant glutathione (liposomal is best for absorption), which helps reduce fatigue and pain, and green tea extract and resveratrol.

SIX QUESTIONS: A NEW WAY TO UNCOVER CHRONIC LYME

Chronic Lyme, which can occur months or even years after infection—often mimicking other chronic diseases such as lupus, fibromyalgia and chronic fatigue—is much harder to diagnose than early Lyme. To improve the odds, I have developed a new questionnaire that checks for six signs and symptoms. The questionnaire is based on a recently validated research study, which is being prepared for publication.

You don't need to have all six markers, but the more that you answer "yes" to, the more likely you are to have Lyme—and should get checked out. *Here they are...*

- **Do you have many different symptoms?** You may have a cluster of symptoms, such as fatigue, joint and muscle pain, headaches, memory problems, poor concentration, mood or sleep disorders.
- **Do your symptoms come and go with no obvious cause?**
- **If you have muscle, joint and/or nerve pain, does it migrate around your body—it could be in your shoulder one day, your knees the next?** (If only your knees ache, for example, it's not necessarily caused by Lyme.)
- **If you're a woman in your child-bearing years, do your symptoms worsen around your period?** For example, while it's normal for any woman to get headaches and mood swings around her period, it's unusual to experience significant increases in fatigue, joint/muscle pain, insomnia and memory/concentration problems around your period.
- **If you've recently taken antibiotics—whether for Lyme or an unrelated infection—did your symptoms get much better or worse?** (With Lyme, antibiotics can make symptoms worse temporarily.)
- **Have you ever had a positive blood test for Lyme or an associated tick-borne infection?** Have you had Lyme (borrelia) specific bands on a Western blot (i.e., 23, 31, 34, 39, 83/93 proteins) indicating exposure? Even if you were treated and declared "Lyme-free," this could be a clue, because Lyme can "hide" in some people after antibiotic treatment.

THE BEST DEFENSE

The new range and infectiousness of deer ticks means it's more important than ever to protect yourself when you're in tick-infested areas. Wear long clothes when you can, apply insect repellent, and when you come inside for the day, take a shower and do a full-body tick check. If you see a tick, remove it with tweezers and a magnifying glass—try to get underneath it and pull it out straight up (don't twist it).

Can a Common Foot Infection Kill You?

Yi Hung Chan, DPM, podiatrist in private practice, West Orange, New Jersey, and lead acupuncturist at Memorial Sloan Kettering Cancer Hospital, New York City.

According to the American College of Foot and Ankle Surgeons, MRSA (methicillin-resistant staphylococcus aureus) infection is an increasing threat among people with foot problems—problems that seem only annoying rather than dangerous. Other common foot conditions that can lead to MRSA infection include dry, cracked skin on the heels (especially in these cold winter months), eczema, psoriasis and athlete's foot.

BLOCK THAT BACTERIA

As you may already know, MRSA is now extremely common in our environment and exists on the skin of about one-third of the population. It becomes harmful only when a break in the skin provides an opportunity for it to enter the bloodstream. But then it can be very harmful, leading to blood-borne infections, multiple organ failure and even death. Therefore, if you have any foot injury or irritation, act immediately to prevent bacteria from entering via a break in the skin.

Treat any problems affecting the skin on your feet by washing with soap and water or, at least, rinsing the area thoroughly with running water as soon as you can, using whatever is most accessible—for instance, if you're hiking and get a blister, pour bottled drinking water on it if nothing else is available. This will remove any MRSA-infested debris that might have entered the area. For further protection, use Bacitracin and cover with a bandage for several days until the skin closes over.

What's even more challenging about the feet is that an infection also can begin in a place where you aren't aware of a skin break, such as in a callus or corn. It's crucial, therefore, to be vigilant about any symptoms of infection. *Be alert to these signs that may indicate an infected foot...*

- **Redness in the area**
- **Swelling**
- **Skin that feels warm to the touch**
- **Pain**
- **Pus**
- **Fever**
- **Difficulty moving,** such as a toe that won't wiggle as usual.

Any of these symptoms may indicate that treatment is needed right away, since MRSA and many other infections can move very fast. Call your doctor, and if you cannot get in that day, go to an urgent-care center or, if no other option is available, the ER. The area will be drained by a health-care professional who may also give you a prescription for antibiotics. Tread carefully...MRSA is a serious matter.

Skin Infections That Are Often Overlooked

Lawrence Eron, MD, associate professor of medicine at the John A. Burns School of Medicine at the University of Hawaii in Honolulu and infectious disease consultant at Kaiser Foundation Hospital, also in Honolulu.

The dangers associated with the highly drug-resistant, sometimes fatal "superbug" known as MRSA (*methicillin-resistant Staphylococcus aureus*) have been widely publicized.

MRSA, once a threat primarily in hospitals, long-term-care facilities and other health-care settings, is now appearing in a slightly mutated form in gyms, schools, military barracks and other settings where people may have skin-to-skin contact and/or share towels, linens or other items that can become contaminated. MRSA may turn life-threatening if the bacteria penetrate the skin, become blood-borne and reach other areas of the body, such as the heart or lungs.

What most people don't realize: The skin can harbor dozens of infectious organisms.

Example: The average handprint on a dinner plate might contain up to 35 species of bacteria, viruses or fungi.

Most of these organisms are harmless—and even those that are capable of causing disease are usually blocked from entering the body by the skin's protective barrier and/or destroyed by immune cells just beneath the skin's surface.

Danger: The skin typically has thousands of microscopic nicks or other openings that provide entry points for harmful germs—even if you don't have an obvious cut. To help prevent harmful bacteria from entering these tiny openings, wash your hands often with mild soap and warm water, and shave carefully. *Infections to avoid...**

CELLULITIS

This skin infection, which can be mistaken for a scrape, bruise or spider bite, is caused by bacteria that enter the body through dry, flaky and/or cracked skin or other skin openings such as those caused by a cut, splinter or surgical wound.

Cellulitis typically occurs on the legs but can occur anywhere on the body—even on your hand. The infection usually originates in the upper layers (the dermis and epidermis) of the skin but can also occur in deeper (subcutaneous) tissues, including the muscles and muscle linings. Infections in deeper tissues are more likely to cause serious symptoms and extensive tissue damage, such as severe swelling and pain, and formation of abscesses. Everyone is at risk for cellulitis, but those with weakened immunity (such as diabetes and dialysis patients) are at greatest risk.

What to look for: The affected area will be red, hot and tender. The redness spreads very quickly, and you may develop a fever (101°F or higher) and body aches. If the infection is severe, confusion or fecal incontinence also may occur. People with any of the severe symptoms described earlier should seek immediate medical care at a hospital emergency department.

Treatment: Oral antibiotics, such as *dicloxacillin* (Dycill) or *cephalexin* (Keflex). These are effective against Streptococcus and about half of the Staphylococcus organisms—common causes of cellulitis—and usually start to relieve symptoms within two days. Patients with more severe infections may require hospitalization and intravenous antibiotics.

To reduce your risk of developing cellulitis: Take a daily shower or bath. People who wash often and use plenty of mild soap are less likely to develop cellulitis or other skin infections.

NECROTIZING INFECTIONS

The media often refer to these infections as "flesh-eating." This isn't entirely accurate. Several bacterial species can cause the necrosis (death) of infected tissue, but the bacteria don't eat the flesh, per se. Rather, they secrete toxins that break it down.

Necrotizing infections are rare—fewer than 1,000 cases occur each year in the US—but the fatality rate is quite high at 25% to 30%. These infections spread very rapidly—if you marked the edge of an infection with a pen, you might see the redness creep past the mark in as little as one hour.

What to look for: Skin redness and/or swelling that's warm to the touch. The initial infection, which can follow even a minor cut or puncture wound, resembles cellulitis. But a necrotizing infection is far more painful. As the infection progresses, you may develop very large, fluid-filled purple blisters (bullae), a high fever (104°F or higher), disorientation and a rapid heartbeat. If you develop any of these symptoms, seek immediate medical attention at a hospital emergency department.

Treatment: Intravenous antibiotics and surgery, sometimes requiring amputation, to remove infected tissue.

To reduce your risk of developing a necrotizing infection: Thoroughly clean even minor cuts and scrapes. Apply an over-the-counter antibiotic ointment, such as Neosporin or bacitracin, and keep the area covered with a clean dressing until the area is completely healed.

*To see examples of the many ways these infections can appear on the body, go to Images.google.com and type in the name of each infection. *Beware*: Many of the images are graphic.

FOLLICULITIS

This skin infection occurs at the root of a hair (follicle) and may produce a small pimple—or, less often, a larger, more painful pimple called a boil. Folliculitis tends to be more common in people with diabetes (which reduces resistance to infection) and those who live in hot, humid climates (excessive perspiration promotes growth of the bacterium that causes folliculitis).

What to look for: A small, white pimple at the base of a hair. Boils, also called abscesses, are larger than pimples (sometimes an inch or more in diameter), with a greater volume of pus. They tend to be warmer than the surrounding skin and can be intensely painful.

Treatment: The small pimples caused by folliculitis often disappear on their own within several days. Applying a topical antibiotic several times a day can prevent the infection from spreading. Apply a warm, moist compress (for 15 minutes four times daily for one to two days) to tender pimples or boils to help them drain.

Painful or unusually large boils should be lanced, drained and cleaned by a doctor. Do not "pop" them yourself. The risk for infection is high—and boils can be caused by MRSA. Antibiotics usually aren't necessary when boils are professionally drained and cleaned.

To reduce your risk of developing folliculitis: Wash your hands several times daily with soap...and take a daily shower or bath. If you have chronic, recurrent boils, use antibacterial soap.

Natural Infection-Fighters

Steven Sandberg-Lewis, ND, naturopathic physician and diplomat of the Homeopathic Academy of Naturopathic Physicians. He is author of *Functional Gastroenterology.*

Antibiotics enable millions of people to survive infections that used to be fatal. However, the widespread use of these drugs has increasingly led to antibiotic resistance—some harmful organisms can keep making people sick even when treated with the newest, most powerful antibiotics.

Little-known fact: Because the immune system of a healthy adult is quite effective at eliminating many types of bacteria, viruses and fungi, many infections can be successfully treated with natural products that strengthen immunity and fight microorganisms.

Important: Always see a doctor if the affected area is becoming more inflamed... seems to be spreading...is accompanied by a fever...or is not improving.

Conditions that typically improve within 24 to 48 hours when treated with natural antimicrobial agents (unless indicated otherwise, all can be found in health-food stores)...*

BRONCHITIS

Bronchitis is inflammation of the lining of the bronchial tubes, which carry air to the lungs. Acute bronchitis is usually due to a virus and often develops in conjunction with a cold or some other upper-respiratory tract ailment.

Natural treatment: Add 10 drops of liquid allicin (an active antibacterial and antiviral compound in garlic) to the reservoir of a portable nebulizer (a device that converts liquid into a fine mist that can be inhaled). Breathe the mist until all of the extract is gone. Repeat the treatment once or twice a day until the infection is gone.

Also helpful: Take eight (180 mg) capsules daily of Allimax, fresh-garlic supplements that can shorten the duration of the illness.

SORE THROAT

Most sore throats are caused by viruses, such as those that also cause the common cold or flu.

Natural treatment: Perform a yoga exercise known as the Lion Pose to increase blood and lymph circulation at the back of the tongue. This movement promotes the migration of immune cells to the area to help fight the infection.

**Caution*: If you have an allergy to a particular natural substance (such as garlic), do not use a remedy that contains the substance.

What to do: Stick out your tongue as far as it will go, and hold it there for three to four seconds. Repeat the movement five or six times daily until your sore throat is gone.

Also helpful: Most people know that gargling with saltwater helps ease sore throat pain.

For better results: Add a few drops of bitter orange oil to a mixture of one-quarter teaspoon salt and one-half cup warm water to help kill bacteria, including some organisms that cause strep throat.

Important: Use a "bass voice" when you gargle the mixture (every few waking hours). The lower-pitched gargling sound causes more of the solution to get into the throat.

SINUSITIS

Infections of the sinus cavities typically cause headache, facial pain or pressure and a loss of smell and taste. Antibiotics can help in some cases, but most sinus infections are caused by organisms, such as viruses or fungi, that aren't killed by antibiotics.

Natural treatment: N-acetylcysteine (NAC), an amino acid that promotes the drainage of mucus and mobilizes infection-fighting white blood cells.

Typical dose: 600 mg, three times daily.

EAR INFECTION

Several studies in children show that most ear infections don't require antibiotics. It's likely that the same is true for adults, particularly for infections affecting the ear canal (swimmer's ear).

Natural treatment for swimmer's ear: Use a clean bulb syringe or eyedropper to administer three to five drops daily of a 50-50 mixture of distilled water and hydrogen peroxide, followed by three to five drops of a 50-50 solution of white vinegar and distilled water.

Also helpful: A combination supplement that includes echinacea, goldenseal and berberis (such as Source Naturals' Wellness Formula), along with a multisupplement containing bioflavonoids, zinc and vitamins C and A. Follow the dosage instructions on the label.

Important: Patients who get frequent ear infections should try eliminating dairy and bananas from their diet. These foods are believed to lead to the production of thicker-than-normal mucus that inhibits normal ear drainage.

Best Ways to Prevent Hospital Infections

Charles B. Inlander, consumer advocate and health-care consultant based in Fogelsville, Pennsylvania. He is the author of 20 books, including *Take This Book to the Hospital With You: A Consumer Guide to Surviving Your Hospital Stay.*

We all know that infection is a very real risk during a hospital stay. And the numbers are staggering—at least 1.7 million Americans develop a hospital-acquired infection each year, and 99,000 people die from it. But aside from being vigilant about asking medical staff to wash their hands, is there really anything a patient can do to prevent infection? Absolutely! *There are several additional—and, in some cases, surprising—approaches...*

- **Start the conversation.** Many doctors never raise the subject of hospital-acquired infection unless the patient brings it up. So, bring it up! Ask your doctor what the overall infection rate is at the hospital where you are going to be treated. If he/she doesn't know, call the facility and ask for the infection control officer (required at every hospital). The infection rate should be below 6%. If it's above that, talk to your doctor about using a different hospital. But keep in mind that your overall medical status is an important factor. For example, people with diabetes are at higher risk for postsurgical infections.

My advice: If you are being hospitalized for a specific health problem, be sure that your doctor is aware of any other medical conditions you may have.

- **Beware of certain procedures.** Research shows that certain procedures have relatively high risks for infection. For example, close to 10% of colorectal surgical patients develop surgical site infections (at the incision). But studies have found that, in some cases, wearing special surgical blankets and hats before—and sometimes during—surgery can help your body fight infection.

My advice: Ask your doctor about steps that can be taken to keep you warm during surgery and/or when you are given IVs.

- **Check out the latest research.** Numerous medical studies have been published on just about all medical procedures. And most discuss infection risk.

My advice: Ask your doctor to discuss what the studies show are the infection risks associated with your procedure. Also ask about infection risks for other procedures that might be appropriate. For example, an open surgical gallbladder removal has a higher infection risk than laparoscopic gallbladder removal.

- **Be alert at home.** Many infections do not become apparent until after you get home. An infection may also be contracted when a nurse or other health-care provider administers care in your home.

My advice: Be watchful for signs of infection, including increasing tenderness, redness or pus at an incision site, unexplained fever or internal pain that was unexpected in the course of your healing. When in doubt, immediately call your doctor.

Childhood Virus Now Targeting Adults

Daniel P. Kelly, MD, pediatrician, Pacific Pediatrics Medical Group, San Francisco.

A virus that normally makes the rounds at day-care centers, preschools and playgrounds during the summer is behaving differently this time around.

Hand, foot and mouth disease (HFMD)—sometimes called coxsackie A16—has been around since about the mid-1900s.

But a new variant of this virus, called coxsackie A6, started hitting the US in 2008...and has entered the news recently with reports of professional atheletes contracting the disease.

The worst part is that the symptoms are more severe than ever before.

Do you know what these symptoms are?

A NEW KIND OF VIRUS

The original A16 virus typically hits children under age five, causing a slight fever, a blister-like rash on the hands and feet and painful sores inside the mouth. These symptoms are usually treatable, and the virus is not considered deadly, plus it can be so mild that many kids who carry it never even have symptoms. (On very rare occasions, it can develop into a serious health problem, such as viral meningitis, myocarditis or encephalitis.) For these reasons, the Centers for Disease Control and Prevention (CDC) hasn't tracked A16.

But in 2008, physicians in Alabama, California, Connecticut and Nevada noticed an illness that resembled HFMD but was affecting people of all ages—with more severe symptoms. The CDC confirmed that the illness was being caused by coxsackie A6, a variant that was reported in Finland and in Japan several years prior. Subsequently, the virus has been identified all over the US, according to the CDC.

To find out more about this awful-sounding virus, we spoke with Daniel P. Kelly, MD, a pediatrician in San Francisco, who was among those first to report cases to the CDC.

AN ANGRIER RASH

So what makes A6 different from A16? For one thing, it's affecting adults and not just children. In his first 25 years of practice, Dr. Kelly saw perhaps three parents catch coxsackie from their children, but over a span of about six months, he has seen at least a dozen such cases—all from this more recent strain.

The A6 virus has not proven deadly, but the symptoms can be severe. Fevers can go higher (up to about 104°F, as opposed to just 101°F with the A16 virus), which can lead to even more dehydration. In rare cases, fingernails and toenails can become separated from the nail beds and fall off. The rashes are considered worse (and more painful) because they can spread out more over the body, affecting the face, arms, legs, buttocks and, specifically, the diaper area for younger children and the back of the knees in people with eczema. No matter which version of the virus you have, the fever tends to last anywhere from one to three days and the rash usually lasts about a week.

MORE MUST-KNOW INFO ABOUT A6

Frequently asked questions...

How is the new version of hand, foot and mouth disease diagnosed?

Although blood tests or throat swabs can detect both the A16 and the A6 virus for sure, those are often expensive and it can take two weeks to get the results. So the diagnosis often is made on the appearance of the telltale blistery rash and where it is located on the body.

How does it spread?

The virus moves from person to person by contact with discharge from the nose or throat, fluid from the blisters or feces. The virus can sometimes remain in the body for weeks after symptoms have gone away, and that's one reason why the virus is so widespread.

How can I protect myself—especially if my child or grandchild gets it?

There are no vaccines to prevent contracting the virus, but you can reduce your chances of infection by avoiding contact with infected people and by washing your hands frequently.

How is it treated?

There is no way to stop the progression of the disease once you've got it—only time and your immune system can do that—but doctors can provide treatments that relieve the pain of the sores, control the fever and help you stay hydrated.

If you (or your grandchild or child) develop symptoms, see a doctor for a diagnosis. It's important to know whether what you have is coxsackie so you can properly treat symptoms and also try not to infect others.

Sudden Rheumatoid Arthritis Symptoms? It Might Be Chikungunya Virus

Jonathan J. Miner, MD, PhD, fellow, rheumatology division, Washington University School of Medicine, St. Louis.

You may not yet have heard of chikungunya virus. It was nonexistent in the Western hemisphere until December 2013, but since then, more than one million cases have been reported, mostly in the Caribbean and South and Central America—and it's here in the US as well. The virus, which is transmitted by mosquitos, can cause symptoms that mimic rheumatoid arthritis—and those symptoms can last for months to years. Plus, treating the infection as if it were rheumatoid arthritis might do more harm than good! Here's what you need to know about this viral threat—and how to tell whether your "arthritis" might actually be a case of chikungunya infection...

RHEUMATOID ARTHRITIS OR CHIKUNGUNYA?

Chikungunya virus, often referred to as "CHIKV," is not a lethal illness. The most common symptoms are joint pain and fever. Symptoms can also include headache, joint swelling and muscle pain in the first seven to 10 days of infection. In most people, the more severe symptoms, such as flu-like fever and achiness, last for about a week or so and pass. But joint symptoms in particular can persist for 12 to 15 months in up to 60% of those infected and up to three years for some.

As mentioned, some CHIKV symptoms, such as joint achiness and swelling, are similar to those of—and easily confused with—rheumatoid arthritis. But unlike rheumatoid arthritis, with CHIKV, joint pain and inflammation occur very suddenly, in the same way flu symptoms occur, in many joints all at once instead of gradually over months or years.

HOW IT GOT HERE

First described in Tanzania in the 1950s, CHIKV spread from Africa to Asia and Europe before hitting the Caribbean and South America and, ultimately, the United States. Most of the nearly 2,500 reported cases in the United States in 2014 were linked to travel to other affected areas, but 11 cases were reported in nontravelers in Florida. This means that mosquitos in parts of the southern United States are now carrying the virus.

The only factor currently limiting the virus's spread in the US is the main type of mosquito that is, so far, carrying the virus—an insect known as the yellow fever mosquito. It is native to the Caribbean, Florida, the Gulf Coast and parts of Texas. According to the CDC, the virus is now also carried by the Asian tiger mosquito, found throughout much of the continental United States, so the number of cases might eventually rival that of West Nile virus, which caused a panic about a decade ago.

Proper diagnosis hinges on giving your doctor appropriate details about your symptoms and travels, such as whether your joint pain and swelling developed slowly over several months...or developed after traveling to places where the virus is actively spreading, such as the Caribbean. If you only visited places such as Canada or most of the United States where CHIKV outbreaks are rare or have not yet occurred, infection is very unlikely, he said.

The problem is that CHIKV, generally speaking, has not necessarily been on an American rheumatologist's radar, which is why you ought to be well informed about it. A rheumatologist might treat the joint symptoms of CHIKV in the same way as rheumatoid arthritis—with immunosuppressive drugs. This may not be so bad when the residual symptoms of joint pain and swelling persist after the body has otherwise fought off the viral infection, but such treatment will thwart your body's natural efforts to fight off the virus during the early stages of infection. And your body's natural efforts are all you've got...there is no medical remedy for CHIKV infection.

Treatment is similar to that of the flu bug, according to the US Centers for Disease Control and Prevention: Get plenty of rest, drink fluids to prevent dehydration and take aspirin, ibuprofen, naproxen or acetaminophen for pain and fever relief.

During the first week of infection, levels of the virus are high in the blood. This is when the body's immune response is extremely important. It has to be allowed to fight off the virus. It's fair to say, therefore, that taking immunosuppressive drugs when symptoms first appear is likely to be dangerous.

In fact, people with weakened immune systems, including infants, people older than 65 and people who have serious medical conditions, such as high blood pressure, heart disease or diabetes, are known to be at greater risk for more severe and prolonged symptoms from CHIKV. And if you already have arthritis, the virus may worsen your condition. On the up side, if you've been infected with CHIKV, your body becomes immune to reinfection if you should happen to again be bitten by an infected mosquito.

SAFE TRAVELS

In addition to keeping yourself protected from mosquitoes (wearing repellent and protective covering), keep abreast of which travel areas are more affected than others. One Caribbean island may be having more of an outbreak than another at any given time. You can find up-to-date information on the number of CHIKV cases by region on the websites of the the Centers for Disease Control and Prevention (CDC.gov) and the Pan American Health Organization (PAHO.org).

CHAPTER 13

Injuries and Surgical Pain

The Secret to Preventing Falls

Each year, about one in every three people over age 65 suffers a fall, a mishap that is far more dangerous than most people realize.

Important new research: In a 20-year study of nearly 5,600 women ages 70 and older, breaking a hip doubled the risk for death in the following year. Men who suffer a broken hip after a fall are also at increased risk for an untimely death.

Most people know the standard recommendations to reduce their risk for falls—get medical attention for balance and vision problems...improve the lighting in and around their homes...and eliminate loose carpets, cords and other obstacles.

What often gets overlooked: Painful feet... foot deformities such as bunions...weak foot and ankle muscles...and improper footwear also can significantly increase one's risk for falls.

Recent scientific evidence: In a study in the *British Medical Journal*, a comprehensive program of foot care reduced falls by one-third among a group of older people with assorted foot problems.

GET A FIRM FOUNDATION

With age, the muscles that support our ankles and feet often become weak—a common problem that contributes to foot pain and reduced activity levels. Structural abnormalities in the feet, such as bunions and hammertoes, undermine stability. And conditions that blunt sensations in the feet, such as nerve damage commonly caused by diabetes, may impair the ability of one's feet to react quickly and adjust to potentially hazardous conditions.

Hylton Menz, PhD, deputy director of the Musculoskeletal Research Center at La Trobe University in Victoria, Australia. He is the author of the textbook *Foot Problems in Older People: Assessment and Management* and a coauthor of *Falls in Older People: Risk Factors and Strategies for Prevention.*

BASIC FALL-PREVENTION WORKOUT

Stretching and strengthening exercises can reduce foot pain—and lower your risk for falls. *Basic exercises to perform daily...*

To increase your ankles' range of motion: Sit in a chair with one knee extended. Rotate your foot in a clockwise, then counterclockwise direction. Repeat 10 times with each foot, in each direction.

To strengthen your toe muscles: Place small stones or marbles on the floor in front of you. While seated, pick up the stones with your bare toes and place them in a box, one by one. Pick up 20 stones with each foot, then repeat.

To stretch your calf muscles: Stand about two feet from a wall, then lean into it with one leg slightly bent at the knee about three inches in front of the other. Then reverse the position of your feet and lean forward to stretch the muscles of the other calf. Hold the stretch for 20 seconds, three times for each leg.

PROPER FOOTWEAR

The right shoes are essential for everyone, but especially those with problem feet.

Most women know to avoid high heels, which make it more difficult to maintain balance. But many people opt for flimsy slip-on footwear, such as flip-flops, which may be comfortable but often become loose or come off the foot altogether, creating a balance hazard. It's far better to wear shoes that fasten to your feet with laces, Velcro or buckled straps.

Surprising fact: Most people assume that thick, cushiony soles, such as those found on most sneakers, help prevent falls because they tend to provide good support for your feet. But thinner, harder soles, such as those on some walking shoes, are safer because thin-soled shoes allow your feet to feel the sensations that help you maintain balance. A trade-off between comfort and safety may be necessary—you may have to wear less cushiony shoes that optimize balance.

Also, be sure that your shoes are the right size. Your feet may slide around in shoes that are too loose, while tight footwear won't allow your toes to respond to variations in the ground to help maintain stability while walking.

Remember: Shoe size often changes with age, as feet swell and spread. So have your feet measured every time you buy shoes.

Slightly more falls occur indoors than outdoors, and the proportion increases with age. Therefore, even when you're at home, proper footwear is crucial.

Important recent finding: When researchers at Harvard's Institute for Aging Research followed a group of older adults for more than two years, they found that more than half of those who fell indoors were barefoot, in their stocking feet or wearing slippers. These injuries tended to be more serious than those of people who were wearing shoes when they fell.

Best to wear at home: Sturdy, thin-soled shoes that have more structural integrity than the average slipper.

DO YOU NEED ORTHOTICS?

Many adults over age 65 could benefit from wearing orthotics—inserts that fit inside the shoe—to help prevent falls by providing additional support.

Properly made orthotics may improve the way your feet move as you walk, distribute your weight more broadly to reduce pressure on sensitive spots and help convey sensory information to your feet, all of which may lessen the risk for falls.

If you have structural foot problems due to diabetes or rheumatoid arthritis, you may need customized orthotics from a podiatrist.

Typical cost: About $400. Insurance coverage varies. But over-the-counter versions (made with firm material, not just a soft cushion) may work as well if your feet are relatively normal and your foot pain is fairly mild. Good brands include Vasyli and Langer. Usually, you will be able to transfer orthotics between shoes.

Most people find that full-length orthotics are less likely to slip inside the shoe than the half-length variety. Full-length orthotics also may feel more comfortable, especially if you have corns or calluses under the toes or on the ball of your foot.

GETTING HELP

If you have foot problems, seek care from a podiatrist or other health professional—and be sure to mention any concerns about falling. Also ask for exercises, in addition to the ones described here, to address your specific foot issues.

Simple Ways to Improve Balance

See how long you can stand on one foot with your eyes closed, and work on improving your time. Rise up on your toes 10 times with your eyes open and then 10 more times with them closed. Balance yourself on one foot for 10 to 15 seconds, then switch legs. Repeat 10 times, then do it again with your eyes closed. Walk in a straight line, placing the heel of one foot in front of the toes of the other foot.

Caution: When doing these exercises, stand near a wall or some other support.

University of California, *Berkeley Wellness Letter,* BerkeleyWellness.com.

An Olympic Trainer's Secret To Improving Your Balance In Just 10 Minutes a Day

Joel Harper, personal trainer in New York City who designs workouts for Olympic athletes, celebrities, musicians and business executives. JoelHarperFitness.com. He is creator of the best-selling DVDs *Firming After 50* and *Slim & Fit.* He is also author of *Mind Your Body* and writes the "Your Personal Mind-Body Coach" blog at BottomLineInc.com.

Health experts have long advocated doing aerobic exercise and strength training on a regular basis, but a new type of activity is now being added to that prescription—balance training.

Startling statistic: Declining balance skills as people age are thought to be a major factor in the 450,000 hospitalizations that occur in the US each year due to falls. Research suggests that up to half of those falls could be prevented with the help of balance exercises.

Good news: Five easy exercises will begin to improve your balance, ankle flexibility, leg strength and overall agility—within days for many people. For best results, spend about 10 minutes performing these exercises every day. If the basic exercises seem too easy, try the advanced versions.

BETTER BALANCE WORKOUT

You can strengthen all the key muscles that are critical to your overall sense of balance by simply using the force of your body weight.

When beginning these exercises, stand next to a sturdy chair for added support when necessary. Keep your stomach taut throughout, pretending there's a string pulling up from the top of your head and lengthening your spine. This helps center your body and engages and strengthens your stabilizer muscles (which support your trunk, limit movement in joints and control balance). Be sure to breathe naturally rather than holding your breath, which can throw off your balance. Also, it's ideal to do the exercises barefoot in order to use the muscles in your feet.

Note: These exercises, designed by leading fitness expert and Olympic trainer Joel Harper, are unique in that they help decrease the imbalance that most of us have—we all carry more tension in one side of our bodies—but also simultaneously strengthen the muscles that support our skeletal structure.*

- **The Hippie**

Purpose: Stretches hips and hamstrings (that run along the back of the thighs).

What to do: Stand with your feet together and bend forward at your waist as far as you comfortably can. Let your arms hang down. If your lower back is stiff or your hamstrings are tight, place your hands on your hips instead of letting them hang down. Let your head hang down to help release tension.

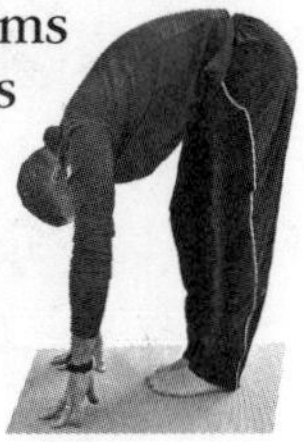

*Consult your doctor before starting this or any other exercise program.

Next, alternate bending one knee slightly for 15 seconds while keeping the other leg straight (keeping both feet flat). Perform a total of three bends per leg. If you feel lightheaded from the blood rushing to your head from this position, put your hands on the ground and look straight ahead.

- **Quad Sways**

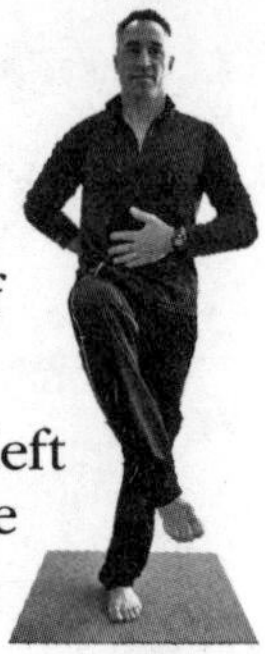

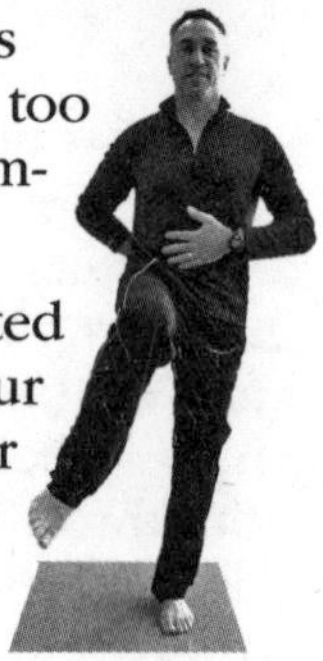

Purpose: Strengthens your core (abdominal and back muscles) and quadriceps (located at the front of the thighs).

What to do: Stand with your left palm flat on your stomach and the top of your right hand on your lower back. Next, lift your right knee in front of you until your thigh is parallel to the floor—if this is too hard, simply go as high as you comfortably can.

While keeping your chest lifted and your stomach pulled in, let your ankle dangle down and sway your lower leg from your knee to your foot from side to side 20 times. Switch legs and repeat.

Advanced version: Do this with your eyes closed.

- **TightRope**

Purpose: Improves mental focus. For this exercise, use a stretched-out, 10-foot string or some other straight line on the floor that you can easily feel and follow with your bare feet, such as a line of tile grout.

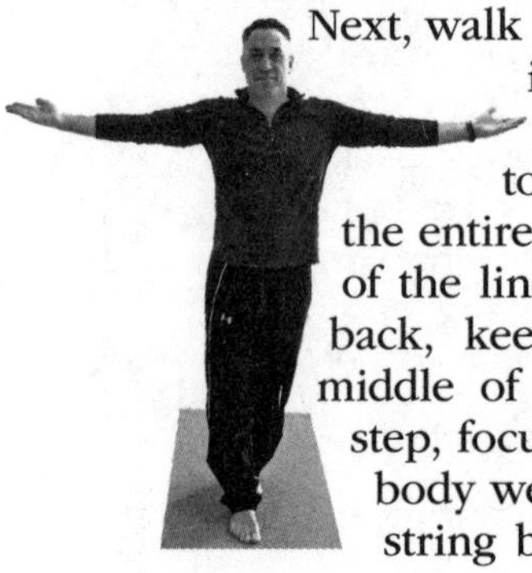

What to do: Stand with arms out to your sides at shoulder height, palms up. Next, walk along the line, imagining that you're walking along a tightrope. Try to look straight ahead the entire time. Walk to the end of the line, then turn and walk back, keeping the line in the middle of your feet. With each step, focus on not shifting your body weight until you feel the string below your foot. Don't move forward until you are centered on the line. Do five times.

Advanced version: Perform the exercise walking backward or with your eyes closed.

- **North and South**

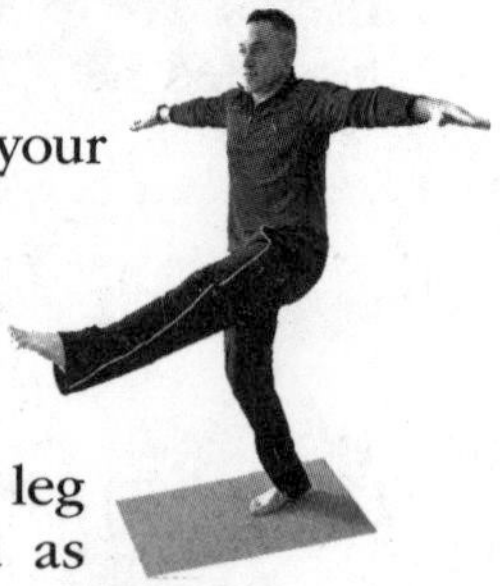

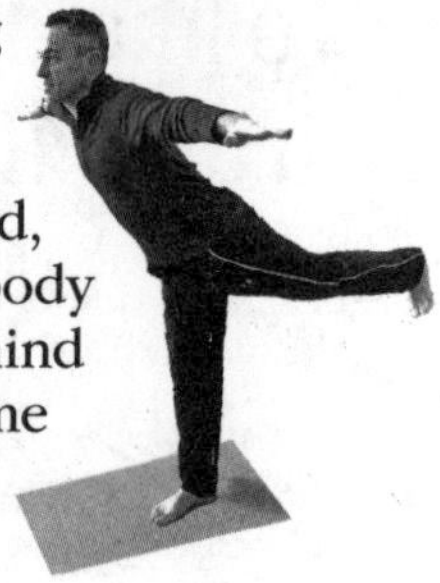

Purpose: Strengthens your legs and core.

What to do: With your arms out to your sides at shoulder height and palms facing down, lift your left leg in front of you as far and as high as you can while holding it straight and keeping your toes pointed forward. Next, without touching the ground, sweep your leg under your body and extend it straight back behind you as high as you can, this time with your foot flexed (your toe pulled in toward your knee). Do 10 times. Then switch legs and repeat.

Advanced version: Reach out your arms and hands at shoulder height directly in front of you while simultaneously reaching your leg directly behind you. Switch directions. Aim to be horizontal while balancing on your supporting leg.

- **Floating Chair**

Purpose: Strengthens lower abdominals, hip flexors (muscles that bring the legs and trunk together in flexion movement) and quadriceps.

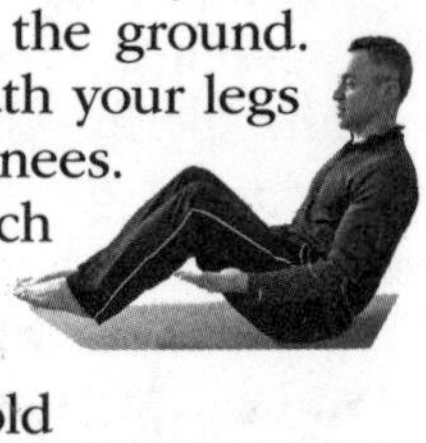

What to do: Sit on the floor with your knees bent and your feet flat on the ground. Place your hands underneath your legs behind the backs of your knees. Next, pull in your stomach and lift your feet off the ground so that you're balanced on your buttocks. Hold for 30 seconds, keeping your back straight and breathing normally.

Advanced version: Perform this exercise with your palms facing up, one inch from the sides of your knees.

Attack the Pain ASAP

Julie K. Silver, MD, assistant professor in the department of physical medicine and rehabilitation at Harvard Medical School, Boston. She is author of *Super Healing: The Clinically Proven Plan to Maximize Recovery from Illness or Injury.*

Injury patients who experience high levels of pain have impaired immunity and more stress. Pain also interferes with sleep, which can further delay healing.

Patients should never tolerate excessive pain. Most doctors aren't trained in sophisticated pain-management techniques, so you may want to see a pain-management specialist (ask your doctor for a referral)...or get a second opinion if you feel your complaints about pain aren't being addressed.

Don't get "behind" the pain. Pain-killing drugs, including mild analgesics such as ibuprofen, are far more effective when taken at the first signs of pain or even before pain starts. They're less effective once pain is under way.

Helpful: Take analgesics in the morning. Patients who treat their pain early in the day tend to get better relief—and often require less medication.

Natural Ways to Feel Much Better After a Fall...

Jamison Starbuck, ND, naturopathic physician in family practice and a guest lecturer at the University of Montana, both in Missoula. She is past president of the American Association of Naturopathic Physicians and a contributing editor to *The Alternative Advisor: The Complete Guide to Natural Therapies and Alternative Treatments.*

Even if you aren't badly hurt, falls are scary. Our inner protective mechanisms become hypervigilant—our muscles become tense and we hold ourselves more rigidly. We also struggle with a lingering sense of unease and begin to mistrust our ability to safely do everyday activities. When a patient falls, I perform a thorough exam to rule out a concussion and possibly order an X-ray to check for fractures. I also treat the patient's nervous system. In addition to the use of ice to treat an injury for the first 48 hours, followed by heat and painkillers, if needed, I've found that natural medicine can help people avoid lasting problems from falls. *My favorite approaches...**

- **Use natural remedies.** Arnica is a well-known homeopathic remedy that is used topically for physical trauma. Arnica lotion, for example, can be applied to bruises or sprains several times a day until they are healed. Along with arnica, I recommend using homeopathic aconite, a remedy that is excellent in treating the fright that follows sudden, violent accidents. Aconite is best taken within 48 hours of a fall. I typically recommend one dose (two pellets of aconite 30C) taken under the tongue. If 24 hours after taking Aconite you remain anxious or scared about your fall, repeat the same dose once a day for up to a week.
- **Try nervine herbs.** Chamomile, valerian and hops are plant medicines that calm the nervous system and help the body recover from a fall by promoting rest and muscle relaxation. Take these herbs alone or in combination in tea or tincture form.

Typical dose for a single herb or mixture: Drink 10 ounces of tea three times a day or take 60 drops of tincture in one ounce of water three times a day for up to two weeks.

- **Get plenty of rest.** Soaking in a warm bath with Epsom salts relaxes muscles and helps you get a good night's sleep. Until you have fully recovered from the fall, it also helps to take 150 mg of magnesium citrate (the form most easily absorbed) twice daily. This mineral promotes relaxation.
- **Consider bodywork.** Soon after a fall, consider getting full-body massage or acupressure treatment several times. These therapies not only promote circulation and healing, but also help people regain trust in their bodies after a scary event.

Caution: If you hit your head, are bleeding significantly or suspect a fracture from a fall, get to a hospital emergency department. If you experience headache, vision changes,

*Check with your doctor first if you have a chronic condition or take medication.

dizziness, confusion, nausea, vomiting or a balance problem (even days after the fall), you may have a head injury and must seek immediate medical help.

You Could Have a Spinal Fracture and Not Know It…

Vinil Shah, MD, assistant professor of clinical radiology and associate program director of the neuroradiology fellowship program at University of California, San Francisco. Dr. Shah's areas of academic interest include assessing clinical outcomes of spine intervention.

Did you know that you can get a spinal fracture from simply stepping off a curb, sneezing, lifting a small pet or even just getting out of bed? Don't assume that an aching back means just a pulled muscle.

Fractures due to osteoporosis are much more common than many people realize. In fact, after age 50, one in two women and one in five men will have an osteoporosis-related fracture in their lifetimes.

The most common type of fracture linked to osteoporosis is a vertebral compression fracture (VCF)—a break in a vertebra of the spine. VCFs are more common than hip or wrist fractures…often are painful…and can lead to loss of height and a stooped back. So why do a shocking two-thirds of VCFs go undiagnosed and untreated?

Osteoporosis can weaken the bones so much that even routine activities or seemingly innocuous movements can cause a spinal fracture. Sudden, nonradiating pain ranging from mild to severe is typically the first sign. But the pain is often mistaken for arthritis or a pinched nerve. And because many people with osteoporosis don't even know they have it, VCFs simply aren't on their radar.

QUICK ACTION IS VITAL

An undiagnosed VCF will often heal on its own, with the pain diminishing in six to eight weeks. But you don't want this fracture to go undiagnosed! One VCF increases the risk for a subsequent VCF fivefold. And multiple fractures result in a loss of height and stooped posture. With each additional untreated VCF, the spine can get a few millimeters shorter. If the vertebrae in the upper back fracture and become wedge-shaped, the spine curves abnormally, causing kyphosis, a rounding of the back better known as a dowager's hump.

If you're a woman or man over age 50 or a postmenopausal woman under age 50 who is experiencing new, unexplained mild-to-severe midline back pain that doesn't go away in a day or two, you need to see a doctor. Your primary care physician will perform a physical exam to check for back tenderness and will likely order an X-ray to confirm the diagnosis, following up with a CT scan or MRI to evaluate the problem further. Your doctor will then advise you on the best treatment for your specific situation.

TREATING THE FRACTURE

If the pain and loss of function from a VCF are mild, conservative treatments are usually recommended…

- **A few days of bed rest.** VCF pain tends to worsen when sitting or standing and improves when lying down.
- **Pain relievers.** Over-the-counter pain relievers, such as *ibuprofen* (Advil) or *acetaminophen* (Tylenol), help reduce mild pain.
- **A hyperextension back brace.** Wearing a rigid hyperextension back brace for a few weeks can help relieve pain and improve function in some patients. Ask your doctor for guidance.
- **Physical therapy (PT).** PT helps strengthen back muscles and can improve posture and prevent the development of chronic pain. It also has a beneficial effect on bone mineral density in osteoporosis patients and may prevent future fractures.

Note: PT can be started once the patient's pain is under control.

Conservative treatment of a VCF is not recommended for more than a few weeks or for those with more severe pain or limited function. Prolonged bed rest may lead to loss of bone mass (up to 1% loss each week) and muscle strength (10% to 15% loss each week). Bed rest can also increase risk for blood clots and bed sores, and painkillers should only be used short term.

OTHER TREATMENTS

Patients whose pain doesn't resolve in two to three weeks with the treatments above may be candidates for a minimally invasive procedure called vertebroplasty. Guided by computed tomography and/or fluoroscopy (a continuous X-ray "movie"), the doctor injects bone cement into the fracture. The outpatient procedure takes about 45 minutes while the patient is typically conscious but sedated. The cement not only stabilizes the fractured vertebra, it also prevents nearby nerve endings from causing pain.

Studies show that 75% to 100% of patients enjoy good-to-moderate pain relief and increased mobility quickly after vertebroplasty, often the next day. The procedure usually doesn't restore much height loss, but it can prevent further height loss and additional fractures.

With kyphoplasty, a modification of vertebroplasty, a balloon is inflated in the fractured vertebra to create a cavity that is then filled with cement. This procedure may offer a better chance of restoring height loss. However, kyphoplasty is more expensive than vertebroplasty, and there is mixed data on its benefit over vertebroplasty.

In general, vertebroplasty and kyphoplasty are safe when done by an experienced doctor. Interventional radiologists and neuroradiologists often do these procedures. Look for a doctor who has experience in using image guidance for spine procedures. Like all invasive medical procedures, these treatments do have risks—such as infection or bleeding. And in rare cases, the cement can leak into the spinal canal, causing nerve compression, or travel into adjacent veins, which can lead to blood clots in the lungs or heart.

The best candidates for these procedures are patients who have pain of at least moderate intensity (rated a five or greater out of 10) that impacts their mobility and daily quality of life. Additionally, those who have fractures that have occurred recently (within a few months prior to the procedure) tend to have more success with vertebroplasty and kyphoplasty than those who have older fractures. The age of a fracture can be determined by an MRI.

PREVENTING FUTURE FRACTURES

Treating the underlying osteoporosis to help prevent future fractures is crucial. Ask your doctor for a bone mineral density test called a DXA (or DEXA)—this low-dose X-ray measures bone density in the hip and spine and can guide your physician in choosing the best course of action for your case. Options include prescription medications such as bisphosphonates (patients should weigh the risks versus benefits of these drugs with their doctors)...calcium and vitamin D supplementation...and weight-bearing exercise to improve bone strength and other exercises to build core strength. Multiple clinical trials have shown that early treatment of osteoporosis can increase bone mineral density by 5% to 15%, reducing vertebral fracture rates by 40% to 70%.

Little-Known Dangers Of Head Injury

Alex B. Valadka, MD, professor and vice-chair of the department of neurosurgery at the University of Texas, Houston, Health Science Center. He directs the neurotrauma services at Memorial Hermann Hospital, also in Houston, and has authored more than 100 papers on brain injury.

Each year, more than one-third of Americans over age 65 fall. Although hip fracture is a well-known consequence, few people are aware of the seriousness of a blow to the head.

Especially in older adults, a head injury—whether it occurs during a fall, a car accident or a sports activity—can trigger potentially deadly bleeding inside the skull. That's because the brain shrinks as we age, increasing tension on the bridging veins, which run from the brain's surface to its outer lining (dura). As a result, the bridging veins become more vulnerable to rupture. The situation is often worsened by the use of blood thinners, which are commonly prescribed to help prevent heart attack and stroke. An estimated 50,000 Americans die each year as a result of head injuries.

Caution: It can be difficult to determine the seriousness of a head injury from outward signs alone. For example, bleeding inside the skull may not cause symptoms until days, or even weeks, after the head injury occurred.

Red flags: Increasing sleepiness...a severe headache that keeps getting worse...confusion...difficulty walking...impaired memory...slurred speech...blurred vision...and/or vomiting.

Important: People who have suffered a minor head injury don't necessarily have to see a doctor—but they should get to an emergency room immediately if any of the above symptoms occur...even if it's days after the injury.

Main types of head injuries...

SKULL FRACTURES

A skull fracture is a break in the skeleton of the head (skull) and typically is caused by a fall or a car accident. A skull fracture is among the most dramatic-looking head injuries because it may be accompanied by copious external bleeding.

In most cases, however, a skull fracture isn't very serious as long as there isn't an accompanying brain injury and/or bleeding. In fact, a skull fracture may protect the brain. When the skull fractures during an accident, it absorbs part of the blow, and less of the trauma reaches the brain itself.

Physical signs of a skull fracture include bruises around the eyes (raccoon's eyes) or behind the ears, or the leaking of clear cerebrospinal fluid from the nose or ears.

Treatment: Many skull fractures heal on their own. Hospitalization may be required for overnight observation. Patients also may be given imaging tests, such as a computed tomography (CT) scan, to check for bleeding inside the skull.

CONCUSSION

A concussion is a head injury that does not cause visible physical damage and is often characterized by headache, confusion and/or amnesia. The brain damage that occurs—which is thought to involve disruptions in blood flow or nerve impulses, or temporary damage to axons (nerve fibers)—may not show up on CT scans or other imaging tests. Doctors rely on a medical history and the concussion symptoms listed above to make a diagnosis.

Most concussions are caused by a fall, car accident or athletic injury. Patients usually recover completely within a few hours—or, at most, a few days.

Treatment: Anyone with concussion symptoms following a blow to the head should get to an emergency room, especially if there is any loss of consciousness, confusion or memory loss.

The patient probably will be given a CT scan to check for bleeding in the skull or brain. If the test is normal—and most are—the patient will be advised to avoid strenuous physical activity, such as heavy lifting or climbing stairs, for a few days to aid healing of the brain. *Acetaminophen* (Tylenol) is prescribed for pain.

CONTUSIONS/LACERATIONS

Contusions (bruises) and lacerations (tears) of brain tissue are potentially more serious than a concussion. Both contusions and lacerations may be caused by a sudden blow to the head, which often occurs during a fall, physical assault or when the head moves very rapidly, causing the brain to hit the inside of the skull, such as often occurs in a car accident.

Symptoms may include severe headaches, dizziness, vomiting, irritability, agitation and/or confusion.

Minor contusions/lacerations usually clear up on their own within a few days.

Warning: Patients who experience severe, persistent headache, decreased alertness or consciousness, weakness in a limb, or one pupil larger than the other may have sustained a serious brain injury and should get immediate attention.

Treatment: Emergency surgery will probably be required if the CT or magnetic resonance imaging (MRI) scan shows significant bleeding/bruising, and the patient is also exhibiting the neurological symptoms described above. The surgeon will make an incision in the skull over the area of the injury. He/she will remove damaged brain tissue, along with any blood/fluids that may be present, to reduce brain swelling and pressure inside the skull.

INTRACRANIAL HEMATOMAS

An intracranial hematoma occurs when blood accumulates inside the brain, or in the area between the brain and the skull, due to an injury.

With a hematoma, the brain may be injured by the pressure caused by a blood accumulation (clot). This pressure can cause neurological problems, such as seizures, visual problems and/or weakness in a limb. Additional symptoms of an intracranial hematoma, including headache, loss of consciousness and one dilated pupil, are similar to those caused by other head injuries.

Treatment: Small hematomas, which can be detected by MRI or CT scans, often clear up on their own without subsequent treatment. Patients with larger hematomas, however, may require emergency surgery to stop bleeding and remove blood that could increase pressure on the brain.

Is It a Concussion?

Diane Roberts Stoler, EdD, neuropsychologist and board-certified health and sport psychologist with a private practice in Boxford, Massachusetts. A brain injury patient herself, she is coauthor, with Barbara Albers Hill, of *Coping with Concussion and Mild Traumatic Brain Injury*. DrDiane.com

With all the recent talk about football players suffering concussions that have caused permanent brain damage, you might think that these brain injuries occur only on sports fields.

But that's far from the truth. Anyone can suffer a concussion. More than 40% of concussions are caused by falls...and 14.3% by car accidents.

IS IT A CONCUSSION OR NOT?

You may assume that you don't have a concussion if you didn't "black out." In fact, a concussion may not cause a noticeable loss of consciousness. You're more apt to be dazed... unaware of where you are...or briefly confused.

Because injuries to the brain can feel minor even when they're life-threatening, I would advise anyone who's been in a car accident that caused significant head movement, taken a hard fall or been hit hard on the head to go to a hospital emergency department.

Doctors can usually diagnose a concussion in a few minutes. You'll be given a quick, in-office neurological exam to assess the degree—and location—of brain damage.

Examples: You might be asked to recite numbers backward and forward...and/or recall what the doctor just said. You will also be given tests to check your balance, reflexes, vision and hearing.

If you have acute symptoms—for example, severe headaches and/or repeated vomiting—you may be hospitalized for further tests, such as an MRI or a CT scan, which also check for conditions that are even more serious, such as hemorrhagic (bleeding) stroke or subdural hematoma (in which blood collects on the surface of the brain).

If these tests are inconclusive and your symptoms suggest a concussion, you can ask your doctor for a specialized test called diffusion tensor imaging. It's a type of MRI that can identify extremely small areas of nerve damage, blood clots or bleeding in the brain.

However, unless you are planning a personal injury or workers' comp claim, you probably don't need to prove your diagnosis with these imaging tests. If you have symptoms of a concussion, your doctor will probably advise you just to wait it out. Symptoms usually subside within six weeks.

LET YOUR BRAIN HEAL

If you suffer a concussion, getting enough rest—including mental rest—is crucial. Until you've recovered, use your television, computer and smartphone only when absolutely necessary and for no more than two hours a day for the first few weeks after a concussion.

Also important...

- **Focus on your sleep.** Many people who have had concussions complain that they sleep fitfully or sleep too little or too much.

To promote sleep: Go to bed and get up at the same time every day...avoid bright lights in your bedroom...and create a soothing atmosphere.

Helpful: Try Bach Flower Rescue Remedy, which promotes the calm and relaxation that's needed to heal the brain.

• **Soothe the inflammation.** Because the brain is inflamed after a concussion, avoid foods that promote inflammation, such as sugar and other refined carbs. Instead, eat plenty of anti-inflammatory foods, such as omega-3–rich salmon and sardines.

Also: Give up all alcohol while a concussion is healing because it can increase the severity of your symptoms.

You Have a Concussion, Do This Now

Study titled "Assessment of Follow-up Care After Emergency Department Presentation for Mild Traumatic Brain Injury and Concussion," by researchers at University of Southern California, Los Angeles, published in *JAMA Network Open*.

You know it as a concussion...doctors call it a mild traumatic brain injury (mTBI)—but don't let the "mild" in that diagnosis fool you into thinking you're free and clear after a knock to the head, even if doctors pronounced you "ok" at the ER. With any concussion, you could be left with symptoms that last weeks or months. Yes, getting checked out immediately is the right first step. But you need to follow up with your doctor—something only 44% of people who get concussions are doing—or you could suffer dangerous consequences. *Here's what should happen for your safety...*

While moderate and severe cases always receive close monitoring, usually in the hospital and possibly in the intensive care unit, doctors don't have a "best practices" protocol for people with mild concussions, and that means these patients may not be getting the care they need after they leave the emergency room. In fact, according to a recent study at the University of Southern California published in *JAMA Network Open*, among people who had mild concussions, did go to the ER for them and continued to experience three or more moderate-to-severe symptoms, only 52% went on to see their doctors about these symptoms. Only 42% of people who went to the ER for a concussion were even sent home with information to help them understand TBI.

WHAT SHOULD HAPPEN AFTER THE ER

A follow-up visit with a physician is key to know when you can safely go back to your normal routine and to make sure that your recovery is on track. Call your own doctor within a day to let him or her know what happened and schedule a visit. Experts at Weill Cornell Medicine suggest asking for physical and cognitive evaluations within a day or two of your injury whether or not you went to the ER—these evaluations can tell you whether you're experiencing any specific problems with thinking or motor skills, what treatment you might need, and when you can get back to everyday activities.

Rest and monitoring may be all you need at that point. Resting your body and brain will help most symptoms go away on their own. Rest is also needed to protect you from potentially catastrophic results if you get a second jolt to your head, because if this happens while your brain is healing, it could result in massive swelling and a life-threatening condition called second impact syndrome. (That's why, if a concussion might have occurred while you are playing a sport, you should never jump back in the game—nor allow a child to—until you've been cleared by doctors.)

If your symptoms don't go away within a week or two or if they get worse, you'll want to see a neurologist. This specialist will do a full assessment and talk to you about treatment for ongoing problems such as headaches, trouble sleeping, cognitive or emotional problems, vertigo and vision issues. For example, cognitive remediation therapy can help improve memory and attention, and rehabilitation with a physical or occupational therapist can help you work on balance. Without this care, daily life will stay challenging.

There was also some positive news in the study to keep in mind: People who initially went to a health-care facility with a TBI department—providers who specialize in concussions—had the best follow-up care. To find facilities near you, check the resource directory at Brainline.org or do an internet search for hospitals with a trauma or TBI department near you.

How to Help Your Brain Heal

Laurie Steelsmith, ND, naturopathic doctor and acupuncturist in private practice, Honolulu.

Don't make the mistake of thinking a brain injury is a problem only for those playing sports. The truth is that a concussion can be the result of banging your head on a piece of furniture, being in a minor car accident or even tripping over your dog in a dark hallway and bumping your head against the wall. About one million concussions occur in the US each year, according to reports of hospital admissions, and there are likely many more people who have them and don't seek help—in short, we're all at risk.

WHAT YOU NEED TO KNOW

First, it's important to review what we should know about concussion, which is like a bruise that results from your brain colliding with your skull. Anyone who has had a blow to the head should consider himself at risk, most especially if there was even a momentary loss of consciousness.

Other signs of concussion: Headache, nausea, difficulty concentrating and/or short-term memory loss. One or more of these symptoms should trigger a call to your doctor, who will determine if further testing is required. Naturopathic medicine can offer natural ways to help the tissues heal after a concussion and help relieve pain. *Here's a protocol...*

- **Load up on antioxidants.** Eat a healthy diet with abundant protein and also eat lots of blueberries during the two weeks following the injury.

The reason: Blueberries contain potent flavonoid antioxidants that help to strengthen blood vessel walls, including in the brain. Supplement the fruit's antioxidants by taking up to 3,000 mg a day of vitamin C, which also helps reduce the oxidative stress in the brain associated with head trauma. Buffered powder (vitamin C combined with small amounts of calcium, magnesium and potassium) is most easily absorbed—it's best to mix the powder with juice.

- **Drink fluids.** Make sure the body is well-hydrated, as that allows the brain to heal more quickly.

How much to drink: Dr. Steelsmith said to drink one ounce of fluid (nonalcoholic and preferably noncaffeinated—water is best) per day per two pounds of body weight, so a person who weighs 100 pounds should drink 50 ounces over the course of the day for the critical two weeks.

- **Take arnica (*Arnica montana*).** You are probably familiar with arnica cream, made from a plant that has served medicinal purposes for more than 500 years and used for sore muscles, sprains and bruises. But arnica also comes in the form of homeopathic pellets, which help to expedite healing of bruised brain tissue. Place three homeopathic arnica 30C pellets (available at health stores and online) under your tongue within 15 minutes of the trauma or as soon as you can get them. Continue this dosage every hour for the rest of the day, reducing frequency on the second, third and fourth days to three doses—one in the morning, one at lunch and one in the evening.

- **Double dose of fish oil—fast.** While the general recommendation for most people is to take one to two grams daily of high-potency fish oil, it is a good idea for people who have suffered head injuries to take up to four grams as quickly as possible after the injury and to continue taking four grams once daily for up to seven days afterward. This advice is based on a recent animal study from West Virginia University School of Medicine reported in the *Journal of Neurosurgery*, which demonstrated that taking high-potency fish oil that contained large amounts of the omega-3 fatty acids EPA and DHA (such as Nordic Naturals Omega-3D, which contains 825 mg EPA and 550 mg DHA per one-teaspoon serving), can assist in healing concussion. This will help decrease brain inflammation and with it the fogginess, memory loss and headaches that are often a part of concussion.

Note: If there is evidence of bleeding in your brain (see page 307), do not take fish oil.

Yoga Can Be Dangerous: Avoid These Common Mistakes

Timothy McCall, MD, a board-certified internist and medical editor at *Yoga Journal*...coeditor of the 2016 medical textbook *The Principles and Practice of Yoga in Health Care*...and author of the best-selling *Yoga as Medicine*. DrMcCall.com

Yoga is good for you, right? Not always.

Troubling recent finding: For one year, researchers tracked more than 350 people who took yoga classes. Nearly 11% of the participants developed a new pain problem, often lasting a few months. And 21% reported that yoga had aggravated existing injuries.

What I tell my patients and clients: As a medical doctor and yoga instructor for more than 20 years, I know that the risk for injury from practicing yoga can be much lower than from many other forms of exercise such as running or tennis—if you avoid making common mistakes. And by staying injury-free, you will enjoy the many benefits of regular yoga practice—relaxation and stress relief...pain relief...a stronger, more flexible body...and a more peaceful mind.

Here's how to bypass the injury-causing errors people often make when they practice yoga...

WRONG TYPE OF CLASS

There are many different styles and types of yoga—from the gentle and restorative to the intense and aerobic. Some of the styles investigated in the new study were intense types in which participants move quickly from pose to pose without stopping. (*Examples*: Vinyasa Flow, Power Yoga and Ashtanga Yoga.)

In my experience, most yoga injuries happen to people doing more vigorous and acrobatic styles of yoga.

My advice: If you are fit and under age 50, more athletically demanding yoga may be fine for you. If you are over age 50 and already practice flowing yoga without problems, you may be fine to continue, but the older you get, the riskier it becomes. If you are not fit or if you have a chronic health problem such as rheumatoid arthritis, poorly controlled high blood pressure or a degenerative disease of the nervous system such as Parkinson's, choose a gentler style of yoga. Examples may be called gentle yoga, restorative yoga or yoga for seniors. Other good choices include Yin Yoga and beginning Iyengar Yoga classes.

Helpful: If you want to practice a fast-paced Vinyasa-style yoga, first take a few classes in which you learn to do the poses slowly and correctly—and then speed up.

Red flag: Anyone who is pregnant, has multiple sclerosis or a chronic inflammatory condition such as lupus or inflammatory bowel disease should avoid hot yoga, including a type of hot yoga called Bikram Yoga—in which the room may be heated to 105°F. The intense heat can aggravate inflammatory conditions or harm a growing fetus.

UNDERTRAINED TEACHER

If possible, find a teacher who has more training, say, 500 hours, or one who has many years of experience. To check the teacher's qualifications, you can call a yoga studio, check online or ask the teacher directly.

If you have a serious medical condition, consider consulting a yoga therapist, a yoga teacher trained to work with students with a wide variety of illnesses. To be certified in yoga therapy by the International Association of Yoga Therapists (IAYT), a teacher needs at least 1,000 hours of training. The IAYT website (IAYT.org) has a search function for finding IAYT members in a growing number of locations.

TRYING TOO HARD

A common cause of injury in yoga is what I call "over-efforting"—trying to stretch more deeply into a pose when your breath and body are telling you that the extra stretch is not a good idea. Sharp pain and/or strained breathing are sure signs that the deeper stretch is a mistake. Over-efforting often happens because of peer pressure—almost everyone else

Danger Zone for Head Injury

It is important to realize that the danger zone following a concussion can last up to 48 hours, with the first 24 hours being the most critical. The danger is that bleeding will occur in the brain (especially likely if a person is taking an anticoagulant medication such as warfarin) or that a blood clot can form. *The following symptoms should be seen as a medical emergency, warranting a call to 911 and a visit to the emergency department of the nearest hospital…*

- **A headache that gets continually worse**
- **Vomiting**
- **Slurred speech**
- **One pupil larger than the other** or other visual disturbances
- **Change in sleeping pattern**—such as sleeping more than normal
- **Seizure**
- **Confusion and restlessness**
- **Amnesia**

Luckily, severe problems are quite rare. Most concussions are much less threatening, and most people can heal safely and completely at home by following these wise, helpful instructions.

Laurie Steelsmith, ND, naturopathic doctor and acupuncturist in private practice, Honolulu.

in class is doing the pose in a certain way, so you want to keep up.

My advice: A yoga pose should be a balance of effort and ease. If the pose is more effort than ease—get out of it. If you get a sharp pain, particularly one in a joint such as the knee—get out of it. Even if the rest of the class is doing the pose…and even if the yoga teacher is telling the class to stay in the pose…if your body is telling you to get out of the pose, get out of it.

RISKIER POSES

There are several common yoga poses that are the most likely to cause injury, and they should be avoided by beginners and many people with chronic medical conditions. *These poses include…*

- **Headstands, which can damage the neck.** When I attend a general yoga class, it often is the case that about half the class should not be doing a headstand—ever. While doing the pose, their faces are red and strained, and they obviously can't wait for the teacher to tell them to come out of the pose. Upside-down poses also can be risky for those with eye problems caused by glaucoma, retinal disease or diabetes.

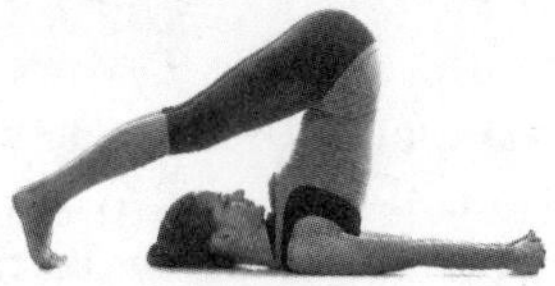

- **Shoulder stands and Plow pose.** These poses can overstretch the back of the neck. If your neck feels tight or uncomfortable, you probably should not be doing the pose.

My advice: It may help to put folded blankets under your shoulders (but not under your head and neck) to take the strain off your neck.

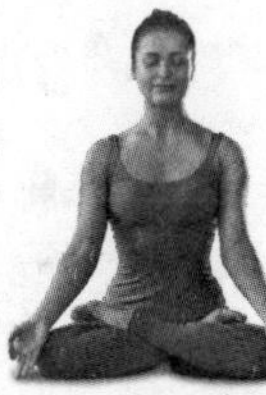

- **Lotus pose,** a sitting pose in which you put the right foot over the top of the left thigh and vice versa. This pose is only for people with flexible hips. If you use your hands to force your legs into this position, you create tremendous torque on your knee joint and you could rip or otherwise injure a knee ligament.

- **Chaturanga (yoga push-ups).** In many athletic yoga classes, students cycle through a series of 12 poses known as a sun salutation. One element is Chaturanga, where you lower your body from Plank pose to a low push-up position. Doing this repeatedly can be murder on your shoulder—particularly if you allow the top of your upper-arm bones to jut forward in the shoulder joint.

My advice: If you can't maintain good shoulder alignment, drop both knees to the ground in Plank pose, which takes some weight off, then descend the upper body to Chaturanga.

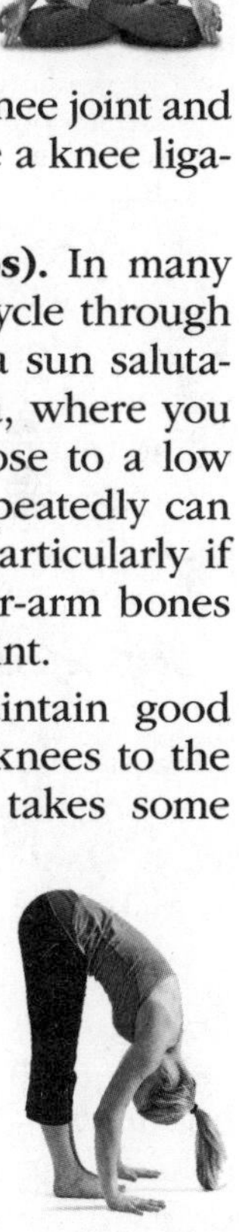

- **Deep back bends, twists or forward bends.** When in doubt, favor less extreme versions of these poses.

Surprising: Less demanding versions of poses confer

most or all the health benefits of the deeper versions.

AGGRESSIVE ADJUSTMENT

Another potential cause of serious yoga injuries is when a teacher aggressively pushes on your body to take you more deeply into a pose (light touching to indicate how or where to move is fine).

My advice: Do not allow an instructor to manually force your body into any yoga position. If you are in a class with an instructor who does that, find a new instructor.

Sprained Ankles Are More Serious Than You Think

Phillip Gribble, PhD, ATC, FNATA, associate professor of athletic training at University of Kentucky, Lexington, and program director for the university's post-professional master's program in athletic training. He is codirector of the International Ankle Consortium, a nonprofit research organization.

A sprained ankle might seem like a temporary inconvenience, but there's growing evidence that the consequences can be serious and long lasting. Recent studies have found that people who suffer one ankle sprain are extremely likely to experience recurrences, with 40% to 70% of first-time sprainers developing "chronic ankle instability."

Self-defense: Whether or not you've had an ankle sprain, do ankle-strengthening exercises regularly. These can include hopping in place or hopping from place to place on one leg or standing on one foot and bending over to pick things up from the floor.

Consider wearing ankle braces when engaging in activities that often cause sprained ankles such as tennis, basketball or hiking on uneven ground, especially if you have sprained your ankle before. Lace-up braces or rigid braces can be equally effective or you can have your ankles taped by an athletic trainer. But avoid slip-on neoprene ankle sleeves, which provide very little support.

If you do sprain your ankle…

- **Resist the urge to "walk it off."** Instead, keep your weight off the ankle as much as possible for at least 24 to 48 hours to give the ligaments a chance to heal.

Use crutches to get around. During these first few days, use ice and keep the ankle elevated as much as possible.

- **When the ankle starts to feel better, try balancing on that side.** If you can do this without pain for 30 seconds, try the ankle-strengthening (balance training) movements such as the hopping and reaching exercises described in the previous column. If you can do those without pain, too, your ankle probably is ready to return to sports or hiking.

Note: It's always a good idea to seek a consultation from a medical professional. He/she can confirm the initial evaluation and determine what additional follow-up is needed.

How to Care for a Sprained Ankle

It's very important to take care of an ankle sprain, even a seemingly "harmless" twisted ankle. Recent research shows that one sprain can cause permanent instability and future sprains (see article below). Don't try to "walk off" a sprained ankle.

Better: Get off the injured foot, prop it up, wrap it in a compression bandage and apply ice over the bandage 20 minutes per hour for the first 24 hours. Do not take a nonsteroidal anti-inflammatory drug such as ibuprofen within the first 48 hours of the injury—it could slow the healing process. If you need something for pain, consider acetaminophen. Have a doctor determine the extent of the injury and the treatment needed.

Recommendations from National Athletic Trainers Association, reported in *The New York Times.*

How NOT to Die of a Broken Hip

John E. Morley, MD, Dammert Professor of Gerontology and director of the Division of Geriatric Medicine at Saint Louis University School of Medicine. He is director of geriatric research at St. Louis Veterans Affairs Medical Center and is coauthor, with Sheri R. Colberg, PhD, of *The Science of Staying Young.*

About 25% of hip-fracture patients 65 years and older die within six months of the fracture...two-thirds die within two years.

Surgery is almost always necessary to repair a hip fracture. Generally, the better your health before a hip fracture, the better your chances for a complete recovery. But for elderly patients, especially those with health problems, a hip fracture can be deadly.

How not to die of a broken hip—plus how to prevent one in the first place...

BASICS TO PREVENT AND HEAL

These measures can help prevent a hip fracture and aid in recovery...

- **Vitamin D.** We've seen a significant increase in hip fractures over the last 20 to 30 years. During this same period, people have been increasingly avoiding the sun or using sunscreen to reduce their risk for skin cancer.

What's the connection? The body synthesizes vitamin D from exposure to the sun's ultraviolet radiation. People who get little sun often are deficient in vitamin D. Low vitamin D decreases bone and muscle strength, increasing the risk for falls as well as fractures.

What to do: Have your vitamin D measured now and also if you suffer a hip fracture. The level shouldn't be less than 30 nanograms per milliliter. Many Americans, including younger adults, have a significant vitamin D deficiency. You can supplement with vitamin D—the recommended dose is 400 international units (IU) to 800 IU daily—but I usually advise patients just to get more sun. About 20 to 30 minutes of sun exposure daily without sunscreen—new research shows that noon is best—will provide adequate vitamin D without increasing the risk for skin cancer.

Eat leafy green vegetables, such as spinach and kale. These are high in vitamin K, which helps calcium in the blood enter the bones. The Harvard Nurses' Health Study found that women who ate at least one daily serving of leafy green vegetables were 50% less likely to suffer a hip fracture than those who ate less. It's not known whether these foods protect the vertebrae, but increasing vitamin K intake as part of a healthy diet is probably helpful.

- **More protein and calcium.** Poor nutrition can impair balance, cognitive abilities and bone and muscle strength. It also can delay healing by impairing tissue repair after surgery.

Recommended: Ask your doctor about taking a balanced amino acid (protein) drink one to three times daily after a hip fracture. I also advise patients to eat eight ounces of yogurt a day. Most yogurts supply about 400 mg of calcium. Combined with the calcium in a normal diet, that's usually enough to promote stronger bones.

MORE HEALING HELP

The following can keep a hip fracture from becoming a death sentence...

- **Treatment for depression.** Depression is extremely common after a hip fracture, partly because patients often feel helpless and dependent.

Why it matters: Patients who are depressed are less likely to exercise and follow through with a rehabilitation program. They also are more likely to get a subsequent fracture because depression increases the body's production of cortisol, a substance that depletes bone calcium.

Most patients with depression do best with medication, alone or in combination with talk therapy.

Caution: Drugs in the SSRI class of antidepressants, such as *paroxetine* (Paxil), can impair alertness and coordination and increase the risk for falls. These drugs also pull calcium from the bones. Some of the older antidepressants, such as *nortriptyline* (Pamelor, Aventyl), are a better choice for hip-fracture patients because they are less likely to impair alertness and balance.

• **Pain relief.** Postsurgical pain is normal—chronic pain that lasts months or years after hip surgery is unacceptable. Chronic pain interferes with exercise and rehabilitation. It also is a leading cause of depression. You should never have chronic pain after hip surgery. Some patients do fine with over-the-counter pain relievers, such as ibuprofen, but others need stronger painkillers. If you're hurting, tell your doctor.

Helpful: The Wong-Baker FACES Pain Rating Scale. Patients look at illustrations of facial expressions (which are accompanied by a number) and choose the one that reflects their pain. During rehabilitation, no one should experience pain greater than a three or four. During daily life, pain should be rated no higher than a one or two.

• **Prevention of clots and pneumonia.** Hospital patients have a high risk of developing deep vein thrombosis, a life-threatening condition in which blood clots in the legs travel to the lungs and cause a pulmonary embolism. They also have a higher risk for pneumonia, partly because being sedentary can allow mucus to collect in the lungs, providing a breeding ground for bacteria.

What to do: In the hospital, move as much as you can, even if it is nothing more than regularly flexing your legs or sitting up in bed.

Patients who have had hip surgery are routinely referred to a physical or occupational therapist. After that, they should continue to be active—ideally, by walking or doing other forms of exercise for 20 to 30 minutes most days. (For more information on hip surgery and pain, see chapter 14, "Knee and Hip Pain.")

Sooner Is Better for Hip Fracture Surgery

Mohit Bhandari, MD, PhD, is a professor of orthopedic surgery at McMaster University in Hamilton, Ontario, Canada, and coauthor of a review of studies on hip fracture patients.

Breaking a hip is a huge health threat for the elderly. In fact, 14% to 36% of seniors die within one year of suffering a hip fracture...many others experience a profound, and sometimes permanent, loss of independence and decrease in quality of life. Some doctors say that risks are minimized when surgery is done as soon as possible after a hip fracture, but other doctors argue that it is safer to optimize a patient's medical condition before subjecting him or her to surgery, even if that takes several days or more. Who's right?

A recent article in *Canadian Medical Association Journal* provides an answer. Researchers analyzed data from 16 studies involving a total of 13,478 hip fracture patients ages 60 and older. Mortality data was adjusted for patients' ages and type and/or severity of illness at the time of surgery.

Findings: Compared with delayed surgery, early surgery (defined as surgery done within 24 to 72 hours of the injury, depending on the study) was associated with a 19% lower risk for death...a 52% lower risk for pressure sores (a complication of prolonged bed rest)...and a 41% lower risk for pneumonia.

A New Incision-Free Surgery

Flemming Forsberg, PhD, ultrasound physicist and associate professor of radiology at the Sidney Kimmel Medical College of Thomas Jefferson University in Philadelphia. His research and clinical interests include ultrasound contrast imaging.

Imagine having a major surgery in which the surgeon uses a light beam to remove a tumor without a single incision. To some, this might sound like science fiction, but believe it or not, this type of surgery has now become a reality.

With high-intensity focused ultrasound, doctors can reach tissues deep within the body—in the bones, brain, blood vessels, etc.—without making a single cut...and often with minimal discomfort.

Focused ultrasound in action: The FDA has currently approved high-intensity focused ultrasound for treating uterine fibroids, prostate problems (cancer or prostate enlargement) and cancer that has spread to the bones.

Focused ultrasound differs from other scalpel-free technologies, such as Gamma Knife, because no radiation is involved and imaging feedback is in real time.

ON THE HORIZON

Focused ultrasound is still at an early stage of development. We're likely to see a rapid expansion of uses beyond those already approved by the FDA within the next five or six years—but a lot of uncertainty remains.

Most procedures are being done only in laboratories or as a part of clinical studies,* and the procedures (and equipment) are very expensive. Even the procedures that have FDA approval may not be covered by insurance. For more information, go to the website of the Focused Ultrasound Foundation, FUSFoundation.org.

HOW IT WORKS

When you were a kid, did you ever use a magnifying glass to burn a hole through a leaf using the sun's rays? The principle is the same with focused ultrasound, except that ultrasound waves (ultrafast vibrating sound waves) are used instead of sunbeams.

These are not the same low-intensity sound waves that are used in diagnostic scans. With high-intensity focused ultrasound, multiple beams of high energy pass through an acoustic lens (instead of a magnifying glass) and then converge to focus on a small area. The beams pass harmlessly through the body until they reach the desired location. There, they generate enough energy to destroy tumors, break down blood clots or create openings in the walls of blood vessels—all without affecting nearby tissues, unlike radiation, which impacts everything in its path.

There's no incision, so recovery times are quicker. And there's little risk of bleeding (the heat of ultrasound closes bleeding vessels) or infection (no external germs are introduced). Patients might experience burning sensations during the procedure, but the discomfort is usually slight.

*To find a clinical trial in your area, go to ClinicalTrials.gov. In the search box, type in "high-intensity focused ultrasound."

Make Sure to Ask Your Surgeon About Post-Op Pain

Make sure pain will be managed aggressively. Postoperative pain inhibits a patient's ability to move, breathe deeply and heal, and it increases the risk for infection and venous thrombosis (blood clots).

Ask your surgeon about his plans to arrange for preoperative medication to preempt pain. You should receive additional medication during the surgery, including injections of anesthetic into the incision. Also, ask your doctor about the possibility of using a patient-controlled analgesic after surgery so that you can manage your own pain by pushing a button. (See chapter 21, "Painkiller Dos and Don'ts" for specific surgery-pain painkillers and warnings.)

Thomas R. Russell, MD, FACS, executive director of the American College of Surgeons, Chicago. He is the author of *I Need an Operation...Now What?*

To Prevent Postsurgery Scarring...

Mayo Clinic Health Letter. HealthLetter.MayoClinic.com

To reduce scarring after surgery, protect the area from the sun for six months to a year. Use sunscreen or cover the area with clothing. Even minimal exposure to sunlight can cause darker pigmentation within a scar.

For the first few days after surgery: Cleanse the wound carefully, and coat it with a thick layer of petroleum jelly—or follow your doctor's instructions if they are different. Contact your doctor if you have any increased pain or tenderness near the wound.

Kitchen Cures for Minor Cuts

Joan Wilen and Lydia Wilen are folk-remedy experts based in New York City. They are authors of several books including *Bottom Line's Treasury of Home Remedies & Natural Cures, Secret Food Cures* and *Bottom Line's Household Magic.*

Ouch! Did you just slice your hand cutting onions (or some other slippery food) and there's not a drop of antiseptic in sight? If you're in the kitchen, you're in the right place to grab one of these items for fast treatment…

First things first: The first thing to do when you get a scratch, small cut or graze is to clean it with warm water and soap.

Spicy remedy: Bleeding caused by shaving mishaps, sport scrapes or superficial cuts from a kitchen knife can be stopped in seconds. How? Cayenne pepper. It's high in vitamin K, a nutrient that's essential for blood clotting. Just sprinkle a little bit of cayenne pepper on the scrape or minor cut, and the bleeding will stop almost instantaneously.

Warning: Don't try this trick on deeper cuts. The burn from the pepper will outweigh the pain from the cut.

Peel some healing: After cleaning your minor wound, put the inside of a piece of banana peel directly on it and secure it with an adhesive bandage. Change the peel every three to four hours. A banana skin on your arm might look funny, but we've seen remarkable and rapid results. This gives you another good reason to pack bananas when you go camping (along with the eating part, of course).

Our favorite for paper cuts: Clean the cut with the juice of a lemon. Then, to ease the pain, dip your cut finger into powdered cloves. Since cloves act as a mild anesthetic, the pain should be gone in a matter of seconds.

Oldie but a goodie: Put honey on the wound and let its healing enzymes go to work. We love how honey stops minor bleeding and pain at the same time.

Caution: If a cut or wound is bleeding profusely, put direct pressure on it with a sterile dressing, or the cleanest washcloth available—and get professional medical help immediately.

Use Whole Milk to Cool Sunburn Pain

Men's Health Magazine. MensHealth.com

The lactic acid in milk reduces inflammation. Dip a washcloth into a bowl of cool milk, then gently place it on the burned areas for about 20 minutes. Rinse off with cool water. Use apple cider vinegar for insect bites and athlete's foot. Dab vinegar onto each bite with a paper towel—it will relieve the itching and reduce swelling. Soak infected feet for 20 minutes in a mixture of three parts water and one part vinegar to kill athlete's foot fungi. This can be done twice daily.

Don't Put Ice on a Burn

The New York Times, NYTimes.com

Don't put ice on a burn. Several published studies have shown that putting ice on a burn can damage the skin further, even causing frostbite. It is much better to run the burn under cold water, take a pain reliever and cover the burn with gauze.

Honey for Burns

Joan Wilen and Lydia Wilen are folk-remedy experts based in New York City. They are authors of several books including *Bottom Line's Treasury of Home Remedies & Natural Cures, Secret Food Cures* and *Bottom Line's Household Magic.*

Ouch! As soon as you burn yourself, mix just enough baking soda with honey to keep it a spreadable solution. Baking soda will help cool the wound, while honey's antibacterial properties will stave off infection and speed up healing. The sooner you apply it to the burn, the better chance you have of preventing it from blistering.

CHAPTER 14

Knee and Hip Pain

Knee Pain: 7 Things You're Doing That Make It Worse, Not Better

Sure, we put a lot of demand on our knees, but knee pain is not an inevitable part of aging.

Yes, over time, wear and tear can lead to arthritis or cartilage problems and, as it progresses, pain, but you can prevent a lot of damage to your knees by avoiding these common lifestyle mistakes, explained Nicholas Sgaglione, MD, director of the Northwell Health Orthopaedic Institute, who has spent 30 years caring for patients' knees.

1. Putting on pounds. With every step, skip and jump you take, your knees absorb the force of your body's weight. Each pound you gain adds exponentially to the amount of pressure exerted on your knees. In fact, each extra pound adds about four pounds of pressure. So if you've gained 20 pounds over the last few years, they feel more like 80 pounds to your knees.

There are three causes of knee problems—injuries, breakdown (of cartilage and other tissues) and deconditioning, the loss of strength in the muscles surrounding the joint. Being overweight puts you at risk for all three. As the obesity epidemic has increased in the US, so has the rate of knee problems. It's all about load on the knee. So the first mistake to avoid is putting on weight. And if you weigh more than you should, use diet and exercise to lose the extra pounds—it's never too late as far as your knees are concerned.

2. Getting weak in the knees. As important as your knee joints are, they depend on surrounding muscles for support. Deconditioning, which leaves knees weak and wobbly, is a setup for knee problems. Avoid this

Nicholas A. Sgaglione, MD, director of the Northwell Health Orthopaedic Institute and chair and professor of orthopaedic surgery at the Donald and Barbara Zucker School of Medicine at Hofstra/Northwell, Hempstead, New York.

mistake by doing twice-weekly strengthening exercises that target the muscles in the fronts of your thighs (quadriceps), the backs of your thighs (hamstrings), your hips and your core.

Options include weight machines and resistance exercises. The best choice for you depends on your current fitness level and the health status of your knees. A physical therapist or orthopedist can tailor a program for you and show you how to do the exercises correctly so that you won't hurt yourself. Start slowly and progress slowly. (See also exercises beginning on page 319.)

3. Letting your knees get stiff. Flexibility helps protect your knees from injury. Once you lose flexibility, it's hard to get it back. The answer is to stretch the muscles that support your knees through their range of motion. Just as with strengthening exercises, an exercise specialist can design a flexibility program for you and teach you the right way to stretch if you're unsure of where to start. Stretching incorrectly, such as not taking time to warm up (with light exercise) first, can cause damage. Also, avoid holding stretches for too long (no more than 30 to 40 seconds) and avoid bouncing. Make flexibility training a part of your daily workout.

4. Doing too much too soon. It's great to get started enthusiastically with exercise, but going from 0 to 60—trying to get into shape too fast or overtraining—is a recipe for an overload injury, particularly of the knees.

5. Being a slave to shoe fashion. One way to help your knees is to add shock-absorbing cushioning to your footwear. Instead of seeing your shoes as a fashion statement, think of them as extra treads for your tires. This is especially important if you already have knee issues. Avoid hard-soled slippers or sandals on weekends—wear supportive sneakers instead. Also consider off-the-shelf orthotics, shoe inserts that add cushioning.

Smart tip: Replace running shoes about every 300 miles. Replace sooner if you start noticing pain anywhere in your body after a workout that typically doesn't cause a problem or if you notice pronounced wear on the heel.

6. Being set in your exercise routine. Doing only high-impact exercise or long-distance running may take a toll on your knees over time. Cross-training will help preserve joints. Alternate between low-impact exercises and high-impact activities, mixing biking or swimming into a running program, for instance.

7. Relying on joint supplements to make up for bad habits. Glucosamine and chondroitin are among the most popular supplements taken by Americans, but it's important not to think of them as a shortcut to knee health or a substitute for the other recommendations here.

Need motivation to put a positive plan into action? Over time, overweight and inactive people with knee pain tend to need knee-replacement surgery while slim and active people tend to avoid it.

Got Knee Pain? How to Choose the Right Treatment

Jordan Metzl, MD, a sports medicine physician at the Hospital for Special Surgery in New York City. He is coauthor of *The Exercise Cure: A Doctor's All-Natural, No-Pill Prescription for Better Health & Longer Life.* DrJordanMetzl.com

Why live with a bum knee when you can have less pain and more mobility with a new one? With such great promises and the relative ease of knee-replacement surgery, it's no surprise that this is now one of the most popular procedures in the US.

It's true that the procedure can be a blessing for those with severe arthritis (the main reason for surgery) that impairs their ability to live an active, pain-free life. But the decision to have surgery should not be made casually—and if you do end up getting a knee replacement, there are facts you should know before choosing between the tried-and-true approach and the newer, less invasive surgical procedure.

TO AVOID SURGERY

If you have mild-to-moderate knee pain, but you're still able to work and do normal activities, chances are you can greatly improve without surgery by following these steps...

• **Stretch and strengthen the muscles.** Studies have shown that simply strengthening the muscles that support the knees (the quadriceps in the front of the thighs and the hamstrings in the backs) can reduce damage, pain and disability.

My advice: Work those muscles three or four times a week for at least six to eight weeks before making a decision about surgery.

• **Try hyaluronic acid.** This naturally occurring substance acts as a lubricant to the joints and may work as well as painkillers and steroids (without the side effects) for some people. It's usually injected into the affected joints once a week for three to five weeks.

My advice: There's no way to predict who will benefit from these injections. Consider them if exercise and weight loss haven't given you adequate relief. Insurance typically covers the cost.

WHAT NEXT?

If you've given the strategies described earlier your best shot and still have serious knee pain, surgery is usually the next step. *What to consider...*

• **Partial knee replacement.** This approach, also known as uni-compartmental knee replacement, is newer than total knee replacement and gets a lot of attention because it is less invasive. The advantages include an incision that is roughly half the size (about three to 3.5 inches) of that used for total knee replacement. Patients also are hospitalized for just a day or two rather than three to five days for a total knee replacement. With the partial approach, the knee may feel more "natural"—for example, it may have less "creakiness" and better range of motion—than it would after a more extensive procedure.

But a partial knee replacement isn't for everyone. To be a candidate for this procedure, the damage is generally isolated to only one part of the knee. Also, the research is not yet clear, but patients who have partial procedures may be more likely to require subsequent "revision" surgery—because of continuing arthritis, for example, or because the first procedure didn't improve pain and/or mobility. For many patients, the risks from repeat surgery could outweigh the benefits of a less traumatic initial procedure.

• **Total knee replacement.** This procedure is called a "total" replacement because the damaged surfaces of the knee bones are replaced—the tibia (shinbone)...femur (thighbone)...and sometimes the patella (kneecap). The surgery requires a large incision (usually seven to eight inches) and typically takes about two hours.

The majority of patients who opt for knee surgery require a total replacement. Surgeons have a lot of experience with the procedure—and there's strong evidence that it works. More than 90% of total knee-replacement patients report that they have a lot less pain...and about 85% of these artificial knees are still going strong after 20 years. While patients who receive total replacements have somewhat less flexibility than those who go the partial route, most are able to do light hiking, ballroom dancing and biking.

THE BOTTOM LINE

No matter which approach your surgeon suggests, make sure you're comfortable with the plan. Some patients will feel best about the decision if they get a second opinion.

Until more is known about the long-term benefits and risks of partial knee replacement, most surgeons advise their patients with severe arthritis to get it over with and have a total replacement.

Patients with osteoarthritis in all areas of the knee and those with inflammatory arthritis (such as rheumatoid arthritis), which tends to affect the entire knee, are not candidates for a partial approach and require a total knee replacement.

Consider a partial procedure only if you mainly have damage in just one part of the knee, you haven't improved after physical therapy, weight loss and the other suggestions described above, and your pain prevents you from sleeping through the night and/or performing your normal daily activities.

Three Nonsurgical Therapies Can Effectively Relieve Knee Pain

David C. Wang, DO, osteopathic physician at The Kaplan Center for Integrative Medicine in McLean, Virginia.

If physical therapy, pain medications and commonly used injections of cortisone or *hyaluronic acid* (Synvisc) no longer relieve your knee pain, don't assume that you need surgery.

Knee replacement is widely known to significantly reduce pain, but 15% of knee-replacement patients still have severe pain several years later. In some cases, scar tissue from the surgery can irritate the surrounding knee structure, which leads to lasting pain.

What's more, the recovery period after knee replacement can be very difficult for some people—for example, it usually takes four to six weeks after the operation before you can drive again, go shopping and do most of your everyday activities. And some knee-replacement patients can never again participate in high-impact sports, such as tennis, jogging or downhill skiing.

Fortunately, there are some highly effective nonsurgical alternatives to knee replacement.

LESS INVASIVE THAN SURGERY

The procedures that show promise for long-term relief are less painful and have a quicker recovery time than knee-replacement surgery. *Nonsurgical approaches...**

- **Platelet-rich plasma (PRP) therapy.** This is rapidly emerging as one of the most popular remedies for knee pain. It's been successfully used by professional athletes, including the golfer Tiger Woods, to improve healing after a knee injury.

How it's done: A small amount of blood is withdrawn from the patient. The blood is then spun in a centrifuge to concentrate platelets, which are then injected back into the knee to stimulate healing. Injections given in the open space inside a joint are only slightly painful... those given directly into a ligament or tendon typically require a local anesthetic to reduce discomfort. The procedure takes about an hour. Moderate to significant soreness lasts a few days.

How it works: Platelets are small cells in blood that initiate clotting. More importantly, they produce growth factors that stimulate, and accelerate, the body's natural healing process. An injection of PRP stimulates the movement of collagen-producing cells to the injured area. The body uses collagen to repair cartilage and other tissues.

My clinical experience: I've found that about 90% of my patients given PRP treatment for knee osteoarthritis report at least a 50% reduction in knee pain after two to four injections given at four- to eight-week intervals. PRP can heal damaged cartilage, but it won't stop the progression of osteoarthritis. Many patients need a booster shot every couple of years.

Best candidates: PRP can potentially be helpful for anyone with mild-to-severe arthritis who wants to avoid knee-replacement surgery, but seems to work best in younger patients with less severe arthritis.

Typical cost: Each injection ranges from $500 to $1,000. Most patients need at least two injections. PRP usually is not covered by insurance. Risks are minimal but include infection and injury to surrounding tissue.

- **Prolotherapy.** Using sugar (dextrose) injections to treat knee pain sounds like a scam. But this approach, known as prolotherapy, has been extensively researched.

Scientific evidence: In a recent study of arthritis patients published in *Alternative Therapies* in Health and Medicine, patients who received dextrose injections had a 44% decrease in pain, 63% decrease in swelling and 85% fewer episodes of knee buckling after one year.

How it's done: Dextrose solution is injected into the painful area. A topical anesthetic can be used to reduce discomfort from the injections. Most patients get several injections during each session. It takes about 15 minutes.

*To find a physician with expertise in evaluating and treating musculoskeletal disorders, click on "Find a Doctor" at the website of the American Association of Orthopaedic Medicine (AAO.Med.org).

Prolotherapy injections are given every three to six weeks. It usually takes one to three months to notice results, which can last for several years.

How it works: The sugar solution stimulates production of collagen fibers, the body's natural healing response. Sometimes other solutions are used, including sodium morrhuate or phenol.

Best candidates: Most effective for patients with mild-to-moderate knee pain from arthritis or ligament and tendon injury.

Typical cost: $150 to $500 per session. The average patient needs five to seven sessions. It probably won't be covered by insurance. Prolotherapy has a small risk for infection, temporary or permanent nerve irritation or injury, or allergic reaction.

- **Stem cell therapy.** Stem cells are undifferentiated cells that have the ability to turn into specialized cells in different parts of the body. They also have the unique ability to repair damaged tissue by dividing and multiplying almost indefinitely. Stem cell therapy is often used to repair damaged cartilage.

How it's done: Stem cells are "harvested" from the patient, often from fatty tissue or from bone marrow. The cells are spun in a centrifuge to separate stem cells and get a high concentration of them. Patients are given a local anesthetic to reduce discomfort, then the cells are injected into the injured/painful area.

How it works: When stem cells are injected into specific parts of the knee, they transform themselves into chondrocytes, or cells that build cartilage. They can also be transformed into cells known as fibroblasts (for soft-tissue repair) or osteoblasts (for building bone).

Unlike PRP and prolotherapy, which mobilize the body's repair mechanisms, stem cell therapy directly repairs damaged areas. I've seen arthritis patients with severe bone damage, who I thought would require joint-replacement surgery, improve dramatically enough from this therapy to not need surgery.

Best candidates: People with severe osteoarthritis who didn't get significant pain relief from PRP or prolotherapy.

Typical cost: About $2,000 to $3,000 per treatment. One treatment might be enough—patients with more severe joint damage may need more. The therapy is not covered by insurance.

Vitamin D for Knee Pain

Low levels of vitamin D may worsen knee pain—especially if you have osteoarthritis and/or are obese, according to a recent analysis.

Explanation: Vitamin D is needed for muscle strength and to fight inflammation and lessen pain sensitivity.

To help prevent knee pain: Ask your doctor to test your vitamin D level. If it's low (under 20 ng/mL), take a supplement and get more sun exposure.

Toni Glover, PhD, assistant professor of nursing, University of Florida, Gainesville.

Insoles for Knee Pain

Howard Hillstrom, PhD, director, The Leon Root, MD, Motion Analysis Lab, Hospital for Special Surgery, New York City.

A recently released study investigated if full-length lateral-wedge insoles worn inside shock-absorbing shoes would diminish the joint pain and stiffness while improving knee function of patients with medial compartment (bowlegged) knee OA.

The conclusion: After four weeks of wearing the insoles, study participants had significantly less pain, less stiffness and better functioning overall.

Knee braces, foot orthoses and shoe gear can be "off the shelf" or custom molded. Again, appropriate health-care specialists can help you decide which are appropriate for your condition. Custom-molded technology generally fits better, but costs more.

Why a Woman Should Sit Like a Man to Prevent Pain

Barbara Bergin, MD, orthopedic surgeon, Texas Orthopedics, Sports & Rehabilitation Associates, Austin. She is currently writing a book based on the SLAM concept. DrBarbaraBergin.com

Ladies, the way you were taught to sit may be polite but could be contributing to a long list of orthopedic problems that cause hip and knee pain.

The solution: SLAM! It stands for "Sit Like a Man," a phrase coined by Texas orthopedic surgeon Barbara Bergin, MD, who believes that the approach is key to treating—even better, *preventing*—painful conditions of the knees and hips that are particularly common in women, especially as they age.

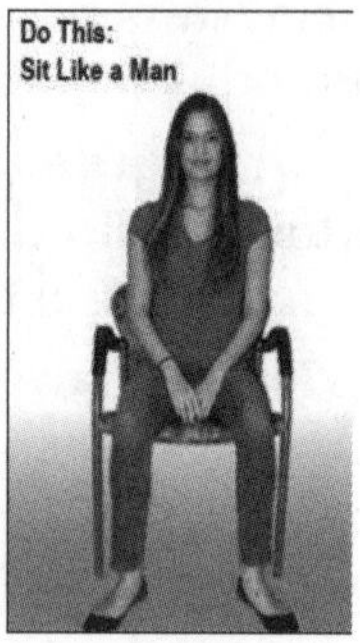

What problems can sitting like a man help prevent? *They include...*

- **Hip bursitis,** caused by inflammation of the tiny fluid-filled bursa near the hips, which serve as cushioning for the hip bones.
- **Patella malalignment,** a kneecap "tracking" condition in which the knee has a tendency to slip out of the "knee groove."
- **Chondromalacia,** sometimes called "runner's knee," in which the cartilage under the kneecap (the patella) deteriorates.
- **Gluteal tendonitis,** an inflammation of the tendons that attach the gluteal muscles on the butt to the thighs.
- **Piriformis syndrome,** in which the piriformis muscle in the butt compresses the sciatic nerve.

If you want to try it, the good news is that you don't need to slouch like a teenage boy with your legs splayed out—aka *manspreading*—to get the benefits of SLAM. It's a subtle change, although it may be easier to get in the habit when you're wearing pants rather than a skirt or dress.

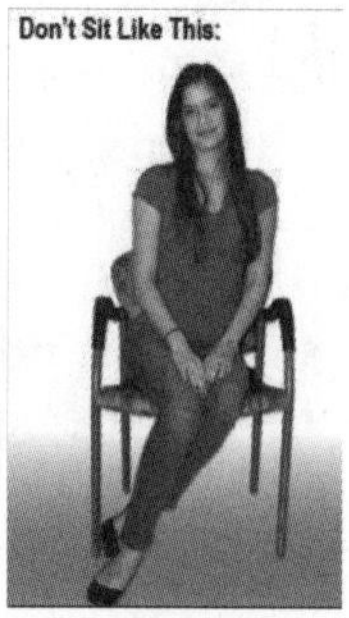

HOW TO SLAM

When sitting, let your knees drop slightly apart, with your knees at about the 11:00 and 1:00 positions. Your knees should align with your feet.

It's a *slight* relaxation of your legs. You may notice that when you sit the way you've been trained, there's a little tension in your legs—when you SLAM, it's a more natural position for your legs. Be especially attentive to using this positioning when you get in and out of your chair, because sitting and standing puts a lot of stress on your kneecaps. When you get up, keep your feet flat on the ground and don't allow your legs to collapse into a knock-kneed position.

While Dr. Bergin's approach hasn't been proven scientifically, she has seen many of her female patients improve from simply sitting differently. "When I have patients start the SLAM program, they start to feel relief in their hips and their knees," says Dr. Bergin. "Most are getting better."

She typically combines the SLAM technique with other recommendations. For kneecap-tracking issues and knee pain, Dr. Bergin recommends also doing physical therapy and avoiding stairs, squats, deep-knee bends and lunges. For hip pain, she recommends physical therapy and avoiding activities that are painful, such as squatting, sleeping on the painful side, power walking and getting in and out of chairs quickly.

Her mission is to help women *prevent* these painful conditions—so they don't have to see

Tai Chi Beats PT for Knee Pain

Tai chi (a traditional Chinese mind-body practice that combines deep breathing with slow, fluid movement) reduced pain and stiffness as well as physical therapy in adults with knee osteoarthritis who did either regimen twice a week for three months.

Bonus: Those who did tai chi reported significantly greater improvements in depression and overall well-being. To find a class near you, go to AmericanTaiChi.org.

Chenchen Wang, MD, director, Center for Complementary and Integrative Medicine, Tufts Medical Center, Boston.

orthopedic experts like her. She understands that it's not always possible to SLAM, but she encourages women to wear pants when they can and to take every opportunity, when seated, to sit like a man. She'd like moms to pass on the new approach to their daughters, too.

Photo credit: Barbara Bergin, MD

Beat Knee Pain Without Surgery—This Is Just as Effective and Safer

Mitchell Yass, DPT, a Florida–based physical therapist and creator of the Yass Method for treating chronic pain. He is also the author of *The Pain Cure Rx: The Yass Method for Diagnosing and Resolving Chronic Pain* and the PBS special *The Pain Prescription.* MitchellYass.com

For most people with knee pain, exercise is at least as effective as surgery—with none of the risks, according to research. *What you need to know...*

MUSCLE PAIN

When you see a doctor because of nagging knee pain, you'll probably be advised to have an X-ray or MRI to look for arthritis, torn cartilage or other structural problems that can cause joint pain. But the tests, more often than not, point doctors in the wrong direction.

Eye-opening research: A study of nearly 1,000 patients with arthritis-related knee pain found that 63% had a damaged meniscus (cartilage that cushions and stabilizes the knee). But the same study also found that 60% of patients without pain had the same type of damage.

Most patients—and many doctors—fail to realize that there's a poor correlation between structural problems and knee pain. That's why I often advise clients not to have imaging tests—or consider surgery—until they've first tried a program of targeted exercise. In my experience, about 90% of knee patients have a muscle imbalance or weakness that causes all or most of their symptoms.

Here is a 30- to 60-minute workout that helps specific types of knee pain. Do the exercises on the side that is painful until the pain subsides—once the pain is gone, do the exercises on both sides. Stop if the exercise hurts.

A resistance band, ankle weight or machine in the gym can be used for resistance, which is key for strengthening muscles.* Start at a level where you feel you are working hard but not in pain, and gradually increase resistance.

The exercises can be performed by anyone, including those who have had knee surgery, but check first with your doctor. The quad stretch should be done daily. For each of the other exercises below, do three sets of 10 repetitions (resting 45 to 60 seconds between sets) and repeat the workouts three times a week (with a day between workouts).

WEAK HAMSTRINGS

The thigh muscles (quadriceps) tend to be a lot stronger than the opposing muscles (the hamstrings) on the backs of the legs. Why? It's because virtually all of our daily movements—including walking and climbing stairs—are "forward."

The problem: Weak hamstrings (they are mainly responsible for knee bending) cannot effectively counteract the force of much stronger quadriceps, causing a muscle imbalance.

Result: The quadriceps shorten and pull up on the kneecap, causing excessive pressure and pain. The majority of people with knee pain will improve when they strengthen the hamstrings and stretch the quads.

***EXERCISE #1:* Hamstring curls.** While sitting in a chair, tie the ends of a resistance band to a doorknob and slip it around the ankle...or try the seated leg curl machine at the gym.

What to do: Begin with the exercising leg pointing straight out, then bend the knee until it reaches 90 degrees. Return to the starting position.

*To increase muscle strength, add resistance (with heavier weights or a stronger exercise band) when the exercises become easy.

EXERCISE #2: **Hip extensions.** This exercise works the gluteus maximus muscles in the buttocks.

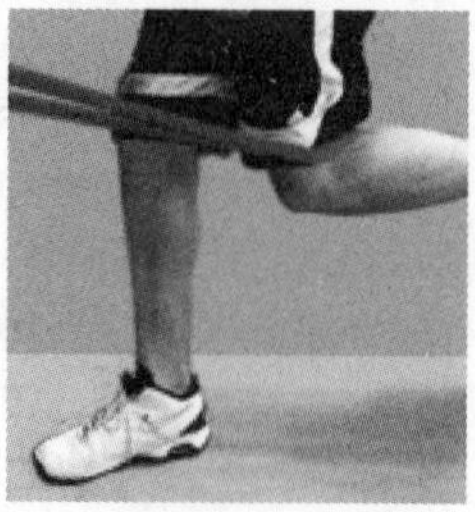

What to do: While standing, place a resistance band behind one knee. Then attach the ends to a fixed point—such as a doorknob. While standing (you can rest your hand on top of a chair or table for extra support), bring the knee about 10 degrees behind the hip, then return to the starting position.

EXERCISE #3: **Quad stretches.** Tight quadriceps pull the kneecap toward the top of the joint and prevent it from moving smoothly. Tight quads can cause both knee and back pain.

What to do: Stand near a wall (or a dresser, bookcase or other solid support), and use one hand for balance. Reach back with your other hand, and grip the ankle.

Pull the heel upward toward the buttock. The knee should be a few inches behind the hip. Keep pulling until you feel a stretch in the front of the thigh. Hold the stretch for 20 to 30 seconds, and do the stretch twice. Pull gently! If it hurts, you've pulled too far (or too quickly).

QUAD STRAIN

Another common cause of knee pain is quad strain. What are the telltale signs? You might notice a "pulling" sensation at the top of the knee or in the thigh when you walk or climb stairs. A weak quadricep can cause the kneecap to shift out of place. *Try this...*

EXERCISE #1: **Knee extensions.** They strengthen the quadriceps and help the kneecap stay in a "neutral" position.

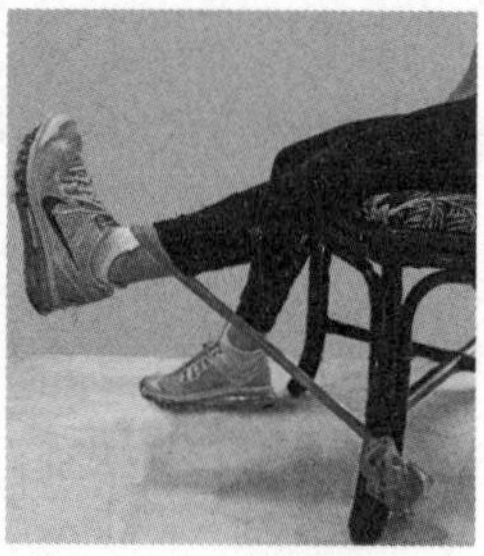

What to do: In a seated position, strap on an ankle weight or tie a resistance band around the front of the ankle and attach the other end to the chair leg. Keep the other foot on the floor. Begin with the knee bent to a 90-degree angle, then straighten it. Return to the starting position.

Important: Make sure that the thigh of the leg being exercised stays on the seat. Raising it will make the exercise less effective.

EXERCISE #2: **Dorsiflexion.** It works the tibialis anterior, a muscle in the front of the shin. Strengthening the muscle can help keep the calf muscle lengthened and allow the knee joint to function properly to prevent knee pain.

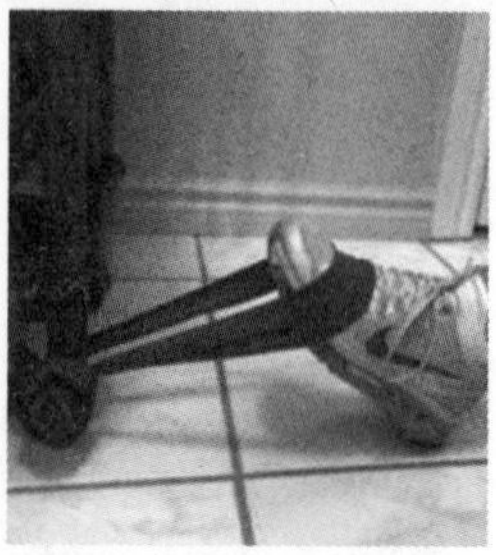

What to do: Sit on the floor with one leg extended. Slip an exercise band over the top of the foot and tie the ends to a sturdy table leg. Start with the ankle angled about 30 degrees forward, then pull the foot toward the upper body until it is 10 degrees past perpendicular. Return to the starting position.

The Ultimate Knee Workout: 4 Must-Do Exercises

Steven P. Weiniger, DC, managing partner of Body-Zone.com, a national online health information resource and referral directory to chiropractors, physical therapists and Certified Posture Exercise Professionals (CPEPs). He is the author of *Stand Taller, Live Longer: An Anti-Aging Strategy.* StandTallerLiveLonger.com

Everyone can benefit from knee exercises. Even if you don't suffer from knee pain now, the following exercises may help prevent problems from developing. People who have received surgery to replace or repair a knee also can benefit by strengthening their muscles to help guard against future knee injuries.

The goal of knee exercises is to work the muscles around the joint. These include the quadriceps (on the front of the thigh)...the hamstrings (back of the thigh)...and the muscles in the calves. Strength and flexibility in these areas support the knees and help keep them aligned. Alignment is critical because asymmetry increases pressure and joint damage.

Perform the following regimen daily—it can be completed in about 15 to 30 minutes. If you have an advanced knee problem due to a condition such as rheumatoid arthritis, your doctor may also prescribe additional exercises that are targeted to address your specific issues.

Important: All of the exercises described in this article should be performed within a range of motion that does not cause pain. If a slight strain occurs with the first repetition, that is acceptable, as long as the pain diminishes with subsequent repetitions. If the pain worsens with subsequent repetitions, stop the exercise.

Four must-do knee exercises...

- **Knee-to-Chest Stretch.** This exercise improves flexibility in the lower back, hips and hamstrings. People who do this stretch will notice an opening of their hips, allowing them to stand taller. This improvement in posture is important for reducing knee stress.

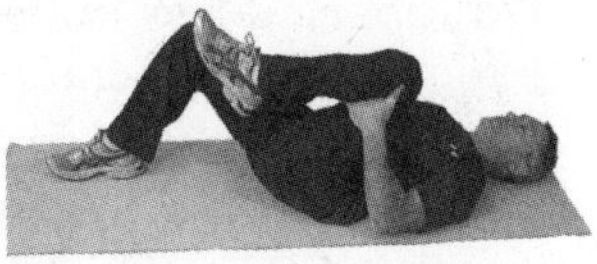

Bonus: You can use this movement to diagnose knee problems. If the knee you're bending doesn't come straight toward your shoulder and stay in line with your foot, you'll know that you have an alignment problem that needs to be corrected.

This knee exercise can be performed in bed if that is more comfortable than doing it on a carpeted floor or on a padded surface.

What to do...

- Lie on your back with your knees bent and your feet flat on the floor (or bed).
- Using both hands, slowly pull one knee toward your chest. (To avoid straining the knee, grip behind it, not on the front.) Go as far as you can without discomfort—you should feel a stretch in your lower back, but no pain.
- Hold the position for 15 to 30 seconds, then slowly lower the leg. Perform the movement eight to 12 times. Repeat with the other leg.

- **Knee-to-Chest Stretch with Resistance.** This is similar to the exercise described above, except that you use a latex exercise band (such as Thera-Band) to increase resistance and strengthen muscles.

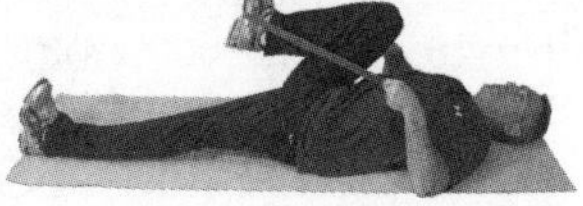

- Lie on your back with your legs straight. Loop the latex band around the bottom of one foot. Grip the loose ends of the band with both hands.
- Use the band to pull your knee toward your chest.
- Hold the position for 15 to 30 seconds, then straighten the leg while pushing against the band—hold the band taut to increase resistance. Do this eight to 12 times, then repeat with the other leg.

- **Standing One-Leg Balance.** This move is more challenging than it looks because you're using the weight of your body to strengthen your legs as well as the "core" muscles in the abdomen. These muscles, which connect the torso and pelvis, help control motions in your whole body. Core weakness is a common cause of asymmetric motion, which often leads to knee problems.

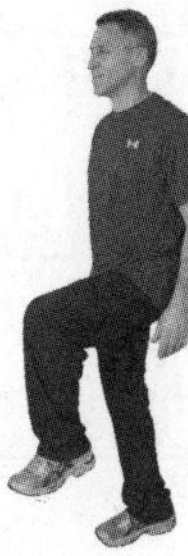

- Stand next to a wall, with your right shoulder just touching the wall.
- Lift your left knee until the foot is off the floor. If you can, keep raising it until the thigh is about parallel to the floor. Make sure that your posture is upright at all times.
- Hold the position for about 15 seconds, then lower your foot. Repeat eight to 12 times, then turn around and do the same thing with the other leg.

Important: If you can't balance for 15 seconds—or if you find yourself using the wall for support or moving your arms or dancing around to balance on one foot—your legs are weaker than they should be. This means you should definitely also do the next exercise.

Note: Even if you can easily perform the one-leg balance above, it's a good idea to do the one below to maintain your strength.

- **Standing One-Leg Balance with Resistance.** This is similar to the exercise that's described above, except that you use a latex band to strengthen muscles in the thighs and hamstrings.

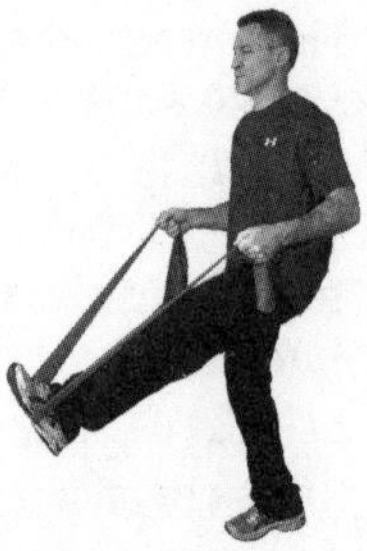

• Stand with your right shoulder barely touching a wall. Loop a latex band under your left foot. Hold the loose ends of the band in each hand.

• With your hands at waist level, raise your left foot until your thigh is about parallel to the floor. Shorten the band by wrapping it around your hands to keep some tension on the band.

• While holding the band taut and your knee elevated, slowly press your foot forward, as though you're taking a big step. Keep the band taut to increase resistance. Maintain your balance!

• Now, pull on the band to return to the bent-knee position. Repeat eight to 12 times, then turn around and repeat with the other leg.

Buff Those Quads

Shreyasee Amin, MD, MPH, rheumatologist, Mayo Clinic, Rochester, Minnesota, and leader of a study of 265 people.

Researchers tested strength in the quadriceps (front thigh muscles) and measured cartilage loss (using MRI scans) in people with arthritis of the knees. Participants' knees were scanned again 15 and 30 months later.

Results: Participants whose quadricep strength measured in the highest one-third had 60% less cartilage loss behind the kneecap than those in the lowest one-third. They also reported less knee pain.

Best: If you have arthritis in your knees, ask your doctor about taking swimming or water aerobics classes to safely build strength in your quadriceps.

Compression Braces and Sleeves for Knee Arthritis

Barbara Bergin, MD, orthopedic surgeon, Texas Orthopedics, Sports & Rehabilitation Associates, Austin. She is currently writing a book based on the idea that women should "Sit like a man." DrBarbaraBergin.com

Wearing a compression brace will not directly prevent your knee from twisting in a way that might injure it. But it may help your brain's awareness of your body in space so that you might avoid moves that could cause further injury and pain.

While compression garments and wraps have no potential to cure disorders of bones and joints for those suffering with arthritis or patients with injuries, they just seem to feel better. That's a good enough reason, if you want to try one of these garments or Kinesio Tape—or even an Ace bandage. See if it helps. And yes, you could even try duct tape, a kind of primitive version of Kinesio Tape. It might work quite nicely—although it's going to hurt like hell and give you a waxing when you take it off!

Knee Replacements Are Getting Younger

Jack Bert, MD, orthopedic surgeon and adjunct clinical professor, University of Minnesota School of Medicine, and medical director, Minnesota Bone & Joint Specialists, Woodbury. He is founder of the Cartilage Restoration Center of Minnesota.

Younger candidates for knee-replacement surgery might want to consider a more conservative treatment that's better for an active lifestyle. It used to be more widely used but has waned in popularity—it's called high tibial osteotomy (HTO).

In younger people—up to around 60 or so years old—arthritis is often limited to one side (compartment) of a given knee, either because that's where the injury occurred or because of gait issues, like being bowlegged or having "knock knees," which tends to put more wear and tear on the inner or outer part of the knee. If you're discussing surgery, your orthopedic surgeon will likely recommend a "partial knee replacement" if your arthritis is confined to just one of the compartments of your knee. But even that may be a bad choice.

When you do a knee replacement in a young person, you've committed that poor patient to having two or three knee revisions (implant redos) in their lifetime. That's because knee implants wear out in 10 to 12 years. In very active people, the lifespan is on the short end of the range. Every time you do a revision, the success rate of the implant drops significantly. That could leave you with painful untreatable knees in your 60s or 70s when you hopefully have many more years to go!

A MORE CONSERVATIVE APPROACH TO KNEE SURGERY

So what about the alternative—the high tibial osteotomy mentioned above? In this procedure, a wedge of bone is cut out of the shinbone (tibia) under the healthy side of the knee. The opening is either closed or opened further, and a bone graft added to fill the space to align your leg better and take pressure off of the arthritic knee joint surface. A plate is then screwed over the repaired bone. By shifting your weight off the damaged side of the joint, the procedure can relieve pain and improve function. Studies have also shown that by reducing the load pressure on the injured part of the knee joint, HTO allows new cartilage to grow back to some extent, providing a little more comfort and protection.

The advantages over a knee replacement are obvious. You're preserving your own knee joint and delaying, or possibly even preventing, the start of a cycle of repeated knee replacement that may not help for your entire life. Even if you eventually need a partial or total knee replacement, you may be able to hold out long enough to take advantage of new techniques being researched that use stem cells or other biological approaches to preserve the joint. Research also shows that the success of a total knee replacement, if you do eventually need one, is just as good in people who've previously had an HTO as in those who go directly to knee replacement.

HTO is also a better choice if you're a runner, play competitive tennis or are otherwise very active, because you really can't resume high-intensity activity at nearly the same level after having a knee replacement.

LONG-TERM GAIN, SHORT-TERM PAIN

HTO can be a tough sell. The main reason is that recovery time is longer than that for knee replacement. Patients are on crutches for six to 12 weeks, or even longer in some cases, because the bone has to heal, versus only a few days after a partial knee replacement for most healthy middle-aged people.

You do need to be committed to the recovery phase if you're going to do this. The operation itself has a low rate of complications, but if you put pressure on the knee too soon, the bone may not heal well.

You may be hard-pressed to find a surgeon who does HTO, too. The main reason is that partial and total knee replacements have become so successful that there's less interest in HTO. It's not being taught universally in orthopedic residency training programs, so some surgeons feel very uncomfortable doing the procedure.

If you're under age 60 (or even 65), and are a candidate for a partial knee replacement, consider nonsurgical options first. Get physical therapy, and work with your doctor, who may prescribe injections, pain meds, knee braces exercises and other short-term approaches to help you stay active.

If it's really time for a knee operation, though, ask your surgeon about HTO before considering a partial or total knee replacement. Make sure any physician you're considering for an HTO has done at least 30 to 40 of the procedures because there is a learning

Knee Replacements Can Lead to Broken Bones

According to a Swedish study, people who have new knees are 19% more likely than others to experience spinal fractures and 4% more likely to break a hip.

Possible reason: Patients become active before they are fully rehabilitated—which increases the risk of falling and breaking a bone.

Self-defense: Ask your physician for balance exercises.

Sabrina Strickland, MD, specialist in knee and shoulder surgery at Hospital for Special Surgery and associate professor of orthopedic surgery at Weill Cornell Medical College, both in New York City.

curve. You may have to head to a large medical center to find an experienced surgeon.

Better Rehab After Knee Replacement: Aquatherapy

Thoralf R. Liebs, MD, attending orthopedic surgeon, department of orthopedic surgery, University of Schleswig-Holstein Medical Center, Kiel, Germany.

According to a recent study, 465 hip and knee replacement patients (average age 69) were randomly assigned to begin aquatic therapy either six or 14 days after surgery. They performed strengthening exercises in a pool for 30 minutes, three days a week, up to the fifth week after surgery. In the knee group, physical function, pain and stiffness improved in those who started therapy six days after surgery. Those with hip replacements, however, did better when they waited 14 days, after the wound had fully healed.

Knee Replacement Works for Those Who Need It

Total knee replacement offers significant pain relief for 90% of people whose knees have been damaged by arthritis. Only 1% of artificial joints fail. About 300,000 Americans get the surgery each year, and that number is expected to increase as the population ages.

E. Anthony Rankin, MD, chief of orthopaedic surgery, Providence Hospital, and clinical professor of orthopaedic surgery, Howard University, both in Washington, DC, and chair, National Institutes of Health consensus development panel on total knee replacement.

Your Knee Pain May Really Be a Hip Problem

Mitchell Yass, DPT, a Florida–based physical therapist and creator of the Yass Method for treating chronic pain. He is also the author of *The Pain Cure Rx: The Yass Method for Diagnosing and Resolving Chronic Pain* and the PBS special *The Pain Prescription*. MitchellYass.com

One of the indicators that the cause of knee pain is muscular is when the pain seems to result from performing activities—but you have no pain when sitting or lying down. Standing up, negotiating stairs, kneeling, walking and prolonged standing are all activities that might bring on knee pain.

What I have been seeing more frequently is knee pain occurring after a hip replacement. In this case, a muscular deficit at the hip region causes knee pain. The gluteus medius muscle sits at the side of the pelvis above the hip joint. It is responsible for creating stability and balance, especially when single-leg standing, such as with walking. This muscle is also responsible for keeping the knee joint under the hip joint when standing.

Here are the red flags that your knee pain may be from a strained hip muscle…

- **Your knee pain has occurred after getting hip surgery.**
- **The thigh with the affected knee seems more angled inward than the unaffected leg.**
- **When you single-leg stand,** your knee feels like it can't support you and that it might cave in.
- **Negotiating stairs seems inhibited** not only because of knee pain but a feeling that your leg won't support you.
- **Tenderness when feeling the gluteus medius for knots or sensitivity.**

These types of causes do not show up on diagnostic tests, and no medical specialty is educated or trained to identify or treat them. (Without identifying the right cause, the symptoms will never be resolved and chronic pain will stay chronic.)

If it appears that the cause of the knee pain is due to a strained gluteus medius muscle, then perform hip abduction. *Here's how…*

Attach a resistance-band loop to the leg of a sturdy table or chair. Stand with the affected leg's foot in the loop farther away from the structure than the unaffected leg. The feet should be close together to start. Turn the foot of the affected leg in so you lead to the side with the heel moving first. Step out so the outside of the ankle meets the line of the hip. Put all your weight on the leg you are stepping out with and then return to the start position. Do a total of three sets of 10 repetitions with a one-minute rest between sets. As the resistance feels easier, either step farther away from the table/chair with both feet to

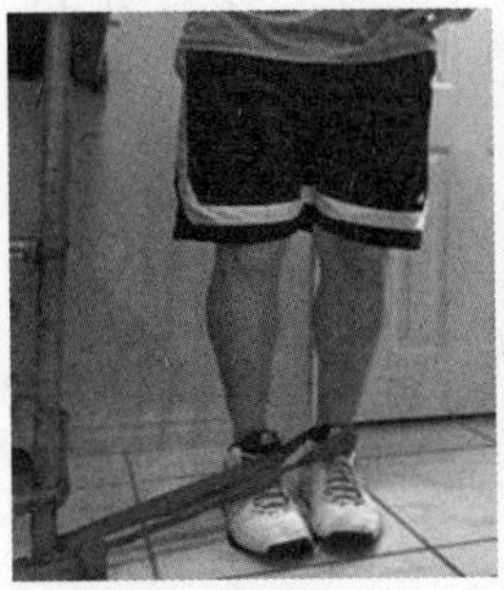

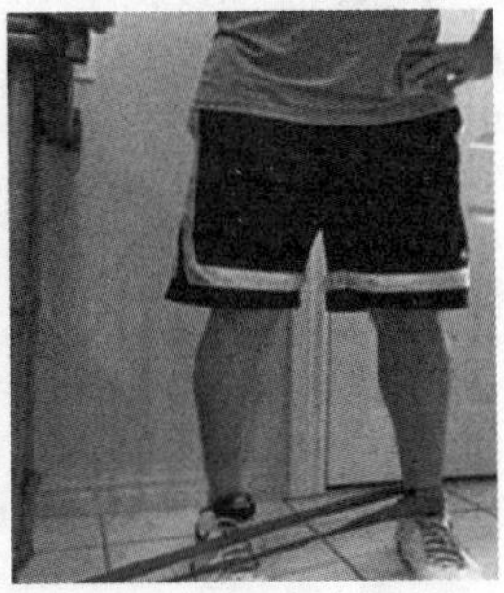

increase the tension of the resistance band or use a more resistive band to continue to build the gluteus medius. Eventually the muscle will become so strong it will be able to support you and prevent the knee from losing alignment under the hip joint.

Keep Your Hips Forever!

Mitchell Yass, DPT, a Florida-based physical therapist and creator of the Yass Method for treating chronic pain. He is also the author of *The Pain Cure Rx: The Yass Method for Diagnosing and Resolving Chronic Pain* and the PBS special *The Pain Prescription*. MitchellYass.com

If you're tired of hobbling around on an aching hip, surgery to replace that failing joint might sound pretty good.

Every year, more than 330,000 Americans get this operation. For those who have severe joint damage (for example, bone-on-bone damage that prevents full range of motion), hip replacement can be an excellent choice.

Here's the rub: Many people who receive a hip replacement aren't in this category. They undergo hip replacement but don't realize that the cause of their pain could be in hip muscles, not joints.

IDENTIFY THE PROBLEM

If you complain about persistent groin pain (one of the most common symptoms of hip dysfunction), your doctor will probably order an imaging test (such as an X-ray and/or MRI scan).

What you need to know: Even though imaging tests can give doctors a great deal of information about the condition of a joint, they aren't as conclusive as you might think. For example, an X-ray can show a decrease in cartilage and less space between the thighbone and hip socket, but doctors differ in deciding at what point surgery becomes necessary. Virtually everyone who's age 50 or older will show some degree of joint damage just from normal wear and tear. A decrease in range of motion at the hip joint is key to the need for surgery.

Does a diagnosis of arthritis at the hip joint mean that you need surgery? Not necessarily. Most hip and groin pain is caused by muscle weakness or a muscle imbalance. People who correctly exercise these muscles can often eliminate—or at least greatly reduce—their discomfort. Strengthening these muscles also can help ease pain in those who have already had hip replacements...and improve balance.

THE BEST WORKOUTS

The following exercises are ideal for hip or groin pain. After getting your doctor's OK, start by trying to repeat each one 10 times. Take a one-minute break, then repeat two more sets. The whole routine, which should be done two or three times a week, takes about 20 minutes.

• **Hamstring curl.** The hamstrings (in the back of the thigh) play a key role in the functioning of the hip joints. However, the hamstrings are weak in most people—mainly because these muscles aren't used much in normal daily movements.

How this exercise helps: It strengthens hamstrings and helps prevent the opposing muscles (the quadriceps, in the front of the thigh) from shortening and causing muscle strain and/or spasms.

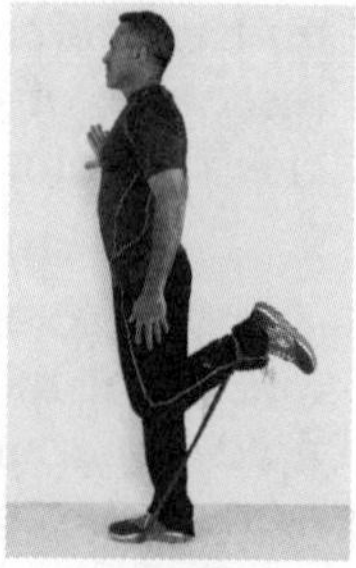

How to do it: Attach one end of a piece of elastic exercise tubing (available in sporting-goods stores and online) to your left ankle. Stand on the other end with your right foot. Leaving more slack will reduce resistance...taking up the slack will increase it.

With your feet a few inches apart and knees slightly bent, raise your left foot and curl it backward toward your buttocks as far as you comfortably can. Then return to the starting position. If you feel unsteady, put one hand (on the side opposite the leg you're working) on a wall. Switch legs and repeat.

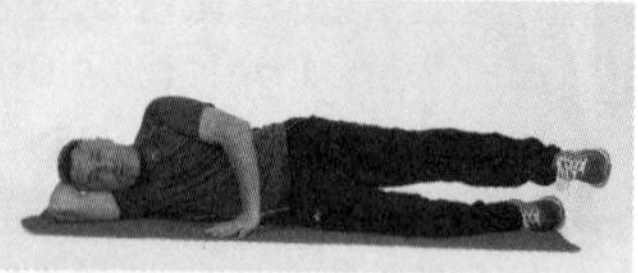

• **Hip abduction.** This is great for hip or groin pain because the abductor muscles (on the outer thighs) tend to be much weaker than the opposing adductor muscles.

How this exercise helps: Weakness in the abductors can allow the pelvis to drop on one side, which can cause groin muscles to tighten and become painful.

How to do it: Lie on the side that's not painful (or less painful) on a mat or a carpeted floor. Your painful side will be on top. Place your arm under your head, and bend your other leg's knee for better support and balance.

Slowly raise your affected leg, keeping it in line with your torso. Keep the knee straight, and don't roll forward or backward. Raise your leg only to hip height (a few inches). Then slowly lower your leg back to the starting position. After performing a set, roll over and repeat the exercise with the other leg, only after pain has eased in the affected leg. Otherwise, focus only on strengthening the painful side.

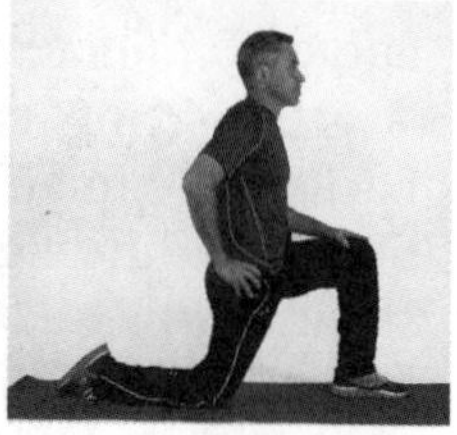

• **Hip flexor stretch.** This exercise is vital. Most of us spend a lot of time sitting, causing these muscles to shorten and tighten.

How this exercise helps: It stretches tight hip flexors, which can stress the low back.

How to do it: Kneel on your right knee on a mat or a carpeted area. (If you need more padding, you can put a folded towel under the knee.) Place your left foot flat on the floor in front of you, with the knee bent. Rest your left hand on your left thigh and your right hand on your right hip. Keeping your back straight and abdominal muscles tight, lean forward so that more of your weight is on the front leg. You'll feel a stretch in your right upper thigh. Hold for 20 to 30 seconds. Switch sides.

• **Quad stretch.** Overly tight quad muscles can pull the pelvis downward—a common cause of low-back and hip pain.

How this exercise helps: Stretching the quads helps distribute weight evenly through the pelvis.

How to do it: Stand near a wall for support. Rest your right hand on the wall, then reach back with your left hand to grip your left foot/ankle. Pull your heel upward toward your buttocks—and eventually behind the hip. Keep pulling, gently, until you feel a stretch in the front of your thigh. Tighten your abdominal muscles. Hold for about 20 to 30 seconds. Repeat on the other side.

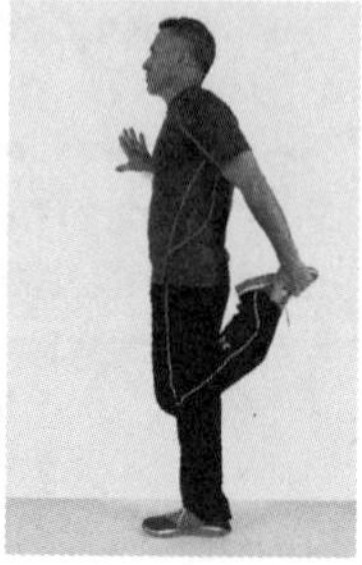

If your pain doesn't improve after a month of performing these exercises, consult your doctor.

How to Have a Successful Hip Surgery

Andrew A. Shinar, MD, chief of the division of joint replacement and an assistant professor of orthopedics and rehabilitation at Vanderbilt University Medical Center in Nashville.

If you suffer from hip pain due to arthritis or some other condition that damages the joints, you may at some point find yourself among the roughly 200,000 adults in the US who opt for a hip replacement each year. This procedure is considered only when other options, such as pain medications, physical therapy and/or the use of a cane or walker, don't provide adequate relief.

Before you or a loved one contemplates a hip replacement: Be sure you're well informed about several recent advances that can help give you the best possible results...*

IS MINIMALLY INVASIVE BETTER?

Most people who are considering hip replacement now assume that minimally invasive surgery, which is reported to cause less pain and allow faster recovery than a traditional operation, is preferable.

With a minimally invasive procedure, the surgeon uses special instruments and one or two incisions (one to six inches long) rather than the one 10- to 12-inch incision most commonly used in the past. It's logical to think that a large incision causes more discomfort than a smaller one. It's not true, however, that hip-replacement patients who undergo minimally invasive procedures automatically do better.

Latest thinking: Studies comparing minimally invasive with traditional hip-replacement procedures have failed to show that one approach is consistently superior to the other. Researchers speculate that other factors, including the choice of painkillers and the type of physical therapy used after surgery, make a bigger difference.

People who are relatively lean are generally the best candidates for a minimally invasive approach... obese patients often require a larger incision because subcutaneous fat makes it difficult for the surgeon to see within the joint. Regardless of the size of the incision, most patients leave the hospital in roughly the same amount of time—minimally invasive, two to three days... and traditional, three to five days. Those who are relatively fit usually resume most of their normal activities within four to six weeks. Older or frailer patients might take three months or more to fully recover.

*When exploring any of the surgeries mentioned in this article, remember that surgeons are best at performing procedures that they do frequently. You may benefit by choosing the approach the surgeon commonly uses when performing hip replacement.

Too Old for a New Hip?

Researchers evaluated 174 men and women (average age 75) with severe osteoarthritis of the hip or knee before and after treatment—either joint replacement surgery or nonsurgical treatment, such as pain medication, physical therapy and/or home exercises.

Result: After one year, patients who had joint replacement surgery had greater improvement in symptoms than those who did not have surgery.

Self-defense: If you have severe osteoarthritis of the hip or knee that has not responded to medication and/or physical therapy, ask your doctor whether joint replacement surgery is appropriate for you.

Caution: Possible complications of the surgery include wound infection and blood clots in the lungs.

Mary Beth Hamel, MD, MPH, associate professor, department of medicine, Harvard Medical School, Beth Israel Deaconess Medical Center, Boston.

BETTER MATERIALS

As the materials used in hip replacements have become more durable—and now that a significant amount of time has passed since the earliest surgeries—it appears that many artificial joints can last the rest of a person's life (20 or more years). In the past, artificial joints generally lasted no more than 10 to 15 years.

In the past, there also was greater concern that vigorous activities and movements could cause the artificial ball to pop loose (dislocate) from the artificial socket— the main complication of hip replacement and a common reason that patients sometimes require a second or even third operation.

Now: Dislocations are rare. At one time, about 3% of patients who had hip replacement would eventually suffer a dislocation. Now, only about 1% do. *Here's why...*

- **Bigger ball joints.** The size of the ball joint has increased from about an inch to an inch-and-a-half in diameter. The larger surface area creates a bigger jump distance—how far the hip can move without the risk that the ball will "jump" from the socket.

New procedure: With anterior hip replacement, the surgeon makes an incision on the front of the hip rather than on the side (lateral) or back (posterior). Studies show that patients who have this type of surgery are only about half as likely to suffer a dislocation as those who don't.

However, the anterior procedure can have a higher risk for other complications, such as nerve injuries or bone fractures. More research must be done before we will know whether the anterior approach is better than other techniques.

POSTSURGICAL ADVANCES

• **Movement.** In the past, people undergoing hip replacement were told to avoid putting pressure on the joint for up to six weeks after surgery.

Now: Within just a few hours of leaving the recovery room, patients are encouraged to stand up and bear as much of their weight as they would by walking.

Resuming activity soon after surgery reduces the risk for potentially deadly blood clots, one of the most dangerous complications. A Swedish study showed that double the number of patients on a fast-track rehabilitation protocol felt well at three months after surgery.

• **Better pain relief.** A decade ago, patients who had undergone hip replacement were given oral and intramuscular narcotics for pain.

Now: More potent combinations of drugs, including slow-release oxycodone (OxyContin) to control pain...and injections or pills of advanced anti-inflammatory drugs—such as *ketorolac* (Toradol) or *celecoxib* (Celebrex)—to reduce inflammation are typically used.

• **Quicker physical therapy.** With hip replacement, physical therapy has traditionally begun the day after surgery. Patients weren't discharged from the hospital until they could perform certain movements, such as a straight-leg raise or getting in and out of bed without help.

Now: The same type of physical therapy is used, but it's often started within four hours of leaving the recovery room. A study reported in the *Journal of Arthroplasty* found that joint-replacement patients who received modified anesthesia and painkillers and quickly started physical therapy were able to complete straight-leg raises in eight hours, compared with 73 hours for those following older protocols.

QUICK FACTS: HIP REPLACEMENT

Most people who undergo a hip replacement are over age 60. That's when the main reasons for the procedure, including hip pain caused by osteoarthritis or a broken hip due to a fall, are most likely to occur.

During a hip replacement, the surgeon removes damaged bone, then presses or cements an artificial hip socket into place. A metal stem with a ball on top is inserted into the top of the thigh bone. The ball is then fitted snugly into the socket. Most artificial hip joints last 20 or more years.

Same-Day Hip Surgery

Matthew S. Austin, MD, orthopedic surgeon and director of Joint Replacement Services at Thomas Jefferson University Hospital in Philadelphia. He is program director of the Joint Replacement Fellowship at the Rothman Institute and a professor in the department of orthopaedic surgery at Sidney Kimmel Medical College at Thomas Jefferson University.

Until recently, people who needed a hip replacement were operated on in a hospital, spent a few nights there and then went home or to a rehabilitation center to embark on a recovery period of up to three months or more.

Now: An increasing number of people are receiving so-called "same-day" hip surgery—you arrive at a hospital or outpatient center in the morning, have the surgery (typically lasting about an hour or so), spend a few hours recovering from anesthesia and then go home at the end of the day.* Even though this approach may sound appealing, it is not necessarily for everyone.

To learn more about same-day hip surgery, we spoke with Matthew S. Austin, MD, a leading orthopedic surgeon who performs both

*If you go to an outpatient center, look for one that's affiliated with a major medical center and/or has accreditation from the Accreditation Association for Ambulatory Healthcare.

traditional and same-day hip replacements and researches optimal recovery methods.

First things first—who needs a hip replacement?

It's mainly done in patients with arthritis- or injury-related hip damage that causes persistent pain. Surgery is recommended when people can no longer do the activities they enjoy and/or when they're suffering from chronic pain that isn't relieved by medications or the risks of taking painkillers outweigh the benefits.

How is a hip replacement done?

In a nutshell, the arthritic joint is cut and removed and then replaced with a synthetic "ball-and-socket" that works much like a natural joint...and much better than an arthritic/damaged joint.

Most hip replacements (including same-day surgeries) are done posteriorly. The surgeon enters the back of the hip to access the hip joint. The incision is typically about six to 10 inches long, although the same procedure can now be done with smaller incisions.

The operation can also be done anteriorly, with an incision on the front part of the hip... or anterolaterally (on the side). With these two techniques (both of which usually require an incision of about four inches or less), the surgeon moves muscles instead of cutting and reattaching them. A surgeon who's experienced in any of these three surgeries can complete the operation in about an hour.

Is there a preferred technique for same-day surgery?

It makes no difference. The different surgeries have similar success rates—roughly 20 years after surgery, about 85% will still have their implant. Same-day surgery is a different process, not a different surgery.

What do you mean by "process"?

It has to do with the care that's given during the time before and after surgery. The same-day approach involves more of a team effort than conventional surgery...and the process begins well before the actual operation.

Patients have to be medically optimized to reduce the risk for complications and allow them to recover at home instead of in the hospital. A diabetic patient, for example, will be encouraged to stabilize his/her blood sugar before having the surgery. Someone who's obese might be advised to lose weight. Even though these recommendations also apply to people having a conventional hip surgery, they are crucial if a patient wants to go home the same day as the surgery.

The same-day approach also requires an extensive support system. Patients having same-day surgery might meet with team members, such as nurses and physical therapists, to learn such things as how to get around on crutches (usually needed for a couple of weeks)...how to safely climb stairs...how to bathe and use the toilet...and how to manage postsurgical nausea. A discharge planner will ensure that they have adequate support at home—for example, a spouse or a friend who can help them with meals, etc.

In addition, you're encouraged to stay in close contact with doctors, nurses and other support staff. A nurse or doctor should be available 24/7 to answer questions.

Isn't this riskier than staying in the hospital?

Not necessarily. As long as patients are ready for the procedure—in terms of overall health, at-home support, etc.—they'll do about the same as hospitalized patients. The overall complication rate—from blood clots, joint dislocation, poor wound healing or infection—is less than 5% in both same-day and conventional hip replacements.

Who should—or shouldn't—have same-day surgery?

A patient who's 85 years old, lives alone, can barely get around the house and has a variety of health problems would probably be advised not to go home the same day.

On the other hand, a 50-year-old who's in great shape will probably be physiologically able to go home the same day—but you have to consider motivation, as well. It may be easier for some in a hospital, where help is a button-push away.

What about recovery?

The evidence suggests that it's about the same regardless of the type of hip replacement. You can expect to walk a bit soon after surgery, while full recovery might take three months or more. Patients may do physical therapy exercises to strengthen the thighs and hips for six weeks or more.

Do all medical centers offer same-day surgery?

It's not available everywhere, so you'll have to ask your primary care doctor or surgeon or call around. Insurance coverage will probably be similar for inpatient and outpatient procedures.

Important: Whether or not you're considering same-day surgery, choose a board-certified surgeon who does at least 50 hip replacements a year. Studies have found that that's the number at which complication rates start to level off.

Also make sure that the surgeon is experienced in the same type of surgery (anterior, anterolateral or posterior) that you are getting.

To find an experienced surgeon: Check the website of the American Academy of Orthopaedic Surgeons, AAOS.org...or the American Association of Hip and Knee Surgeons, AAHKS.org.

Is Hip Resurfacing for You?

William Macaulay, MD, professor of clinical orthopedic surgery, director of the Center for Hip and Knee Replacement, NewYork-Presbyterian Hospital at Columbia University, all in New York City.

A procedure that "resurfaces" worn-out hip joints rather than replacing them is available in the US. Known as hip resurfacing, the technique can be as durable as hip replacement with less pain during recovery and greater long-term mobility. Originally introduced in England in 1997, the Birmingham Hip System (one of the products used for hip resurfacing) was approved by the FDA in May 2006.

For several years, Americans who wanted to try an alternative to hip replacement have traveled to England, India or one of the other countries that have offered hip resurfacing. Now this procedure is available at more than 100 medical centers throughout the US.

With hip resurfacing, the round head of the femur (thighbone) is reshaped and covered with a metal cap about the same size as the natural femoral head. The reshaped head moves within a smooth metal socket that is implanted into the pelvic bone. Enough bone is left in place to allow for a future hip replacement, if necessary.

Hip resurfacing is a good option for patients age 55 and younger...people of any age who have relatively healthy bones or who are highly active.

Hip resurfacing may take slightly longer than the hour to hour-and-a-half required for a standard hip replacement surgery. The incision is often two to three inches longer than the six- to 12-inch incision required for conventional hip replacement. As with traditional hip replacement, a two- to three-day hospital stay is usually required following hip resurfacing, and healing is more than 90% complete within six to eight weeks.

Editor's note: Resurfacing is not risk free and can have a high failure rate. Speak with your doctor about risks and improved procedures.

Better Hip Surgery

If you're considering hip replacement, you may want to put it off for a few months if you've just received a steroid shot in your hip.

New study: Infection rates jumped 40% in hip replacement patients who received a steroid injection in the three months prior to surgery...but those who received an injection earlier showed no increased risk. Steroids may weaken the immune system, which could account for the higher infection rate. Although rare, an infection in the hip joint could require additional surgery, intravenous antibiotics and a prolonged recovery.

William Schairer, MD, orthopedic surgeon, Hospital for Special Surgery, New York City.

CHAPTER 15

Muscle Cramps and Weakness

Kitchen Cures for the Ouch Of Muscle Cramps

Muscle cramps are a common problem—medically speaking, a muscle cramp is a sudden, involuntary contraction of one or more muscles that can be very painful, sometimes leaving tenderness for up to 24 hours after the cramp subsides. Aging and overuse of the muscles are two common causes, but other triggers can include dehydration...low blood sugar...calcium, sodium and/or magnesium deficiency...underactive thyroid...kidney or liver dysfunction...peripheral vascular disease (which restricts blood flow to the legs)...nerve compression...Lou Gehrig's disease (ALS)...brain tumors/cancer...multiple sclerosis...well, you get the picture. You probably really get the picture the day after a long workout in the garden or with your grandchildren.

WHAT YOU NEED TO KNOW

There is no surefire, works-every-time solution for muscle cramps. First, be sure to differentiate a run-of-the-mill (if excruciating) cramp from one that you must tell your doctor about.

Here's a list of questions to ask yourself...

- **Are my cramps random?** A cramp that comes on suddenly and inexplicably is usually not a problem. Since the majority of random cramps are no big deal, it's fine to try the "old standby" cures, including eating a banana (for potassium)...drinking more water to counter dehydration...light stretching of the affected area...self-massage...and heat packs to relieve pain and tenderness.
- **Are my cramps becoming more frequent and/or following a pattern?** Cramps that begin to establish themselves in a predictable pattern—such as at a particular time of day or when you walk—may be a worrisome sign that you should discuss with your doctor.
- **Did I do something that might explain this cramp?** If you realize that you are getting cramps often, even predictably in certain

Barry Wiese, DC, board-certified chiropractic neurologist in private practice in Rochester, New York.

situations, start a log of when they strike including time of day...what you've eaten...how long they last...how painful they are (consider a score between one and 10)...and what you were doing before and during the episode. Share this information with your doctor.

• **Should I see my doctor?** With persistent or worsening muscle cramps, you need to see your doctor to discuss potential causes and treatments. Though muscle cramping represents abnormal function, it's only rarely serious. However, many disease processes include cramping in their list of symptoms...and for many of those, the earlier you get treated, the better the outcome—so it pays to follow a conservative, cautious route until proven otherwise.

You'll be asked about your medical history, and your doctor may suggest some tests, including blood work, to find the root cause. Treatment options could range from vitamin B supplementation...to prescription medications, such as diltiazem (a calcium-channel blocker) and baclofen (a potent muscle relaxant sometimes used to treat muscle spasms in patients with MS and ALS)...and possibly even quinine, the malaria treatment, though it's used only in extreme cases because of the potential for adverse side effects.

KITCHEN CURES

Even if your muscle cramp falls into the "random and not worrisome" category, it's still pretty painful. So here's the secret kitchen cure...pickle juice! (You could also just eat a pickle.) No, we're not kidding, and you may be surprised that eating mustard, too, can help muscle cramps. Both contain acetic acid, salts and other ingredients that help neutralize the compounds or electrolyte deficiencies that may cause cramps. Other helpful remedies you may be able to pull out of your kitchen cabinets include apple cider vinegar (mix two teaspoons with one teaspoon of honey into a glass of warm water), which works much like the pickle juice...and chamomile tea, which contains glycine, an amino acid that helps relieve muscle spasms.

A Surprising Cure for Joint and Muscle Aches

Mitchell Yass, DPT, a Florida-based physical therapist and creator of the Yass Method for treating chronic pain. He is the author of *Overpower Pain: The Strength Training Program That Stops Pain Without Drugs or Surgery*, *The Pain Cure Rx: The Yass Method for Diagnosing and Resolving Chronic Pain* and *The Yass Method for Pain-Free Movement: A Guide to Easing through Your Day without Aches and Pains* and host of the PBS special *The Pain Prescription*. MitchellYass.com

When you hear the term "weight lifting," you may think of body builders with bulging muscles. Only in the past few years has it become more widely known that weight lifting—often called strength training—also helps control body weight and increase bone mass.

What most people still don't know: Weight lifting can play a significant role in relieving muscle and joint pain. Even though doctors often overlook muscle weakness as a cause of pain, it is the culprit in an estimated 80% to 90% of my patients, many of whom are ages 60 to 90 and suffer from aching joints and muscles.

Surprisingly, muscle weakness contributes to pain even in people who have been told by a physician that a structural problem, such as a torn ligament or arthritis, is responsible for their symptoms.

WHY DO STRONG MUSCLES FIGHT PAIN?

Exercises designed to strengthen muscles improve joint function and overall body mechanics in two important ways. When the muscles of a joint are weak, the bones can move out of position, causing bone surfaces to rub together and leading to irritation and pain at the joint. Also, because muscles work together to produce movement, if one is underdeveloped, other muscles can easily become strained.

The following exercises target areas that are especially prone to pain-causing muscle weakness that often goes undetected.

The exercises require hand weights or ankle weights. Both are available at sporting-goods stores.

Typical cost: Hand weights—$10 a pair... ankle weights—$20 a pair.

Helpful: When choosing weights, select ones that you can lift about 10 times without straining. If your muscles are not tired by the time of the last repetition, choose a heavier weight.

For each exercise, perform three sets of 10 repetitions two to three times a week.* As you lift the weight, breathe out and count to two... as you lower it, breathe in and count to three.

Important: See a doctor if your pain was caused by a traumatic injury, such as a fall...if your discomfort is constant and/or severe...or if you have limited range of motion (less than 50% of your normal range). In these cases, the pain may be due to a problem that cannot be improved with exercise.

Best exercises to relieve...

SHOULDER AND ELBOW PAIN

What's targeted: The rotator-cuff muscles, which hold the humerus (upper arm) bone in place when you lift your arm. Building the rotator-cuff muscles also alleviates the strain on forearm muscles that leads to elbow pain. Rotator-cuff muscles can be strained during such activities as driving or using a computer for long periods without supporting the arms.

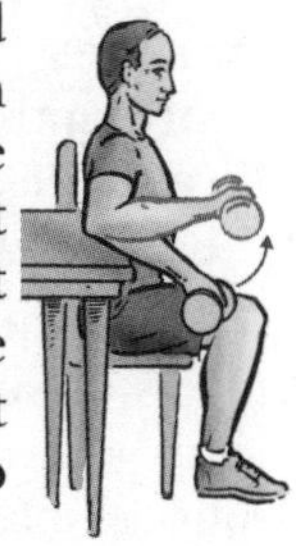

What to do: Sit in a chair placed at the front edge of a table with your left side a few inches from the corner of the table. Hold a weight in your left hand and rest your left elbow on the front edge of the table. Your hand should be about three inches below the table top with your palm facing down.

Raise your forearm, keeping your wrist straight, until your hand is about three inches above the table. Lower the weight to the starting position. Reposition the chair so that your right side is next to the table, and repeat the exercise with the weight in your right hand.

SHOULDER PAIN

What's targeted: The posterior-deltoid muscles located at the back of the shoulders. These muscles tend to be weaker than the front shoulder muscles due to our natural tendency to hold and carry objects in front of our bodies, which makes the chest, front shoulder and bicep muscles work harder. This imbalance can throw off bone alignment in the shoulder joints, causing pain.

What to do: Stand with your feet a little more than shoulder width apart. Position yourself so that your knees and elbows are slightly bent and your back slightly arched. Hold a weight in each hand in front of your thighs, palms facing each other. Using your shoulders, extend your arms out to the side until the weights are about six inches from your thighs, stopping the motion before your shoulder blades begin to come together. Return the weights to the starting position.

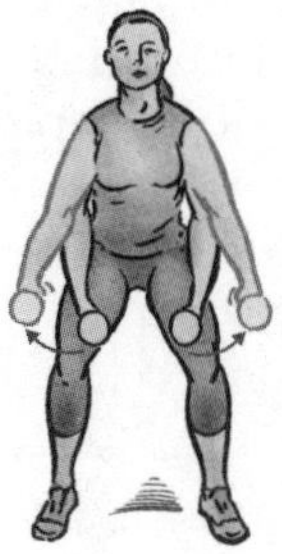

ELBOW PAIN

What's targeted: The wrist-extensor muscles, which run along the top of the forearm. Building these muscles relieves strains caused by gardening, playing tennis or other activities involving repetitive wrist movement, gripping or squeezing.

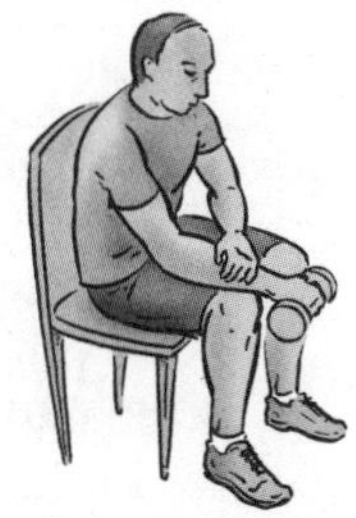

What to do: Sit with your feet flat on the floor directly under your knees. While holding a weight in your right hand, rest your right forearm on the top of your right thigh with your wrist about three inches directly in front of your knee and your palm facing down. Place your left hand on your right forearm to keep it steady. Using your wrist muscles, lift the weight until your wrist is fully flexed. Return to the starting position. Repeat the exercise on your left thigh, using your left hand.

HIP, KNEE AND HEEL PAIN

What's targeted: The hip-abductor muscles, which support your legs when you walk and climb stairs. Strengthening these muscles can relieve muscle strain at the hip joint and prevent the knee and foot from rotating toward the midline of your body when you walk

*Consult your doctor before starting any new exercise program.

(causing knee pain and heel pain)—instead of staying in line with your hip.

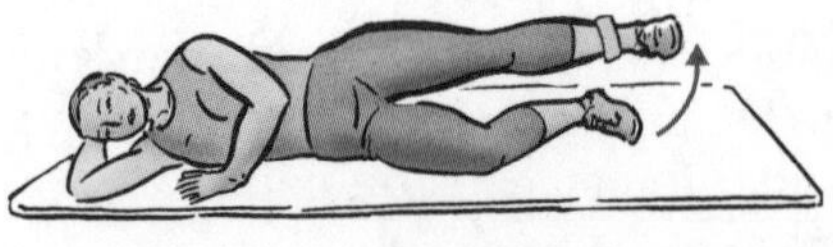

What to do: Lie on your right side on a carpeted floor or a mat with an ankle weight strapped to your left leg. Fold your right arm under your head and bend your right leg. Place your left hand on the floor in front of you for support. Flex your left foot (as if standing on it) and raise your straightened left leg to hip height, keeping it in line with your torso. Lower your leg to the starting position. Lie on your left side and repeat the exercise raising your right leg.

Illustrations: Shawn Banner

More Natural Remedies for Painful Muscle Cramps

Jamison Starbuck, ND, naturopathic physician in family practice and a guest lecturer at the University of Montana, both in Missoula. She is past president of the American Association of Naturopathic Physicians and a contributing editor to *The Alternative Advisor: The Complete Guide to Natural Therapies and Alternative Treatments.* DrJamisonStarbuck.com

As a kid, I loved the funny sound of "charley horse." Somewhere along the line, I learned that the term may have originated from a baseball pitcher who played in the late 1800s—Charley "Old Hoss" Radbourn—who evidently suffered from excruciating muscle cramps while playing baseball. Nowadays, I know how painful a muscle cramp can be, and as a naturopathic physician, I disagree with my medical doctor colleagues who believe that a muscle cramp is just one of those things you must "learn to live with." The truth is, muscle cramps usually result from one of three causes—dehydration, muscle overuse or mineral deficiency. *To protect yourself...*

- **Get enough fluids.** If you don't get enough fluids, your risk for muscle cramps increases, especially while exercising. Soda, juice, coffee, diet drinks and even sweetened electrolyte-replacement beverages are no substitute for plain water.

For adequate hydration: I recommend drinking one-half ounce of water per pound of body weight per day.* So, if you weigh 150 pounds, you should drink 75 ounces. It's wise to increase your total daily water intake by 16 to 32 ounces if you are doing vigorous exercise (such as hiking, biking or running)...are out in hot weather (above 80° F)...are pregnant (a risk factor for muscle cramps)...are flying long distances (through two or more time zones)...or if you are starting a new project, such as gardening or house painting, involving physical activity that stresses the muscles in new ways.

- **Stretch your muscles properly.** Sometimes we can't avoid overusing our muscles. But we can stretch. This should be done before overusing your muscles, but if you forget, then do so afterward and again before bed.

What to do: Immediately after vigorous activity, spend 10 minutes elongating the muscles you used, especially those of the thigh, calf and low back, which are most likely to suddenly spasm. For example, try forward bends (bend from the waist to touch the floor, if possible—use a table edge for support if you feel unsteady)...and calf stretches (put your hands on the wall while standing about three feet away from it—lean in, elongating the calf muscles).

- **Get the right minerals.** Inadequate blood levels of such minerals as magnesium, potassium and sodium will increase your risk for muscle spasms. Most people get plenty of sodium in their diets but lose much of it when they perspire during exercise and/or are out in hot weather. Potassium and magnesium in vegetables, whole grains, beans, nuts, seeds and fresh fruit are most readily available for absorption. However, if you suffer from muscle spasms, talk to your doctor about taking daily mineral supplements of potassium and magnesium to ensure adequate levels. Be sure to consult your doctor first if you have kidney or heart disease or take any type of medication.

*Talk to your doctor before significantly changing your daily water intake.

• **Try homeopathy.** The homeopathic remedies Mag phos (6X) and Kali phos (6X), taken together, often relieve muscle cramps. The remedies, manufactured by Hyland's/Standard Homeopathic, are available in stores selling natural medicines. Dissolve two pellets of each remedy (four pellets total) under the tongue. Repeat the same dose every 10 minutes for up to one hour until the pain is gone.

Muscle Weakness Is Not Inevitable: How to Fight Sarcopenia

John E. Morley, MD, director of the division of geriatric medicine and the Dammert Professor of Gerontology at Saint Louis University School of Medicine. He is coeditor of the textbook *Sarcopenia* and editor of the professional publication *Journal of the American Medical Directors Association*. Dr. Morley is also a recipient of the American Geriatrics Society's Lascher/Manning Award for Lifetime Achievement in Geriatrics.

If you're age 50 or older, you've probably noticed that your suitcases and grocery bags have gotten mysteriously heavier. It's hard to admit it, but your muscle power is not what it used to be.

Unfortunately, far too many people assume that this age-related condition known as sarcopenia, which literally means "loss of muscle or flesh," is an inevitable part of aging. But that's simply not true. New and better ways to prevent and diagnose this condition now are available—and there's more reason than ever to not ignore it.

The dangers of sarcopenia are more serious than experts once thought—and may involve other crucial elements of your health such as your risk for diabetes, dementia and other chronic conditions.

MORE THAN MUSCLE LOSS

With advancing age, our muscles shrink because the body loses some of its ability to convert protein into muscle tissue. By age 50, the average adult loses about 1% to 2% of muscle mass every year.

That's bad enough, but the real problem is what results from this muscle loss. Over time, it becomes more difficult to stand up from a chair...climb a flight of stairs...or even open a jar. People with sarcopenia are far more likely than stronger adults to suffer falls and/or bone fractures. They're also more likely to be hospitalized or admitted to a nursing home—and even die during a given period of time.

An increasing body of evidence shows that people with weak muscle strength have a higher risk of developing type 2 diabetes—a disease that can also double your risk for heart attack and stroke.

Recently discovered danger: People with sarcopenia are at increased risk for cognitive decline, including brain atrophy and dementia, according to research published in *Clinical Interventions in Aging*. In this study, people with sarcopenia were six times more likely to suffer from physical/cognitive impairments than those without this condition.

What this means to you: Collectively, the risks associated with sarcopenia are so great that clinicians from a variety of disciplines assess signs such as weight loss (from shrinking muscles)...fatigue...and a loss of strength to determine which patients are at highest risk for frailty and to work toward intervention.

THE 4-STEP PLAN

As scientists learn more about sarcopenia, the better your odds are of fighting it—if you take the appropriate steps. *What works best if you have sarcopenia...*

STEP 1: **Load up on protein.** Everyone needs protein to increase muscle size/strength. People with sarcopenia need a lot of protein. The recommended daily allowance (RDA) for protein is 0.8 g per kilogram of body weight. (That's about 54 g for a 150-pound woman.) If you've been diagnosed with sarcopenia, you need much more (about 1.2 g per kilogram of body weight).

My advice: Whenever possible, get most or all of your protein from natural foods rather than from protein-fortified foods—the nutrients in natural foods work synergistically to provide greater benefits than supplements. (For example, a small, 3.5-ounce serving of lean pork has about 26 g of protein...one-half cup of pinto beans, 7 g...and a large egg, about 6 g.)

Note: If you have kidney disease, you may have been told to limit your protein intake. Ask your nephrologist for advice on optimal protein levels for you.

Helpful: If you find it difficult to get enough protein from food alone, try whey protein supplements. You can buy these milk-based supplements in powder and liquid forms. Products such as Ensure typically provide 12 g to 20 g of protein per serving, while some protein powders deliver up to 60 g in two scoops mixed in a smoothie, for example. An advantage of whey protein supplements is that they contain leucine, an amino acid involved in muscle synthesis. If you can't have dairy, ask your doctor about taking an essential amino acid supplement enriched with leucine.

STEP 2: **Get enough vitamin D.** You need vitamin D for both muscle and bone strength. Depending upon the time of year and where you live, you can get all you need from 10 or so minutes of daily unprotected sun exposure. But many older adults don't spend that much time in the sun...and those who do are probably covering up or using sunscreen to protect against skin cancer.

My advice: Consume at least 1,000 international units (IU) of vitamin D daily. You can get some of this from D-fortified cereal, milk or juice. If you don't eat a lot of these foods, you may find it easier to take a 1,000-IU vitamin D supplement.

STEP 3: **Eat fish.** There's good evidence that two to four weekly meals of fatty fish (such as salmon, mackerel or sardines) will improve blood flow to all of the body's muscles, including the heart. In theory, this should help people with sarcopenia maintain or gain muscle mass, but the evidence that it helps isn't conclusive. Even so, I still recommend fish because it's a good protein source and has many other health benefits.

STEP 4: **Exercise the right way.** Exercise is the only way to build muscle, even if you consume plenty of protein. Aerobic exercise (such as brisk walking) is good—everyone should get some because it improves both muscle and cardiovascular health. But strength training is the real ticket for building muscle. As an added bonus, it also appears to promote brain health.

Important recent finding: When Australian researchers had 100 people age 55 or older with mild cognitive impairment (a condition that often precedes Alzheimer's) do weight-lifting exercises twice a week for six months, the stronger the study participants' muscles got, the greater their cognitive improvement, according to a study published in 2016 in *Journal of the American Geriatrics Society.*

Even if you are not able to use weight-lifting machines at a gym, there are plenty of ways to do strength training. The American College of Sports Medicine recommends lifting weights (hand weights are fine) or using elastic resistance bands two to three days a week. Unfortunately, that's too ambitious for many people.

My advice: Just do some exercise, whether it's 10 minutes every day or an hour once a week. If you feel too weak to start with "real" exercise, you can keep things simple.

Example: A chair-stand exercise, in which you sit in an armless chair...extend your arms in front of you...slowly stand up...then slowly lower yourself back down. Do this five to 10 times, twice daily.

For arm strength: Hold the ends of a large elastic resistance band in each hand, and stand with both feet on the middle of the band. Keeping your body straight and your elbows by your side, slowly curl your hands up toward your shoulders. You can raise both hands together or one at a time. Try to repeat the movement eight to 12 times, twice daily.

For leg strength: Sit on a chair. Keeping your back straight, slowly extend your right leg straight out in front of you and hold for several seconds before lowering it slowly back down. Repeat with the left leg. Do 10 repetitions on each leg. When this becomes easy, strap on an ankle weight that's heavy enough so that you cannot do more than 15 repetitions per leg.

If you tend to get bored with exercise...

Research shows that people who work with an exercise coach or personal trainer—at home or at a health club—are more likely to stick with regular exercise. In a program that my colleagues and I supervise, patients with sarcopenia first attend physical therapy to help restore flexibility, balance and endurance, then attend weekly sessions led by exercise coaches who are enthusiastic and keep people motivated.

My advice: Consider using an exercise coach. It may be one of the best things you do for your overall health! To find an exercise coach near you, consult the American Council on Exercise, ACEfitness.org.

The Secret Muscles That Can Cause Chronic Pain

Jo Ann Staugaard-Jones, MA, advanced Pilates and Hatha yoga instructor based in Andover, New Jersey. She is a former professor of kinesiology, exercise science and dance at County College of Morris in Randolph, New Jersey, and the author of *The Anatomy of Exercise & Movement* and *The Vital Psoas Muscle.* Move-Live.com

Most people have heard plenty about the core—that band of muscles in the abdomen, low back, hips and pelvis. But what if there were some far less well-known muscles that could be causing all your trouble? Say hello to the psoas (pronounced SO-as) muscles! Ignoring these crucial muscles can lead to low-back pain and poor posture.

What you need to know...

WHERE ARE THEY?

Located deep within the center of the body, the psoas major muscles are the only muscles that connect the upper and lower extremities of your body. As a pair of muscles on both the right and left sides, they run from the lower spine, past the front of the pelvis, through either side of the groin and attach to the inside of the femurs (thighbones).

So what exactly do these muscles do? The psoas muscles help with the transfer of weight when you're walking or running. When you extend your leg back, for example, the psoas on that side lengthens...when you lift your knee, it contracts. The psoas muscles also act as stabilizers of the lower spine, the pelvis and the legs, aiding body alignment and posture.

What goes wrong: If the psoas muscles are shortened for long periods of time—as occurs when sitting, for example—they can tighten on one or both sides. If the psoas on one side of the body is tighter than the other (from leaning to one side while sitting, for instance), it can also torque the spine, affecting your posture and gait. An imbalance on one or both sides can lead to inflammation and pain while walking.

Unlike toned abs, you can't see the psoas muscles. Because you can't touch your psoas muscles either, it can be difficult to tell if they're the cause of your back pain and poor posture.

There are some clues, however, that may indicate that these muscles are tight or weak—for example, you may also feel discomfort in the hip sockets, the glutes or even the sacroiliac joints, which are in the back of the pelvis. The pain can be in one spot or travel throughout the path of the muscle.

KEEPING YOUR PSOAS MUSCLES IN SHAPE

The first step to keeping the psoas muscles in top shape is to stand up. Instead of sitting for long periods of time, get up and move around at least every hour. To help prevent or relieve psoas-related pain, also do these three exercises every other day (as with any exercise program, check with your doctor first)...

Exercise #1: **Lunge.** Also known as the "runner's stretch," the lunge strengthens and stretches the psoas and thigh muscles.

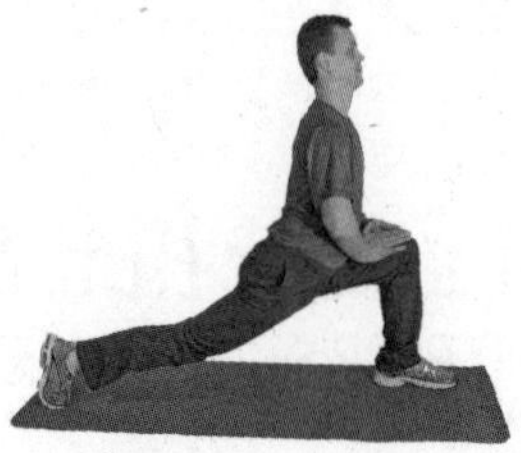

What to do: Stand with your left foot forward and right leg back (about three to four feet apart). Bend your front knee until it's directly over your toes, at about a 90-degree angle. Slide your right leg straight back until it is almost parallel to the floor. Keep your feet facing forward, and don't let your front knee extend beyond your toes. Your spine should be straight, and you can rest your hands on the floor or the front of one thigh. Hold for up to 30 seconds, then repeat on the other side.

***Exercise #2:* Teaser or Boat pose.** This position, used in both Pilates and yoga, works the psoas muscles and several other core muscles.

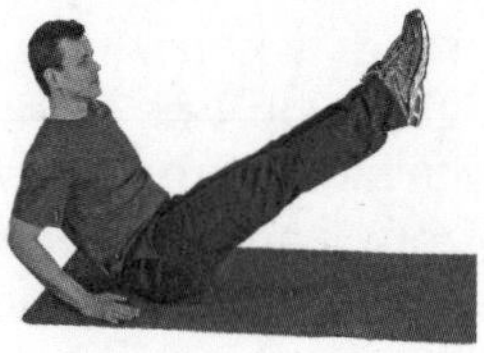

What to do: Sit on the floor with your legs extended out in front. While keeping your hands on the floor behind your hips, lean back slightly and balance just behind your "sit" bones (beneath your buttocks). Then gently raise one leg and then the other as high as possible, so that your body is in a "V" position. Hold for 10 seconds while keeping your chest lifted and your torso long. If you're able, extend your arms forward for added challenge. Repeat three times, or hold longer.

***Exercise #3:* Windmill.** This exercise strengthens and stretches the psoas muscles and oblique (side abdominal) muscles.

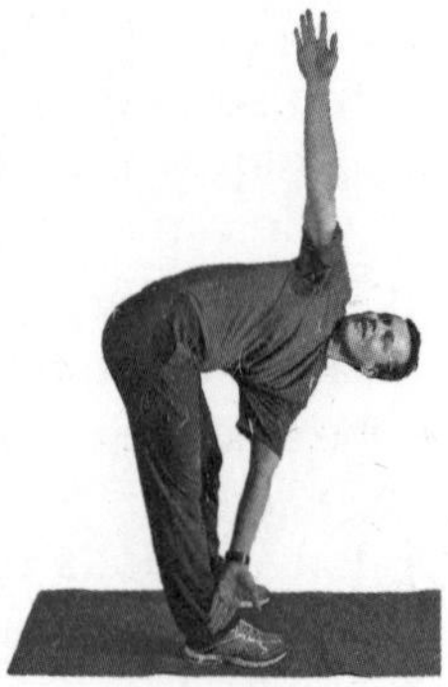

What to do: While standing with your arms extended out to each side and your knees slightly bent, lean forward and touch your left hand to your right ankle as you extend your right arm upward and look up toward the ceiling. Return to the original standing position and repeat on the other side. Do five reps, without rushing, for maximum benefit.

It's Your Butt Muscles!

Chris Kolba, PhD, PT, sports medicine physical therapist and clinical instructor at The Ohio State University Wexner Medical Center in Columbus. He developed The Ohio State Tactical Rehab and Conditioning Program to meet the needs of firefighters, police officers and other tactical operators.

Want to get to the bottom of your persistent back, knee or hip pain? Look behind you, and you'll find the likely cause.

Dormant butt syndrome is the name that I've coined for a serious problem that affects millions of Americans, especially those who spend most of the day sitting. Weak gluteal (butt) muscles are often the common link. A lack of strength in this area forces other muscles to compensate and do jobs that they're not designed to do alone, resulting in pain in unexpected parts of the body.

THE NEGLECTED CORE

Dormant butt syndrome strikes people who are generally sedentary—whether they're sitting behind a desk, driving a car or watching their favorite sitcoms. When you're positioned on your derriere for hours on end, the glutes aren't "firing" and there's more tightness in the hip flexor muscles, which can lead to hamstring injuries or back, hip or knee pain. Runners and other athletes who do repetitive motion can also get tight hip flexors.

When I evaluate clients who have lower-body pain, I always check for adequate glute strength. To do this, I ask the patient to lie on his/her stomach and do a leg lift against resistance from my hand to determine how strong his glutes are.

I also put my fingertips lightly on the hamstring and gluteal muscles of the lifted leg to evaluate the "firing pattern" of muscles. Normally, the gluteal muscles will fire (or activate) first, followed by the hamstrings. If the pattern is reversed, I'll know that the gluteal muscles are weaker than they should be.

MORE BANG FOR YOUR BUTT

I advise clients to spend the majority of their waking hours standing, if possible. Since this isn't always practical, at least make an effort to increase your amount of upright time—staying on your feet when watching TV, for example, or standing (and pacing) when talking on the telephone. Six other movements that help—do each one twice a week (except for the hip flexor stretch, which should be done daily)...*

*Consult your doctor before beginning this regimen—or any other new exercise program, especially if you've had knee, hip or back surgery.

• **Glute Bridge.** It is among the best exercises for targeting the glutes. It gives the abdominal core muscles a bit of a workout, too.

What to do: Lie on your back with your knees bent and your feet flat on the floor. Contract your abdominal muscles slightly. Next, raise your hips up about six inches and hold for a few seconds...then slowly lower yourself back down. Repeat this movement 10 to 12 times.

• **Lunges.** They strengthen the gluteal muscles, along with muscles in the hips and thighs.

What to do: Stand with your feet together and your hands on your hips. Take a step forward with your left leg, while simultaneously bending that leg until the thigh is parallel to the floor. Keep your front foot flat on the floor as you bend your knee (most of the weight should go onto your heel), and don't let the front knee extend farther forward than the toes. Return to the starting position, then repeat with the other leg. Work up to 12 to 15 reps on each leg.

Note: If a deep knee bend is painful, don't go down as far.

• **Wall squats.** Squats are popular because they increase both gluteal and thigh strength. This exercise is easier than traditional squats because it requires only body weight and a wall for support.

What to do: Lean back against a wall with your feet shoulder-width apart and out a foot or two. Keep your back and hips against the wall.

Slide down until your thighs are parallel to the floor. Hold the position until your thighs start to say "enough," then rise back up. In the beginning, your thighs might start shaking after just a few seconds. Over time, try to work up to holding the position for 30 to 60 seconds.

If you're out of shape or have weak knees, you can lower yourself about halfway to the parallel position. Don't let your knees collapse inward, and stop if you feel any pain. Work your way toward the full bend as you build strength.

• **Side planks.** For those with dormant butt syndrome, it's important to stretch/strengthen surrounding muscles as well as the glutes themselves. This exercise activates muscles in the midsection, including the hips.

What to do: Lie on your right side, with your legs extended and "stacked" on top of each other. Prop up your upper body by supporting your weight on your forearm, keeping your shoulder aligned with your elbow. Contract the ab muscles and lift your hips and knees off the floor. Hold the position for 10 to 30 seconds, then lower back down. Repeat on the other side. Start with two to three sets, holding the position for 10 seconds, and gradually work up to one minute per set.

• **Single Leg Balance.** Most people lose some strength, balance and rotational motion (the ability of their joints to rotate) as they get older. This exercise is a good way to improve hip and core stability while challenging balance.

What to do: Stand on one leg, with your arms held slightly away from your body for balance.

Important: For safety, stand next to a counter to catch yourself if you start to topple over. Try to hold the position (without swaying) for 30 to 60 seconds. Then try it on the other leg. It's challenging at first! Once it gets too easy, lift the leg a bit higher and/or try to do it with your eyes closed. This is harder because vision helps the body orient itself.

• **Hip flexor stretch.** Tight hip flexors cause dormant butt syndrome. When these muscles are tight, there's compensatory movement throughout the lower back, which can lead to pain as well as disk damage in the lower back.

What to do: Kneel on your left knee, with your left hand on your hip and your right foot flat on the floor in front of you—the right knee should be bent and the right thigh should be roughly parallel to the floor. Move your left hip forward until it extends beyond the left knee. Don't bend forward during the movement. Hold the position for 20 to 30 seconds, then repeat for three or four reps. Change position and repeat on the other side.

Muscle Tightness Could Be Causing Your Pain

Donna Finando, Roslyn Heights, New York–based licensed acupuncturist (LAc) and massage therapist (LMT). She is the author of the *Trigger Point Self-Care Manual for Pain-Free Movement.*

When any one of the more than 200 muscles in your body suffers from overuse or an injury, it can develop a trigger point—a tiny knot in which a strand of the muscle becomes constricted, making the muscle stiff and weak.

Left untreated, this condition can persist for years, causing pain to recur repeatedly. Fortunately, you can relieve this type of pain with a simple technique known as trigger-point therapy. It involves locating the associated trigger points and compressing them for 20 to 30 seconds several times a day. Press only hard enough to feel the tightness of the muscle and the soreness of the trigger point. Stretches for each condition also should be repeated several times daily.

Helpful: Whenever possible, also apply 20 minutes of moist heat once or twice a day to the affected muscle. Moist heat brings blood and body fluids to the muscle, increasing circulation. (Moist heating pads by Cara, Sunbeam or Thermophore can be purchased at most drugstores for $20 to $50.)

If you've worked on your muscles for several days and felt little or no relief, check with your doctor to make sure there is no other source of pain, such as arthritis.

Conditions often caused by trigger points—and how to treat them…

STIFF NECK

Stiff neck frequently occurs after sleeping with your head turned all the way to one side, or as a result of holding a phone between your ear and shoulder. The condition is often due to a trigger point in the levator scapulae muscle, which runs from the inner edge of the shoulder blade to the neck.

To find the trigger point: Reach the hand that is on your pain-free side over to touch your shoulder on the painful side. Locate the inside edge of the shoulder blade, then move your hand a bit closer to your spine, feeling for a hard band the size of a pencil running up toward your neck. While bending your neck toward your pain-free side, use your fingers to locate a tender spot along this band, then press it for 20 to 30 seconds.

Helpful stretch: Turn your chin 30 degrees away from the affected side, then drop your chin down slightly toward your chest. Hold for a slow count of 20.

HIP, BUTTOCK AND LEG PAIN

Pain in the hips, buttocks or legs is often diagnosed as sciatica (pain in your back that radiates into your buttocks and legs) when it actually may be caused by trigger points in the muscles of the back and buttocks. One of these muscles, the gluteus medius, lies midway between the top of your pelvis and the top of your thighbone.

To find the trigger point: Lie on the floor on your pain-free side with your knees slightly bent, and use your fingers to massage your hip under the top of your pelvis and down toward the top of your thighbone. If trigger points are present, you'll feel taut bands and tender spots. Once you've located a tender spot, roll onto your painful side and place a tennis ball between this spot and the floor. Then let your weight press the ball into the tender area for 20 to 30 seconds.

Helpful stretch: Stand facing a wall with your arms raised and the backs of your hands pressed against your forehead. Cross your pain-free leg in front of your other leg. Bend the knee of your rear leg into the back of your pain-free leg while shifting your weight onto your painful hip. This should create a stretch between your pelvis and the top of your thighbone. Hold for a slow count of 20.

CALF PAIN

If you're experiencing pain or soreness in your calf or the back of your knee, it may be caused by trigger points in the gastrocnemius muscle (the large muscle that gives the calf its characteristic shape).

To find the trigger point: Sit in a chair and place the sole of the foot of your affected leg on a footstool or coffee table in front of you. Place one hand on the outer side of this leg and the other on the inner side of this leg—in both cases, just above the ankle. Run your fingers along your Achilles tendon (the large tendon at the back of your heel) and work your way to the middle of the calf, feeling for tender spots. Continue upward, toward the back of the knee. When you find a tender spot, compress it with your fingers for 20 to 30 seconds.

Helpful stretch: While standing about 12 inches from a wall, facing the wall, place your hands on the wall at chest level. Keeping your feet hip-width apart and the toes of both feet facing the wall, move your painful leg 18 inches behind the other leg. Bend your front knee, keeping your rear leg straight. Your weight should remain on the front leg. Hold for a slow count of 20.

TENNIS ELBOW

Inflammation of the tendon on the outside of the elbow, known as "tennis elbow," can cause sharp pain down the back of the forearm into the wrist, making it hard to grip objects. However, sometimes the condition may not be an inflammation but a result of trigger points in the extensor muscles of the hand and fingers, which can be caused by repeated or forceful gripping, such as when holding a tennis racket—or even a coffee cup.

To find the trigger point: Rest the elbow and forearm of your sore arm on a table, with your palm facing up. Use your opposite hand to feel along the muscle on the outside (thumb side) of your elbow crease, then follow this muscle down toward your hand. When you find a tender spot, press down and hold for 20 to 30 seconds.

Helpful stretch: Sit on a chair, and keeping your elbow straight, place the back of the hand on the affected arm flat on the seat beside you, palm up, feeling a stretch in your forearm. Hold for a slow count of 20.

Do-It-Yourself Pain Relief With a Tennis Ball

Mark H. LaBeau, DO, physician of osteopathic medic, Encinitas, California. DrLabeau.com

There's a simple home remedy for muscle pain—self-massage with tennis balls. It is remarkably easy to do and effective. It is based on bodywork techniques such as myofascial release and acupressure, in which pressure is applied at the point or points of tenderness.

WHICH BALL IS BEST?

While using a tennis ball is more common, patients can experiment with a golf ball, which often is easier to use because it's smaller. Try both—and see which works best for you. To relieve discomfort in two nearby areas, place two balls in a sock and arrange them at the points of tenderness.

So easy to do...

Even though we're using the word "massage," the technique actually involves just lying on or pressing on a tennis ball (not rolling over it). As you'll see, the pressure of your body's weight on the ball is all you need to relieve tension. The back, neck and feet are the places most helped by tennis ball massage, but you can place a ball under any muscle or muscle area in which there is tenderness or a knot.

Repeat each exercise multiple times a day, but limit the duration of each time to no more than 10 minutes. Doing it longer than that can irritate the tissue.

Caution: Ongoing muscle discomfort that lasts for about a week or more may be a sign of a more complex condition, such as a muscle tear or tendonitis, and should be evaluated by your doctor.

FOR THE BACK

Lie comfortably on the floor, and position the ball under the area or areas where you are experiencing any tenderness or pain. Adjust as needed. You should feel relief of some or all of the pain within five minutes. Remain with the ball in place for up to 10 minutes.

FOR THE NECK

Lie on the floor or a bed, and position the ball in the natural curve at the back of the neck...at the base of the neck...or on either side of the neck that is sore. You should feel relief of some or all of the pain within five minutes. Remain with the ball in place for up to 10 minutes.

FOR THE FOOT

Sit in a comfortable chair with your feet on the floor in front of you. Place a ball under your arch or any place that you feel pain. You can either press your foot into the ball—or roll over the tender point. (This is one time when rolling over the ball can help!)

What to Do with Persistent Muscle Pain and Weakness

Mark Stengler, NMD, naturopathic doctor and founder of the Stengler Center for Integrative Medicine in Encinitas, California. He is author or coauthor of numerous books, including *The Natural Physician's Healing Therapies* and *Bottom Line's Prescription for Natural Cures*, and author of the newsletter *Health Revelations*. MarkStengler.com

Each morning, I'm so stiff and achy that I can hardly get out of bed. All day long my neck and shoulders hurt, so I have to take pain pills every few hours," said Brian, 68, on his first visit to me.

Two years earlier, Brian had been diagnosed with polymyalgia rheumatica (PMR), an inflammatory disorder characterized by severe pain and stiffness in the muscles of the neck, shoulders, upper arms, low back, hips and/or thighs. PMR can come on literally overnight, as it did with Brian, or develop gradually. It usually appears after age 50 and is more common in women. Though the cause of PMR is unknown, the pain may result from swelling of blood vessels in the muscles. Diagnosis is based on patient history, symptoms and blood tests for markers of inflammation.

I advised Brian to minimize use of over-the-counter painkillers, such as *acetaminophen* (Tylenol) and *ibuprofen* (Advil), because they can cause gastrointestinal bleeding, cardiovascular problems, and/or kidney or liver damage. I also cautioned him that steroid medication—the conventional treatment for severe PMR, which he had used several times—can cause weight gain, high blood pressure, brittle bones, high blood sugar and cataracts. As a safe alternative, I suggested methylsulfonylmethane (MSM), a nonprescription sulphur-containing supplement that reduces pain and inflammation.

Brian also suffered from muscle weakness, low energy, night sweats and erectile dysfunction—all signs of low testosterone. Sure enough, a week later, test results revealed that Brian had very low testosterone levels—a fairly common condition in men over age 60, especially those who have used steroid medication. I prescribed a bioidentical (natural) testosterone cream. Transdermal testosterone is less likely than oral testosterone to cause liver problems or enlargement of the breasts or prostate.

Three months later, Brian's muscle pain was 90% better—a very good response for a relatively short period of time on MSM. The testosterone cream, which has anti-inflammatory effects, also helped to alleviate his PMR pain. In addition, thanks to the testosterone, Brian's muscle strength was much improved, his energy had soared, and his night sweats and erectile problems were gone. We decided that he should continue indefinitely on the MSM and testosterone cream, given how well they had worked.

CHAPTER 16

Mystery Illness: What's That Pain Mean?

Unraveling the Mystery of Pain

Anyone who lives with unexplained chronic pain knows that it can be depressing. In fact, of the more than 47 million American adults who suffer from chronic pain—often with no identifiable cause—at least two-thirds also have depression.

It's no coincidence, according to Gary Kaplan, DO, a pain expert who believes that the two disorders may be an important symptom of the same underlying condition—inflammation in specific cells of the brain. To learn more about his theory, we recently spoke with Dr. Kaplan.

What actually causes chronic pain?

There are many possible causes, including joint or nerve damage and cancer. However, if a doctor cannot identify the origin of chronic pain or pain persists beyond the point of expected healing, inflammation in the brain could be the cause.

What role does brain inflammation play in causing pain?

The brain contains different kinds of cells, among them microglia, which make up about 10% of brain cells. These cells act as the immune system of the central nervous system. If threats (see below) make it into the brain, microglia go into attack mode—they become upregulated—to destroy the threat.

While upregulated, microglia secrete inflammatory chemicals to create swelling that helps to protect the healthy brain cells. Even in relatively tiny amounts, inflammatory chemicals make us feel sick, even though the

Gary Kaplan, DO, founder and medical director of the Kaplan Center for Integrative Medicine in McLean, Virginia. He is also clinical associate professor of family medicine at Georgetown University School of Medicine in Washington, DC. Dr. Kaplan, who is board-certified in both family medicine and pain medicine, is the author of *Total Recovery: Solving the Mystery of Chronic Pain and Depression.* KaplanClinic.com

body is fighting illness. Signs of inflammation include fever, fatigue, headaches and pain virtually anywhere in the body.

What causes microglia to become upregulated?

Infections (such as meningitis or Lyme)...toxins (including heavy metals, mold or excessive alcohol)...loss of oxygen to the brain, which occurs in sleep apnea...autoimmune disorders such as celiac disease...physical traumas... surgery...and chronic use of narcotics. In addition, emotional traumas—experienced due to long periods of stress, a physical assault or a car accident, for instance—can turn on the microglia. That explains why a person who grew up in an emotionally or physically abusive household is more likely to suffer chronic pain as an adult—an association that has been shown in numerous studies.

With enough repetitive assaults, the microglia can become so hyperreactive that they constantly spew inflammatory chemicals. Constant inflammation in the brain can result in not only chronic pain but also depression, anxiety disorders and other health issues.

Why does chronic pain affect only certain people?

Each of us has a different level of resilience (due to genetics and environmental factors such as emotional nurturing). Some people can take a huge number of physical or mental blows and remain healthy...others can be physically affected by just a few assaults.

So how do we "turn off" the microglia that are making us sick?

That's still being researched. In my practice, however, we try to address each of the factors provoking the inflammation in the brain.

My advice for people who are suffering from unexplained chronic pain...

1. Create a time line of life and health. On one sheet of paper, write down the major traumas of your life—physical and emotional—along with the dates (or approximate dates) they happened. On another sheet, write down the dates your pain, depression or illnesses began. By comparing the two, you should be able to see a correlation between them.

2. Consider psychotherapy. If you recognize a pattern in your time line, some of your pain could be due to unresolved feelings about the traumas. Unresolved guilt, shame, resentment and anger inflame neurons in the central nervous system. But resolving these issues can reduce or reverse inflammation.

MRIs of patients who have post-traumatic stress disorder (PTSD) have shown that with cognitive behavioral therapy or eye movement desensitization and reprocessing—in which certain eye movements and discussion of the trauma are combined—neuron function can return to normal.

3. Avoid NSAIDs. Occasional use of nonsteroidal anti-inflammatory drugs (NSAIDs), such as Aleve or Motrin, is fine, but frequent use (three or more times a week) can, over time, lead to chronic intestinal inflammation, which can spread to other organs, including the brain.

4. Ask about medication. I sometimes prescribe low-dose (1.25 mg to 4.5 mg) naltrexone (a medication that is used to treat addiction), which can return microglia to a noninflammatory state. Other drugs that may help include minocycline, an antibiotic, or an angiotensin receptor blocker, a medication that relaxes blood vessels. If you have chronic pain, ask your doctor about these.

EXTINGUISH YOUR INFLAMMATION CYCLE

Certain lifestyle factors can promote pain-causing inflammation. *What helps...*

- **Test your diet.** For six weeks, avoid all foods with wheat, soy, milk and milk products (foods that often trigger allergies or sensitivities that promote inflammation). Eat only fresh fruits, vegetables, brown rice, fish, chicken and eggs—these foods, in general, are the least likely to cause inflammation.

After six weeks, add back one category of food—such as dairy—per week. Note whether these foods have a negative effect on your energy, mood or level of pain. If so, eliminate that food from your diet entirely.

- **Try meditation.** Research shows that meditation builds new neuronal tissue and helps create a natural resilience to future trauma. Your meditation doesn't have to be a formal program—you can start by simply sitting quietly in a room for 20 minutes each day, allowing your body to gradually relax while you focus on your breathing. Aerobic exercise and adequate sleep also help control inflammation.

---

5 Hidden Causes of Pain: Find the Real Culprit...

Vijay Vad, MD, sports medicine specialist at the Hospital for Special Surgery and assistant professor of rehabilitation medicine at Weill Cornell Medical College, both in New York City. He is author of *Stop Pain: Inflammation Relief for an Active Life.*

Do you have arthritis, backaches or some other type of nagging pain that just won't go away?

Why pain often persists: For a significant number of people who chalk up their pain to a creaky joint, muscle aches or some other common problem, the true culprit actually has never been properly diagnosed.

But don't give up. One of the following conditions may be at the root of your pain—or at least making it much worse. *The good news is that there's plenty you can do to treat these hidden causes of pain...*

VITAMIN D DEFICIENCY

What does your backache have to do with the amount of vitamin D in your body? More than you might think, according to recent research.

Here's why: Vitamin D is needed for normal bone metabolism. People who don't produce enough are especially susceptible to low-back pain, possibly because the vertebrae become weakened. Low vitamin D levels also have been linked to hip pain and knee pain.

My advice: Get your vitamin D level tested once a year, particularly if you live in the Northeastern US or the Pacific Northwest. Limited sun exposure in these areas can make it difficult for the body to synthesize enough vitamin D, and it is difficult to get adequate amounts of this vitamin from food.

If your vitamin D level is low (most experts put the optimal blood level between 20 ng/mL and 36 ng/mL), take a daily supplement that provides 1,000 international units (IU) to 2,000 IU...and continue to get tested annually.

LOW THYROID

Underactive thyroid gland (hypothyroidism) is more common than most people realize. Even though the condition is most often found in women, it can affect men, too. The blood tests used to detect the condition are simple and inexpensive, yet few doctors order the testing routinely, as they should.

Thyroid hormones are real workhorses in the body—for example, they help regulate how many calories you burn, your heart rate and body temperature. If you have low thyroid levels, you're likely to suffer from fatigue, sensitivity to cold and unexplained weight gain.

What's not so well known is that people with hypothyroidism tend to have nagging muscle and joint pain. This is because low thyroid can accelerate the loss of cartilage in those who already have a touch of arthritis.

My advice: If you have arthritis or any type of joint or muscle pain that has unexpectedly worsened, ask your doctor for a thyroid test. This advice applies to men, too. A thyroid function panel measures blood levels of thyroid stimulating hormone (TSH), along with levels of different thyroid hormones. A normal TSH level is typically between 0.4 mIU/L and 4.0 mIU/L.

Even if your TSH level is "borderline," your thyroid may be contributing to your pain, so ask your doctor about medication. Thyroid-replacement hormones, such as Synthroid or Levothroid, mimic the effects of natural thyroid hormone and can start to relieve symptoms, including thyroid-related arthritis pain, within a month.

NOT ENOUGH ESTROGEN

Women tend to experience more pain overall once they go through menopause—not necessarily because of pain-causing conditions, but because the body's drop in estrogen lowers their pain tolerance.

Example: Knee pain that you might have rated as a 5 (on a 1-to-10 scale) before menopause might now feel like an 8. Pain sensitivity is higher in postmenopausal women who also have low thyroid.

My advice: Try supplemental curcumin. This potent anti-inflammatory reduces pain and improves joint flexibility. Most postmenopausal women (and men, too!) notice an improvement when they take it.

Dose: 2,000 mg daily. This supplement is generally safe for everyone to use, but consult your doctor first, especially if you take any medication (it can interact with some drugs, such as anticoagulants)...or if you have gallstones, since it could increase painful symptoms.

Good product: Northeast Natural's Triple Curc, ActiveBodyActiveMind.com.

If this doesn't give you adequate pain relief, you may also want to consider estrogen replacement. It decreases pain sensitivity and reduces the loss of joint cartilage.

Important: Estrogen replacement can increase risk for heart disease, stroke and breast cancer in some women, so ask your doctor to help you sort out the pros and cons.

LYME DISEASE

This tick-borne illness can be easily treated (usually with a three-week course of antibiotics)—if it's detected early. But many people don't know they have it, in part because the test isn't always accurate.

What happens: The bacterium that causes Lyme can destroy joint cartilage. Many people with Lyme know that something's wrong, but it often takes months—and multiple visits with different specialists—to get an accurate diagnosis.

My advice: If you live in an area where ticks and Lyme disease are common, do not wait to get help. The symptoms might include muscle or joint pain, unexplained fatigue and/or a burning sensation that affects your whole body. Treating Lyme disease quickly reduces the risk of lingering joint pain and other symptoms.

If you test negative but still suspect that your pain may be caused by the disease, consider seeing a doctor who specializes in diagnosing Lyme for a second opinion. To find such a specialist near you, consult the International Lyme and Associated Diseases Society at ILADS.org.

POOR SLEEP

People who have chronic pain often don't sleep well. But it also works the other way—less deep sleep lowers your tolerance to pain.

Even if you think that you sleep well, you may not be getting enough rapid eye movement (REM) sleep—the more time you spend in this stage of sleep, the better equipped your body will be at tolerating pain.

My advice: Get at least 30 minutes of aerobic exercise every day. This type of exercise increases levels of deep sleep, which is needed for you to get adequate REM sleep.

Mystery Illness: When Pain and Bloating Won't Go Away

Leo Galland, MD, founder and director of the Foundation for Integrated Medicine (MDheal.org) in New York City, specializing in the diagnosis and treatment of complex illnesses. He is the author of *Power Healing* and *The Fat Resistance Diet*, as well as numerous scientific papers on a range of medical topics.

Life changed quite suddenly for Judith at the age of 52, when she developed a serious episode of abdominal pain and diarrhea. Her doctor diagnosed food poisoning and ulcerative colitis, and her pain resolved within three weeks, but the diarrhea continued. She soon found that most of the foods she loved, such as bread and fresh fruit, increased her bouts of diarrhea and caused uncomfortable swelling of her abdomen.

When Judith consulted me for a fresh opinion, my first impression was that the diagnosis of ulcerative colitis had been made perhaps too quickly, without taking into account all the features of her case that are not typical of this condition...

• **Sudden onset at the age of 52.** Ulcerative colitis usually begins at a younger age, although it may be triggered by an acute gastrointestinal infection, which is what happened in Judith's case.

• **Lack of response to anti-inflammatory drugs.** Most patients with ulcerative colitis will show at least partial improvement with medication, but Judith did not.

• **Intolerance to multiple foods.** Although many patients with ulcerative colitis experience intolerance to some foods, Judith was far more sensitive to a wide variety of common foods than most people.

Based on these inconsistencies, my first decision was to test Judith for a chronic intestinal infection using stool testing. During the past two decades, I have evaluated scores of patients with "ulcerative colitis." In all of these cases, I have found that thorough testing for an intestinal infection was crucial to identifying the root cause of the problem. About one-quarter of these patients tested positive for intestinal infection. In almost half of these cases, the intestinal infection was the real cause of their symptoms. In the other half, the diagnosis of chronic ulcerative colitis was correct, but the infection had produced an acute flare-up of symptoms. In either case, curing the infection relieved the symptoms.

Judith's lab results showed that she was infected with two intestinal parasites—*Entamoeba histolytica*, which causes a form of colitis that is very hard to distinguish from ulcerative colitis...and *Giardia lamblia*, which may cause severe food intolerance. Parasites are organisms that survive by living on or inside another organism. They generally enter the body via the mouth or skin—for example, through exposure to contaminated food or water.

After treatment with the appropriate antibiotics, Judith's diarrhea cleared up and her sensitivity to foods began to decrease. Six months later, she was able to eat a varied diet (she still avoids sweets and dairy products). A follow-up colonoscopy showed no evidence of inflammation in her large intestine.

Correct diagnosis: Intestinal parasites.

Lesson for all: Just because your illness has been given a name, it does not mean that its cause has been found. If you suffer sudden gastrointestinal symptoms, such as diarrhea, pain, bloating and/or constipation, do not accept a diagnosis until you have been tested for parasitic infection.

What Your Foot Pain May Really Mean

John M. Giurini, DPM, Harvard Medical School, with Rebecca Shannonhouse, editor, *Bottom Line Health.*

Foot discomfort can precede a diagnosis of diabetes by as many as five years.

Problem: This telltale symptom is frequently overlooked. Burning, tingling or numbness in the feet often is due to diabetic peripheral neuropathy, a type of nerve damage that can lead to foot ulcers (sores).

Sensory neuropathy (no sensation) occurs with almost all diabetic foot ulcers, which can become as large as several inches and an inch or more deep. About 20% of patients who get these ulcers will require amputation.

Neuropathy can be a serious problem even without ulcers, explains John M. Giurini, DPM, of Harvard Medical School. About 15% of diabetic patients develop painful (nonulcerous) neuropathy, which can impair mobility, decrease fitness, interfere with sleep and increase obesity as well as depression.

Never ignore foot symptoms. See a foot and ankle specialist right away. Even if tests for neuropathy are negative, you already may have diabetes or prediabetes (a precursor to diabetes). *To be safe...*

• **Get a blood glucose test as part of your annual exam** if you have any of the symptoms described above or a family history of diabetes.

• **Examine your feet if you have diabetes.** Look for sores, blisters or redness every day. If you have neuropathy, you may not feel pain, so a visual check may be the only way to detect ulcers.

• **Get treated immediately if you have a foot sore.** Diabetes impairs immunity as well as wound healing. The sores can progress very rapidly—and the damage may be irreversible.

A Charley Horse…or a Deadly Blood Clot?

Daniella Kadian-Dodov, MD, assistant professor of medicine in the department of vascular medicine at the Zena and Michael A. Wiener Cardiovascular Institute and the Marie-Josée and Henry R. Kravis Center for Cardiovascular Health at the Icahn School of Medicine at Mount Sinai Hospital in New York City.

If you've ever been stopped cold by a charley horse, you know just how excruciating these muscle spasms can be. But are you sure it's just a muscle spasm? Or is that leg pain due to something far more serious?

What can cause leg pain…

PERIPHERAL ARTERIAL DISEASE (PAD)

This is one to worry about. Even though the pain usually isn't intense, it can triple your risk of dying from a heart attack or stroke.

What it feels like: About 10% of people with PAD suffer leg cramps, leg aching and leg fatigue that occur only during physical activity involving the legs (any type of activity can trigger it—even just walking). When you rest your legs, the discomfort goes away, usually in 10 minutes or less. As PAD becomes more severe and blood circulation worsens, pain can occur during rest and result in leg ulcers and even gangrene.

What to do: See a doctor. PAD is usually caused by atherosclerosis, the same condition that leads to most heart attacks. Your doctor will compare the blood pressure in your arms to the pressure at your ankles. If there's a significant difference, that could mean that you have PAD and you'll need an ultrasound of the legs to determine the extent and location of arterial obstructions.

Next steps: The same practices that protect your heart—such as not smoking, controlling diabetes, maintaining healthy blood pressure and getting plenty of exercise—will help stop PAD from worsening and could even reverse it.

Important: You must walk—even when it hurts. Walking ultimately reduces pain and improves circulation by stimulating the growth of blood vessels that bypass the damaged ones. With your doctor's OK, walk five times a week, for 30 to 45 minutes each time. I usually advise my patients to walk fast for two blocks or until they feel moderate pain, then rest a moment and walk fast for two blocks again, repeating until the end of their workout.

DEEP VEIN THROMBOSIS (DVT)

It doesn't always cause leg pain, but if pain occurs, this warning could save your life. DVT means that you have a blood clot—most often deep in a leg vein. It can be fatal.

What it feels like: You might notice a sudden, pulsating or aching pain deep in your calf or thigh, sometimes accompanied by redness and/or swelling. DVT usually occurs after you've been immobile for a long time—you're laid up in bed after surgery, for example, or following a long car or plane trip.

What to do: Get to an emergency department or a physician's office where you can get an immediate ultrasound. The clot could break free, travel to the lungs and cause pulmonary embolism, a clot in the lungs that's fatal in up to 30% of cases.

If you have a DVT, your doctor will probably give intravenous or injectable heparin, a blood-thinning drug that prevents the clot from growing. After a day or two, you'll be switched to oral blood-thinning medication, such as *warfarin* (Coumadin) or *dabigatran* (Pradaxa). You'll need to take the medication for about six months. If the clot is not entirely dissolved after treatment, it should be monitored with ultrasound—and if you have had one clot, you might get another one. Prevention is critical.

Everyone—whether you've had a DVT or not—should flex the ankle and calf muscles for about 30 seconds every 20 or 30 minutes when sitting for longer than four hours. Stand up and move around at least every hour or so.

If you have risk factors for blood clots—you're over age 40, obese, have a family history of blood clots or use hormone replacement therapy—ask your doctor about such precautions as taking aspirin before travel and/or wearing compression stockings while you're immobile.

SCIATICA

This back condition is typically caused by a herniated spinal disk. The legs become involved because the disk exerts painful pressure on the sciatic nerve, which runs down the backs of the legs.

What it feels like: Intense, shooting and/or knifelike pains may extend through the buttocks and into one leg. Sciatica also can cause leg and/or ankle weakness.

What to do: See your doctor. If you do have sciatica, you may get better within eight weeks by doing physical therapy and using a nonsteroidal anti-inflammatory medication such as ibuprofen (Motrin)—90% of sciatica patients do.

Next steps: Consider surgery for a herniated disk/sciatica only when the pain is too intense to handle...you have responsibilities that don't permit extended downtime...or you're having additional symptoms such as muscle weakness or a loss of bowel/bladder control.

WHEN IT REALLY IS A CHARLEY HORSE

A muscle spasm, including the infamous "charley horse" of the leg, can occur after hard exercise or for no obvious reason. It can cause sudden, localized pain (usually with sharp contractions) that often hits the calves.

If you're getting muscle spasms with any sort of regularity, see your doctor. Muscle spasms have a variety of causes—for example, you may have overworked your legs by doing yard work...you may be dehydrated (without enough water, muscle cells can spasm)...or a medication you're taking, such as a diuretic, may be the culprit.

Helpful: Because most muscle spasms are caused, in part, by tight hamstrings (the muscles in the backs of your upper legs), I recommend doing a standing hamstring stretch on a regular basis. Start in a standing position with your knees straight...bend at the waist...and reach for your toes or the floor until you feel a stretch in your hamstrings. Hold for a few seconds, and repeat a few times a day.

How to Tell If That Lump or Bump Is Cause for Concern

Ellen Warner, MD, MSc, medical oncologist, associate scientist, Odette Cancer Centre, Ontario, Canada.

Childhood is full of lumps and bumps as kids jump, climb, leap and, yes, fall. But as people grow up and slow down, lumps and bumps become more unusual so any appearance of one can be cause for alarm. Why that peculiar lump on my arm? Why do the glands in my throat seem bigger today? What's the bump on the back of my neck? In truth, lumps and bumps are almost never anything to worry about. But that said, some are definite cause for concern and should prompt a call to the doctor because certain lumps and bumps might signal one of several types of cancer. How do you know what's what? When to worry and when to ignore it and wait for it to go away?

LYMPH NODES ARE KEY

Ellen Warner, MD, a medical oncologist and researcher at the Odette Cancer Centre in Ontario, Canada, says the type of lump or bump (or in this case actually a swelling) that is the most common cause for concern has to do with lymph nodes. These nodes exist throughout the body and in numerous locations the head and neck, under the arms, in the chest and abdomen, in the groin area and in the legs. They also appear in approximately the same place on either side of the body. Lymph nodes are part of the body's immune system and swell in response to any type of infection and inflammation as part of their role in helping to fight it off or resolve it.

However, if a node swells and stays swollen on just one side or in several lymph nodes, and if there is seemingly no reason, such as a sore throat or other recent illness, Dr. Warner cautions that it must be checked out. Cancer of the lymph nodes (as opposed to cancer that metastasizes to nodes from another location) can be one of two types Hodgkin's or non-Hodgkin's lymphoma. Dr. Warner explains that the difference between the two mostly has to do with cellular structure that shows up under the microscope. But they also have different survival rates. Hodgkin's is the more curable of the two with an 85% survival rate while the non-Hodgkin's rate is 60% after five years. This year it is estimated that there will be about 8,200 cases of Hodgkin's lymphoma diagnosed in this country as opposed to approximately 66,120 of non-Hodgkin's lymphoma diagnosed in the same year. Hodgkin's tends to be more common between ages 15 and 34 and at age 60 and over, though non-Hodgkin's is more common in older adults, 50 plus, and people who have compromised immune systems.

What to watch for: A considerable (not slight) swelling in a lymph node that may or may not be tender or possibly painful on one side, or in several lymph nodes, especially in the neck, and less commonly in the armpits or groin, when there has been no recent illness. Usually the swelling is under the chin, along the side of the neck. While there is no way to detect internal swelling of lymph nodes, there are symptoms such as itching, fatigue, coughing, fever, night sweats, weight loss and chest or abdominal pain, says Dr. Warner.

CANCEROUS BUMPS

Another frightening but even less common cause of dangerous lumps and bumps is cancer of connective tissue, a form of sarcoma called soft-tissue sarcoma. Fortunately, this type of cancer is extremely rare, accounting for less than 1% of malignancies diagnosed in this country each year. However, it can appear in numerous places in the body and is subclassified according to which soft tissue it develops. Do not confuse soft tissue sarcoma with fatty nodules called lipomas, which are benign. These are extremely common, usually appearing just under the skin in the arms, legs and trunk of the body.

Dr. Warner says lipomas are generally round and smooth with what she calls a roly-poly feel to them...they grow slowly and can become quite large, even several inches in diameter, and they are not malignant. Soft tissue sarcomas, on the other hand are almost always malignant and the tumor can grow quickly, most often appearing on the limb. But it can show up on the abdomen or in other parts of the body as well, including the head, neck and trunk.

What to watch for: A sudden swelling that may or may not be tender or painful, beneath the surface of the skin, usually over a fairly large and diffuse area and a lump that does not have distinct borders. Do not hesitate to see a doctor immediately since the survival rate for soft tissue sarcoma that is diagnosed while the tumor is still small and shallow is over 80%.

CANCER PATIENTS PAY ATTENTION

Finally, anyone who already has cancer should be alert for any lump or bump that appears elsewhere on the body seemingly unrelated to the primary site. As is true with any mysterious lump or bump one that cannot be explained for ordinary, everyday reasons such as a recent infection or fall, go to the doctor and insist on getting it checked, especially if it seems to grow quickly or change character, or becomes itchy.

No need to panic. Just be aware of your body and its changes. Careful observation can make a big difference in the long run.

Unexplained Pain Or Numbness? It Could Be Spinal Stenosis

David Borenstein, MD, clinical professor of medicine at George Washington University Medical Center and in private practice at Arthritis and Rheumatism Associates, both in Washington, DC. He is author of *Back in Control.*

If you have pain or numbness in your legs, back, neck, shoulders or arms, you may have spinal stenosis. Most spinal stenosis cases are due to osteoarthritis. After decades of friction—most sufferers are over age 50—cartilage breaks down, causing bone to rub against bone. The body tries to repair the damage by stimulating growth of extra bone, called spurs, which may protrude into the spinal canal and press against nerves or the spinal cord.

Other causes...

- **Shrinking.** As we age, the spinal vertebrae may break down, causing us to "shrink." When this happens, the thick ligament inside the spinal canal may fold over and exert nerve pressure.
- **Tumors in the spinal canal can press against the nerves or spinal cord.**
- **Injuries from accidents.**
- **Congenital defect.** Some people are born with very narrow spinal canals. They may start to have symptoms in their teens.

SYMPTOMS

Leg pain or cramping—known as neurogenic intermittent claudication—is a common symptom of spinal stenosis.

Self-test: While standing, bend forward to open up space in the spinal canal. If your leg pain disappears, you probably have spinal stenosis.

Other symptoms include back or hip pain, pain in the neck and shoulders and/or a persistent backache. Pressure in the neck also can result in a loss of balance. In rare cases, patients may lose bowel or bladder function due to severe nerve pressure in the lower back.

Spinal stenosis usually is diagnosed with an MRI or CT scan.

TREATMENT

Surgery may be required to remove bone or soft tissue that is pressing against nerves. In the majority of cases, however, symptoms can be relieved with nonsurgical methods...

- **Changing posture.** Standing ramrod straight narrows the spinal canal and worsens symptoms. People who have spinal stenosis should slouch a bit to keep the back flexed. Bending forward slightly when you stand or walk often will relieve pain.
- **Over-the-counter nonsteroidal anti-inflammatory drugs (NSAIDs),** such as aspirin and *ibuprofen* (Advil), taken up to four times daily may reduce inflammation in the spinal canal.

Note: *Acetaminophen* (Tylenol) relieves pain but has little effect on inflammation.

- **Steroid injections.** In some cases, a series of steroid injections into the spinal fluid can reduce inflammation. People usually get one or two initial injections and "maintenance" injections every two to 12 months.

PREVENTION

- **Exercise regularly to maintain strength and flexibility.** Combine aerobic activities, especially biking and walking, with weight training and stretching.
- **Strengthen your midsection with abdominal exercises, including crunches.** Strong abdominal muscles make it easier to maintain a tilt in the pelvis, which creates more space in the spinal canal.
- **Don't smoke.** It decreases the amount of oxygen available to the spinal cord. Diminished oxygen increases the risk and severity of nerve pain.

What to Do When an Imaging Test Finds an Unexpected Abnormality

Stella K. Kang, MD, MS, assistant professor of radiology and population health at NYU Langone Medical Center in New York City. She is the author or coauthor of more than two dozen scientific papers published in the *Journal of the American College of Radiology, Clinical Oncology* and other leading medical journals.

You're having abdominal pain and visit your primary care physician. As part of the workup, your doctor orders a CT scan of your abdomen and pelvis to rule out possible causes, such as an infection. The results arrive two days later, and there's nothing obviously wrong with your bowels. *But...*

In the report accompanying the scan, the radiologist noted an incidental finding (IF)—a spot on your kidney that was "too small to characterize."

Is it a harmless cyst...or a tumor that might grow and spread if left untreated? Should your doctor ignore it for now...or order more tests, possibly opening a medical Pandora's box that could perhaps entail a biopsy and raise radiation exposure? More and more patients and doctors are facing such questions.

Incidental findings—when a physician investigating a specific problem finds another possible problem (known in doctor-speak as an "incidentaloma")—are on the rise, in part because scanning technology is more precise than ever before.

Eye-opening statistics: On average, about 40% of all scans reveal an incidental finding. For two common imaging tests—CT of the abdomen and pelvis...and CT of the thorax (below the neck and above the abdomen)—IFs are now detected 61% and 55% of the time, respectively. *Basic types of IFs...*

• **High risk.** This type could cause real harm, even death, if it's not discovered and dealt with.

Example: A large cancerous kidney tumor.

• **Intermediate risk.** This type has some potential to cause future harm, with a need for medication or other treatment.

Example: A kidney stone that is asymptomatic.

• **Low risk.** This type has a greater than 99% chance of never causing harm.

Example: A benign kidney cyst, which does not interfere with kidney function.

Why it gets tricky: Even though the discovery of an abnormality can sometimes be lifesaving (when an asymptomatic malignancy is found, for example), there are few medical standards for reporting and managing IFs—often leading to unnecessary testing and treatment of low- and intermediate-risk IFs.

BEST STRATEGIES

Here are ways to increase the likelihood that IFs are responded to safely and effectively—but unnecessary follow-up is avoided...

• **If your doctor orders any type of imaging test (X-ray, CT, PET or MRI scan, for example), ask about the likelihood of an IF.** You should know before the test whether or not it's likely to uncover an IF—so you're less apt to be surprised and frightened if an IF is found.

Helpful: Before the test, ask your doctor to give you a quick overview of high-, intermediate- and low-risk IFs commonly produced by the test.

To ensure that you are made aware of any IFs from an imaging test, ask to receive a copy of the radiologist's report so that you can discuss it with your doctor.

• **Partner with your primary care doctor.** With its array of specialists and subspecialists, medical care is increasingly fractured—making it more likely that specialist-ordered testing will follow the discovery of any IF, including those that are intermediate- and low-risk.

Best: Even if a specialist ordered the test, talk over the results with your primary care physician. He/she is likely to have a sense of your overall health and preferences regarding medical interventions such as testing.

• **If there's an IF, get an accurate description of the risk.** Sometimes a doctor will talk in vague terms about the risk from an IF—for example, "It's probably not going to hurt you." But that's not enough information to effectively partner with your doctor in deciding if more testing is appropriate.

Best: Ask for a statistical estimation of risk. Is the likelihood of harm (such as cancer that could metastasize or an enlarged blood vessel that could rupture) from the IF one out of 10? One out of 1,000? If the numerical level of risk is hard to understand, ask the doctor to explain it another way.

• **Ask if the American College of Radiology (ACR) recommends further imaging for this type of IF.** The ACR, the professional organization for radiologists, has guidelines for further investigation of some of the most common IFs, such as thyroid nodules, ovarian nodules and IFs discovered during abdominal CTs.

Best: Ask your physician if there are ACR guidelines for your IF and if he is following them.*

• **Ask your doctor to consult with the radiologist.** When certain IFs don't fall under ACR guidelines, radiologists don't always agree about their significance or management. One radiologist might recommend further testing. Another might say no additional testing is necessary. A third might not make a recommendation, letting the primary care physician decide what to do next.

Best: If your test has an IF with unclear implications for management, your doctor might schedule a joint consultation with the radiologist so the three of you can talk through your options—a strategy that is effective but underutilized.

• **Get a second opinion.** When a lesion is indeterminate (unclear in importance), consider asking your doctor to have another radiologist take a look at the result.

Best: Ask your doctor to recommend a consultation with a subspecialist—for instance, if the IF is on the kidney, talk to a radiologist who is expert in examining the kidney.

WHEN FOLLOW-UP IS NEEDED

Some IFs require follow-up testing and medical care. *Discuss follow-up options with your doctor for...*

• **Lung nodules**—a risk factor for lung cancer—found during a CT of the thorax.

• **Coronary artery calcification**—a risk factor for a heart attack—detected during a CT of the chest or a CT of the abdomen and pelvis.

• **A solid lesion on an ovary,** which could be a tumor, revealed by an abdominal and pelvic CT.

• **Enlarged lymph nodes,** which may be related to infection or malignancy, found during a pelvic MRI.

• **Enlarged aorta (aneurysm) found by an abdominal CT.** If this major blood vessel is enlarged, you could be at increased risk for it to break open and cause severe bleeding that could be fatal.

*To read the American College of Radiology's guidelines on incidental findings, go to ACR.org/Clinical-Resources/incidental-findings

Solving Your Mystery Pain and Illness

Keith Ablow, MD, psychiatrist in private practice in Newburyport, Massachusetts, and an assistant clinical professor of psychiatry at Tufts University School of Medicine in Boston. He is the author of *Living the Truth: Transform Your Life Through the Power of Insight and Honesty.* KeithAblow.com

If you suffer from a chronic ailment for which no doctor has been able to find a cause or effective treatment, it's possible that hidden emotions may be to blame. Perhaps you have chronic back pain or frequent digestive upset. Or you may have had chest pains that doctors can't explain or skin eruptions that keep coming back despite treatment.

What's often overlooked: Sometimes a mysterious physical malady has a secret source—repressed emotions. These hidden feelings often have their roots deep in your personal past—for example, in events, situations and people who were important to you as far back as your childhood but are still haunting you.

WHAT YOU CAN'T HIDE

How well your body functions depends, in part, on your emotional health. Unfortunately, many people spend years or even their entire lifetimes running from realities that seem too painful to face.

How we fool ourselves: You may have had selfish, neglectful parents, but it's easier to tell yourself that they were loving and generous... or you may have convinced yourself that the lonely adolescence that you experienced was not a problem because it made you stronger.

Research shows that this relentless cover-up of painful emotions exacts a physiological toll. All the energy you expend to keep "safe" from difficult memories leaves your body with little resilience to cope with the demands of daily life—your immune system may misfire, hormones may become imbalanced, your muscles may become chronically tense and your cardiovascular system may behave erratically.

WHAT AN AILMENT REALLY MEANS

If you have a medical ill that is linked to buried feelings, the connection to your past trauma is rarely obvious.

Example: A 60-year-old man suffered from excruciating back pain that persisted despite physical therapy, chiropractic treatment and even surgery. With a psychotherapist's encouragement, he started exploring his past, which included things he "didn't want to think about," such as physical and sexual abuse. But when he did think about them—and remembered the terrible emotions of the time—he started to experience relief from his back pain. Although there was no direct evidence of a cause-and-effect relationship between the man's psychotherapy and reduced symptoms, there was no mistaking that his back pain improved when he finally accepted and came to terms with the psychic pain he had suffered.

THE QUESTIONS TO ASK YOURSELF

If you have an unexplained physical problem and wonder whether repressed emotions may play a role, ask yourself: *If I were to change three things about my life, what would they be?* Write them down.

Be sure to be specific. If you wish your marriage were better, what's missing? Would you like more honest communication? More time together (or more time alone)? More sex? *Then...*

- **Sit quietly and tune in to the emotions your statements arouse.** I can't talk to my spouse about my real needs and fears because I know she won't really listen.
- **Connect to the past.** Spend time with your statements about today's dissatisfactions. Ask yourself: Why do I feel this way? What do this situation and these feelings remind me of from my past? What events, people and/or family relationships aroused the same emotions?

For example: Your older brother was the family star. You admired him and gladly lived in his shadow while your parents showered him with praise. If you had any other feelings about it—resentment and hurt that you counted for so little—you buried them.

Is it any wonder that you are now afraid to speak up in your marriage?

Important: This process typically involves thinking at length about things that you have tried not to think about at all. For example, your painful memories may be related to the death of a family member, humiliating events that occurred at your school or even some form of physical or sexual abuse that you experienced.

If your efforts to go through the process described above don't help your physical symptoms, become too emotionally painful—or make you feel worse physically or emotionally—then see a therapist. You don't have to commit to years of psychoanalysis. Most types of shorter-term therapy, such as cognitive behavioral therapy, include discussion of past feelings, thoughts and behaviors to help you gain insight and make connections that may improve your physical ailment. When seeking a therapist, ask close friends who they would recommend—and consider visiting a few therapists before selecting one. (For more information on using your mind and emotions to heal your pain, see chapter 25, "Mind-Over-Body Pain Relief.")

Little-Known Skin Cancer Sign

Pain or itching can be signs of skin cancer. People often are told to be on the lookout for visual changes to their skin, but it is important not to overlook changes in how skin feels.

Recent findings: More than one-third of skin cancer lesions itch—these can be a sign of basal cell carcinoma. About 30% are painful, and these can indicate squamous cell carcinoma.

Gil Yosipovitch, MD, chair of dermatology at Temple University School of Medicine and director of Temple Itch Center, both in Philadelphia, and leader of a study published in *JAMA Dermatology.*

Hidden Parathyroid Disease Can Wreak Havoc

Shonni J. Silverberg, MD, professor of medicine, division of endocrinology, Columbia University College of Physicians and Surgeons, New York City. Her research has focused on investigation and management of disorders of bone and mineral metabolism, including the treatment of primary hyperparathyroidism.

You get a painful kidney stone and get treated, and your doctor tells you to drink more water to prevent another one.

You break a bone, and it turns out that you have osteoporosis, so your doctor talks to you about diet, exercise and prescriptions.

You're feeling nauseous, don't feel like eating and are experiencing constipation and diarrhea. Your doctor suggests various tests to see if you have a gastrointestinal condition.

You have trouble concentrating, find that your memory isn't as good as it used to be and, in general, feel like you're experiencing brain fog. Your doctor asks if you've been sleeping well lately.

But what if all these symptoms were caused by a little-known disease...one that's entirely curable with surgery?

It's called primary hyperparathyroidism, a disease of the parathyroid glands, and it can cause havoc to the bones, kidneys and even the brains of sufferers.

A DISEASE WITH TERRIBLE SYMPTOMS...OR NO SYMPTOMS AT ALL

In a sense, you're lucky if you have symptoms. Some people have no symptoms at all even as the disease is causing serious harm. Fortunately, a common blood test for calcium levels that your regular doctor may routinely order can pick up the earliest signs. That's the first step to identifying the condition.

Unless you have symptoms, however, your doctor may not suggest surgery right away. Some physicians recommend watchful waiting for asymptomatic patients. But waiting while the disease may be damaging your body is controversial, even among experts.

Fortunately, the most current guidelines make it clear exactly who should get treated right away. Here's what you need to know.

A TINY GLAND CAN TURN YOUR WHOLE SYSTEM UPSIDE DOWN

About one in 1,000 Americans have primary hyperparathyroidism, three times as many women as men. It's becomes increasingly more common over age 60. (Primary means it's not caused by another disease.)

A little background: Primary hyperparathyroidism is not a problem with the thyroid gland. Rather, it affects the tiny pea-size parathyroid glands on or near the thyroid. There are four of them, but usually only one is overactive, signaling excessive release of parathyroid hormone. That hormone's purpose is to maintain the right level of calcium in the blood, and when it's overactive, it signals the body to pull too much calcium from the bones into the bloodstream. That can weaken bones and lead to osteoporosis and fractures...cause kidney stones...and create neurological issues that affect concentration and memory and lead to depression.

Until the 1970s, people with primary hyperparathyroidism would be diagnosed when they went to their doctors with serious complaints—bone pain, broken bones, abdominal pain and kidney stones. (Other symptoms of severe disease may include nausea, vomiting, loss of appetite, constipation and an increased need to urinate.) Since that time, the disease is generally caught earlier through calcium tests, which are now part of the routine blood test you get during an annual physical.

If you have any of the symptoms or conditions mentioned above and you haven't had a checkup recently, ask your doctor for a blood test. If the result shows a high calcium level in your blood, your parathyroid hormone level will be tested...and if it is high, you'll likely be diagnosed with parathyroid disease. It's usually caused by a noncancerous tumor on one of the glands.

Although medication is sometimes prescribed to manage the disease, there are no medications that can cure it or treat all of its effects. The only way to cure it is through surgical removal of the overactive gland or glands. Within the first year, your bones become stronger, kidney stones wane and you may find that the brain fog and mood issues get better, too.

But what if you get the diagnosis after a regular checkup but don't have any symptoms? Should you still get your diseased parathyroid gland removed?

THE SURGERY DECISION

Most people who show up at the endocrinologist with primary hyperparathyroid disease don't have any obvious symptoms. When the calcium test was added to routine blood tests in the 1970s, patients began to be diagnosed when they were asymptomatic. The number of people diagnosed with the disease rose by a factor of four to five times.

Experts disagree about what to do if you don't have symptoms. Some recommend waiting because not everyone does develop clinical problems, and the disease progresses at different rates in different people...and more slowly in older adults. Other experts are concerned that those who don't receive surgery are needlessly putting themselves at risk for complications down the road.

Recently updated guidelines from an international group of experts can make that decision easier. *Unless you are too frail for surgery, even if you have no clear symptoms, you should have surgery if you are diagnosed with primary hyperparathyroidism and have any of these factors...*

- **Very high blood calcium levels.** A normal blood calcium level for an adult ranges from 8.5 milligrams per deciliter (mg/dL) to 10.2 mg/dL, although there are slight variations based on different labs. If your calcium level is 1 mg/dL above the normal range, it's not just slightly but significantly elevated.

- **Silent kidney stones.** If you have kidney stones, you should have the surgery. When they're painful, you'll know you have them. But the new guidelines acknowledge that some people may have "silent" stones, meaning that they're there but not causing any symptoms. One study found that 15% of patients had kidney stones that were not causing symptoms. An ultrasound or other imaging test is recommended to detect any silent stones, and if any are found, you would be a candidate for parathyroid surgery.

- **Kidney trouble.** If your kidneys are not working well (impaired kidney function) for any reason, that's another reason to have surgery. This can be detected by a routine blood test as well.

- **Osteoporosis or fractures.** Patients with osteoporosis have low bone density and are at risk for fracture. Primary hyperparathyroidism can affect your bones, making them weaker. If you have low bone density, you should have surgery. Your physician can use a bone densitometry machine to noninvasively measure the density of your bones. The new guidelines now also recommend imaging of the spine to look for compression fractures, which can go undiagnosed but indicate that the bones are already fragile enough to have fractured...and support the need for surgery.

- **Early onset.** If you're under 50, you should have surgery because you are likely to develop symptoms in your lifetime.

Unlike many illnesses, primary hyperparathyroidism can be cured with surgery more than 95% of the time, so experts tend to recommend it. In most cases, you can go home the same day that you have the surgery, although it takes between one and three weeks to heal fully. Most of the time, you won't need any medication or further treatment (since you'll still have some working parathyroid glands) although you will have to have your blood calcium levels checked regularly and may need to take calcium/vitamin D supplements.

If you do opt for surgery, finding an experienced surgeon is key. The area is delicate and sometimes the glands are hard to find (or more than one is involved), so surgeons need to know how to respond in those circumstances. In general, a surgeon should do more than 50 parathyroid operations a year to be considered an expert.

Dangerous Painful Symptoms Women Should Never Ignore

Marie Savard, MD, medical contributor for ABC News. A board-certified internist, she is the author of *How to Save Your Own Life.* DrSavard.com

Conditioned to be care-givers rather than care-getters, women frequently downplay their own seemingly insignificant symptoms, such as bloating and headaches. Many doctors trivialize women's complaints, too.

Example: Among patients with chest pain, men are more likely than women to be given a screening test for heart disease, while women are more likely than men to be offered tranquilizers—even though heart disease is the number-one killer of Americans of both sexes.

Self-defense: Familiarize yourself with the conditions that a new or persistent symptom could signal, then see your doctor as soon as possible and insist on being given the appropriate diagnostic tests.

1. Swelling could be due to fluid retention from your period, varicose veins, eating too much salt or sitting too long. *But watch out for...*

• **Chronic kidney disease**—especially if swelling is severe enough to leave indentations when the skin is pressed. This common condition, which often goes undiagnosed, increases the risk for heart attack, stroke and kidney failure.

Action: Diagnosis requires a urine test for the protein albumin...a blood test for the waste product urea nitrogen...and a glomerular filtration rate calculation based on blood and urine levels of the waste product creatinine and other factors.

• **Heart failure,** in which the heart's pumping action is insufficient to meet all of the body's needs. Other telltale symptoms include shortness of breath and rapid pulse.

Action: Get blood tests and imaging tests—most importantly, an echocardiogram (heart ultrasound).

• **Blood clot**—if swelling appears in only one leg and the area is tender. A clot that breaks off and travels to the lungs can be fatal.

Action: Go to the emergency room. You need an ultrasound or computed tomography (CT) scan.

2. Breast changes, such as lumps and tenderness, often are signs of benign breast cysts (fluid-filled sacs). *But watch out for...*

• **Breast cancer**—particularly if you also have nipple discharge, puckered or pitted skin, redness or a change in breast contours. Don't dismiss symptoms just because your last mammogram was negative—mammograms miss up to 20% of breast cancers. An aggressive type called inflammatory breast cancer is especially hard to detect with mammography because it forms no lumps, but instead causes tenderness, painful swelling, itching and/or redness.

Action: If you notice something abnormal or different, a biopsy is almost certainly warranted. Your doctor also may order magnetic resonance imaging (MRI). When a woman's symptoms or high-risk status indicate a medical need for a breast MRI, insurance generally pays.

3. Headache may occur because you are prone to tension headaches or migraines, which are more common in women. *But watch out for...*

• **Brain tumor**—if you recently started having headaches, especially in the mornings, or have experienced a change in headache patterns.

Action: Call your doctor immediately. An MRI or CT scan can rule out a brain tumor.

• **Meningitis**—if the headache is accompanied by a fever and stiff neck. This deadly infection causes inflammation of the membranes around the brain and spinal cord.

Action: Go to the ER immediately. You need a lumbar puncture (spinal tap) to check for white blood cells and bacteria in the cerebrospinal fluid.

• **Bleeding in the brain**—particularly if head pain is sudden and extremely severe. Possible causes include a cerebral aneurysm (a bulging, weakened area in a brain artery)...

subarachnoid hemorrhage (bleeding beneath the tissues covering the brain)...or hemorrhagic stroke.

Action: Call 911. You need magnetic resonance angiography (MRA), which produces detailed images of blood vessels...and a lumbar puncture to check for red blood cells in the cerebrospinal fluid.

4. Chest pain frequently can be a symptom of heartburn. *But watch out for...*

• **Heart disease.** Although chest pain is more typical in men with heart disease, it also is a common sign of heart trouble in women. Be especially vigilant if you have high blood pressure, high cholesterol, a history of smoking or a family history of heart problems.

Action: If you are at risk for heart disease, ask for an ultrafast heart CT scan, a noninvasive test that measures calcium buildup in coronary arteries. Chest pain with fatigue, shortness of breath, dizziness or back pain could signal a heart attack so call 911.

CHAPTER 17

Neck and Shoulder Pain

Easy, Daily Yoga Moves to Relieve Neck Pain

About 15% of US adults endure the misery of neck pain at some point each year. When neck pain occurs, the sufferer will do almost anything to get relief—whether it's popping strong painkillers, paying for massages or seeing a chiropractor.

While these and other approaches may be appropriate in some cases, one of the most effective—but underutilized—therapies for neck pain is yoga. Almost all causes of neck pain, including arthritis, can benefit from yoga, which is a great adjunct to medical treatment. It is also helpful to relieve neck pain stemming from poor posture.

Why yoga? Key yoga moves not only stretch tight muscles and strengthen weak ones, but also help create proper body alignment and posture—crucial steps in both preventing and treating neck pain.

To alleviate neck pain and keep it from coming back, practice these steps every day—but be sure to see your doctor first if you're experiencing severe pain...*

HOLD YOUR HEAD RIGHT

The adult head weighs about 10 pounds—roughly the same as a medium-weight bowling ball. So it is important to correctly balance that weight to avoid strain on the neck.

Many daily activities, including sitting at a desk, working at a computer and talking and texting on the phone, cause our shoulders to round...bodies to lean forward...and heads to protrude in front of the shoulders. This pos-

*Check with your physician before doing any physical activity, including yoga poses, if you have neck pain that is accompanied by numbness, tingling or weakness in your arm or hand...the pain was caused by an injury or accident...you have swollen glands or a lump in your neck...or you have difficulty swallowing or breathing.

Carol Krucoff, a yoga therapist at Duke Integrative Medicine in Durham, North Carolina. She is author of *Healing Yoga for Neck & Shoulder Pain* and *Relax into Yoga for Seniors*. HealingMoves.com.

ture puts extreme pressure and tension on the neck and shoulders.

What to do: For correct head posture whether sitting or standing, your ears should be directly over your shoulders and your shoulders directly over your hips. Check yourself several times a day to make sure you're doing it. This posture may feel strange to you when you first try it, but learning to keep your head balanced over your shoulder girdle can make you feel better and will eventually seem natural.

CHECK FOR "BODY ARMOR"

When stressed, many people tighten the muscles in the upper back, shoulders and neck. As this physical response becomes habitual, we develop a "body armor" of tight, overused muscles in the neck and shoulders. The pattern becomes so ingrained that we don't even notice that we hold this tension constantly in our bodies.

To break this cycle, it's important to consciously consider how tension is affecting your neck muscles.

What to do: Set your wristwatch alarm or phone alarm to sound once every waking hour. When you hear the alarm, take a moment to identify any areas of discomfort or tension in your body, including your back, shoulders and neck. Close your eyes, take a deep breath and relax these muscles. With practice and patience, it is often possible to get substantial release of muscle tension.

Also helpful: Repeat a simple mantra, such as "Lips together, teeth apart," throughout the day to avoid clenching the teeth and help relax the jaw, a common site where tension resides. Jaw tightness often radiates downward and exacerbates neck pain.

STRETCH AND STRENGTHEN

Don't worry if you have never done yoga—these are easy poses that will improve your body alignment and gently stretch the shoulders and neck. Practice the following yoga poses throughout the day, while at your desk, a table, while waiting for coffee to brew, etc. The seated mountain pose can be done anytime you're sitting. The other poses can be done once a day. It should take about five minutes to do them all.

- **Seated mountain pose.**

What to do: Sit tall in your chair, with your feet on the floor. Use your hands to gently move the fleshy part of your buttocks aside and allow your "sit bones"—the two rounded knobs at the base of your pelvis—to press down onto the chair seat.

Extend the crown of your head up toward the sky, lengthening your spine. Relax your shoulders down away from your ears, and let your hands rest on your thighs. Be sure your chin is parallel to the ground and neither tilted up nor tucked in.

What helps: Imagine that you have a headlight in the center of your chest at your breastbone—and shine that light forward. Relax your face, and look straight ahead. Linger here for five to 10 slow, easy breaths.

- **Shoulder shrugs.**

What to do: Inhale and lift your shoulders up toward your ears and then exhale as you drop them down. Repeat five to 10 times, moving with the breath—inhale as you lift, then exhale (with a sigh if you like) as you release. Be sure to keep your arms as relaxed as possible.

- **Shoulder circles.**

What to do: Lift your shoulders straight up as high as they will comfortably go. Then bring them behind you as far as is comfortable. Next, release the shoulders down toward your hips, then bring them forward as far as you comfortably can and finish the circle by bringing them up toward your ears.

Continue circling your shoulders, and avoid holding your breath. Let the movement be easy and get as much motion as possible in your shoulders. Circle five times in this direction, then circle five times in the opposite direction. When you've finished, relax your shoulders and take three to five easy breaths.

- **Head turn.**

What to do: Inhale and extend the crown of your head toward the sky. Exhale and turn your head as far to the right as comfortably possible, keeping your shoulders still. Allow your eyes to turn also so you can look toward whatever is behind you. Inhale and turn back to center. Exhale and turn to the left. Repeat the set three to six times, moving with the breath.

• **Ear to shoulder.**

What to do: Sit tall with your hands on your thighs. Inhale and lift the crown of your head toward the sky. Then exhale and drop your right ear down toward your right shoulder, trying not to lift that shoulder toward the ear. Keep your left shoulder down and relax the left side of your neck.

Keep your breath flowing as you take your left hand off your thigh and let your left arm dangle at your side. Stay in this pose for a few breaths while relaxing. Bring your head back to the center and pause. Then repeat on the other side.

Quick Relief When You Hurt Your Neck

Gerard P. Varlotta, DO, associate professor of rehabilitation medicine and director of sports rehabilitation at the Rusk Institute of Rehabilitation Medicine at New York University Medical Center in New York City.

There are very few upper-body movements that don't require use of the neck. That's why neck injury is one of the most common problems treated by orthopedists and physiatrists (doctors who specialize in rehabilitation medicine).

Most neck injuries are due to "onetime overload"—for example, putting too much strain on the neck by not keeping it in a neutral position while lifting a heavy object. Neck pain also can be caused by strain due to repetitive motions, such as twisting and turning the neck while exercising...muscle tension from stress...arthritic changes...or whiplash. Also, neck pain can be "referred" pain stemming from shoulder or elbow injuries or gallbladder disease.

Good news: Since neck pain usually includes muscle inflammation, it responds well to self-care. Even chronic pain usually can be relieved—and prevented—with simple exercises. Surgery is recommended in rare cases, such as those in which neck pain is accompanied by radiating arm pain and compression of a nerve.

REASONS FOR NECK PAIN

Severe neck pain usually comes on suddenly, but often there's an underlying irritation and/or weakness in the muscles. In most cases, the sufferer reports that the neck feels a little weak or sore, then suddenly worsens—after turning the head abruptly, for example.

When to get help: Neck pain that doesn't begin improving within 48 hours or is accompanied by neurological symptoms—tingling in the arms, hand weakness, loss of muscle strength, etc.—indicates a more serious problem. *Examples...*

• **Disk damage.** A herniated disk (the gelatinous material inside a disk pushes through the outer coating and presses against nearby nerves) can be excruciatingly painful and, in severe cases, cause permanent spinal cord damage.

Red flag: A loss of bowel and/or bladder control or any of the above neurological symptoms. See a doctor immediately.

• **Arthritic changes.** The joints in the neck can deteriorate or stiffen due to osteoarthritis or rheumatoid arthritis.

• **Whiplash.** Injury results when the head is jerked violently forward and backward, as can occur during a car accident.

The above problems are diagnosed during a physical exam, often in conjunction with an X ray and/or magnetic resonance imaging (MRI) scan. Treatment involves controlling inflammation and restoring strength and range of motion.

RAPID PAIN RELIEF

In the absence of neurological symptoms, arthritis or traumatic injury, patients can assume that neck pain is probably due to muscle strain. *To reduce muscle inflammation and pain...*

• **Apply ice immediately.** It's the quickest way to reduce inflammation as well as pain—but only if you apply it within the first 24 to 48 hours. Hold a cold pack or ice cubes wrapped in a towel or washcloth to the painful area for 20 minutes once an hour throughout the day.

> **When Neck Pain Means a Serious Problem**
>
> Seek medical attention if neck pain precedes or accompanies a headache—it could indicate an impending stroke or heart attack...when the pain radiates to your shoulders or arm or is accompanied by leg weakness or difficulty walking—this may be a sign of a herniated disk...if the pain worsens at night or is accompanied by fever or weight loss—this may indicate an infection or another serious condition, such as cancer.
>
> *Mayo Clinic Health Letter.* HealthLetter.MayoClinic.com

Important: Do not apply heat during the first two days after an injury. It relieves stiffness but can increase inflammation and pain.

- **Take the proper anti-inflammatory drug.** Over-the-counter *ibuprofen* (Advil) and *naproxen* (Aleve) are equally effective at relieving muscle pain and inflammation.

Main difference: Ibuprofen is a relatively short-acting drug—generally lasting four to six hours. Naproxen lasts eight to 12 hours. *Acetaminophen* (Tylenol) may help, but it mainly eases pain, not inflammation.

Caution: Ibuprofen and naproxen can cause stomach upset...acetaminophen can cause liver damage when combined with alcohol. Don't take any of these drugs for more than a week without consulting your doctor.

- **Stretch muscles often.** Stretching lengthens muscle fibers and reduces the tension caused by neck-related ergonomic problems, such as how you sit at a computer or hold a telephone. *Helpful...*

While standing or sitting, slowly lower your ear toward your shoulder. Stop when pain significantly increases. Hold the stretch for a few seconds, then relax. Switch to the other side. Repeat eight to 12 times, five times a day.

Bring your chin toward your shoulder, following the directions above.

Although chiropractic treatment can help alleviate pain that emanates from the neck joints, its effects are not long-lasting. Acupuncture also may be helpful but needs to be repeated until the pain dissipates.

LONG-TERM NECK CARE

Most people with chronic neck pain need to perform strengthening exercises (consult your doctor first) and change their posture.

Important: Don't sleep on your stomach—and don't raise your head too high with pillows. Both put excessive pressure on the neck.

Better: Sleep on your side with your head level—propped just high enough to keep your nose in line with your navel. The pillow (when compressed) should be just thick enough to support the side of your head without elevating it.

If you spend a great deal of time on the telephone, use a headset. Cradling a phone between the neck and shoulder is one of the most common causes of neck pain. Choose a headset that is comfortable for you. Good ones, such as those made by Plantronics, are available for $40 to $100 at electronics stores.

If you spend time at a desk, adjust your workstation. The center of a standard computer monitor should be directly at eye level (a bit lower if it's a large monitor)...your knees should be slightly lower than your hips...and use your chair's armrests when possible to avoid hunching forward.

Strengthen your neck and shoulders—they share some of the same muscles. Keeping these muscles strong makes them more flexible and less prone to injury. Perform eight to 12 repetitions of each of the following exercises three times, two to three days a week. Once you can do 12 repetitions easily, gradually increase the weight lifted.

- **Shrugs.** While standing straight with your arms down at your sides, hold a two-pound dumbbell (or a household object, such as a can of soup) in each hand. With palms facing your thighs, shrug your shoulders as high as possible, keeping your head straight. Hold for five seconds, then return to the starting position.
- **Flies.** Lie on your back on an exercise bench, with a two-pound dumbbell in each hand. Hold your hands out to the sides so that the weights are about even with your chest. Keeping your back straight, raise your arms over your chest in a semicircular motion until the weights touch in the middle over your

chest. Lower them back to chest level in the same semicircular motion.

• **Side deltoid raise.** While standing straight with your arms down at your sides, hold a two-pound dumbbell or other weight in each hand, with your palms facing your thighs. Keeping your elbows slightly bent, raise your arms up and out to your sides until they're shoulder level (your palms will be facing the floor in this position). Hold for five seconds, then slowly lower the weights.

Reflexology for Neck Pain

Bill Flocco, reflexology teacher and researcher, founder and director of the American Academy of Reflexology, based in Los Angeles and author of several books on reflexology.

Locate the flap of cartilage at the top of your earlobe, then feel where this flap and the earlobe meet. Move your finger slightly above the small, hard cartilage flap at the top of your earlobe and find a ridge of cartilage running up and down the ear. Place the tips of your index fingers on the lower inch of this ridge on both ears while resting your elbows on a table or desk. Squeeze gently but firmly between your index fingers and thumbs, with your thumbs behind the ears. Continue for five to 10 minutes.

Whiplash? Here's the Real Way to Relieve Your Pain for Good

Mitchell Yass, DPT, a Florida–based physical therapist and creator of the Yass Method for treating chronic pain. He is also author of *The Pain Cure Rx: The Yass Method for Diagnosing and Resolving Chronic Pain* and the PBS special *The Pain Prescription*. MitchellYass.com

You get into a car accident and end up with neck pain. You seek medical care and you are told it is whiplash. You may get chiropractic care, physical therapy and/or take medications all under the diagnosis of whiplash. It may or may not help. Why?

Because there is a problem with this diagnosis: The term "whiplash" merely describes the fact that upon impact, your head was jerked forward and back. It doesn't attempt to define the tissue in distress that is eliciting your pain. It is not a diagnosis.

Think about it...if you tripped and fell and bruised your knee, you wouldn't say that your wound was a trip, right?

SO...WHAT DOES HAPPEN WITH WHIPLASH?

The most-common tissue that is affected by the quick, jerky motions of whiplash is muscle. Muscle has a certain tone to it. If it is forced to stretch excessively in a quick manner, the tone in the muscle will try to prohibit the stretching. This can lead to muscle strain and pain.

In the neck region, the muscles that support the head attach from the skull and top of the cervical spine to the shoulder blades. If these muscles are quickly stretched they could strain and elicit pain at the neck and between the shoulder blades. This type of muscular deficit does not show up on diagnostic tests so conventional practitioners won't treat it. It will continue to elicit pain...and could lead to chronic pain.

EXERCISES TO RELIEVE (OR PREVENT) THE PAIN FROM WHIPLASH

You need to strengthen the rhomboids/midtrapezius (muscles in the upper back between the shoulder blades), lower trapezius ("trap"), posterior deltoids (muscles in the back of the shoulders), rotator cuff (muscles that stabilize the shoulders) and triceps (muscles in the backs of the upper arms).

For each exercise, perform three sets of 10 repetitions with a minute rest in between each set. Perform the series three times a week with a day of rest between. Resistance should be progressed to eventually get the muscles strong enough to perform all functional tasks without straining and eliciting symptoms.

1. Lat Pulldown (*interscapular muscles*: midtraps and rhomboids).

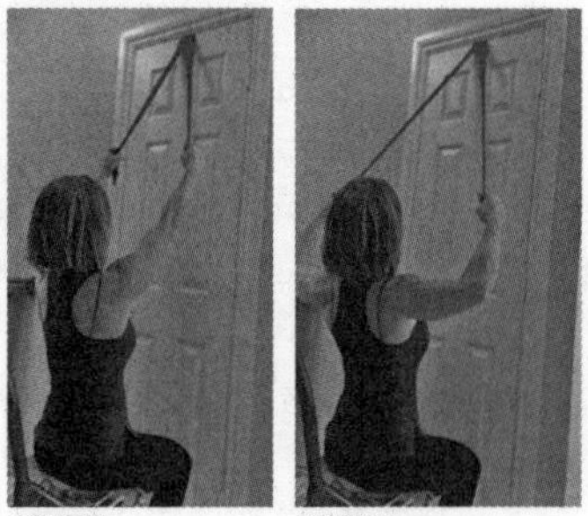
START FINISH

Tie a knot in the center of a resistance band and secure it in place at the top of a closed door. Sit in a sturdy chair facing the door and lean back with an angle at the hip of about 30 degrees. Reach up for the ends of the band so that the start position begins with the arms nearly straight and the elbows just unlocked. Pull the band down keeping your arms wide and bringing the elbows just below shoulder height and slightly behind the line of the shoulders. At this point, you should feel the shoulder blades squeeze together (the elbows will barely reach behind the line of the shoulders if performing this exercise correctly). Then return to the start position.

Important: If the elbows start to drop so they are lower than the shoulders, you are using the incorrect muscles to perform the exercise.

2. Lower Trap Exercise (lower trapezius muscle).

Sit in a sturdy chair with a back and lean back slightly—about 10 degrees. This posture will prevent the resistance from pulling you forward. Step on one end of the resistance band to secure it and hold the other end in your working hand. Start with your arm halfway between pointing straight forward and pointing straight to the side, with your hand at shoulder height and your elbow just unlocked. Begin to raise the resistance until the arm reaches about 130 to 140 degrees (about the height of the ear). Then return to the start position at shoulder height.

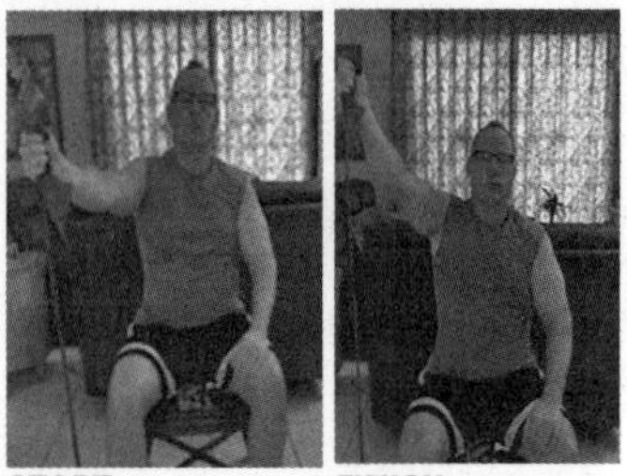
START FINISH

3. Posterior Deltoid Exercise.

Stand with your feet more than shoulder width apart, knees slightly bent, and your butt pushed behind you. Your weight should be mostly on your heels. Step evenly on the band and hold the ends in front of your thighs with your palms facing in and your elbows unlocked. Begin to move the resistance out to your sides from the shoulders like a pendulum. Go out until you feel the shoulder blades start to move inward (about 60 degrees), and then return to the beginning position.

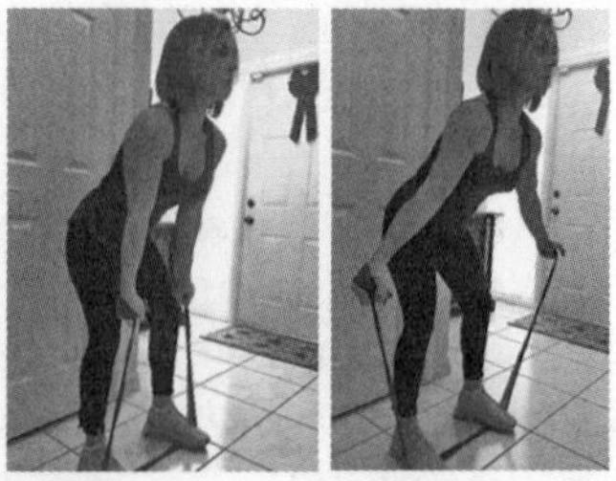
START FINISH

4. External Rotation Exercise (rotator cuff.)

You can do this exercise using a dumbbell or resistance band. With the elbow supported at the end of a surface so that the elbow is just below shoulder height, the elbow should be maintained at a 90-degree angle through the whole motion. The elbow of the arm performing the exercise should be in a line with both shoulders (if the elbow is in front of this line, the rotator cuff will have difficulty performing the exercise). The start position is with the forearm facing about 20 degrees below parallel. The resistance is pulled upward until the forearm is facing about 20 degrees above parallel. Then return to the start position.

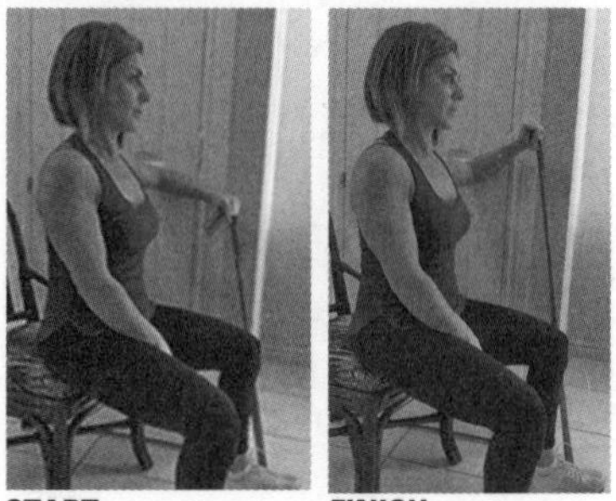
START FINISH

Careful: This is an exercise where people want to go through too much range of motion. If excessive range of motion is performed, there is a chance of straining the rotator cuff.

5. One-Arm Triceps Extensions Exercise.

This exercise is done sitting in a chair. If you are using a resistance band, secure one end at the top of a closed door and sit with your back to the door. If you are using a hand weight, hold it over your head, with your arm straight up and your elbow close to your head. Bend your elbow and lower the weight just behind your neck, then raise it back up. Repeat with the other arm.

I have treated patients who had pain for years after a car accident and they continued to say the cause of their pain was whiplash. If you continue with this thought process the odds of resolving your pain diminishes because you are focused on the mechanism that led to your pain. Unless you identify the tissue in distress eliciting the pain and treat that tissue, it will continue to elicit pain indefinitely.

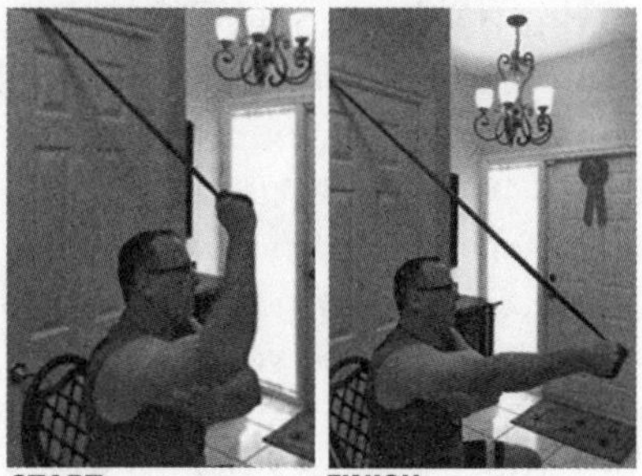
START FINISH

Remember: Whiplash is not diagnosis, it is a mechanism.

Simple Stretches to Ease a Stiff Neck

Natalie Thomas, PT, DPT, doctor of physical therapy, managing director, In Motion O.C., Irvine, California. InMotionOC.com

Let's say you're sitting at a computer for a while—it could be for an hour or more. You get up out of your chair—and ping, your neck aches and feels stiff. You can barely turn to look over your shoulder. Ouch! This type of pain can happen when we've been working at a desk...driving...even doing something relaxing such as working on a puzzle or craft.

Reason: Many of us sit with poor posture, and this affects the connecting muscles that control the position of the spine, including the neck. Stay in this position for a while—and muscles become tight, resulting in pain and stiffness.

Stretching the neck muscles during and after you have been sitting for a while can help, so try the five stretches below. These five moves are easy to do—and feel great. For all of these exercises, sit up straight and comfortably in a hard-backed chair that has no armrests. To make them easier to do, you can watch them atVimeo.com/57019333/.

Note: If you have constant neck pain (that does not appear to be related to how much time you spend sitting), don't do these exercises for pain relief. While they might help you, it's much better to speak to a doctor or physical therapist, who can help determine the root cause of your pain.

HEAD STRETCH

This move stretches the large muscle that connects the base of the skull to the upper back, collarbones and shoulder blades.

Place your right arm behind your back at waist level. Place your left hand over the top of your head and gently grasp the right side of your head. With your left hand, gently pull your head toward your left shoulder. Your left ear will be close to your left arm. Hold for one minute...or hold for 30 seconds, relax and then repeat the move. Switch hands and repeat on the other side.

DOWNWARD HEAD STRETCH

This move eases tightness of the muscle that runs between the upper part of the shoulder blades and neck. You will really feel this stretch in the back of your neck.

As you did in the first exercise, place your right hand behind your back at waist level. Put your left hand on the top of your head. Turn your face toward your left armpit and gently push your head toward the armpit (it's OK if your left hand slides back down your head to get a good stretch). Hold for 30 seconds and repeat. Or hold for one minute and only do one repetition. Repeat on the other side.

SHOULDER PINCH STRETCH

This move helps you maintain good posture. You will feel a stretch across your pectoral muscles in the upper chest.

Sit up tall. With your arms by your sides, bend your elbows at a 90-degree angle, hands palm-up. Position your arms so that the backs of your palms are a foot or so above your thighs. Pull your shoulder blades together and as you do so, let your arms rotate out to your sides, keeping elbows bent. Repeat the rotating movement 20 times.

TORSO ROTATION

This move increases upper- and lower-back flexibility.

Cross your arms in front of you and place your right hand on the front of your left shoulder and your left hand on the front of your right shoulder. Gentle rotate your torso and head to one side as far as you can go—and return to center. Then rotate to the other side. Repeat 10 times on each side.

SITTING KNEE PILLOW SQUEEZE

This move strengthens the hip flexors and solidifies your core muscles and the foundation upon which your neck depends. You will feel this move in your hips and inner thighs.

Sit straight up in your chair—and place a thick pillow between your knees. Roll your hips forward. Hold the pillow with your thighs—squeeze and release. Repeat 20 times—and work up to three sets.

How to Use Your iPad to Avoid Neck Strain

Jack T. Dennerlein, PhD, director, Occupational Biomechanics and Ergonomics Laboratory, senior lecturer on ergonomics and safety, Harvard School of Public Health, Boston.

You bought an iPad or another electronic tablet or received one as a gift, and now you feel pain in your neck and upper back.

There's no doubt that tablet computers are fun and useful gadgets (in fact, approximately 350 million have been sold since 2010). But depending on how you position an iPad when you use it, you could be seriously straining your neck and upper back.

So how are you supposed to use your tablet without straining your neck?

If you're watching a video: The best thing to do is to put the tablet on a table or other surface in front of you in a case that lets you keep the tablet perpendicular or nearly perpendicular (at its high angle)—as if it were a laptop screen. That way, your head will stay in a more neutral position, putting less strain on your neck and back. If you don't have a case, you can put the tablet on the surface and prop it up with whatever's handy—a rolled-up coat, a purse, a backpack.

If you're touching the screen: While sitting, instead of holding the laptop flat on your lap, try putting your bag or a few pillows on your lap and then putting the tablet on top of those things (ideally in its case at its low angle). That way, the tablet will be higher up so you don't have to slump over as much to use it. While standing, try to hold the tablet like a clipboard, or rest it on a high counter if you can, as opposed to holding it horizontally at waist level.

But no matter which posture you choose, try to switch it up every 15 minutes if you can—that way you'll vary which muscles you're using and avoid straining one particular set.

Is Your Phone Causing Neck Strain?

Shani Soloff, manual orthopedic physical therapist and founder of The Posture People, Stamford, Connecticut, reported by Rebecca Shannonhouse, editor, *Bottom Line Health*.

If you've got neck pain, you know all too well the misery it causes.

In your search for relief, don't forget to consider this: How much time do you spend on the phone? Even if it's just a few calls a day, using a handheld landline or cell phone causes you to hold your body in ways that nature never intended.

When you're talking, you naturally tip your head toward the phone—and get even more contorted when your hands are busy and you raise a shoulder to prop the phone in place. It's no wonder that these movements were widely cited in a landmark study that found more than 45% of office workers had frequent episodes of neck pain!

You may think that you've solved the problem if you've switched to a speakerphone. But chances are you haven't. A speakerphone may not be a good alternative, because many people tend to move their necks forward—and lean toward the speakerphone.

Fortunately, the solution is often as simple as investing in a good headset. Shani Soloff, a manual orthopedic physical therapist and founder of the Stamford, Connecticut–based ergonomics firm The Posture People, advises everyone who uses a phone to do this. It will help you maintain proper posture—with your body straight and your shoulders square—while talking on the phone.

It doesn't really matter what style you choose, as long as it's comfortable and easy to use. You can start by checking online at such sites as Headsets.com, BestBuy.com or Staples.com. Headsets come in corded and wireless versions...prices range from about $15 to $350. Your neck will thank you!

Text Much? Unkink Your Neck and Shoulders with These 3 Simple Moves

Peter Scordilis, DC, CCSP, CSCS, a certified chiropractic sports physician and a partner in Scordilis Chiropractic in Clifton, New Jersey. He is an avid triathlete and certified triathlete coach.

Unless you've been hiding under your office desk, you've undoubtedly heard that laboring over your laptop (or desktop) can wreck your posture. But constantly checking your phone or tablet can lead to a different set of posture problems—which need different solutions.

Here's the position...

- **Head jutting forward**
- **Shoulders hunched**
- **Upper back curved into a hump**

Recognize it? Sports medicine science even has a name for the postural muscle imbalance it often causes—upper crossed syndrome. The name refers to a phenomenon in which tightness in muscles in the back and sides of the neck and chest crosses with weakness in the deep-neck muscles and upper arm muscles. You may find that you can't turn your head fully from side to side—your range of motion is reduced. "These imbalances in strength and flexibility can lead to pain and even breathing problems because of the restricted position of the rib cage," says Peter Scordilis, DC, a chiropractic sports medicine physician in Clifton, New Jersey, who treats patients with this condition.

He often prescribes three easy moves that you can do at home. They're designed to help lengthen the specific muscles that get shortened, and strengthen those that get weakened when you're spending too much time hunched over your phone.

Try to incorporate these exercises into your daily routine. Do at least three sets of 15 repetitions of each (set the alarm on your computer or phone as a reminder to take a movement break), and you'll go a long way toward repatterning your body to do the right thing.

NECK RETRACTION

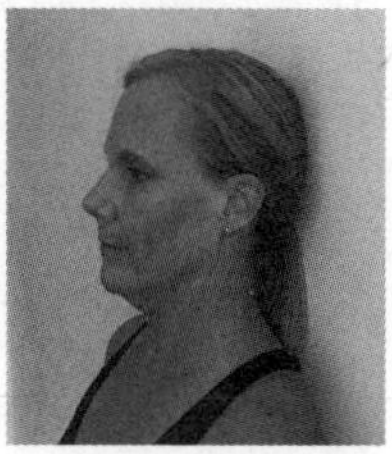

What it does: Stretches the muscles in the back of your neck and strengthens the muscles in the front of your neck (deep cervical flexors).

How to do it...

- **Stand with your back flat against a wall, arms by your sides.**
- **Keeping your chin parallel to the floor** (in other words, don't tuck it under or lift it up), press the back of your head into the wall. Hold for a few seconds, release and repeat.

CORNER STRETCH

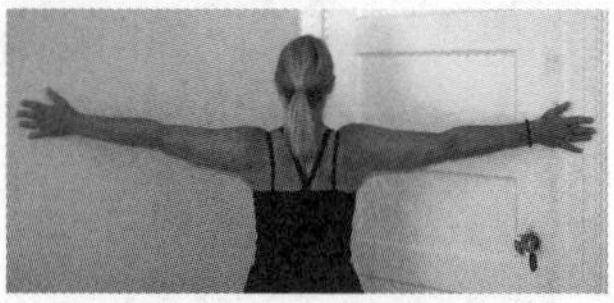

What it does: Loosens and lengthens the muscles in the chest.

How to do it...

- **Stand facing a corner of the room,** about one foot away from where the walls meet.

• **Stretch both arms straight out to the side toward the wall until your palms lie flat against each wall.**

• **Without hunching your shoulders, lean forward until you feel a stretch across the front of your chest.** Hold for a few seconds, release and repeat.

STANDING ELBOW CURLS

What it does: Strengthens upper back and shoulder muscles to counter forward hunch.

How to do it...

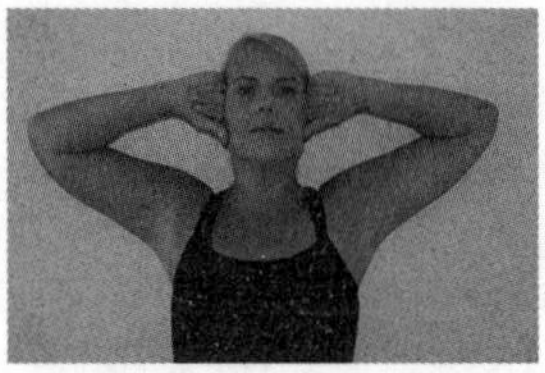

• **Stand with your back against a wall, feet parallel and hip distance apart.** Your heels, butt, upper back and the back of your head should touch the wall throughout the exercise.

• **Make loose fists with both hands,** and place your knuckles against your temples, with your thumbs pointing down.

• **Spread your elbows as wide as you can.** Touch the wall if possible.

• **Squeeze your elbows toward each other,** allowing your knuckles to roll against your temples, until your elbows touch (or come as close as they can).

• **Spread your elbows apart to the starting position.** That's one rep.

HOW TO PREVENT UPPER CROSSED SYNDROME EVERY DAY

While Dr. Scordilis finds that these exercises can really help, he emphasizes that they're not miracle cures. To undo this common syndrome, you also need to pay attention to how you stand—and text—all day long. "It doesn't matter how much you stretch at the gym," he says. "If you're bent over your desk or phone for eight hours a day, your chest and neck muscles are going to tighten up. Flexibility is a function of what you do throughout the day."

So pay attention to your posture. Notice when you're hunched forward, and train yourself to sit or stand up straight instead. Move around frequently. Instead of staying hunched over your computer or your phone, let your body move and stretch frequently throughout the day. Doing these exercises daily will help you experience the kind of healthy posture that you'll want to carry throughout your day.

Don't Let Your Computer Ruin Your Posture

Gregory Thielman, PT, EdD, assistant professor of physical therapy at the University of the Sciences in Philadelphia.

The fact that so many of us spend time sitting in front of computers, whether for work or leisure, has led to an increase in the number of posture-related concerns. We slump or hunch our shoulders as we work, and we sit in unnatural positions. The design and placement of our desks, chairs and computers may not be doing us any favors, either, encouraging us to position our bodies incorrectly.

The potential consequences cannot just be shrugged off—because they can affect our comfort, health, safety and quality of life as we get older. Poor posture can contribute to chronic neck, back and shoulder pain...headaches...muscle stiffness, tension and fatigue...joint degeneration...and kyphosis, an excessively rounded or humped upper back.

Self-defense: If you sit at a computer for hours, at home or at work, here's what to do to protect your posture...

WORKSTATION MAKEOVER

I've conducted numerous workstation evaluations for fellow university employees and found that many posture-related problems can be minimized or prevented with some simple adjustments. The goal of these adjustments is to keep the body in a comfortable and neutral position, leaning neither too far forward nor too far backward.

Take a look at your office and home workstations with the following recommendations in mind. If any of your furniture or equipment doesn't pass muster, adjust or replace it. *Check your...*

• **Desk chair seat and arms.** At the proper seat height, your thighs are parallel to the ground...your knees are bent at a 90° angle so that they are directly above your ankles...and both your feet are flat on the floor (as they ideally should be to minimize the stress on your joints). The chair seat should be long enough to support three-quarters of the thigh (yet still allow feet to be flat on the floor) when your hips are all the way back in the chair. The chair should have armrests that allow the elbows to be supported when bent at 90°.

• **Chair back.** This should come at least three-quarters of the way up your back.

Exception: If you have chronic neck pain, the chair back needs to be high enough and the headrest aligned in a way that allows you to sit with your neck straight and the back of your head resting against the headrest.

• **Computer monitor height.** The top of the monitor should be at your eye level so you don't have to sit with your neck bent too far forward or backward to see the screen. If your monitor is too low, put a book underneath it to raise it. If it is too high and has no mechanism for adjusting it, you may need to get an adjustable monitor or a lower desk.

• **Keyboard position.** As you type, your upper arms should hang straight by your sides from shoulder to elbow...elbows should be bent at about a 90° angle and supported by the armrests of the chair...and your forearms should be roughly parallel to the floor. If your desk is too high for this, you can affix a keyboard tray to the underside of the desktop.

Laptop users: People tend to use laptop computers when they are in a relaxed position, paying no mind to body mechanics—so at least use a lap desk to hold the computer at an appropriate height, and try to remain conscious of the recommendations above.

OFFICE-FRIENDLY EXERCISES

When you spend hours sitting at a computer, it is important to periodically stop what you're doing and change your position—gently roll your shoulders, turn your head from side to side, stretch your arms overhead, stand up and walk around for a minute. *Also, every hour or so, do these easy exercises...*

• **Chin tuck.** This helps counteract the tendency to sit with your head jutting forward. Sit up straight in your chair. Put your index finger on your chin, and gently push straight back, so that your entire head moves back and realigns with your spine. Continue pressing your chin back for three seconds...relax...do 10 times.

• **Pelvic tilt.** This strengthens the abdominal muscles that help support the spine. Sit up straight in your chair and place a tissue at the small of your back...then use your abs to tilt the bottom of your pelvis forward, so that your lower back presses the tissue firmly against the back of the chair. Hold for three seconds...relax...do 10 times.

• **Back stretch.** This helps combat a tendency to slump forward. Stand tall with feet shoulder-width apart and place your hands on your lower back. Gently arch your back so that your hips come forward a bit, keeping your head aligned with your spine and taking care not to push too far so you don't strain your neck or back. Hold for 10 seconds...relax...do 10 times.

Have a Pro Take a Look at Your Posture

Steven P. Weiniger, DC, focuses on posture rehab and biomechanics in his private practice in Atlanta. His books include *Stand Taller—Live Longer: An Anti-Aging Strategy* and *Posture Pictures: Posture Assessment, Screenings, Marketing and Forms.* BodyZone.com

Are you plagued by the curse of the curved back? You may not realize it if you do, because it can creep up over the years. What's more, spinal straightness is just one aspect of overall postural health—so even a straight-backed person may have another type of posture problem, such as an uneven gait, that contributes to pain and loss of function.

The first step toward solving a posture problem is to recognize that a problem exists. To that end, it's a good idea to get a posture assessment by a chiropractor, physical therapist or massage therapist who is specially trained in posture therapy.

A professional posture assessment includes analysis of your...

• **Alignment.** Various methods may be used to check this. I use "posture pictures." Whole-body photos are taken from the front, back and side, then superimposed onto a computerized grid. The vertical and horizontal lines make it easy to pinpoint alignment problems, such as one shoulder that is higher than the other...one arm that is held closer to the body...a head that juts too far forward...or feet that turn in too much.

• **Balance.** To assess this, you may be asked to perform certain balancing exercises. For instance, you may need to stand on one foot with the other foot held off the ground, thigh parallel to the floor. It's a good sign if you can balance for at least 30 seconds without waving your arms, twisting or putting your foot down. Poor balance suggests weakness in the core, the band of muscles that encircle your midsection to connect and support the upper and lower halves of your body. Women are particularly prone to problems with core strength because pregnancy overstretches the muscles in this area.

• **Gait.** The posture professional observes how you walk, either visually or using a computerized video analysis device. He or she checks how each foot strikes the ground... how the knees flex...and whether the head, torso or pelvis shifts to the side. Asymmetry of motion trains the muscles on one side differently from the other, resulting in uneven posture.

To find a posture professional: Ask your doctor for a referral...or check the practitioner locator at BodyZone.com. A posture assessment typically takes about 10 to 15 minutes and costs $20 to $35. Based on the results, the practitioner can then develop an individualized posture improvement program to help you sit erect, stand tall and move gracefully—so you can look and feel your very best.

The Right Way to Carry a Purse

Karen Erickson, DC, a chiropractor in private practice in New York City. She is a faculty member at the Center for Health and Healing of Beth Israel Medical Center, also in New York City, and a spokesperson for the American Chiropractic Association. ACAtoday.org

Backaches, headaches, neck and shoulder pain often have a common cause—that too-heavy handbag you habitually carry. It throws your posture out of alignment...causes spasms of the trapezius muscle that runs from the base of your skull to your midback...and speeds arthritic degeneration of the spine.

Solution: Lighten your load, and relieve the pain.

• **Weigh your purse.** It should weigh no more than 10% of your body weight. That's 14 pounds for a 140-pound woman.

Ideal: No more than two pounds.

Choose a bag made of lightweight material. Avoid heavy leather and canvas, buckles and embellishments.

• **Switch shoulders every few minutes...** place the strap diagonally across the chest... or use a backpack that distributes weight evenly.

• **Edit your bag daily.** Weed out water bottles, magazines, seldom used keys and loose change. Carry only what's essential.

• **Get multiples of heavy items**—gym gear, makeup, hairbrush, etc. Keep the spares in your desk or car instead of carrying them around.

• **Stretch muscles.** With hands on your shoulders, trace slow, wide circles with your elbows, five in each direction. Next, shrug your shoulders up toward your ears, then drop them down. Repeat five times. Do several times daily.

• **Get a deep-tissue massage** to increase circulation to muscles and remove lactic acid, a chemical that causes soreness.

Referrals: American Massage Therapy Association (877-905-2700, AMTAmassage.org).

• **Realign your spine.** A chiropractor can help to restore the normal alignment of your spine and shoulders. Relieving purse-related pain typically takes no more than a few visits.

Referrals: American Chiropractic Association (800-986-4636, ACAtoday.org).

When Shoulder Pain Won't Go Away

Beth E. Shubin Stein, MD, associate attending orthopedic surgeon at the Hospital for Special Surgery and associate professor of orthopedic surgery at Weill Cornell Medical College, both in New York City. DrBethShubinStein.com

When you've got a painful shoulder, you're reminded of it many times each day. As many as half of all Americans suffer from shoulder pain each year. For a significant number of these people, the problem lingers on…for weeks, months or even longer.

There is hope: Whether the pain stems from an injury, overuse or some unknown cause, chronic shoulder pain can be dramatically improved—and usually eliminated. The treatments may also help those whose shoulder pain is caused by arthritis. *Here are the latest approaches for the most common shoulder problems…*

ROTATOR CUFF PROBLEMS

Most people are quick to chalk up shoulder pain to tendinitis, a nagging form of inflammation. But that's usually a mistake.

New thinking: The shoulder pain thought of as tendinitis is typically a result of tendinosis, a related condition that occurs when the tendons (ropelike cords connecting muscle to bone) begin to deteriorate. Tendinosis can usually be diagnosed with a physical exam and an X-ray and/or MRI.

Red flag for the patient: The pain may be barely perceptible while the arm is at rest—but if you extend the arm outward, in front of the body or overhead, the pain can range from dull to excruciating.

Rotator cuff tendinosis develops when tendons in the rotator cuff (a group of tendons and muscles that attach the upper arm to the shoulder joint) break down over time. This can occur due to age…repetitive use…or weakness of the rotator cuff muscles.

What works best: During the first week or two, to "quiet" the inflammation around the tendon, apply ice (for 15 to 20 minutes several times daily)…and take a nonsteroidal anti-inflammatory drug (NSAID), such as *ibuprofen* (Motrin).

If pain continues, your doctor should also refer you to a physical or occupational therapist, who can recommend exercises (such as those on the next page) to strengthen the rotator cuff and shoulder blade (scapula) muscles. If pain worsens or lasts longer than a week or two, a cortisone injection into the bursa surrounding the rotator cuff tendons can help.

Red Flags for Shoulder Injury

If you experience any of the following signs of shoulder injury—or any kind of acute shoulder pain and/or restricted movement for more than a few days—see an orthopedic physician…

• **Pain when you are putting on a coat** or when you're reaching around to the backseat of a car could be signs of impingement or rotator cuff irritation.

• **Inability to lift your arm from your side** and raise an object above shoulder height without arching your back. This can indicate a serious rotator cuff tear.

• **Inability to sleep on one shoulder due to pain.** It is often a sign of early-stage rotator cuff damage.

• **Pain when reaching for objects overhead.** This can indicate impingement or other shoulder problems.

Caution: If you experience severe shoulder pain, go to the hospital right away. You could have a dislocated shoulder.

Kevin D. Plancher, MD, Plancher Orthopaedics & Sports Medicine, Cos Cob, Connecticut.

Good news: Within six weeks, this nonsurgical regimen alleviates the pain 90% of the time.

Beware: Chronic use of cortisone can damage tendons, so surgery (see below) should be considered if two or three injections (given no more than every three months) have not relieved the pain.

If you don't get relief after six weeks or the pain returns after cortisone therapy wears off, you may want to consider surgery. Arthroscopy (inserting a tiny camera via small incisions) allows the surgeon to assess the shoulder joint and correct the damage that has led to rotator cuff tendinosis. When performed by an experienced surgeon, the procedure has a high success rate. Complications are rare but may involve infection or stiffness.

To find an experienced surgeon, consult The American Orthopaedic Society for Sports Medicine, SportsMed.org.

Two approaches that are less invasive than surgery...

- **Platelet-rich plasma (PRP) injection involves the use of platelets from a patient's blood.** The platelets are separated from the blood with a centrifuge and reinfused into the affected tendons. The platelets are rich in growth factors that aid healing, and the technique is considered safe, since the patient's own cells are used.

A small study published in 2013 in *Global Advances in Health and Medicine* found that a single PRP injection significantly improved pain and function at a 12-week follow-up. More research is needed, however, for definitive evidence of its effectiveness. Some patients opt to have a series of PRP injections. Insurance rarely covers the cost—typically about $1,500 per injection.

- **Stem cell treatment.** With this therapy, which is currently experimental, certain bone marrow cells are reinjected into the shoulder area, where they can help replace degenerated tendon tissue. Though promising, this therapy is not yet widely available. Several clinical trials are now ongoing. To find one, go to ClinicalTrials.gov.

FROZEN SHOULDER

Frozen shoulder (or adhesive capsulitis), which usually occurs for unknown reasons, develops when the capsule surrounding the shoulder joint gets inflamed and then stiffens. A dull ache in the shoulder can come and go, slowly worsening to a ferocious pain that may awaken you during sleep or hurt even when your arm is at your side.

In the past, doctors recommended physical therapy to "thaw out" the joint and restore range of motion. But the physical therapy typically aggravated the condition—and it often did not improve for more than a year.

New thinking: With a two-part approach—a cortisone injection given early on into the joint and gentle exercises—sufferers can get pain relief and restore their range of motion within a matter of weeks to months.

Surgery is rarely needed if frozen shoulder is promptly diagnosed and treated at this stage. Cortisone injections are usually not helpful when frozen shoulder has progressed to severe stiffness, but physical therapy may help restore mobility.

After receiving a cortisone injection, the following exercises should be performed on the recovering shoulder three times a day. *Gently hold each for five seconds and do 10 reps of each exercise...*

- **Overhead stretch.**

What to do: Lie on your back and lift the arm that's affected by frozen shoulder as high as possible. Use your other hand to gently press the arm upward for 10 seconds. Rest for a few seconds and repeat three times.

- **Cross-body reach.**

What to do: Stand and lift your arm to the side until it's a bit below shoulder height, then bring it to the front and across your body. As it passes the front of your body, grab the elbow with your other arm and exert gentle pressure to stretch the shoulder.

- **Towel stretch.**

What to do: Drape a towel over the unaffected shoulder, and grab it with your hand behind your back. Gently pull the towel upward with your other hand to stretch the affected shoulder and upper arm.

SLEEPER STRETCH

What to do: Lie on your side with the affected arm outstretched in front of you. Bend the elbow so that the wrist is in the air. Using the other arm, pull the wrist down toward the floor. Hold for 30 seconds. Rest for a few seconds and repeat three times.

If these measures don't help within eight to 12 weeks, talk to your doctor about noninvasive or minimally invasive procedures to break up scar tissue and "unfreeze" your shoulder. Manipulation and/or capsular release surgery both are done while under anesthesia. The procedures may be covered by insurance—but check with your carrier, including whether you need prior authorization before having the procedure.

Important: Once the pain is relieved and range of motion improves, you should continue doing the stretches described above every other day to help prevent a recurrence.

"Thaw" Your Frozen Shoulder with Acupuncture

Fred Lisanti, ND, LAc, naturopathic physician and licensed acupuncturist specializing in pain management. He also is trained in clinical hypnosis, botanical medicine and neurolinguistic programming and is the attending doctor at Integrative Med Solutions in Eastchester, New York. IntMedSolutions.com

---

The Chinese call it the 50-years shoulder…doctors call it adhesive capsulitis…in the US, folks usually say frozen shoulder.

With frozen shoulder, extending the arm—to reach, lift, get dressed, style hair, etc.—becomes not only increasingly painful, but nearly impossible. The shoulder literally feels locked in place as the inflamed connective tissue around the joint thickens, contracts and loses elasticity. Keeping the shoulder still only makes matters worse by reducing production of lubricating fluids and allowing scar tissue to form. The condition most often develops in midlife (hence the "50-years" moniker), and almost 70% of those affected are women. The exact cause is unknown, but people with a thyroid disorder, Parkinson's disease, diabetes or a history of shoulder injury are at increased risk.

Left untreated, frozen shoulder usually heals on its own—but this can take years! And typical conventional treatments may not help much…can have side effects (for instance, corticosteroid injections can lead to infection, loss of skin color and tendon damage)…and, in the case of physical therapy, can be effective but time consuming.

Good news: Acupuncture can help. It helps loosen tight connective tissues, muscle fibers and scar tissue in the shoulder. It also increases blood flow, and where blood goes, nutrients go—and these help scavenge inflammatory particles, thus promoting healing.

Recent scientific evidence supports the use of acupuncture for frozen shoulder. For instance, in one study, 86% of frozen shoulder patients who received acupuncture showed improvement. Acupuncture may be especially helpful when combined with physical therapy, another study showed. In that study, patients who got acupuncture alone experienced better pain control than those who did only physical therapy exercises…those who got physical therapy alone experienced more improvement in range of motion…and those who got both treatments benefited most.

What to do: If you have symptoms that suggest frozen shoulder, see your doctor to rule out other possible causes, such as arthritis, dislocation or a rotator cuff tear. If you decide to try acupuncture, alone or as a complement to physical therapy and/or other treatments, you can find a licensed practitioner through the American Association of Acupuncture and Oriental Medicine (AAAOMonline.org, 866-455-7999).

What to expect: Based on a thorough exam, the acupuncturist chooses the appropriate acupuncture points. The hair-thin needles cause little or no discomfort and are left in place for about 30 to 40 minutes. Patients are usually seen two or three times a week for six to eight weeks. Some patients also benefit from periodic follow-up sessions. Acupuncture sessions range from $75 to $200 apiece and often are covered by insurance.

While acupuncture cannot guarantee a 100% cure for frozen shoulder, Dr. Lisanti reported that at least half of his patients start feeling better and enjoying increased range of motion after just a few treatments.

Don't Shrug Off Shoulder Replacement Surgery

Peter J. Millett, MD, MSc, director of shoulder surgery, Steadman-Hawkins Clinic, Vail, Colorado.

Joint replacement is almost ho-hum these days—at least when it comes to knees and hips. But only about a tenth as many shoulder replacements are done as hip or knee replacements. One reason for this is that even among physicians, the buzz is that shoulder replacement is difficult and not very successful, something it's best to avoid. But the buzz couldn't be more wrong. A new study from Johns Hopkins in Baltimore revealed that shoulder replacement surgery actually has fewer complications and shorter hospital stays than either knee or hip replacement. As to the success rate, the study concludes that most patients who have shoulder replacement are only sorry they didn't do it sooner.

ARM YOURSELF WITH FACTS ON SHOULDER REPLACEMENT

Fewer shoulder replacements are performed in large part because the need for them isn't as great.

The reason: Arthritis, the malady that erodes joints and often makes them unbearably painful, doesn't affect the shoulder as frequently as it does hips and knees...since we don't walk on our hands, we don't wear down the shoulder as much as we do our lower joints. But also, shoulder replacements may be rarer because many people don't realize it's an option or they lack access to doctors who perform shoulder replacement surgery...and there aren't as many different repair options, such as partial replacements. Furthermore, few doctors have the training to perform the surgery and many have not seen the excellent results that can be achieved, so they are often reluctant to advise it for their patients.

As with all joint replacements—indeed, all surgeries—having an experienced surgeon vastly improves the odds that the operation will be a success. This is a particularly complex surgery, so it is mandatory to find a highly skilled surgeon working at a major medical center or a medical center specializing in orthopedics only, who does a significant volume of shoulder replacements each year.

ABOUT THE SURGERY

The reason total shoulder replacement is such a challenging operation is that it involves removing the humeral head (the top of the upper arm bone)...replacing it with a new prosthetic ball...and then resurfacing the shoulder socket (the glenoid) by affixing a second dish-shaped plastic component to the shoulder blade. The shoulder is smaller and more complex than knees and hips, so it is more difficult to place the prostheses exactly right. Access to the joint is complicated by the numerous nerves, tendons and blood vessels in the area. Also, the anatomy of this joint varies considerably from person to person so standardized parts don't fit well. Prostheses today are more flexible and can adapt to the individual's structure, but placement of the implant is still very demanding from a surgical standpoint. Done properly, shoulder replacement

Shoulder Replacement for Rheumatoid Arthritis

In a recent finding, 93% of rheumatoid arthritis (RA) patients who had a total shoulder replacement... and 88% of those who had a partial replacement had pain relief and improved function. RA patients with severe shoulder pain and stiffness that are not relieved by medication or physical therapy may want to consider the surgery.

Note: Rehabilitation after shoulder surgery can take many months.

John Sperling, MD, an orthopedic surgeon at the Mayo Clinic, Rochester, Minnesota, and leader of a study published in *Journal of Shoulder and Elbow Surgery.*

reliably eliminates the arthritis pain—patients often wake up from surgery pain-free for the first time in years.

After surgery, patients can begin to move their shoulder immediately, though they generally remain in the hospital for two days. Several months of physical therapy will be necessary to gain full functioning and range of motion. Most patients can raise their arm by six weeks and resume full activities after three or four months. Although patients experience the most dramatic improvement in the first four months, progress continues for a full year—by then patients can return to their previous activities, including, for some, doubles tennis, skiing and golf. Excessive overuse of the joint will wear it out faster, but many patients can return to jobs that require repetitive overhead lifting without relapse if care is taken.

WHO SHOULD CONSIDER REPLACEMENT

You may be a candidate for shoulder replacement if you have significant arthritis with pain that is disabling or interfering with sleep and functioning of the shoulder. Since arthritis is often age-related, the surgery is also mostly for older patients, who must, of course, be healthy enough to withstand it. Since prostheses currently are expected to last an average of 15 to 20 years, it's best to wait until at least age 50—or even 60 or more if possible. While second-time joint replacements can certainly be done if and when the implants fail, those surgeries are riskier and more complex so younger patients might do better starting out with other procedures to relieve pain. For example, surgeons can arthroscopically clear debris from the joint…readjust tendons…resurface…or stimulate new growth of the cartilage that cushions the shoulder joint. In some cases patients even choose to have their shoulder fused to eliminate pain—but there's significant compromise in that option. It stops the pain, but also severely limits shoulder function.

People who've done their homework to find a highly qualified surgeon and who commit themselves to healing properly and working hard on their physical therapy have described the operation as being "truly life-altering."

Don't Use Just Any Old Pillow

William J. Lauretti, DC, an associate professor in the department of chiropractic clinical sciences at the New York Chiropractic College in Seneca Falls, New York, and spokesperson for the American Chiropractic Association in Arlington, Virginia.

Plenty of people agonize about buying a mattress—you can easily spend $1,000 or more, and there are all those features to choose from (such as pillow toppers and coil counts).

The truth is, there's no unbiased research showing that any of these features will reduce pain. The best mattress for you is simply the one that feels best for you. (For best sleep positions to accommodate pain, see page 457 in chapter 22, "Drug-Free Protocols for Pain Relief.")

The features offered in pillows, however, do matter. That's why pillows should never be selected as an afterthought. *How to select a pillow based on where you need support and how you sleep…*

PILLOWS FOR NECK PAIN

I usually advise people to sleep on their sides because it's a neutral position that's easy on the back, shoulders and knees.* But side-sleeping leaves a large gap between the downward-facing shoulder and the head. A too-thin pillow will allow your head to dip down, which puts a lot of stress on the neck.

Best pillow for side-sleepers: One that's thick enough to fill the space between your ear and the mattress. It will support your neck and head and keep them in line with your spine. A firm foam pillow is ideal because the weight of your head won't compress it very much while you sleep.

Good products: BackJoy SleepSound Pillow, $99.99, BackJoy.com/sleep. Or you could try a water pillow so you can customize your pillow height. Chiroflow Premium Water Pillow, $46.17, Amazon.com.

*We all have a preferred sleep position, but certain positions are better for various types of pain than others. I have found that patients can adopt a new sleep position if it helps their pain.

Best pillow for back- and stomach-sleepers: A feather pillow. You can shape a feather pillow and make it thicker under the neck for better support and thinner under the head so that it remains flat.

Good product: 700-Fill-Power Sateen White Goose Down Pillow, $199, LLBean.com.

If you like the feel of a feather pillow but are allergic, try the Grand Down All Season Down Alternative Standard Pillow Set, $34.40, Amazon.com.

Another option for neck pain is a thin conventional pillow with a "neck bone" support pillow placed under the neck.

Good product: Original Bones NeckBone Chiropractic Pillow, $14.99, Amazon.com.

You can also try a specialized pillow that is thicker at the ends, with a slight cavity in the middle and built-in neck support. These pillows help keep the head at the right height while supporting the neck. In addition, they provide flexibility for people who like to change from back-sleeping (when they would use the thinner middle part of the pillow) to side-sleeping (when the thicker end would be appropriate).

Good product: Core Products Core 200 Tri-Core Pillow Standard Support, $37.99, Amazon.com.

PILLOWS FOR BACK PAIN

For back pain, the usual advice is to sleep on your back on a superfirm mattress. Back-sleeping does give good support, but many people aren't comfortable in this position, and it tends to increase snoring.

I have found that back pain patients tend to do better when they sleep on their sides. It keeps the spine straight and is generally less stressful than stomach- or back-sleeping.

Stomach-sleeping tends to produce a forward curve in the low back, jamming the joints together and causing pain. Back-sleeping can be better, but if the mattress is too soft, it causes a forward curve in the low back. And if the mattress is too firm, it flattens the low back, which can lead to tight muscles.

Best pillow pick: When sleeping on your back, use a feather pillow that's "fluffed" to provide more lift under the neck, and flattened out a bit under the head. When sleeping on your side, use a fairly thick and firm foam pillow to support the head and fill the gap between the head and bottom shoulder. See feather pillow and foam pillow recommendations mentioned earlier.

PILLOWS FOR SHOULDER PAIN

It's a challenge to find a comfortable position when you have shoulder arthritis or a history of shoulder injuries. If you sleep on your stomach, you would have to keep your head turned all night, which could make shoulder pain worse. Of course, sleeping on the "bad" shoulder can be painful as well, but lying with the bad side up is also tricky because the shoulder isn't supported by a pillow or the mattress.

Best pillow pick: A large body pillow. While on your side, hug the pillow to your chest and rest your top-side arm (with your painful shoulder) on top of it. It will support the shoulder and keep it from "folding" while you sleep.

Good product: Dreamland Body Pillow, $21.20, Amazon.com.

PILLOWS FOR KNEE PAIN

Back-sleeping is ideal when your knees hurt, but as mentioned earlier, few people can comfortably sleep on their backs. And stomach-sleeping is a problem because it overextends the knees. Side-sleeping is less stressful to the knees, but this position can be uncomfortable when the bones of the knees press together.

Best pillow pick: While sleeping on your side, placing a pillow between your knees will prevent them from rubbing against each other and keep your upper hip at a comfortable angle.

Good product: Remedy Contoured Memory Foam Leg Pillow, $17.99, Walmart.com.

You can also put a body pillow between your knees.

HELPFUL RESOURCE

For reviews of additional types of pillows, go to SleepLiketheDead.com/pillow-reviews.html.

CHAPTER 18

Neuropathy and Other Nerve Pain

Put a Stop to Tingling And Numbness

If you experience occasional tingling, numbness or weakness in your fingers, arms or feet, it may be tempting to shrug it off as a minor complaint. That's a mistake.

Peripheral neuropathy is a nerve disorder that affects 15 million to 20 million Americans—and often it is one of the first signs of a serious medical condition. For example, 60% to 70% of patients with diabetes have peripheral nerve disease.

WHAT IS PERIPHERAL NEUROPATHY?

Peripheral neuropathy refers to damage, disease or dysfunction of nerves outside the brain and spinal cord. The condition, which affects an estimated 20 million Americans, has more than 100 known causes, including diabetes, autoimmune disorders, tumors, heredity, nutritional imbalances and infections.

If identified early, neuropathy may disappear with proper treatment.

THE HIDDEN CULPRIT

The majority of people with neuropathy have an underlying disease that affects multiple nerves. *Main causes...*

- **Diabetes (or prediabetes,** a precursor to diabetes) is the most common cause of peripheral neuropathy. Although it is not known exactly how diabetes triggers neuropathy, it is thought that episodes of elevated blood sugar (glucose) can overwhelm mitochondria (the power plants inside cells that convert glucose to energy), resulting in accumulations of molecules (such as free radicals) that damage nerve cells.

Red flag: Persistent foot pain and/or numbness is often the first symptom of diabetes. If

Eva L. Feldman, MD, PhD, Russell N. DeJong Professor of Neurology and director of the Juvenile Diabetes Research Foundation Center for the Study of Complications in Diabetes and the Amyotrophic Lateral Sclerosis (ALS) Clinic at the University of Michigan in Ann Arbor.

you experience these symptoms, see a doctor right away.

• **Autoimmune diseases** (such as lupus and rheumatoid arthritis) can lead to peripheral neuropathy. That's because the body's immune system attacks the layers of tissue, known as the myelin sheath, that wrap around peripheral nerves.

• **Medications can cause toxic neuropathy**—particularly the chemotherapeutic drugs used to treat cancer. Other drugs that can cause peripheral neuropathy include certain antibiotics, such as *nitrofurantoin* (Macrodantin) and *metronidazole* (Flagyl). Exposure to workplace or environmental heavy metals, such as arsenic and mercury, also can cause neuropathy.

• **Vitamin deficiencies**—particularly a deficiency of vitamin B-12—can lead to a form of neuropathy most prevalent in older adults. These people are particularly at risk because they are more likely to have insufficient levels of intrinsic factor, a substance secreted in the stomach that's required for vitamin B-12 absorption.

GETTING THE RIGHT DIAGNOSIS

Neuropathy usually can be diagnosed in the doctor's office with a complete medical history, blood work and the following tests...

• **Nerve conduction study (NCS).** With this noninvasive test, electrodes are placed on the surface of the skin—on the hands and feet, for example—and mild electric shocks are delivered to help measure the speed of nerve signals. Some types of neuropathy, such as Charcot-Marie-Tooth disease (a hereditary disorder), strip the nerves of their protective coating (myelin), causing nerve impulses to travel more slowly.

• **Pinprick.** The doctor will very lightly touch the patient's bare foot in several places with a pin. A patient with neuropathy—particularly when it's caused by diabetes—might not feel the pin.

• **Tuning fork.** Neuropathy patients may not feel the vibrations when it's held against the big toe.

• **Reflex tests.** Rapping the ankle, knee or other affected body part with a small rubber hammer helps determine whether muscles are responding properly to nerve signals.

In addition, the doctor might perform an electromyography (a test of electrical activity in the muscles) and/or a nerve conduction study, in which electrodes are placed on the patient's skin and nerves are stimulated via an electrical pulse. The test measures the speed at which the nerves carry electrical signals.

BEST TREATMENT OPTIONS

Because neuropathy is almost always a symptom of another condition, the main goal is to identify and treat the underlying problem. Once that's achieved, the nerves will gradually start to heal—and the neuropathy will usually improve significantly—and even disappear.

For example, patients with prediabetes or diabetes who achieve good blood sugar control—with diet, regular exercise and/or the use of medication—often will have a complete reversal of neuropathy within one year.

Nerves that are severely damaged or entirely dead—as a result of chemotherapy, for example—may continue to cause pain or other symptoms indefinitely.

Most effective pain treatments...

• ***Pregabalin*** **(Lyrica) or** ***gabapentin*** **(Neurontin)** are used for treating diabetic neuropathy. Both drugs were originally developed for the prevention of epileptic seizures. Taken orally, the drugs are thought to work by affecting electrical activity in the brain and inhibiting pain sensations. Both drugs reduce pain by 20% to 30% in most patients.

Main side effects: Dizziness, sleepiness and/or peripheral edema (swollen ankles).

• ***Duloxetine*** **(Cymbalta),** an antidepressant, was approved by the FDA in 2004 for treating diabetic neuropathy—even in patients who aren't depressed. This medication increases levels of the brain chemicals serotonin and norepinephrine, which appear to work, in part, by increasing feelings of well-being. Like pregabalin and gabapentin, it reduces pain by 20% to 30% in most patients.

Main side effects: Nausea, dry mouth and/or constipation.

• **Opioid analgesics,** such as *dextromethorphan* (Neurodex), *oxycodone* (OxyContin) and codeine, are very effective painkillers. These drugs commonly cause sedation (and also pose a risk for addiction), so they're recommended only for patients with severe pain that does not respond to the therapies described above.

Main side effects: Nausea, sleepiness and/or dependency.

• **Nondrug therapies,** such as acupuncture and transcutaneous electrical nerve stimulation (TENS), are often used with or without medication. Many patients report that acupuncture helps relieve the pain related to neuropathy.

TENS, in which tiny electrical signals are transmitted through the skin, appears to block pain signals. In patients who respond to TENS treatment (typically performed by physical therapists), it can reduce pain by 50% to 70%.

For more information on peripheral neuropathy, contact the Neuropathy Association, 212-692-0662, Neuropathy.org.

Hidden Causes of Peripheral Neuropathy

Janice F. Wiesman, MD, FAAN, associate clinical professor of neurology at New York University School of Medicine and adjunct assistant professor of neurology at Boston University School of Medicine. She is also the author of *Peripheral Neuropathy: What It Is and What You Can Do to Feel Better.*

Tingling, burning, numbness and weakness. The symptoms of peripheral neuropathy are usually obvious, painful—and potentially debilitating. Yet the disorder is not always easy to diagnose.

About 20 million people in the US have peripheral neuropathy, a condition caused by damage to the peripheral nervous system. Most of these cases are linked to diabetes. But there are millions of other people who suffer from this condition and don't know why.

In fact, for about 30% of people with peripheral neuropathy, the cause remains mysterious. In these cases, it's diagnosed as "idiopathic" neuropathy—the same as saying "unknown cause."

The problem: Without identifying and treating the underlying cause of peripheral neuropathy, the symptoms will only get worse. At its most extreme, neuropathy can lead to difficulty standing or walking, as well as nonstop agony from dying nerves. While symptoms can be treated without knowing the cause, addressing the root of the problem is far more effective and may eliminate the neuropathy.

THE BASICS

Our peripheral nerves are in constant communication with our central nervous system (brain and spinal cord). Communication signals are transmitted to and from the central nervous system and all the distant (peripheral) parts of the body, such as the hands and feet.

Peripheral neuropathy occurs when the peripheral nerves become damaged—as a result of diabetes…or a less commonly recognized issue (see examples below). Those impaired nerves send pain or pins-and-needles tingling sensations…or they can fail to transmit physical signals, leading to numbness or muscle weakness. There's also the risk for injury when damaged nerves prevent you from feeling pain in dangerous situations.

THE BEST-KNOWN CULPRIT

Most people realize that neuropathy is commonly caused by diabetes (type 1 or type 2). It accounts for nearly two-thirds of all peripheral neuropathy cases.

What happens: High blood sugar damages cells lining the blood vessels that transport nutrients and oxygen to body cells, which in turn harms nerves.

What you may not realize: When it comes to peripheral neuropathy, prediabetes (a precursor to diabetes) may be just as hazardous as full-blown diabetes. Nerve cell damage starts early. About 20% of patients newly diagnosed with diabetes already have neuropathy.

SURPRISING CAUSES

Besides diabetes, dozens of conditions can lead to neuropathy, including some that pri-

What is SCIATICA?

Sciatica is a common form of low-back pain that radiates along one of the two sciatic nerves, each of which runs down the back of the thigh and calf and into the foot. Most cases of sciatica occur when one of the spinal disks—gel-filled pancakes of cartilage between the vertebrae—swells, tears (ruptures) or herniates (part of the interior of the disk bulges out), exerting painful pressure on a sciatic nerve. About 1 million Americans suffer from sciatica, and up to 300,000 a year have surgery to relieve the pain.

Eugene Carragee, MD, professor of orthopedic surgery and director of the Orthopedic Spine Center at Stanford University School of Medicine in Stanford, California.

mary care physicians often don't consider, such as...

• **Celiac disease.** This autoimmune disorder causes the body to mount a powerful defense against gluten, a protein found in wheat, rye and barley. Eat a slice of wheat bread, and the body creates antibodies that attack the small intestine. The antibodies also cause general inflammation, which is thought to cause nerve damage.

Important: Neuropathy may be an early sign of celiac disease. And contrary to common belief, it can begin at any age. Celiac disease should always be considered when peripheral neuropathy is present. A blood test can be used to check for celiac antibodies. If tingling and numbness improve after going gluten-free, it's likely that celiac is the cause of the neuropathy.

• **Bariatric surgery.** Bariatric surgery for extreme weight loss is becoming more common, but it can cause a vitamin deficiency. This is partly because the surgery alters the digestive system in a way that can prevent nutrients from being properly absorbed. For example, some surgeries remove the part of the stomach responsible for creating a protein called intrinsic factor, which allows the body to absorb vitamin B-12. Severe B-12 deficiency leads to neuropathy.

Important: Neuropathy due to vitamin B-12 deficiency is also more common in people who follow a strict vegan or vegetarian diet. Long-term use of the medications metformin (for blood sugar control) or proton pump inhibitors (for acid reflux) also block B-12 absorption. A fasting blood test can determine your B-12 level. If it's less than 200 pg/mL, a B-12 deficiency may be causing your neuropathy.

• **Kidney disease.** If your kidneys can't properly filter toxins from your blood, the buildup of toxins can harm your nerves. Left untreated, even mild chronic kidney disease can result in peripheral neuropathy. Kidney disease is diagnosed with blood and urine tests.

• **Hepatitis C.** This virus causes white blood cells to create substances in the blood called cryoglobulins, abnormal proteins that damage nerve cells. A blood test can determine if you have hepatitis C.

• **Paraneoplastic syndrome.** When battling cancer, our bodies create antibodies to the cancer cells. Paraneoplastic neuropathy occurs when there is a cross-reaction between tumor cells and components of the nervous system. It can come on quickly, progress rapidly and is often extremely painful.

Important: In some cases, neuropathy may be the first outward sign of cancer—and may be a vital diagnostic clue. This is especially true with lung cancer.

Since there are so many conditions that can cause neuropathy, in most cases your physician will determine the cause only after a thorough medical exam and after ruling out unlikely conditions.

WHAT YOU CAN DO

Neuropathy damage isn't necessarily permanent. Our bodies naturally repair our nerve cells all the time. However, the only way to halt the damage and repair your nerves is to get control over the original disease process. For diabetes, maintain tight control over blood sugar levels...for celiac disease, avoid gluten...seek care for kidney disease or hepatitis C...and get appropriate medical vitamin supplementation for a B-12 deficiency. Unfortunately, treating cancer with chemotherapy may cause neuropathy, which may improve if the chemotherapy regimen is changed.

If you smoke: Neuropathy is one more reason to quit. Nicotine constricts blood vessels, which can starve nerves of the oxygen they need and increase injury to nerves that are already damaged.

Also: Alcohol is one of the most common causes of neuropathy in the US. If you drink heavily or have neuropathy due to an underlying condition, cut down on alcohol use or stop drinking altogether.

Is Your Medication Causing You Pain?

Janice F. Wiesman, MD, FAAN, clinical associate professor of neurology at New York University School of Medicine in New York City and adjunct assistant professor of neurology at Boston University School of Medicine. She is author of *Peripheral Neuropathy: What It Is and What You Can Do to Feel Better.*

When your foot goes numb after a few hours of couch time or you wake up at night with a tingling (or even painful) arm crooked beneath your head, you're experiencing what people with neuropathy live with...every day.

Peripheral neuropathy is a mysterious condition. Many patients never discover what is causing their nerve-related numbness, pain, tingling or other sensations.

Often-overlooked culprit: The medicine cabinet. After diabetes, medication is one of the most common causes of neuropathy. Dozens of medications—even those that you would think are totally safe—can cause nerve damage that's often slow to appear and equally slow to heal...if it ever does. *What you need to know...*

THE LEADING CULPRITS

Nerve-related side effects, known as drug-induced neuropathies, are tricky to identify because they often appear months or even years after starting a medication—although there are exceptions.

Example: Some of the drugs used in chemotherapy are notorious for causing neuropathy. These cases are easy to identify because the symptoms show up quickly—typically within a week or a few months of starting the chemotherapy. Up to 75% of cancer patients given the chemotherapy drug *vincristine* (Oncovin) will experience neuropathy. *Paclitaxel* (Taxol), discussed later, is another common offender.

In general, about one-third of patients who have drug-induced neuropathy will completely recover when they stop—or at least lower the dose of—an offending drug. One-third will stay the same, and another third might get worse. *Drugs to suspect...*

- **Statins.** Cholesterol-lowering statins—including *atorvastatin* (Lipitor), *rosuvastatin* (Crestor) and *simvastatin* (Zocor)—are among the most commonly prescribed medications in the US. According to research published in *Neurology*, statin users were four times more likely to develop neuropathy than people not taking statins.

Experts aren't sure why statins often cause neuropathy. The good news, however, is that most people with statin-related nerve symptoms will recover when they stop taking the drug, though it may take months in some cases. But how do they manage their cholesterol without the medication?

My advice: Switching to a different statin might be the solution—but it's impossible to predict if (or when) a new drug will cause similar problems. To help control your cholesterol levels, your doctor should advise you to exercise more and eat a lower-meat (or even vegetarian) diet.

Even if you can't completely control cholesterol with lifestyle changes, diet and exercise can lower it enough that you might be able to take a lower statin dose—important because the higher the statin dose, the greater the risk for neuropathy.

Note: Case reports have shown that people taking supplements containing red yeast rice, a naturally occurring statin, have also developed neuropathy.

- **Antibiotics.** A number of antibiotics can lead to neuropathy. *Ciprofloxacin* (Cipro) is a widely used broad-spectrum antibiotic. Along with other drugs in this class, known as fluoroquinolones—such as *levofloxacin* (Levaquin) and *moxifloxacin* (Avelox)—it's a common cause of nerve symptoms.

Important: If you notice neuropathy symptoms while taking one of these drugs, don't ignore them. The discomfort usually involves tingling and/or numbness that starts in the feet, moves up to the knees and then starts to affect the hands and fingers.

My advice: If you experience such symptoms, promptly contact your doctor. Ask him/her whether you can switch to a safer antibiotic, such as penicillin, tetracycline or doxycycline. Neuropathy symptoms usually subside when a person goes off a fluoroquinolone but, in rare cases, may not.

In my opinion, Cipro or another fluoroquinolone antibiotic should be used only when you have an infection that won't respond to one of the safer antibiotics mentioned above.

• ***Nitrofurantoin*** **(Macrobid)** is an antibiotic that's used both to treat urinary tract infections (UTIs) and to help prevent recurrent UTIs in patients who are particularly susceptible, such as nursing home patients and those with spinal cord injuries using urinary catheters.

Unlike most other drug-induced neuropathies, the ones caused by Macrobid usually occur quickly—within a week, in some cases. The discomfort usually begins in the feet and legs and moves upward (as described earlier) and can be irreversible if the drug isn't stopped quickly enough.

Most UTIs can be treated with newer, safer drugs or drug combinations, such as *trimethoprim* and *sulfamethoxazole* (Bactrim or Septra). Patients should tell their doctors immediately if they notice neuropathy symptoms, such as numbness, tingling, etc., to determine whether they can be switched to a different antibiotic.

• **Taxol.** About 30% to 40% of cancer patients who are treated with chemotherapy will develop neuropathy. Taxol, commonly used for breast cancer, is a common offender because many women take it for years after their initial diagnosis and treatments.

Important finding: More than 40% of women taking Taxol or similar drugs continued to experience numbness and/or tingling in their hands or feet two years after starting treatment...and 10% rated the discomfort as severe, according to a report in *Journal of the National Cancer Institute.* Neuropathy symptoms should subside when Taxol is changed or stopped, but this might take months or years.

You're more likely to get foot tingling/numbness (the so-called "Taxol toes") or other symptoms, such as sensations of burning in a hand or loss of touch sensation, if you're also obese... have a preexisting history of neuropathy...have had a mastectomy...or if a large number of your lymph nodes harbored cancer cells.

My advice: Be sure to tell your oncologist (if he doesn't ask) if you've had neuropathy in the past. You might be advised to undergo treatments that have about the same survival benefit but are less likely to have this side effect.

• ***Amiodarone*** **(Cordarone).** This drug is one of the most frequently prescribed for heart-rhythm abnormalities (arrhythmias).

Up to 10% of patients who take Cordarone over a period of years will develop neuropathy...and some will develop optic neuropathy, which can cause blurred vision, abnormalities in the visual field (such as "halo vision") or even progressive (and painless) vision loss.

Note: Certain other drugs, including Cipro, the cancer medication *tamoxifen* (Nolvadex) and the erectile dysfunction drug *sildenafil* (Viagra), also can cause optic neuropathy.

My advice: Tell your doctor right away if you notice visual symptoms after starting any of these medications. "Ocular toxicity" usually begins within one year, with vision changes occurring in as little as six months. The vision changes usually will clear up once you stop the drug and switch to a different one, but in rare cases they may not.

• ***Phenytoin*** **(Dilantin).** This antiepilepsy drug is sometimes used, paradoxically, to treat neuropathic pain. Up to half of patients who take Dilantin for 15 years will develop neuropathy. Many patients experience neuropathy sooner.

Shingles Vaccine Reduces Long-Term Nerve Pain

Shingles vaccine reduces long-term pain in women. Shingles patients often develop postherpetic neuralgia (PHN), long-term pain that is a complication of the condition. PHN is characterized by intense nerve pain that lingers for months or years after the blisters themselves have healed. More than 10% of unvaccinated women developed PHN. But only 4% of vaccinated women developed PHN. (Vaccinated and unvaccinated men had a roughly 6% chance of developing PHN.) The US Advisory Council on Immunization Practices recommends that all people age 60 and older be vaccinated against shingles. (For more information on shingles and PHN, see chapter 12, "Infectious Diseases.")

Study of 2,400 people over age 60 who developed shingles by researchers at Kaiser Permanente Southern California, Pasadena, published in *Journal of Infectious Diseases.*

Neuropathies caused by the drug tend to be minor. These might include diminished (or absent) tendon reflexes in the legs that are barely noticeable, although some may observe that they're a bit unsteady when they walk.

My advice: Be sure to tell your doctor about your neuropathy symptoms. If they are mild, he may feel that the benefits of the drug outweigh the risks. More likely, your doctor will advise switching to one of the newer (but more expensive) antiepilepsy drugs, such as *lamotrigine* (Lamictal) or *topiramate* (Topamax), which do not cause neuropathy. If the medication is changed, neuropathy symptoms may or may not subside.

Blood Sugar Levels for Neuropathy

Larry Deeb, MD, president for medicine and science, American Diabetes Association, Tallahassee, Florida.

Up to 70% of diabetes patients have some form of neuropathy. The most common is peripheral neuropathy, in which nerves in the feet, legs, arms and/or hands are damaged. Symptoms include numbness that results in a reduced ability to feel pain. The first step in treating diabetic neuropathy is to bring blood glucose (sugar) levels within the normal range—high levels can injure nerve fibers throughout the body. Blood sugar levels should be 90 mg/dL to 130 mg/dL before meals and less than 180 mg/dL two hours after meals. Consistently keeping blood sugar within this target range can help delay progression of diabetic neuropathy and may improve existing symptoms.

Relieve the Pain of a Pinched Nerve

David Borenstein, MD, clinical professor of medicine at George Washington University Medical Center, Washington, DC. He maintains a private practice at Arthritis and Rheumatism Associates in Washington, DC, and is author of *Back in Control: Your Complete Prescription for Preventing, Treating, and Eliminating Back Pain from Your Life.*

Nerve pain is one of the worst kinds of pain. People with a pinched nerve (sometimes called a "stinger") may experience sharp, burning pain for anywhere from a few seconds to a few days or longer. The pain usually comes on suddenly and may disappear just as fast—only to return. There also might be temporary numbness or slight weakness.

A nerve gets "pinched" when surrounding tissue presses against it and causes inflammation of the nerve. Causes include repetitive motions, traumatic injuries and joint diseases, such as rheumatoid arthritis. The most common pinched nerves occur in the wrist, elbow, shoulder and foot. Nerve roots in the spinal canal also are vulnerable.

Red flag: Nerve pain that is accompanied by significant weakness or that doesn't improve within a few days needs to be checked by a physician. Excessive pressure on—or inflammation of—a nerve can result in loss of function and permanent damage.

SELF-HELP

To reduce the pain...

- **Stop repetitive movements.** A pinched nerve that's caused by performing the same movements over and over again usually will improve once the offending activity—leaning with your elbows on a counter, typing, working a cash register, etc.—is stopped for a few days. Avoiding these activities (or changing work position and practice) can help prevent a pinched nerve.

Example: Raising the back of a computer keyboard (most are adjustable) will enlarge the carpal tunnel in the wrist and reduce pressure on the nerve.

- **Ice the area.** Applying cold in the first 24 to 48 hours after nerve pain starts can reduce tissue swelling and nerve pressure. Use a cold pack or ice cubes wrapped in a towel. Hold cold against the affected area for about 15 minutes. Repeat every hour or two for a day or two.

- **Take an anti-inflammatory.** Over-the-counter analgesics that have anti-inflammatory properties, such as aspirin, ibuprofen and naproxen, reduce the body's production of chemicals that cause inflammation and swelling. Don't use acetaminophen. It will reduce pain but has little effect on inflammation.

- **Wear looser clothes.** It's fairly common for women to experience a pinched nerve in the outer thigh (meralgia paresthetica) from too-tight jeans or skirts...or foot pain (tarsal tunnel syndrome) from tight shoes.

MEDICAL CARE

Nerve pain that's severe or keeps coming back—or that's accompanied by other symptoms, such as a loss of bowel or bladder control—requires immediate medical care. Customized splints or braces can be used to minimize pressure on a nerve from repetitive movements. *Also helpful...*

An injection of a corticosteroid into the painful area—or a short course of oral steroid therapy. These drugs reduce inflammation very quickly and provide short-term relief. The pain may disappear after a single treatment, but most patients need repeated courses. Sometimes, if pain is not relieved, acupuncture may be used in addition to medication and physical therapy.

Surgery is recommended when the pain is severe or keeps coming back. The procedures vary depending on the part of the body affected.

6 Natural Fixes for Neuropathy

Janice F. Wiesman, MD, FAAN, associate clinical professor of neurology at New York University School of Medicine in New York City. She is author of *Peripheral Neuropathy: What It Is and What You Can Do to Feel Better.*

Nerve damage can be both mysterious and maddening. It's mysterious because about one-third of those with neuropathy never discover what's causing the pain, tingling and numbness. It's maddening because damaged nerves recover slowly—if they recover at all. Even when an underlying cause of neuropathy is identified (diabetes, for example, is a big one) and corrected, the symptoms may persist for months, years or a lifetime.

Other common causes of neuropathy: Heavy alcohol use, rheumatoid arthritis, vitamin deficiencies (including vitamin B-12) and certain medications, especially some chemotherapy drugs.

Important finding: One-third to one-half of patients with neuropathies of unknown origin have inherited neuropathies—that is, they're genetically susceptible to nerve damage, even in the absence of a specific disease/injury, according to research conducted at Mayo Clinic.

NATURAL TREATMENTS

It can be a challenge for doctors (usually neurologists) to identify what is responsible for neuropathies. But it's worth making the effort because treating the cause early can stop ongoing damage and potentially allow injured nerves to regenerate. When nerves repair there may be some increased sensitivity, but this is usually temporary.

When the cause of neuropathy can't be identified, the symptoms can still be treated. If your symptoms make you very uncomfortable, there are medications that can help. The drugs that have been FDA-approved for neuropathic pain include *pregabalin* (Lyrica), also often used for seizures...and *duloxetine* (Cymbalta), also used for depression. Lyrica can cause drowsiness and weight gain...and Cymbalta can cause drowsiness as well as sweating in a small number of people. *Gabapentin* (Neurontin) and tricyclic antidepressants, such as *amitriptyline* (Elavil) and *nortriptyline* (Pamelor), are used off-label for neuropathy. Neurontin is similar to Lyrica with the same side effects...and the antidepressants can cause sedation, dry mouth and, in high doses, arrhythmias.

My advice: If you'd describe your symptoms as uncomfortable and annoying—but not debilitating—you might want to start with nondrug treatments. They probably won't eliminate the discomfort altogether, but they can make it easier to tolerate. Plus, if you do decide to use medication, these treatments may enable you to take it for a shorter time and/or at a lower dose. *Try one or more of the following at a time...*

• **Natural fix #1:** *Vibrating foot-bath.* Most patients will first notice tingling, numbness or other symptoms in the feet. Soaking your feet in a warm-water vibrating footbath (available in department stores, pharmacies and online) for 15 to 20 minutes dilates blood vessels and increases circulation in the affected area. More important, the vibrations are detected and transmitted by large-diameter sensory nerve fibers. Because of their large size, these fibers transmit signals very quickly. The sensations of vibration reach the spinal cord before the pain signals from damaged nerves, which blunts the discomfort.

The pain relief is temporary but reliable. You can soak your feet as often as you wish throughout the day.

Helpful: Soak your feet just before bed—the pain relief you get will help you fall asleep more easily. For discomfort in other parts of the body, you can get similar relief from a whirlpool bath or a pulsating showerhead.

Important: Some people with neuropathy are unable to sense temperatures and can burn their feet in too-hot water. Test the temperature with your hand first (or have someone else test it).

• **Natural fix #2:** *Menthol cream.* The smooth muscles in arterial walls are lined with receptors that react to menthol. When you rub an affected area with menthol cream (such as Bengay), the blood vessels dilate, create warmth and reduce discomfort. Creams labeled "menthol" or "methyl salicylate" have the same effects. These creams can be used long-term as needed.

• **Natural fix #3:** *Transcutaneous electrical nerve stimulation (TENS).* This therapy delivers low levels of electric current to the surface of the skin. It's thought that the current stimulates nerves and sends signals to the brain that block the discomfort from damaged nerves.

How well do the devices work? The research is mixed. In 2010, a meta-analysis of TENS in patients with diabetic neuropathies found that the treatment led to a decrease in pain scores. Other studies, however, have shown little or no benefit.

Battery-powered TENS units cost about $30 for low-end models. The treatment is largely without side effects, and some people have good results. Treatments are typically done for 30 minutes at a time and can be repeated as needed throughout the day. Treatments should not be done on skin that is irritated.

My advice: If you want to try TENS at home, start using it under the direction of a physical therapist so that he/she can suggest the appropriate settings and amount of time for treatment.

• **Natural fix #4:** *Percutaneous electrical nerve stimulation (PENS).* Percutaneous means that the electric current is delivered under the skin, using short needles. Studies have shown that the treatments, done in rehabilitation/physical therapy offices, decrease pain, improve sleep and may allow patients to use smaller doses of painkilling medication. After each treatment, the pain relief can potentially last for weeks or longer.

The treatments take about 30 minutes per session and are generally repeated three times a week, until the patient achieves the desired amount and duration of pain relief. The risks are minimal, although you might have mild bruising or a little bleeding. Infection is possible but unlikely. Most patients have little or no pain during the treatments. PENS is not advised for those with pacemakers and should not be done on areas of irritated skin. The treatments might or might not be covered by insurance—be sure to ask.

• **Natural fix #5:** *Self-massage.* Firmly rubbing and/or kneading the uncomfortable area is another way to block pain signals. You don't need to learn sophisticated massage techniques—but you (or a loved one) must use enough pressure to stimulate the big nerves that carry the pressure sensations. A too-light touch won't be helpful.

Caution: If you have a history of deep vein thrombosis, ask your doctor before massaging your legs.

• **Natural fix #6:** *Relaxation techniques.* Stress and anxiety do not cause neuropathy, but patients who are tense may feel pain more intensely. A multiyear study found that patients with chronic pain who completed a mindfulness/stress-reduction program reported significantly less pain—and the improvement lasted for up to three years.

Helpful: Meditation, yoga and other relaxation techniques. Most large medical centers offer programs in anxiety/stress management. Excellent guided meditations are also available on YouTube.

Socks for Neuropathy

Neuropathy—the tingling, burning pain or numbness that's often a side effect of diabetes, medications or autoimmune disease—is caused by nerve damage. Foot-warming socks can help soothe this type of nerve pain. Some foot-warming socks are heated in the microwave, while others are battery-powered. Prices range from $20 to $40.

To prevent burns: Test microwaved socks before putting them on, and do not sleep in battery-powered socks.

Janice F. Wiesman, MD, FAAN, associate clinical professor of neurology at New York University School of Medicine, New York City.

What to Do About Sciatica Pain

Mark Stengler, NMD, a naturopathic doctor and founder of the Stengler Center for Integrative Medicine in Encinitas, California. He is author or coauthor of numerous books, including *The Natural Physician's Healing Therapies* and *Bottom Line's Prescription for Natural Cures*, and author of the newsletter *Health Revelations*. MarkStengler.com

I have had many patients tell me that they experience a combination of lower back pain and an unpleasant radiating tingle down one leg and sometimes into the foot or toes. These symptoms are called sciatica, and they typically stem from a disc problem in the lower back.

Debbie, a 57-year-old writer and mother of two, experienced constant lower back pain, a sharp pain down her right leg, plus numbness in her right foot and toes. Also, her left hip felt as if it were constantly about to "go out." The pain caused her to limp, and she used a cane to help her walk.

A doctor prescribed painkillers, which helped to alleviate Debbie's discomfort. A chiropractor provided some relief, but the pain and numbness remained. Debbie's back pain had accelerated after she spent two days in a hospital bed, being treated for complications related to her diabetes.

After examining Debbie, I told her I was concerned that she had a compression of one or more of the discs (collagen and gel pads that cushion the bones of the spine) in her lower back. I referred her to a neurologist, who ordered a magnetic resonance imaging (MRI)

scan to view the spine. Sure enough, she had two bulging discs that were squashing the nerve roots as they exit the spine. The pressure was causing her back pain and sciatica. Additional nerve tests showed that there was decreased nerve sensation to the right foot.

I suggested Debbie try spinal decompression, a procedure that is gaining popularity among chiropractors and some osteopathic doctors. The treatment works by creating negative pressure—essentially, a vacuum—inside the disc to pull in the bulge or herniation (when a disc has actually broken open), relieving pressure on the affected nerves. Spinal decompression also increases the flow of blood and nutrients back into the disc, allowing the body to heal the injury.

How it works: The patient lies down fully clothed on his/her back or stomach, with pads comfortably securing the upper body and pelvis. Computer-controlled tension gently stretches the lower back, separating the vertebrae by miniscule increments and creating the vacuum effect.

The treatments are completely painless. Each lasts 15 to 30 minutes, and patients usually require a series of 15 to 30 visits, one to three per week.

Cost: $80 to $100 per visit. You can find a practitioner through the American Spinal Decompression Association (888-577-4625, AmericanSpinal.com).

Note: Spinal decompression is not advised for people with severe osteoporosis or nerve damage, pregnant women or those who are very obese.

Debbie noticed great relief after just five treatments. After her 20th treatment, she reported a substantial improvement in her back pain and sciatica. She also began to feel sensation in her right toes and foot again. She is 80% improved and continuing the treatments.

Tai Chi Can Relieve Neuropathy

Peter M. Wayne, PhD, assistant professor of medicine at Harvard Medical School and research director of the Osher Center for Integrative Medicine, jointly based at Harvard Medical School and Brigham and Women's Hospital, both in Boston. He has trained in tai chi for more than 35 years and is the author, with Mark L. Fuerst, of *The Harvard Medical School Guide to Tai Chi.*

Perhaps you've seen people performing the graceful, seemingly slow-motion movements of tai chi in a nearby park. If you've never tried it before, you may think that this form of exercise is easy to do and provides little more than a mild workout.

The truth: Even though tai chi consists of slow, gentle movements, this exercise is no pushover. Long known for its stress-reducing benefits, it also gives you an aerobic workout that's as intense as walking at a moderate pace...increases muscle strength and flexibility...improves breathing...improves posture and balance (to help prevent falls)...and focuses the mind.

What's new: Tai chi, which was developed centuries ago in China as a means of self-defense, is now linked to a number of new health benefits, including improved cardiovascular health and bone density...and reduced back and neck pain.

Even better: Tai chi is safer than many forms of exercise because of its 70% rule: You never move your joints or exert yourself beyond 70% of your maximum potential.

To remedy neuropathy: Millions of people with diabetes and other conditions have peripheral neuropathy, nerve damage in the hands and/or feet that causes numbness, tingling or pain. The condition is particularly troublesome because reduced sensations in the feet can impair balance and increase the risk of falling.

Research has found that people with peripheral neuropathy who practiced tai chi had improved sensitivity in the soles of the feet. They also had better balance and walking speed.

It's easy to get started: Tai chi classes are commonly offered at health clubs, YMCAs and even some hospitals. Classes are particularly useful because of the feedback given by the instructor and the group support, which helps keep you motivated.

Good goal: Two one-hour tai chi classes a week—plus at-home practice for at least 30 minutes, three times a week.

You can find a tai chi expert in your area at AmericanTaiChi.net.

The Supplement That Soothes Sciatica

Gad M. Gilad, PhD, Department of Physiology and Pharmacology, Sackler Faculty of Medicine, Tel Aviv University.

The pain of sciatica ranges from mild tingling to electric agony, and parallels the path of the nerve, shooting from the low back to the buttocks and down the back of (typically) one leg. Other symptoms can include numbness and weakness in the affected leg and foot.

An estimated 3 to 5 million Americans have sciatica, and most get better in a few weeks or a few months. But in the meantime, the nerve pain is very difficult to treat.

Solution: A study shows you can soothe sciatica by taking a nutritional supplement of *agmatine*, a compound produced when your body breaks down the amino acid arginine, a component of protein found in small amounts in meat, fish and plants.

FOUR TIMES MORE PAIN RELIEF

Sixty-one people who had suffered with sciatica from two to four months took either agmatine or a placebo for two weeks.

The agmatine group had a 28% improvement in pain levels—compared with 7% for the placebo group.

The researchers also used an extensive questionnaire to measure the participants' "general health status." The agmatine group improved by 70%, compared with 20% for the placebo group.

Suggested dosage: Taking a supplement of the compound can help a person with sciatica avoid the painful "pins and needles," burning and tingling sensations, and numbness and weakness that characterize the problem. AgmaSet, the agmatine supplement used in the study, contains G-agmatine, a unique form of the compound.

Start with two capsules twice a day, for four days. If there is no decrease in symptoms, take three capsules twice a day for as long as needed for reduction of pain and other symptoms—it may take two to three weeks before you see an effect. Once the symptoms are reduced, switch to two capsules, two times a day, for a maintenance dose.

Resource: You can order AgmaSet at ForNerveHealth.com or call 888-484-4523. *E-mail:* info@fornervehealth.com.

4 Best Nondrug Remedies For Diabetic Nerve Pain

Michael Murray, ND, naturopathic physician and educator based in Scottsdale, Arizona. He serves on the Board of Regents of Bastyr University in Seattle, and is author of more than 30 books, including *How to Prevent and Treat Diabetes with Natural Medicine* and *The Encyclopedia of Natural Medicine.* DoctorMurray.com

If you have diabetes, or even prediabetes, you don't have to accept that neuropathy is inevitable—and if you have diabetic neuropathy, you don't have to just live with its variety of terrible symptoms. Besides diet and exercise, there are certain supplements and one proven topical treatment that can help prevent, delay and even possibly reverse the cascade that ultimately causes neuropathy.

Here are four remedies—three supplements and one topical pain treatment—for diabetic neuropathy that I recommend. With the supplements especially, it's important to talk with your doctor before you start them.

ALPHA-LIPOIC ACID

My top recommendation for people with diabetic neuropathy is alpha-lipoic acid (ALA).

It's a powerful antioxidant, a natural compound produced by our cells that helps convert blood glucose into energy. Yet it's often deficient within the nerve cells in patients with diabetes. By improving nerve blood flow and nerve conduction velocity, ALA is associated with improvements in pain, tingling, numbness, sensory deficits and muscle strength.

Scientific studies back this up. The strongest evidence is for intravenous ALA, which has been shown to provide substantial short-term relief from pain and numbness. But oral supplements have also had positive effects. In a randomized, double-blind study of 181 patients with diabetic neuropathy, those who took 600 mg of ALA once daily for five weeks had a 51% reduction in their "total symptom score," which measured symptoms such as stabbing pain, burning pain, a prickling sensation and foot numbness, compared with 32% in the placebo group. In a very small (45 participants) randomized study, those who took 600 mg of ALA for four weeks had a similar reduction in painful symptoms. For those who continued ALA for a total of 16 weeks, there was a further reduction in symptom severity. For those who stopped taking ALA after four weeks, however, symptoms showed no further improvement—and they wound up taking more pain medications than those treated with ALA.

In the longest trial to date, four-year treatment with oral ALA in mild-to-moderate diabetic retinopathy resulted in a clinically meaningful improvement and prevention of progression of impairment in nerve function and was well tolerated.

The typical oral dosage of ALA is 400 mg to 600 mg daily. There are no known complications or drug interactions with the use of ALA, although at higher doses (e.g., greater than 1,200 mg per day), some people may experience nausea and dizziness. Since ALA also may lower blood sugar, if you are taking a diabetic medication, discuss taking ALA with your doctor.

To enhance the effectiveness of ALA supplementation, consider combining it with 600 mg of benfotiamine, a synthetic form of vitamin B-1 that is fat-soluble and easily absorbed and may have a beneficial effect on several biological pathways that contribute to diabetic neuropathy. It has been shown in preliminary trials to be helpful in some cases of diabetic neuropathy, and one clinical trial suggests that use with ALA is an effective combination.

Animal studies suggest that another way to make oral ALA more effective is to combine it with my next recommendation—GLA.

GAMMA-LINOLENIC ACID (GLA)

Another supplement that I recommend for diabetic peripheral neuropathy is gamma-linolenic acid (GLA), one of the omega-6 fatty acids. Normally, most of the GLA that we need to maintain nerve function and other functions comes from vegetable oils that contain an essential fatty acid that the body converts to GLA. But diabetes is known to substantially disturb fatty acid metabolism. A key part of that disturbance is impairment in the ability to convert this fatty acid to GLA.

Supplementing with GLA can help bypass that disturbance.

Example: In a randomized, double-blind study of 111 people with diabetic neuropathy, those who took 480 mg a day of GLA had a statistically significant improvement in 13 out of 16 measures of diabetic neuropathy severity after one year, compared with the placebo group that didn't get ALA. Participants who had good glucose control had bigger improvements than those with poor glucose control.

GLA is found in some plant-based foods and herbs, including oils of borage, evening primrose and black currant seed. Most GLA supplements are derived from these oils. Just remember that the dosage is based upon the

Ginkgo for Nerve Pain

Neuropathic pain—in which damaged nerves send erroneous pain signals in response to harmless stimuli such as a light touch—is hard to treat. Common causes include diabetes and shingles. Among rats with neuropathic pain, those given a ginkgo biloba herbal extract showed significantly lower pain responses to cold and pressure than those given a placebo. Human studies are needed.

Hae-Jin Lee, MD, chief/professor of anesthesiology, Catholic University of Korea, Seoul, Republic of Korea, and leader of an animal study.

level of GLA, not the amount of the source oil. The GLA content of these oils is usually stated on the label—look for a GLA dose between 360 mg and 480 mg.

Important: If you are taking a supplement or medication that thins the blood or that may affect bleeding time (ginkgo biloba, aspirin, warfarin, clopidogrel, etc.), talk to your doctor before taking GLA. It may increase the risk of bleeding, so the combination can be dangerous. Don't take GLA if you have a seizure disorder, as there have been case reports of the supplement contributing to seizures in people with such disorders. It can interact with other prescription medications as well, so be sure to talk with your doctor before taking GLA.

TOPICAL CAPSAICIN

You may already know that hot peppers can provide pain relief—you can find pepper-based topical pain creams on the shelves of any drugstore. And in fact, I recommend topical capsaicin, the active component of cayenne pepper, for many patients with diabetic neuropathy. When applied to the skin, capsaicin works by stimulating and, ultimately, desensitizing, the small nerve fibers that transmit the pain impulse. Numerous double-blind studies have shown capsaicin to be of considerable benefit in relieving the pain of diabetic neuropathy. In those studies, roughly 80% of participants experienced significant—often tremendous—pain relief.

Topical capsaicin is available in both prescription and over-the-counter forms. Prescription patches with 8% capsaicin can provide surprisingly long-term relief—studies find that a single 60-minute application can reduce pain for weeks. This high-dose capsaicin works just as well at reducing pain as *pregabalin* (Lyrica), the commonly used oral medication for nerve pain, and it avoids the systemic adverse effects associated with oral nerve-pain medications, including drowsiness, blurry vision, constipation and an increased risk for infection.

Capsaicin is also available over-the-counter as a cream and a patch. My recommendation is to use the cream so that it can be applied more liberally. Look for a concentration of 0.075% capsaicin, and apply it twice daily on the affected area. (Be sure to cover your hand with plastic wrap to prevent capsaicin from later coming in contact with your eyes, nose, mouth or lips, where it can be especially irritating.) It takes a few days for the nerve fibers to become desensitized, so the capsaicin cream can produce a tingling or burning sensation initially. After a few days, however, the nerve fibers will no longer transmit the pain signal. At these lower doses—as compared with the prescription patches—capsaicin works only with regular application. Capsaicin does not interfere with normal nerve function—it only affects the perception of pain.

Above all else: Although the nondrug remedies in this article can help with neuropathy, the primary goal for everyone with diabetes is to keep blood sugar in the healthy range. Reducing excess blood sugar—with a healthy diet, weight loss, regular exercise and managing stress—improves many of the consequences of diabetes, including neuropathy.

ALC for Hereditary Peripheral Neuropathy

Mark Stengler, NMD, naturopathic doctor and founder of the Stengler Center for Integrative Medicine in Encinitas, California. He is author or coauthor of numerous books, including *The Natural Physician's Healing Therapies* and *Bottom Line's Prescription for Natural Cures*, and author of the newsletter *Health Revelations*. MarkStengler.com

People with peripheral neuropathy, damage to the nerves in the extremities, often experience pain and numbness in their hands and/or feet. Studies show that the nutrient acetyl-l-carnitine (ALC) can increase and repair nerve fibers. Although not studied for hereditary peripheral neuropathy, I have seen ALC reduce the symptoms of other types of neuropathy. I recommend 1,000 mg of ALC three times daily between meals. Acupuncture also can help to reduce your symptoms. A holistic doctor can provide you with other natural therapies, such as injectable or intravenous vitamin B-1, which can help the neurological system.

CHAPTER 19

Teeth, Face and Mouth Pain

When Your Head Pain Is a Dental Problem

I have found in my more than 30 years as a dentist that head pain (including headaches and facial pain) can be linked to problems in the mouth.

Example: My receptionist had been getting daily headaches for years. When I removed her impacted wisdom teeth, the headaches stopped. An impacted tooth can cause no local symptoms but still can affect nerves and cause chronic headaches.

Other dental problems that can lead to head pain…

- **Misaligned bite.** It's among the main causes of "tension" headaches, which cause tightness and/or dull pain in the temples, across the forehead or on the back of the head.

What happens: An uneven bite prevents jaw muscles from completely relaxing. Chronic muscle tension produces excess lactic acid, a metabolic by-product that can lead to head pain.

Few people have perfectly aligned teeth. For genetic reasons, some people's teeth are crooked or overlap. The upper and lower jaws might be different sizes or malformed. Poor dental restorations, such as crowns and fillings, also can cause an uneven bite.

Dentists can make various types of appliances that fit over the teeth and allow the muscles to relax. I advise patients to wear the appliance for several days. If the headaches disappear, the bite probably needs to be permanently realigned. This usually is done by slightly grinding/reshaping certain teeth.

- **Temporomandibular dysfunction (TMD)** —formerly known as TMJ syndrome—can cause severe headaches, often accompanied

Mark A. Breiner, DDS, holistic dentist and founder of Breiner Whole-Body Health Centre, in Trumbull, Connecticut. He is a Fellow of the International Academy of Oral Medicine and Toxicology and a member of The National Center for Homeopathy. He is author of *Whole-Body Dentistry.* WholeBodyDentistry.com

by pain in the jaw, neck, shoulders or back, as well as dizziness and ringing in the ears.

What happens: The temporomandibular joint, in front of the ear, where the lower jaw rests in the skull-bone socket, gets a lot of stress. It moves when we talk, eat or swallow. It experiences even more pressure in those who grind their teeth at night...clench their jaws...have misaligned bites...or chew gum constantly. Continuous pressure can produce chronic pain.

Most patients with TMD will require bite adjustments, and sometimes braces, to achieve normal jaw movements and teeth alignment. (A bite appliance, as described above, can enable your dentist to tell if your symptoms are related to TMD.)

Also helpful: Natural remedies, such as hypericum, magnesium phosphate and calcium phosphate.

• **Trigeminal neuralgia (TN)** typically causes sudden severe pain that starts at one side of the mouth and then "shoots out" to different parts of the same side of the face. It lasts only a few seconds and often is caused by previous dental work.

What happens: Dental procedures, such as a tooth extraction or root canal, may produce a small hole (cavitation) in the jawbone that can become a repository for pain-causing toxins and inflammatory chemicals—and a site of persistent infection.

A dentist can drill a hole into the cavitation and inject a few drops of anesthetic. The pain will disappear almost instantly when a cavitation is surgically debrided (cleaned). Patients also may improve with the injection of homeopathic remedies into the cavitation.

Important: Anyone with chronic head pain should be seen by a doctor to rule out conditions such as high blood pressure and tumors.

Oh, My Jaw! You Can Get Relief for Hard-to-Treat TMD

Noshir R. Mehta, DMD, professor and chair of the department of general dentistry, and director of the Craniofacial Pain Center at Tufts University School of Dental Medicine in Boston. He is the chief editor of *Head, Face and Neck Pain Science, Evaluation and Management: An Interdisciplinary Approach.*

Some dentists are quick to recommend surgery for people who suffer from the often painful conditions known as temporomandibular disorders (TMD).

But that's a mistake. Surgery should be the last resort for the vast majority of patients who suffer from these disorders, which affect the jaw joint and/or facial muscles that allow us to chew, speak and swallow.

Good news: Roughly 95% of the 10 million Americans who have TMD can get relief without surgery—if they use the right treatments. What you need to know...

RED FLAGS TO WATCH FOR

Contrary to popular belief, people with TMD do not always suffer jaw pain. In fact, these disorders often go undiagnosed because they can cause symptoms in other areas of the body, including in the neck, head, face or ears.

When jaw pain does occur, it's usually related to the temporomandibular joint (TMJ)—there's one on each side of the head, and it acts as a hinge connecting the lower jaw to the skull. These joints are almost constantly in motion—when we chew, yawn, speak or tighten or relax our facial muscles.

This constant movement means that even slight misalignments of the jaw (the bite) or other problems can produce painful inflammation that can persist for years or even indefinitely without treatment.

Many TMD patients—with or without jaw pain—first complain to their doctors about headaches, earaches or sinus pain. About 75% of my TMD patients also have neck pain. Most people with TMD eventually experience pain in the jaw. *Common TMD symptoms...*

• **Headaches,** particularly tensionlike pain on the sides or the back of the head. Headaches in the morning indicate that the TMD might be related to bruxism, nighttime tooth-grinding, gnashing or clenching. Headaches during or after meals indicate a problem with bite alignment.

• **Aching facial pain or face fatigue,** especially after meals. This can be due to an uneven bite or teeth making premature contact, which stresses the jaw and causes fatigue.

• **Ear pain and stuffiness** (meaning the ears feel clogged) are common symptoms because the same nerves that carry signals to the chewing muscles also connect to muscles in the middle ear. People who clench their teeth often report ear discomfort as well as jaw pain.

• **Clicking or popping sound in the jaw,** with or without pain. Clicking means that something within the joint is binding (so that the cartilage is slipping back and forth).

DIAGNOSIS AND TREATMENT

Most cases of TMD can be diagnosed by a dentist who takes the patient's medical history, followed by a hands-on evaluation of the movement of the joints and/or jaw muscles, listening for clicking, popping or grating, looking for limited jaw motion and examining the bite. Main causes...

• **Disk displacement.** Each temporomandibular joint has a ball-and-socket that is held together with a shock-absorbing disk. When this disk slips out of place, the cushioning between the joints is gone, causing clicking.

Two possible treatments...

• Disk manipulation. During this in-office procedure, the dentist will inject a local anesthetic, then manipulate the jaw to push the disk back into the normal position. This can eliminate pain and/or unlock the jaw, but it's a temporary solution because the disk will still have a tendency to move out of position.

• Bite plate appliances, such as bite guards or mouth guards, are usually custom-made for each patient and fit over the teeth and keep the jaw stable. This prevents the disk from slipping. Most patients will need to wear the plate continuously for the first few days. This allows inflammation and muscle tightness to subside. After that, they need to wear the guard only while sleeping to prevent tooth grinding, a common cause of displacement.

Important: A custom-made dental guard from your dentist, which typically costs $250 to $1,000, is more durable than an over-the-counter mouth guard.

• **Bruxism is a common cause of TMD** because the jaw is in continuous—and forceful—motion when a person grinds his/her teeth during sleep. Most patients with this condition have only minor, occasional pain, but it can cause long-term damage to the teeth and, secondarily, the gums unless it's treated.

Stress management is critical because stress can exacerbate the grinding or trigger it. Relaxation techniques such as massage therapy and biofeedback can be helpful. These patients should also wear a dental guard at night.

• **Teeth alignment.** Patients with missing teeth, or changes in how the upper and lower teeth come together, will often experience neck pain and other symptoms of TMD.

Self-test: When you bring your teeth together, the bite should close without any shifting of the jaw. If your lower teeth slide against the upper teeth to achieve a "normal" bite, there's a misalignment that may be causing excessive pressure.

A dentist can evaluate your bite height and tooth positions and make the necessary adjustments—by removing tooth material in some places, for example, or by adding height with a crown.

SELF-CARE FOR TMD

Most people with TMD can significantly reduce their discomfort and avoid the need for medical procedures with self-care. *Helpful...*

• **Apply ice (wrapped in a washcloth)** to the painful area for a few minutes at a time two to three times throughout the day.

• **Eat soft food during painful episodes.** Avoid any food that requires opening the mouth wide (such as a whole apple).

• **Gently exercise the jaw with up-and-down and side-to-side movements even when it's tender.** Movement will help prevent subsequent stiffness in the joint.

Eat This Before You Go to the Dentist

Who doesn't love going to the dentist for some heavy-duty tooth-and-gum work? Here's a bit of natural help to heal your sore mouth after all the drilling is done.

Three days before you go to the dentist, start eating pineapple. Have a serving of fresh pineapple or a cup of canned pineapple in its own juice, and drink a cup of 100% pineapple juice every day. The enzymes in pineapple should help reduce pain and discomfort. They can also help speed the healing process.

Continue the pineapple regimen for a day or two after the dental work is completed.

Joan Wilen and Lydia Wilen are folk-remedy experts based in New York City who have spent decades collecting "cures from the cupboard." They are authors of *Bottom Line's Treasury of Home Remedies & Natural Cures* and *Bottom Line's Household Magic.*

- **Don't chew gum and/or ice.** Limit excessive stretching of the jaw—with big yawns, for example—during painful episodes.
- **Take over-the-counter anti-inflammatory medications,** such as *ibuprofen* (Advil), as needed, following the directions on the label.

Quick Relief for Jaw Pain

Rob E. Sable, DDS, a restorative dentist in private practice in Alpharetta, Georgia.

Waking up with a sore jaw or a headache may indicate that you grind your teeth in your sleep. This condition, called bruxism, is primarily caused by stress. Symptoms include tooth sensitivity to hot and cold food and drinks as well as pain while chewing. Sinus congestion can cause severe pressure on dental roots, leading sufferers to grind their teeth or clench the jaw. Misaligned dental work can also trigger bruxism, leading to unconscious grinding. This grinding causes noticeable noise in only 30% of patients.

Your dentist can diagnose the problem by feeling muscle tension in the jaw and face...observing if teeth are worn or cracked...and viewing X rays. Treatments include reshaping and polishing of tooth enamel to improve tooth alignment and/or the use of a mouth guard during periods of excessive grinding.

To ease jaw pain: Place your palm or fist under your chin and push up while barely opening your jaw against resistance. Hold for one to two seconds. Repeat 30 times, twice a day. This will stretch and strengthen jaw muscles, which helps alleviate pain.

Best Natural Cures for Canker Sores and Fever Blisters

Jamison Starbuck, ND, naturopathic physician in family practice and a guest lecturer at the University of Montana, both in Missoula. She is a past president of the American Association of Naturopathic Physicians and a contributing editor to *The Alternative Advisor: The Complete Guide to Natural Therapies and Alternative Treatments.* DrJamisonStarbuck.com.

When he came to see me, Dave complained of painful sores in his mouth and on his lips. When I took a look, I found many circular, yellow-white sores inside his mouth and on his gums and tongue (canker sores) and two large red ulcers on his lower lip (oral herpes). Many people suffer from one or both of these common lesions at some time in their lives, but fortunately, the following remedies can be used individually or simultaneously to help them heal—see what works best for you...*

Canker sores are small, painful, noncontagious lesions that occur inside the mouth. They can be caused by trauma to the mouth (such as biting yourself), dental procedures, digestive problems, food allergies, excess sugar, acidic foods or emotional stress. Canker sores can hurt for seven to 10 days and may take weeks to heal. *To speed the healing process, try...*

**Caution:* If any mouth sore lasts for more than two weeks, see a doctor to rule out a cancerous lesion. Also, check with your doctor if you take medication or have a chronic health condition, such as diabetes, before using these remedies.

• **Licorice root paste.** Licorice root is soothing and reduces local inflammation.

What to do: Make a paste of powdered licorice root (use deglycyrrhizinated licorice, or DGL, if you have high blood pressure—the ingredient that can raise blood pressure has been removed) and water. If you can't find licorice root powder, purchase capsules and open several of them to make the paste. With your finger or a Q-tip, apply the paste to each canker sore several times a day for immediate, though short-lived, pain relief.

• **Chamomile tea.** The tannins in chamomile help with wound healing, including canker sores.

What to do: Steep two chamomile tea bags in 16 ounces of hot water for five minutes. A mouth swish with warm, strong chamomile tea offers pain relief and speeds healing. Swish as often as you like.

Note: Avoid chamomile if you are allergic to plants in the ragweed family.

Also: Avoid coffee, sugar and citrus foods to help heal canker sores.

Oral herpes lesions, commonly referred to as "cold sores" or "fever blisters," most often occur on or near the lips. However, these red, ulcerated sores can spread to other parts of the face, including the eyes, so they should not be touched. Lasting for seven to 10 days, they are caused by the herpes simplex virus and are transmitted by skin-to-skin contact (kissing or touching) or by sharing objects (lip balm, eating utensils, razors, etc.) with a person who has the virus but not necessarily the sores. After the initial outbreak, the virus remains dormant in the body. Future outbreaks can be triggered by stress, illness, sun exposure and allergies. *What helps these sores heal...*

• **Lemon balm.** This herb is a potent antiviral that's highly effective against herpes.

What to do: Use one tablespoon of dried lemon balm in 16 ounces of hot water. Steep, covered, for five minutes. Discard herbs. Apply the tea directly to the lesions with a Q-tip or washcloth four to seven times a day, and drink 16 ounces of lemon balm tea a day for up to a week.

Note: Lemon balm tea can be sedating.

• **Lysine.** This amino acid also helps fight oral herpes. I recommend 3,000 mg of lysine daily while the herpes outbreak is present.

Also: Avoid chocolate and nuts—these foods feed the herpes virus.

A Possible Cause of Stabbing Facial Pain

Janice Wiesman, MD, FAAN, clinical associate professor of neurology, New York University School of Medicine, New York City.

Trigeminal neuralgia (TN) refers to facial pain caused by the compression or irritation of the trigeminal nerve, which crosses the face. TN often develops when the nerve is compressed by an overlying blood vessel, tumor or—more rarely—an infection. The result may be intermittent stabbing pain or constant aching or burning pain.

Anticonvulsant drugs are generally the first medications used, but there are others. Treating TN with *Botulinum toxin* (Botox) is common but is not always effective.

Other treatment options: Results are often excellent with decompression surgery. Nerve ablation (a procedure to kill the nerve using medication, radio waves, heat or nerve compression) or stereotactic radiosurgery (such as Gamma Knife), a noninvasive procedure that focuses radiation at the nerve, are also effective.

Blame Menopause for Your Burning Mouth

Gary D. Klasser, DMD, associate professor in the department of comprehensive dentistry and biomaterials at Louisiana State University School of Dentistry in New Orleans. Dr. Klasser has authored or coauthored numerous textbook chapters and peer-reviewed journal articles, including a recent study on burning mouth syndrome.

Did you know that the hormonal changes of menopause could lead to degenerative alterations in certain small nerves in the mouth? Known as "burning mouth syndrome (BMS)," our taste buds (of which we have thousands) receive information from both pain fibers and from specialized taste fibers—so nerve damage can trigger the erroneous firing of pain messages in addition to transmitting abnormal taste sensations. Thanks again, menopause.

Hormone therapy (which is often prescribed to ease hot flashes and other troublesome menopausal symptoms) does not relieve chronic BMS, probably because it cannot correct the nerve damage. While early studies suggested that supplementing with alpha-lipoic acid (ALA) might improve symptoms, follow-up research did not find ALA to be effective in relieving BMS.

Good news: By some estimates, in as many as 50% of cases, BMS does eventually improve or entirely go away on its own, typically within three to six years.

In the meantime, for relief: BMS sufferers commonly report experiencing temporary relief while eating...sipping a beverage...sucking on hard candy...or chewing gum. This stimulates saliva, which in turn causes nerve fibers to function more normally, if only for as long as there is actually something in your mouth. Of course, you cannot eat, drink or chew gum all the time, so ideally this strategy should be used at times when your discomfort is worst. For many BMS patients, pain peaks in the late afternoon or early evening.

The types of foods, beverages and gum flavors that most effectively alleviate pain vary among individuals, so you need to experiment to find those that work for you. To protect your teeth from decay, choose water or another sugar-free noncarbonated beverage, sugar-free hard candy or sugar-free gum.

What to avoid: Some BMS patients report that burning pain worsens when eating hot, spicy and/or acidic foods...drinking alcohol... using mouthwash that contains alcohol...or using toothpaste that contains sodium lauryl sulfate (a surfactant) or cinnamon flavoring.

Pemphigus: The "Canker Sore" You Can't Ignore

Neil J. Korman, MD, PhD, professor of dermatology at Case Western Reserve University School of Medicine and clinical director of the Murdough Family Center for Psoriasis and director of the Dermatology Clinical Trials Unit at University Hospitals Case Medical Center, all in Cleveland. He specializes in autoimmune blistering diseases, psoriasis and atopic dermatitis and has published more than 120 articles in peer-reviewed literature.

Eating a bowl of chili one night, a woman felt a burning pain as if she had bitten the inside of her cheek. Oddly, the pain lingered. The next day, she looked in a mirror and saw what appeared to be several canker sores inside her mouth. She shrugged them off at first, but then more sores appeared. No sooner would some heal than others would form. Within a few weeks, her mouth was filled with a multitude of blisters that were so painful she could barely eat a thing.

Her primary-care doctor, dermatologist and dentist were all completely mystified. Finally her periodontist did some digging and came up with the answer—it was an autoimmune disease called pemphigus. Yet even with a diagnosis, the afflicted woman had to contact numerous dermatologists before finding one who was familiar with the condition and its treatment.

This story is typical of pemphigus patients, since the disorder is uncommon enough that doctors often don't think to check for it. Yet early diagnosis and treatment are crucial because they make this potentially serious condition much easier to control, according to Neil J. Korman, MD, PhD, a professor of dermatology at Case Western Reserve University School of Medicine who specializes in autoimmune blistering diseases.

What is this weird disease? With pemphigus, the immune system makes antibodies that mistakenly attack the proteins in skin cells that keep adjacent cells adhering to one another. This causes cells to separate from each other—to become "unglued," so to speak. Fluid collects between the layers of tissue, forming numerous fragile blisters that rupture easily, shearing away the top layer of skin and leaving open sores.

Of the several types of pemphigus, the most common is pemphigus vulgaris, in which blisters usually appear first in the mouth. Later, blisters may erupt in the mucous membranes of the nose, throat, eyes and/or genitals, as well as on the skin.

Pemphigus occurs most frequently in middle-aged adults and seniors, and women are at somewhat higher risk than men. The disease can develop in people of any ethnicity, though it is more common in those of Mediterranean, Middle Eastern or Ashkenazi Jewish descent.

Getting help: If you have mouth sores that do not heal, seek out a dermatologist or otolaryngologist (ear, nose and throat doctor) who is familiar with pemphigus. If your primary-care physician cannot provide a referral, check the website of the International Pemphigus & Pemphigoid Foundation, Pemphigus.org. Diagnosis is based on a physical exam, biopsy of affected tissue and a blood test that measures antibody levels.

Pemphigus patients of yesteryear often died when their mucous membranes or skin became so severely damaged that life-threatening infection set in. Today, fortunately, the disease can be controlled with one or more medications. Options include corticosteroids (such as prednisone)...oral immunosuppressants such as *mycophenolate mofetil* (CellCept), which help keep the immune system from attacking healthy tissues...biological therapies such as *rituximab* (Rituxan), which target the white blood cells that produce antibodies...and antibiotics or other drugs as necessary to combat infection.

Because pemphigus is a chronic condition, patients may need to be on medication for life—yet all these drugs can have side effects, so the goal is to find the lowest effective dose. In some cases, patients achieve remission and can withdraw from medications. But as Dr. Korman cautioned, "A remission is not a cure. The blisters can come back."

Your doctor also may advise taking supplements to help minimize medication side effects. Typical recommendations include calcium with vitamin D for patients on steroids and probiotics for patients taking antibiotics.

To minimize mouth pain during a flare-up...

- **Drink beverages at room temperature (not hot or cold),** using a straw so you can guide the liquid away from the sides of your mouth and down your throat.
- **Avoid hard foods in favor of soft ones.** Cook vegetables until they are tender...dip foods in sauces to soften them...accompany each bite of food with a sip of liquid.
- **Keep a list of foods that worsen your pain.** For instance, the woman mentioned earlier quickly learned to steer clear of spicy foods, Italian salad dressing and anything with cinnamon. Some pemphigus patients report problems with foods containing thiols (such as chives, garlic, leeks, onions and shallots)...isothiocyanates (found in broccoli, cabbage, cauliflower and turnips as well as mustard)...phenols (in bananas, mangoes, potatoes, tomatoes and milk)...or tannins (in ginger, berries, coffee and tea).

When It Hurts to Eat Ice Cream...

What's going on when your teeth ache after eating ice cream, but pretty much nothing else? The brief pain you experience may be due to the effect that the cold and sugar in the ice cream have on exposed roots, tiny cracks in your enamel and/or early decay forming on a tooth. If the pain is not due to decay, the sensitive exposed root(s) can be made less sensitive to cold and sweets by medications applied to your teeth by your dentist. I also recommend using a soft toothbrush to minimize continued abrasion to the teeth. In addition, you may want to try a toothpaste, such as Sensodyne, that is designed for sensitive teeth. Another option you may want to consider is bonding, a procedure in which a dentist applies a tooth-colored material to the teeth to fill in cracks in the enamel. If the pain lingers after you eat ice cream, the teeth's nerves may be stressed due to factors such as gum recession and deep fillings. Your dentist is the best person to recommend the appropriate treatment.

Alan Winter, DDS, periodontist in private practice, New York City.

• **Dental hygiene can be difficult when mouth tissues are sore and fragile, but remember, it's still important.** Rinse your mouth out with water after eating to remove bacteria...and use a small, soft toothbrush to clean your teeth.

• **Use over-the-counter anesthetic mouth lozenges as needed to reduce discomfort.**

• **For some patients, stress worsens symptoms**—so consider practicing meditation or some other relaxation technique.

Herbal Relief for Painful Mouth Sores

Eric Yarnell, ND, is an associate professor in the department of botanical medicine at Bastyr University in Kenmore, Washington, and a private practitioner at Northwest Naturopathic Urology in Seattle. He is the author or coauthor of 10 books on natural medicine, including *Nature's Cures: What You Should Know*. DrYarnell.com

The inside of your mouth hurts like crazy, so you stand in front of a mirror and open wide. Do you see white, lacy, raised patches...red, swollen, tender spots...and/or open sores? If so, you may have oral lichen planus (LIE-kun PLAY-nus), an inflammatory disease that affects more women than men and often arises in middle age. Lesions usually appear on the inside of the cheeks but also may develop on the tongue, gums, inner lips and throat. The disorder causes burning pain...a metallic taste in the mouth...sensitivity to spicy foods...dry mouth...and/or bleeding gums.

Oral lichen planus is not contagious. It occurs when the immune system attacks the cells of the mucous membranes in the mouth. The exact reason for this attack is unknown, but outbreaks can be triggered by allergies (for instance, to a food or dental product)...a viral infection (such as hepatitis C)...certain vaccines and medications (including nonsteroidal anti-inflammatory drugs)...or stress.

When outbreaks are linked to an allergy or drug, identifying and avoiding the offending substance can resolve the problem. However, in many cases, oral lichen planus is a chronic condition in which flare-ups continue to come and go indefinitely, with lesions lasting for days, weeks or even months. Since there is no known cure, treatment focuses on alleviating discomfort and promoting the healing of lesions.

Problem: Steroid medication helps, but has potentially serious side effects. Topical steroids can lead to thrush (a fungal infection of the mouth) and suppress adrenal gland function, while oral and injected steroids increase the risk for osteoporosis, diabetes, high blood pressure and high cholesterol. And once steroid treatment is halted, lesions may return.

Intriguing alternative: Herbal treatments. While the herbs below have not been proven to cure oral lichen planus, they can ease discomfort...and some patients who use herbal treatments experience quick resolution of symptoms and remain free of recurrences for long periods of time.

Important: Certain herbs can have side effects, so work with a health-care provider knowledgeable about herbal medicines, such as a naturopathic doctor, who can devise a safe and effective protocol for you and determine appropriate dosages. A swish-and-swallow approach (taking a mouthful of a diluted herbal extract and swishing it in the mouth before swallowing it) is often effective. The herb acts topically as well as systemically—your own practitioner can advise you on this. You can use one or more of the following herbs, depending on the specific symptom (or symptoms) that bothers you the most. *Ask your health-care provider about using the following...*

• **For pain—aloe vera (*Aloe barbadensis*).** The gel inside the leaves of the aloe plant contain complex carbohydrates, including glucomannan, that soothe painful tissues and modulate the immune response.

• **For inflammation—turmeric (*Curcuma longa*).** This spice contains substances called curcuminoids that reduce inflammation via multiple pathways. Turmeric doesn't dissolve well in water, so it's best to blend in soymilk, nut milk or animal milk.

Caution: People who are prone to kidney stones should not use turmeric (which is high in oxalic acid)—for them, curcumin extract is better.

- **For easily irritated tissues—tormentil (*Potentilla tormentilla*).** Used in the form of a tincture (a medicinal extract in a solution of alcohol), this herbal preparation coats lesions, protecting them from irritation by food or compounds in saliva. This remedy should not be used within 30 minutes of taking any other medications, as the herb may block absorption of other drugs.

Caution: People who want to avoid alcohol should not use tormentil tincture.

- **For stress—licorice root (*Glycyrrhiza glabra*) or deglycyrrhizinated licorice (DGL).** This is an adaptogen that helps patients handle the anxiety and stress that can contribute to oral lichen planus...it also modulates the immune system. It often is used in tincture form, though patients who want to avoid alcohol should use chewable DGL tablets instead.

Caution: Licorice root remedies should not be used by patients who have uncontrolled hypertension or who are taking corticosteroids or other drugs that can deplete potassium.

Note: Oral lichen planus may increase the risk for oral cancers, so it is important for patients to get regular oral cancer screenings from a doctor or dentist.

Facial Acupuncture

Laurie Steelsmith, ND, LAc, naturopathic physician and acupuncturist in Honolulu and author of *Natural Choices for Women's Health*.

Facial acupuncture can treat many kinds of pain in the face and head, including pain in the eyes, ears and sinuses, headache, temporomandibular joint disorder (TMD), dental conditions or hard-to-treat conditions such as trigeminal neuralgia, a facial nerve disorder.

Some acupuncturists also offer cosmetic acupuncture to tighten skin and reduce wrinkles. Typically, patients will have weekly treatments for at least four weeks to obtain the best results.

In all facial acupuncture treatments, up to 15 very small, thin needles are left in place for approximately 20 minutes. Most patients report that the procedure is nearly pain-free and that they feel only a slight pricking sensation.

Acupuncture is sometimes covered by insurance. To find an acupuncturist, go to the website of the American Association of Acupuncture and Oriental Medicine (AAAOM online.org) and click on "Find a Practitioner."

Natural Cures for Toothache

C. Norman Shealy, MD, PhD, founding president of the American Holistic Medical Association, and a leading expert inthe use of holistic and integrative medicine. He is the author of numerous books, including *The Healing Remedies Sourcebook* and *Living Bliss: Major Discoveries Along the Holistic Path*. Norm Shealy.com

Victor Zeines, DDS, a holistic dentist with practices in New York City and Woodstock, New York. He is a founder of the Institute for Nutritional Dentistry in Los Angeles and author of *Healthy Mouth, Healthy Body: The Natural Dental Program for Total Wellness*. Natdent.com

Few things are more painful than a toothache—and it always seems to erupt on weekends or late at night, when you can't get to a dentist.

Most toothaches are caused by an infected nerve. Conventional dentists usually treat the infection with antibiotics and/or a root canal procedure—but that may not be necessary.

Decay can come close to the nerve chamber but not affect the nerve itself, causing a toothache. Ask your dentist if a sedative filling is appropriate. A sedative filling relieves pain and stimulates the formation of secondary dentin—tissue that can prevent bacteria from damaging the nerve. It works only in the earliest stages of tooth decay and is a temporary restoration intended to relieve pain. The sedative filling will eventually need to be replaced with a permanent filling, but you may have avoided the need for a root canal procedure.

Be aware that once decay enters the nerve chamber and the nerve is infected, root canal therapy is needed to save the tooth. See

This Tea Helps Toothache Pain

You bite down on your usually reliable teeth and there it is, a shooting pain that now won't go away. *Until you get to the dentist for the drilling, filling and billing, try this remedy to ease the toothache pain...*

Make a cup of stronger-than-usual sage tea, which means steeping a tablespoon of dried sage leaves in a cup of just-boiled water for five minutes. If your teeth are not sensitive to "hot," hold the hot tea in your mouth for 30 seconds, then swallow and take another mouthful. (Let the tea sit and cool to lukewarm if the heat makes the pain worse.) Keep doing this until you finish the cup of tea, and by then, you should have no more pain.

Lydia Wilen and Joan Wilen, folk-remedy experts based in New York City. They are coauthors of many books, including *Bottom Line's Household Magic.*

a dentist whenever you have discomfort from a tooth.

Until you can get to a dentist, the following can reduce toothache pain...*

- **Clove oil.** Available in most pharmacies, it's a fast-acting pain reliever. Clove oil can irritate gums, so dilute it with an equal amount of olive or vegetable oil. Soak a small piece of cotton with the oil mixture, and apply it to the affected area. The pain relief lasts about an hour—repeat as needed.

Press firmly on the lower part of the "web" between your thumb and index finger, on the top of the hand on the side of the body with the toothache. This often gives temporary relief.

- **Cinnamon oil.** Dip a cotton ball in the oil and apply it to the painful area. The oil often curbs pain almost instantly. It's also an antimicrobial that kills oral bacteria and can reduce inflammation and swelling.

If cinnamon oil doesn't help after five to 10 minutes, add crushed garlic. Like cinnamon, it's a natural antibiotic with analgesic properties. If it doesn't hurt too much, you can carefully chew a whole clove. Or you can crush a clove and apply the pulp to the painful area.

*Consult your doctor before trying any of these remedies if you take medication or have a chronic medical condition.

What Really Works to Clear Your Sinuses

Study titled "Medical Therapies for Adult Chronic Sinusitis: A Systematic Review" by Luke Rudmik, MD, MSc, director of the Endoscopic Sinus and Skull Base program, and colleagues, University of Calgary, Canada, published in *The Journal of the American Medical Association.*

If you're one of the millions of Americans who suffer from chronic sinusitis, with that nasal discharge, painful pressure and congestion that builds up in your head and just won't go away, you may have tried just about anything to get relief—antibiotics, decongestants, pain relievers, saline sprays, steroid sprays, steroid pills...you name it. You may have even considered surgery.

You can stop now. We know what really works.

A MISUNDERSTOOD CONDITION

Sinus passages are small, hollow air-filled spaces in your face that drain into your nose. After a cold, you might feel nasal congestion for a few days or a week, and then it goes away. But for some people the condition turns into a constant stuffy nose, pain and pressure in the face, postnasal drip, and a reduced sense of smell. You have trouble sleeping, which makes you tired during the day. You're just miserable. When this lasts three months or more, it's chronic sinusitis. It affects 3% to 7% of the population.

When you just can't take it anymore, you might run to your doctor for an antibiotic. It's a common treatment that many doctors still rely on. But most of the time, antibiotics just don't work.

Here's why: While chronic sinusitis was until recently believed to be basically an infection, it's now recognized as primarily an inflammatory disease...similar to asthma.

To find out what works best, researchers at University of Calgary in Canada and the Medical University of South Carolina performed a systematic review of more than 40 clinical studies. They found out that antihistamines, antibiotics and other common treatments didn't work very well.

Here's what probably will: A combination of saline nasal irrigation and prescription corticosteroid sprays.

A GREAT COMBINATION

Saline irrigation doesn't mean those low-volume saline nasal sprays or mists you can buy in the pharmacy—which only help a little—but a product such as a neti pot. These vessels look like tiny teapots or squeeze bottles, and they make it easy to pour salt water into one side of your nose and let it drain out the other side. They've been used for centuries but have only recently become a part of mainstream Western medicine. Saline irrigation helps clean the sinuses by removing mucus and irritants that contribute to inflammation. According to the new analysis, saline irrigation improves sinusitis symptoms—and quality of life.

Cortocosteroid nasal sprays are prescription-only topical medicines that reduce inflammation and reduce symptoms such as nasal congestion and nasal discharge. Steroid sprays by themselves have been shown to be more effective than nasal irrigation by itself.

While there haven't been studies of the two approaches together, these were the only two treatments that scored the highest rating (A-1) based on the American Heart Association Grade of Evidence and Recommendation Grading Scale. They also work in a true complementary fashion—nasal irrigation clears out the sinus passages while corticosteroids fight the inflammatory process.

Based on the strength of the evidence, the researchers recommend a combination of the two treatments as the best first therapy for most people with chronic sinusitis.

WHAT WORKS FOR YOU

Since several other conditions can mimic sinusitis, including sinus migraines, if your symptoms don't improve after about two to three months, check back in with your doctor to rule out other conditions. If you're seeing your primary care doctor, he or she may send you for a CT scan of your sinuses or to an otolaryngologist for more detailed evaluation.

Finally, no one study can replace individualized medical care. For example, many people with chronic sinusitis have nasal polyps—noncancerous, teardrop-shaped growths that form in the nose or sinuses. For them the best treatment is often to take an oral corticosteroid pill (such as prednisone) for one to three weeks, to take a course of the antibiotic doxycycline for three weeks or to use a leukotriene receptor antagonist (such as montelukast/Singulair), a drug that blocks inflammation.

If you don't want to use any medications at all, there's no harm in trying a neti pot for a few weeks and seeing if that works for you. Make it part of your preventive strategy. Since sinus infections typically follow a cold or other upper respiratory infection, use your neti pot at the first sign of an infection coming on. Avoid cigarette smoke, which can irritate nasal membranes, and consider getting a humidifier at home to increase the moisture in the air.

But if preventing colds plus saline irrigation isn't enough help for a chronic sinus condition, talk to your doctor about adding a corticosteroid spray to the mix.

Witch Hazel for Sinusitis

Jamison Starbuck, ND, a naturopathic physician in family practice and a guest lecturer at the University of Montana, both in Missoula. She is a past president of the American Association of Naturopathic Physicians and a contributing editor to *The Alternative Advisor: The Complete Guide to Natural Therapies and Alternative Treatments.* DrJamisonStarbuck.com.

To soothe irritated nasal passages due to allergies and to reduce the copious mucus that can accompany sinusitis, add one-quarter to one-half teaspoon of witch hazel to four ounces of saline solution to use in a neti pot. The witch hazel will make OTC saline solution more astringent to help dry mucus. Use this solution for nasal irrigation and rinse whenever you have allergy or sinusitis symptoms.

Hum to Relieve Sinus Pain

Murray Grossan, MD, is an otolaryngologist and head and neck surgeon with Tower Ear, Nose & Throat Clinic at Cedars-Sinai Medical Towers in Los Angeles. He is the author, with Debra Fulghum Bruce, of *The Sinus Cure and Free Yourself from Sinus and Allergy Problems—Permanently.* Grossan.com

Chronic sinusitis is the most common long-term respiratory disease in the US. Acute sinusitis, which lasts just one to two weeks and causes similar symptoms, such as congestion and headache, is even more common.

Doctors routinely treat sinusitis with antibiotics, but this is rarely effective because the majority of cases are caused by viruses, not bacteria. Even when the infection is caused by bacteria, it will often clear up on its own without medication.

Simple home remedy: Humming to relieve sinusitis symptoms—and to prevent the condition. Humming also helps relieve congestion due to a cold or allergies.

When you hum, you produce vibrations that accelerate the movement of nasal cilia, hairlike projections that sweep bacteria, dust and mucus out of the nose. Fast-moving cilia also remove bacteria before they multiply and cause infection.

Humming vibrates the mucus layer and breaks up the thick accumulations. This makes mucus thinner and easier to eliminate. Five minutes of humming several times a day may be all you need to breathe easier—and stay healthier.

Important: Hum deeply. Lower sound frequencies break up mucus more effectively than a higher-pitched hum. Put your fingers on the tip of your nose (or on your cheek or upper lip) and hum at different frequencies to feel the vibration. If you have trouble feeling the vibration, you can try using a kazoo instead.

CHAPTER 20

Very Personal Pain

How to Cure Chronic Pelvic Pain—Women and Men Can Finally Get Relief

It is one of the most common but least talked about medical conditions. Chronic pelvic pain (CPP)—dull aching, cramping and/or sharp pains in the area between the navel and the hips—is mostly thought of as a woman's disorder. But men account for approximately 20% of the 11 million Americans who suffer from CPP.

It's a tricky condition to diagnose because the symptoms—which in women and men may include painful intercourse, difficulty sleeping, low energy and/or alternating constipation and diarrhea—can be caused by many different conditions, such as endometriosis in women...or prostate enlargement in men. In both women and men, infection of the urethra or bladder and food sensitivities can trigger CPP.

And even though the condition is chronic—that is, lasting for six months or longer—it might wax and wane daily...or you might have a weeklong flare-up after a pain-free month.

WHERE TO START?

Every woman with CPP symptoms should see a gynecologist, who will perform a thorough pelvic exam to look for such problems as abnormal growths and tension in the pelvic muscles. Men affected by CPP symptoms should be seen by a urologist. Specific testing will depend on what your physician finds—or suspects—during the initial exam as the underlying cause of CPP.

Examples: Ultrasound to examine the organs for abnormalities such as ovarian cysts in women and prostate enlargement in men...and laboratory tests to look for infections. In

---

Geo Espinosa, ND, LAc, IFMCP, CNS, naturopathic doctor and clinical assistant professor of integrative and functional urology at New York University. Dr. Espinosa is the author of *THRIVE Don't Only Survive! Dr. Geo's Guide to Living Your Best Life Before & After Prostate Cancer.* DrGeo.com

some cases, a woman may also undergo laparoscopy, the insertion of a thin tube into the abdomen to look for endometriosis.

Some patients get relief once the underlying problem is identified and treated, but many patients don't.

Reason: Within just months, CPP can trigger sometimes permanent changes in the spinal cord that allow the persistent passage of pain signals to the brain—even when the underlying cause of the pain has been corrected.

THE NEXT STEP

Patients with CPP can improve with conventional treatments (such as the use of painkillers or surgery to remove growths), but these approaches won't necessarily give them the greatest odds of adequately relieving their pain.

Better: Taking a complementary approach that combines conventional and alternative treatments.

Best therapies to try—in addition to mainstream treatments...

- **Relax trigger points.** Most women and men with CPP have one or more trigger points (areas of knotted muscle) somewhere in the pelvic area—for example, on the lower abdomen or on the upper thighs. Trigger points themselves can be excruciatingly painful and can transmit pain throughout the pelvic region.

Example: Vaginal pain could be caused by a trigger point elsewhere on the pelvis.

Massage therapists are typically trained to identify and treat trigger points. Simply pressing on one of these points for 20 to 30 seconds—and repeating the pressure several times during an hour-long massage—can relax the tension and help ease the pain. Having a weekly massage for several months sometimes can eliminate symptoms of CPP.

To find a massage therapist who specializes in trigger point treatment, go to AMTAmassage.org/findamassage/index.html, and enter "trigger point therapy" for keyword, along with your city.

Drawback: Pressure on a trigger point can be painful. You can get the same relief, with less discomfort, with electroacupuncture. Two or more hair-width acupuncture needles are inserted into the skin above the trigger point. Then, a mild electrical current is administered, which causes the muscle to relax.

- **Treatment for CPP will typically require about six to 20 sessions of electroacupuncture.** Many acupuncturists are trained in electroacupuncture. However, because the technique is less well-studied than standard acupuncture, it may not be covered by your health insurer. Electroacupuncture typically costs about $70 to $100 per session.

Electroacupuncture should not be used on patients who have a history of seizures, epilepsy, heart disease, stroke or a pacemaker.

- **Try standard acupuncture.** Even if you don't have trigger points, acupuncture is among the most effective treatments for CPP. A study of 67 women who had bacterial cystitis (infection of the bladder wall that commonly causes CPP) found that 85% of them were virtually pain-free after receiving 20-minute acupuncture sessions, twice weekly for four weeks. Reinfection rates were also reduced.

Acupuncture is believed to help block the transmission of pain signals. It's also an effective way to reduce muscular as well as emotional stress, both of which increase all types of chronic pain. Most CPP patients will need 10 to 20 treatments. Acupuncture is often covered by insurance.

- **Identify food sensitivities.** Many women and men with CPP are sensitive to one or more foods, particularly wheat and dairy.

What happens: When these patients eat "problem" foods, they have increased intestinal permeability, also known as "leaky gut" syndrome. Large, undigested food molecules that are normally contained within the intestine pass through the lining of the intestine to reach immune cells, where they trigger the release of inflammatory chemicals that can cause pain throughout the body, and in the pelvic region in particular.

Blood tests known as leukocyte reactivity assays can identify specific food sensitivities. Although reasonably reliable, these tests usually aren't covered by insurance because they're considered "alternative" diagnostic tools. Cost is usually $400.

Another option: An elimination-challenge diagnostic diet.

What to do: Quit eating wheat, dairy and other likely food triggers, such as soy, wine and sugar, for 21 days. If your symptoms improve, at least one of the foods was a problem. Then, reintroduce the foods, one at a time over a period of weeks, to see which food (or foods) causes symptoms to return.

Patients may get frustrated, initially, because they feel like there are few foods left to eat, but many of the foods that they give up during the test will turn out to be harmless. Foods found to cause problems should be given up indefinitely.

- **Take probiotics.** Because infections, such as those described earlier, are a common cause of pelvic pain, patients often receive multiple courses of antibiotics. Antibiotics eliminate infection, but they also kill beneficial bacteria in the intestine. This can lead to digestive problems such as irritable bowel syndrome and leaky gut syndrome—both of which are linked to CPP.

Helpful: A daily probiotic supplement with a mix of at least 10 billion live, beneficial organisms, such as *Acidophilus* and *Lactobacillus*. A probiotic supplement should be taken indefinitely.

Also helpful: Glutamine—100 mg to 200 mg, taken twice daily until symptoms improve. It nourishes the cells that line the intestine and can help prevent leaky gut syndrome. People with liver or kidney disease should not take glutamine.

Caution: Do not take a B-complex nutrient if you're suffering from CPP. In my practice, patients who take B vitamins have more CPP symptoms for reasons that aren't clear.

- **Learn to relax.** Emotional stress doesn't cause CPP, but people who are stressed and anxious tend to be more aware of their pain. Women and men who practice stress-reduction techniques—such as deep breathing and meditation—report about a 50% reduction in CPP symptoms, on average.

Very helpful: Yoga. It is probably the best workout if you have CPP. That's because it relaxes muscle tension as well as trigger points...increases levels of painkilling endorphins...and promotes overall relaxation.

Ahhh...Safe, Quick Relief From Hemorrhoid Pain

Mark A. Stengler, NMD, a naturopathic doctor and founder of the Stengler Center for Integrative Medicine in Encinitas, California. He is author or coauthor of numerous books, including *The Natural Physician's Healing Therapies* and *Bottom Line's Prescription for Natural Cures*, and author of the newsletter *Health Revelations*. MarkStengler.com

According to the National Institutes of Health, an estimated 50% of American adults develop painful hemorrhoids by age 50. However, when you speak with proctologists (medical doctors who specialize in diseases of the rectum, anus and colon), they will tell you that everyone has at least some hemorrhoidal tissue, even though many people don't experience symptoms. Problematic hemorrhoids are found equally in men and women, and the prevalence of this condition peaks between ages 45 and 65.

Hemorrhoids, also known as piles, occur when veins and soft tissue around the anus or lower rectum become swollen and inflamed as a result of pressure from straining or carrying extra body weight and/or irritation due to diet. The most common culprits are constipation (especially when a person strains to pass stools)...obesity (extra body weight bears down on veins in the lower rectum, causing pressure)...and pregnancy/childbirth (the fetus increases pressure on the pelvic and rectal tissues, and hormonal changes make blood vessels more lax). Diarrhea associated with inflammatory bowel diseases, such as Crohn's disease and ulcerative colitis, can cause irritation that predisposes sufferers to hemorrhoids.

Hemorrhoids are often the cause of bleeding from the anus. This is due to the rich network of veins in tissues of the rectum and anal canal. Besides pain, other common hemorrhoidal symptoms include itching and burning in the anal area.

Caution: If you experience excessive or recurrent rectal bleeding, discuss it with your doctor.

CONVENTIONAL TREATMENT OPTIONS

There are a variety of conventional therapies for hemorrhoids. They include ointments, creams and suppositories, all of which provide temporary relief from rectal pain and itching. Common over-the-counter topical treatments include ointments and suppositories, such as Anusol and Preparation H, as well as Tucks medicated wipes. Stool softeners such as *docusate sodium* (Colace) are commonly recommended. These treatments can provide temporary relief, but they don't address the root causes of hemorrhoids.

Internal hemorrhoids that are confined to the anal canal become a problem if they prolapse and bulge from the anus. If this occurs, they are candidates for several procedures, each of which destroys the affected tissue and leaves a scar at the treatment site. The procedures include ligation (putting a rubber band around hemorrhoids so that the tissue dies)...sclerotherapy (injecting chemicals into the hemorrhoid, causing shrinkage)...heat coagulation (using heat from lasers to destroy hemorrhoidal tissue)...and cryotherapy (freezing of hemorrhoidal tissue).

Large hemorrhoids that protrude from the anal canal and/or cause bleeding that is difficult to control are commonly removed by surgery. Hemorrhoidectomy involves surgical removal of internal and/or external hemorrhoids from the anal canal by cutting out the hemorrhoidal tissue and stitching the site. Postsurgical pain is a major problem with this procedure, and strong pain medications are required for days to weeks. Patients are also told to sit on a large, soft "donut" to ease pressure after the surgery. Other complications may include painful bowel movements, difficulty urinating, hemorrhaging, infection, narrowing of the anus (due to scarring) and bowel incontinence. Obviously, this type of surgery should be used only as a last resort.

AN IMPROVED DIET TO THE RESCUE

Hemorrhoids are yet another result of the typical Western diet. People who live in countries where fiber intake is high, such as Japan, have a very low incidence of hemorrhoids. The problem is that the average American consumes only about 15 g of fiber daily. For efficient bowel movements, a person should consume about 25 g to 30 g of fiber daily.

Insoluble fiber, which is found mainly in whole grains and vegetables, bulks up the stool and allows for better elimination. In addition to increasing your intake of these foods, it is imperative that you drink enough water, which allows for easier bowel movements by preventing dryness and adding weight to stool. If you are prone to constipation, drink 64 ounces of water daily, spread throughout the day. Ground flaxseed is an excellent source of insoluble fiber. I recommend using one to two tablespoons daily of ground flaxseed (grind fresh flaxseed in a coffee grinder for five seconds or buy preground flaxseed, known as flaxmeal) on cereal, yogurt, salads, etc. It adds a delicious, nutty flavor. Drink at least 10 ounces of water immediately after consuming flaxseed.

Not surprisingly, certain foods can aggravate hemorrhoids. These include coffee and other caffeine-containing products, alcohol, spicy foods and high-sugar products. In addition, patients who are prone to repeated hemorrhoidal flare-ups usually do better when they reduce or eliminate their intake of tomatoes, cow's milk, citrus fruit, wheat and peanuts. No one knows exactly why these foods and drinks are problematic, but they most likely cause veins to swell.

SOOTHING SUPPLEMENTS WORK WONDERS

I consistently find the following nutritional supplements to be effective in treating and preventing hemorrhoids. If you have an acute flare-up, I recommend taking the first two or more supplements for quicker healing. After symptoms subside, continue taking them for two months to prevent a recurrence. If your symptoms don't improve after using the first two supplements for 30 days, consider taking the others listed below (individually or in a combination formula) for a more aggressive approach. All of the products are available at health-food stores and some pharmacies.

Horse chestnut improves circulation to the rectal area and reduces swelling of hemorrhoidal tissue. Take 400 mg to 600 mg of horse chestnut three times daily. Choose a product that contains 40 mg to 120 mg of aescin per capsule.

Important: Because horse chestnut may have a mild blood-thinning effect, it should not be used by anyone taking a blood-thinner, such as *warfarin* (Coumadin).

Butcher's broom is an herb that reduces hemorrhoidal symptoms, such as bleeding and pain. Take a total daily dose of 200 mg to 300 mg of butcher's broom with 9% to 11% ruscogenins. This supplement is very safe, with only rare reports of nausea.

Bilberry helps hemorrhoids most likely because it strengthens blood vessel walls and improves circulation. I recommend taking 320 mg daily of a 25% anthocyanoside extract. Bilberry can be used during flare-ups or on an ongoing basis for prevention.

Psyllium seed husks are used as a supplement to treat constipation. Some people find that taking psyllium capsules is more convenient than adding flaxseed to food. Take 3 g to 4 g of psyllium in capsule form with 8 ounces of water twice daily. People who are prone to digestive upset should start with 1 g and slowly work up to 3 g over a period of three weeks.

Caution: Do not use psyllium within two hours of taking a pharmaceutical medication—it can hinder absorption of the drug.

Witch hazel, an astringent derived from the bark of the witch hazel shrub, works well as a topical treatment to soothe inflamed, bleeding hemorrhoids. It's available in cream and liquid forms. Use a cotton ball to dab it on the hemorrhoid three or four times daily and after bowel movements during flare-ups.

A SECRET HEMORRHOID CURE

Steve Gardner, ND, DC, and a limited number of doctors (mostly naturopathic and chiropractic physicians) use a procedure known as the Keesey Technique, where the doctor touches the protruding hemorrhoids with an electrode that conducts a galvanic (electrical) current for hemorrhoids. Wilbur Keesey, MD, developed this technique in the 1930s and never reported a severe complication in more than 700 individual treatments. Dr. Gardner has performed this therapy several thousand times. The technique is not FDA approved, but it has a strong history of clinical efficacy.

To find a doctor who uses the Keesey Technique, visit the American Association of Naturopathic Physicians website, Naturopathic.org. Or see Dr. Gardner or one of his colleagues at his Sandy Blvd. Hemorrhoid Clinic East in Portland, Oregon, 503-786-7272, Hemorrhoid help.com.

Help for Problem Hemorrhoids

Michael Epstein, MD, a gastroenterologist in Annapolis, Maryland, and a founder and board member of Macedonia, Ohio–based MAX Endoscopy. MaxEn doscopy.com

---

Hemorrhoids can make life miserable... and that's especially so if you have the ones that are internal, because these can cause problems that range from being very uncomfortable to actually being dangerous. Some people who have internal hemorrhoids don't even realize it (they may be found during a colonoscopy or blood in the stool may reveal their presence), but other people experience a great deal of pain.

Internal hemorrhoids may cause constipation, pain, itching, bleeding and even soiling. If they get large enough to extend through the anus (a condition called prolapse), they sometimes bleed. This type of hemorrhoid can be difficult to treat, but a new technology uses infrared energy to shrink them. Michael Epstein, MD, a gastroenterologist in Annapolis, Maryland, and one of the founders of the company that makes the medical device, MAX Endoscopy, explained how it works.

NEW AND IMPROVED TECHNOLOGY

The improved form of treatment for internal hemorrhoids is easier for both doctor and patient. It's a procedure performed with a fiber optic tool (with a lamp and a tiny video camera) that gets passed into the rectum, where it delivers bursts of infrared light to the tissue above the vein, coagulating the blood and thereby shrinking the tissue. The patient feels some heat and sometimes some minor discomfort, but it's over in just a few minutes. This can be done as outpatient surgery, even in the doctor's office (or as part of a colonoscopy, if the hemorrhoids are discovered that way and/or a patient is scheduled to have one), and the patient can go home immediately afterward and resume normal activities. Treatment typically costs about $300 and usually is covered by Medicare and most insurance companies.

Naturopath Andrew L. Rubman, ND, explained that while the new device may indeed work quite well, it doesn't solve the root problem—why a particular patient suddenly has developed internal hemorrhoids. He said that it's important to recognize that even a small change in the digestive environment—like taking antibiotics or experiencing an unusual amount of stress—can indirectly lead to hemorrhoids. He often prescribes a botanical suppository (such as the ones manufactured by Earth's Botanical Harvest), which can be very soothing...and only then, if that doesn't resolve the complaint, proceed to treat the tissue with either electrical current or ultrasound (the appropriate therapy depends on the particulars of each situation) if needed.

Chronic Rectal Pain—Treatment That Works

William E. Whitehead, PhD, professor of medicine and adjunct professor of obstetrics and gynecology, University of North Carolina at Chapel Hill.

A surprisingly common problem not often talked about in polite company, as they say, is levator ani syndrome. An estimated 6% of the US population suffers this chronic pain in the rectal area, and while the joke potential is obvious, the situation is no laughing matter. It's a dull ache high in the rectum that results in discomfort variously described as fullness, pressure and sometimes burning. The discomfort is caused by spasm in the levator ani, a pair of muscles that stretch across the pelvic cavity and help support the pelvic organs. (Incidentally, these are the muscles dogs use to wag their tails.) Sufferers say that sitting can hurt so much that they often choose to stand instead. Recent research has identified a solution.

There seems to be more than one cause for levator ani syndrome, and few treatments that help. Some people find that walking alleviates the pain, but beyond that, doctors have only three therapies to offer—biofeedback, electrogalvanic stimulation (EGS) and deep digital massage followed by a warm bath.

A recent study verifies that biofeedback training is by far the most effective—with a total of 57% of patients reporting adequate relief from biofeedback versus 26% for EGS and 21% for massage. The study was conducted by Giuseppe Chiarioni, MD, at the University of Verona, Italy, in collaboration with William E. Whitehead, PhD, professor of medicine and codirector at the University of North Carolina Center for Functional GI & Motility Disorders.

HOW DOES THIS WORK?

According to Dr. Whitehead, the biofeedback used focuses on the pelvic floor. The technique teaches patients how to relax their muscles and to avoid excessive straining, reducing tension or "spasm" in the pelvic floor muscles and—usually—making the pain go away.

The biofeedback involves five to nine training sessions of up to an hour each, and patients report that the relief is long-lasting. In a typical session, the doctor or nurse will insert a small plastic cylinder that is about three inches long and three-quarter inches wide into the anal canal and connect it to the biofeedback machine. The plastic cylinder has metal plates in it that pick up electrical impulses from the pelvic floor muscles and display them as a measure of muscle tension. With guidance and encouragement from the therapist, patients use this feedback to learn how to relax the muscles. They also do exercises at home, including squeezing and relaxing the pelvic floor muscles 20 to 50 times a day.

WHO DOES THIS HELP?

Researchers found that 87% of the patients who reported tenderness when a doctor pressed on the levator ani muscles during a digital rectal exam found relief from the biofeedback training...and also that these were the only patients helped by this therapy. Dr. Whitehead said that there is likely a different mechanism causing the pain for the other patients—he recommends talking to your doctor to see if another problem (such as IBS) might be the cause, in which case different treatment might help.

Hospitals with pelvic floor biofeedback programs offering this therapy include the Mayo Clinics in Rochester, Minnesota, and Scottsdale, Arizona...the Cleveland Clinic in Fort Lauderdale, Florida...and the University of North Carolina, where Dr. Whitehead works. Dr. Whitehead also suggests checking the website of the American Gastroenterological Association (Gastro.org) for a list of gastroenterologists in your area—you can call around to find one who is familiar with this therapy.

No More UTIs!

Tomas L. Griebling, MD, MPH, the John P. Wolf 33° Masonic Distinguished Professor of Urology at The University of Kansas (KU) School of Medicine in Kansas City.

Anyone who has ever had a urinary tract infection (UTI) knows that it's extremely unpleasant. The first clue may be that your urine is smelly and/or looks cloudy. You could also suffer burning or pain during urination, have blood in your urine and a fever or chills. To make matters worse, many people suffer repeated UTIs, and some doctors don't do much more than prescribe an antibiotic each time.

Good news: Studies now show that there are some surprisingly simple steps you can take to help guard against UTIs—whether you have suffered them repeatedly or never even had one.

WOMEN AND MEN GET UTIS

Even though UTIs are commonly considered a "women's problem," men develop them, too.

What men need to know: About 12% of men will suffer a UTI at some point in their lives, but men over age 50 are at increased risk. Common causes include prostatitis, a bacterial infection of the prostate gland that can also enter the urinary tract...and the use of urinary catheters in medical procedures.

What women need to know: More than 50% of women will experience a UTI at some point in their lives, and one-third of them will suffer recurring infections. Women are more prone to infection around the time of sexual activity due to the spread of *E. coli* bacteria to the vagina. In postmenopausal women, lower levels of estrogen decrease the amount of *Lactobacillus*, a "good" bacterium that grows in the vagina and serves as a natural defense against UTIs.

Symptoms are sometimes puzzling: Diagnosis of a UTI can be difficult in older men and women because they often don't suffer the classic symptoms but instead have atypical symptoms such as lethargy, confusion, nausea, shortness of breath and/or loss of appetite. If you suspect a UTI, ask that your doctor perform a urine culture.

STOP A UTI BEFORE IT STARTS

When a woman or man suffers from recurring UTIs (three or more infections in a one-year period), these steps will help break the cycle...

- **Go to the bathroom often.** Many people hold their urine longer than they should. This is a bad idea because the bladder may distend, making it more difficult to empty the bladder and preventing bacteria from being flushed out. To protect yourself, try to urinate roughly every four waking hours.

Helpful: When you think you are finished, give yourself another moment to see if there's any urine remaining before leaving the toilet.

• **Drink a lot of water.** You probably know that drinking water is a good way to help flush bacteria from the urinary tract. However, few people drink enough—you need to consume eight to 10 eight-ounce glasses of water each day. Water is best because it's pure and has no calories. Caffeine, soda and alcohol can aggravate the bladder.

Other preventives include...

• **Yogurt.** A 2012 study suggested that lactobacilli, found in probiotic supplements and yogurt, may be an acceptable alternative to antibiotics for the prevention of UTIs in women (with recurring infections, medication may be used for this purpose). The additional lactobacilli are believed to displace E. coli and stimulate the immune system to fight back against the infectious bacteria.

My advice: Consume a cup of yogurt each day—it should be low in sugar (avoid any yogurt that lists sugar as the first or second ingredient) and make sure it contains live cultures. Or take two probiotic capsules each day containing *Lactobacillus rhamnosus GR-1* and *Lactobacillus reuteri RC-14*—the probiotic strains used in the study mentioned earlier. Probiotic supplements with these strains include Pro-Flora Women's Probiotic from Integrative Therapeutics, IntegrativePro.com...and Ultra Flora Women's from Metagenics, Metagenics.com.

• **Cranberry juice or cranberry supplements.** Research has been mixed, but several studies have shown that drinking at least one to two cups of cranberry juice daily may help prevent UTIs. Just be sure to drink real cranberry juice—not cranberry juice cocktail, which has lots of sugar.

You may want to try a cranberry supplement if you have diabetes (even real cranberry juice contains carbohydrates) or if you don't like cranberry juice. Do not exceed label instructions on dosage—research suggests that high doses may increase the risk for kidney stones.

• **Estrogen creams.** For postmenopausal women, a small amount of estrogen cream applied inside the vagina several times per week has been shown to significantly reduce the risk for recurrent UTIs. The cream thickens the walls of the urinary tract, making it more difficult for bacteria to penetrate.

Important: Most women who take estrogen in pill or patch form can safely add an estrogen cream—the amount absorbed into the bloodstream is negligible. Women with a history of uterine cancer or certain breast cancers may not be suitable candidates for any form of estrogen therapy. Ask your doctor.

WHEN YOU NEED AN ANTIBIOTIC

If the steps above do not prevent recurring UTIs, you may need a long-term course (six months or longer) of a low-dose antibiotic. To minimize the development of bacterial resistance, it's wise to start with a milder antibiotic, such as *sulfamethoxazole* and *trimethoprim* (Bactrim), if possible. However, more powerful antibiotics, such as *ciprofloxacin* (Cipro), may be needed to help prevent or treat stubborn infections.

Important: Many women self-diagnose a UTI, call up their doctors and receive a prescription for an antibiotic when in fact they may have a condition, such as vaginitis, that mimics UTI symptoms. Urinalysis and/or a urinary culture is necessary to get an accurate diagnosis.

WOMAN PAIN

When It Hurts to Make Love

Barbara Bartlik, MD, a psychiatrist in private practice in Manhattan and assistant professor of psychiatry and sex therapist at NewYork–Presbyterian Hospital/Weill Cornell Medical College in New York City.

When it comes to sex, sometimes the spirit is willing but the flesh says, "Ow!" If lovemaking has become painful, see your gynecologist. *Possible causes...*

• **Dryness.** Insufficient vaginal lubrication can be caused by dehydration...side effects of birth control pills or antidepressants...and decreased levels of the hormone estrogen after menopause.

What helps: Drink 64 ounces of water daily. Try an over-the-counter (OTC) lubricant, such as Replens, available at drugstores. Extend foreplay to give your body time to create lubrication.

Prescription topical estrogen also can help. It is less likely than oral estrogen to increase risk for cardiovascular problems and breast cancer. Options include a vaginal estrogen cream or an estrogen-containing ring inserted into the vagina.

Recent research: A low-dose vaginal estrogen suppository or ring (about 10 to 25 micrograms) is as effective as a higher-dose product for relieving dryness yet is less likely to cause side effects, such as headache and breast pain.

- **Endometriosis.** When tissue from the endometrium (uterine lining)—which should stay inside the uterus—instead attaches itself to organs outside the uterus, it causes pelvic pain and inflammation for women in their reproductive years.

Options: Take an OTC nonsteroidal anti-inflammatory drug (NSAID), such as *ibuprofen* (Advil) or *naproxen* (Aleve), starting the day before your period is due and continuing until bleeding stops. To halt disease progression, your doctor may prescribe oral contraceptives. In severe cases, surgery to remove endometrial tissue and adhesions can relieve pain while preserving fertility—though symptoms may recur. If pain is extreme and you are done having children, you may want to consider a hysterectomy.

- **Pelvic inflammatory disease (PID).** A bacterial infection of the reproductive organs, PID results from a sexually transmitted disease (such as chlamydia or gonorrhea) or other vaginal infection. Repeated douching and using an IUD (intrauterine device for birth control) can increase risk. PID symptoms include painful intercourse, vaginal discharge and abdominal or back pain.

Caution: PID can cause scarring that leads to infertility and chronic pain. Antibiotics cure the infection but cannot reverse damage.

Your partner: He must see his doctor, even if he has no symptoms of infection (such as pain or discharge from the penis)—without treatment, he could reinfect you.

- **Trichomoniasis.** This parasitic infection usually is transmitted sexually but in rare cases can occur if genitals come in contact with an object that harbors the parasite, such as a wet towel. It causes vaginal odor, yellow-green discharge, sores on vaginal walls, genital itching and pain during sex.

Cure: One large dose of an antibiotic, such as *metronidazole* (Flagyl), can work as well as a seven-day lower-dose course of treatment—but it increases risk for side effects, such as nausea and vomiting. Your partner also must be tested.

- **Uterine prolapse.** This occurs when weakened muscles and ligaments of the pelvic floor allow the uterus to drop into the vagina, creating pressure in the vagina or a lump at the vaginal opening. Contributing factors include pregnancy, childbirth, obesity, chronic constipation and decreased estrogen.

Self-help: Kegel exercises strengthen the pelvic floor. Contract vaginal muscles as if to stop the flow of urine...hold five seconds...relax...repeat. Aim for 30 repetitions daily.

Treatment: Your doctor may fit you with a pessary—a flexible plastic device worn in the vagina to reposition the uterus. Some pessaries can be worn during sex. If a bulge protrudes from the vagina, your doctor may recommend surgery to repair the pelvic floor...or a hysterectomy.

- **Vaginismus.** Involuntary spasms of the pubococcygeus (PC) muscles surrounding the vagina make intercourse extremely painful. Possible causes include pelvic or vaginal infection or injury...lingering pain (or fear of pain)...hormonal changes...or psychological issues.

Relief: Treat any underlying physical cause—with medication to cure an infection or with hormone therapy for low estrogen. Kegel exercises, physical therapy and biofeedback help relax the PC muscles.

In the privacy of your home: Your doctor may recommend vaginal dilators, phallic-shaped rods of various sizes. Starting with the smallest (tampon-size), you gently insert the dilator into your vagina, working up to larger dilators over time until you can comfortably accommodate penetration by your partner.

• **Vulvodynia.** This chronic condition is characterized by stinging or stabbing pain in the vagina or vulva. The cause may be related to genetics...infection...or injury to vulvar nerves, such as during childbirth, especially if you had an incision or tear at the vaginal opening. There is no known cure.

What helps: Medication options include an anticonvulsant or tricyclic antidepressant to block pain signals...and injections of the anesthetic lidocaine. Physical therapy and biofeedback help relax pelvic muscles.

Avoid: Hot tubs, tight underwear, scented toilet paper and perfumed soaps.

For more comfortable sex: Apply a topical anesthetic, such as lidocaine cream, 30 minutes before intercourse. This will diminish sensations of pain (and also, unfortunately, of pleasure). Use a vaginal lubricant...and apply cold compresses after lovemaking.

Help for Clitoral Pain

Barbara Bartlik, MD, sex therapist in private practice and clinical assistant professor of psychiatry and obstetrics, Weill Cornell Medical College, New York City. She is past-president of the Women's Medical Association.

Women with clitoral pain, itching or burning may have a fungal problem. Flare-ups of the yeast *Candida*, a common fungus, can be triggered by antibiotics or certain other drugs, alcoholic drinks or a diet with too much sugar or gluten.

Self-defense: Reduce consumption of sugar, starch and alcohol. Eat plenty of garlic. Treat the affected area with coconut oil (three or four times daily) or drink three drops of oil of oregano daily in a glass of water.

Also helpful: Swallow one olive leaf capsule twice daily after meals. Insert a gauze-wrapped garlic clove in the vagina for 30 minutes a day.

If the problem persists for more than a week, consult a physician, who may suggest using nystatin, tioconazole or another pharmaceutical.

Natural Cures for Women's Vexing Health Problems

Tori Hudson, ND, a naturopathic physician, medical director of A Woman's Time Health Clinic in Portland, Oregon, and program director of the Institute of Women's Health & Integrative Medicine. She is the author of *Women's Encyclopedia of Natural Medicine.*

Across America, millions of women have been suffering for years from two common health problems that can be cured or at least dramatically improved.

If you're a woman with one of these conditions, you may mention it to your gynecologist, but chances are slim that you will get long-lasting relief from medication or other treatments prescribed by most MDs.

What I see in my practice: Every day, I treat women who are suffering unnecessarily from interstitial cystitis (also known as "painful bladder syndrome") and painful and/or lumpy breasts. Frequently, women actually give up on ever getting relief from these problems.

While anyone who has never endured these conditions may think that they are "not that big a deal," the truth is, these problems can greatly interfere with a woman's ability to go about her daily life and may even cause difficulties in her sexual relationship.

A natural approach: As a naturopathic physician, I look for the root cause of these conditions and help women use natural therapies that rely on the body's inherent ability to restore good health.

Here's how I treat my patients who have one of these vexing problems...

INTERSTITIAL CYSTITIS

Researchers are now finding that interstitial cystitis (IC) is much more prevalent than originally thought, affecting as many as eight million women in the US.

What it feels like: IC causes pelvic and/or perineal pain (the area between the anus and vagina). It can range from mild burning or discomfort to severe, debilitating pain that can also affect the bladder, lower abdomen, low back and/or thighs.

Along with the pain there can be urinary problems including a constant urge to urinate...frequent urination (more than eight times a day)...and needing to urinate several times overnight.

What MDs typically prescribe: Drugs, including painkillers, antidepressants and the medication *pentosan* (Elmiron), which is FDA approved for IC. Pentosan may take up to four months to relieve pain and six months to improve urinary frequency.

Other procedures, such as stretching the bladder and administering medication directly into the bladder, are sometimes also used.

All of these approaches have potential side effects, including gastrointestinal damage and liver problems and, most importantly, work less than 50% of the time.

My natural approach: Using several of the following natural treatments at the same time, my patients find that their symptoms of pain and urinary urgency and/or frequency typically improve within about three months—sometimes even faster.

Here's what I recommend...

• **Avoid acidic foods and beverages.** In one study, 53% of IC patients linked a flare-up of their symptoms to specific foods, especially citrus fruits, tomatoes, chocolate and acidic beverages such as alcohol and coffee. To see whether this is true for you, avoid these foods for two weeks. If your symptoms improve, avoid these foods indefinitely.

If you need more relief, try adding the following supplements (you may be able to reduce the doses as your symptoms start to improve)...*

• **Glycosaminoglycans (GAGs).** These two related natural compounds strengthen the lining of the bladder (epithelium), which may be more permeable in people with IC, leading to irritation and pain.

Typical dose: N-acetyl glucosamine—500 mg, twice daily...glucosamine sulfate—750 mg, twice daily.

• **Vitamin A.** This nutrient can help IC by decreasing inflammation and stimulating epithelial repair.

Typical dose: 5,000 international units (IU) daily.

• **L-arginine.** This amino acid helps regulate levels of nitric oxide in the blood, relaxing the muscles of the bladder and improving circulation. It also improves urinary frequency and sometimes helps reduce the pain associated with IC.

Typical dose: 500 mg, twice daily.

• **Kava extract.** This herb from the South Pacific acts in several ways to relieve the symptoms of IC, including balancing potassium levels (high potassium can increase pain sensitivity).

Typical dose: One capsule, three times daily. Don't exceed 280 mg daily of kavalactones (an active ingredient).

PAINFUL AND/OR LUMPY BREASTS

Painful and/or lumpy breasts are one of the most common reasons women see a gynecologist. The good news is that this condition rarely accompanies breast cancer—cancer occurs as a painful, firm lump in only about 5% of cases.

What it feels like: Breasts that are painful and/or have one or more grape-size (or smaller) soft, rubbery lumps that can be moved are often due to hormonal changes during a woman's menstrual cycle. The breast pain can also be caused by an old injury or an acute infection (mastitis).

What MDs typically prescribe: When breasts are painful and/or lumpy due to hormonal changes, conventional doctors typically refer to it as fibrocystic breast disease.

Drug treatments that are frequently prescribed, such as birth control pills, can cause serious side effects, including headache, nau-

*Check with your doctor before starting a new supplement regimen—especially if you have a chronic medical condition and/or take medication.

sea and a slightly increased risk for stroke and deep vein thrombosis.

My natural approach: Because most women have some lumps or lumpy areas in their breasts all the time, as well as occasional pain, I don't consider this a disease.

Here's what I recommend...

- **Start with your diet.** Though scientists aren't sure why, research shows that simply eating more fruits and vegetables and avoiding caffeine (in all forms, including food sources such as chocolate and certain over-the-counter medications such as Anacin) can help prevent lumpy breasts.

In a one-year study, increasing daily soy intake also reduced breast tenderness and fibrocystic changes. Soy does not increase breast cancer risk, as some researchers had theorized, or pose danger to women who have had or have the disease.

Recommendation: One to two servings daily (a serving equals one cup of soy milk, for example, or four ounces of tofu). *Also, consider taking the following...*

- **Vitamin E.** Two studies show that vitamin E relieves breast pain and tenderness regardless of whether they are linked to a woman's menstrual cycle.

Typical dose: 400 IU to 800 IU daily of the d-alpha tocopherol form of vitamin E.

- **Evening primrose oil.** The linoleic and gamma linolenic acid in the oil help the body produce compounds that reduce pain and balance hormones.

Typical dose: 1,500 mg, twice daily.

If your condition doesn't improve in two to three months, consider...

- **Iodine.** Studies suggest that iodine deficiency plays a role in fibrocystic breasts. Without an adequate amount of iodine, breast tissue becomes more sensitive to estrogen, producing lumps.

Typical dose: 3 mg to 6 mg daily of aqueous iodine (by prescription).

Also helpful: Consume more iodine-rich foods, such as shellfish, seaweed, Swiss chard and lima beans.

Don't forget: In addition to undergoing an annual breast exam by a physician and any imaging tests he/she recommends, every woman should conduct a monthly breast self-exam. If any new, unusual changes, thickenings or lumps are detected, they should be promptly evaluated by a physician.

When It Hurts "Down There"

Elizabeth G. Stewart, MD, assistant professor of obstetrics and gynecology at Harvard Medical School, Boston, and director of the Vulvovaginal Service at Harvard Vanguard Medical Associates, Burlington, Massachusetts. She is author of *The V Book: A Doctor's Guide to Complete Vulvovaginal Health.*

The use of euphemisms such as "nether regions" and "privates" keeps women from speaking openly and knowledgeably about their genitals. That's one reason why many patients just say "It hurts down there," with no idea what is causing their problem or what to call it. The word to learn—vulvodynia.

Vulvodynia (VVD) means chronic pain, irritation, burning and/or stinging sensations of the vulva (external female genitalia). Typically, pain is most severe around the vaginal opening, but it can extend from the pubic bone to the anus or thigh. Women with VVD may find it uncomfortable if not excruciating to wear slacks, ride a bike or have sex. Some feel pain even when nothing is touching the vulva. Discomfort may be constant but vary in severity...or symptom-free intervals may alternate with periods of intense pain lasting hours, days or weeks.

A TRICKY DISORDER

The exact cause of VVD is not yet known.

Basic theory: Due to a central nervous system glitch, nerve endings don't work properly and neurological messages get mixed up. *There are two types of VVD...*

- **Provoked VVD.** This is the type I see most often. It occurs when inflammation in the genital area makes nerve endings supersensitive to contact. Clinicians are not sure what type of inflammation this might be. Possible triggers include a vaginal infection...immune system problem, such as a chronic skin disorder or semen allergy...or malfunction of the nerve endings.

• **Unprovoked VVD.** Characterized by continuous pain, this develops when there is a malfunction of the pudendal nerve, which serves the entire genital/anal area and urinary tract. It may arise from childbirth, vaginal or pelvic surgery, injury or herpes infection... then for unknown reasons, the nerve may continue to send pain signals even after the original trigger has healed.

If you have symptoms of VVD, see a gynecologist who specializes in vulvovaginal disorders.

Referrals: National Vulvodynia Association, 301-299-0775, NVA.org.

With VVD, a physical exam typically reveals little—at most, there may be slight redness and mild swelling. There are no lab tests to confirm VVD. Diagnosis is made by testing for and ruling out other possible causes of vulvar discomfort, including a vaginal infection... sexually transmitted disease...shingles (a rash caused by the chickenpox virus)...or a skin disorder, such as eczema, lichen sclerosus or lichen planus.

OPTIONS FOR RELIEF

Once VVD is properly diagnosed, symptoms often can be eased or eliminated within a few weeks or months. With provoked VVD, it is critical to eliminate the root cause of the inflammation—for instance, with antifungal or antibiotic medication to clear up infection.

Physical therapy is rapidly becoming a mainstay of VVD treatment. Soaking in a warm tub or applying an ice pack to the area may bring temporary relief. *In addition, symptoms may improve with one or more of the following...*

• **Analgesic cream.** A pea-size dab of prescription lidocaine can be used topically up to four times daily. Often, patients apply it 15 minutes before sex. Though it stings at first, it quiets the nerves' response in the painful area (such as at the vaginal opening) without interfering with sensation in nonaffected areas (such as the clitoris).

• **Antidepressants.** A daily oral tricyclic drug, such as *amitriptyline* (Elavil), may help by raising levels of brain chemicals that affect nerve messages. The dosage for VVD often is lower than that used for depression. Side effects may include dry mouth, sedation and increased heart rate. This drug may not be right for patients with cardiac or liver problems or glaucoma.

• **Antiseizure medication.** Some patients are alarmed by the idea of taking these drugs. However, the newer ones—*gabapentin* (Neurontin) and *pregabalin* (Lyrica)—have fewer side effects than older anticonvulsants. They block pain by occupying conduction channels on nerve fibers and often are effective for VVD at lower doses than those used to prevent seizures. Some patients use medication until pain is under control, then taper off...others use it indefinitely. Side effects may include sleepiness, dizziness and vision problems.

• **Oral pain medication.** Because antidepressant and antiseizure drugs take a few weeks to take effect, your doctor may suggest a short course of a prescription painkiller.

• **Topical estrogen therapy.** This can ease the postmenopausal vaginal dryness that contributes to vulvar discomfort and pain during sex. Topical estrogen therapy—a cream, vaginal ring or suppository—carries fewer risks than oral estrogen.

TRIGGER ELIMINATION

Certain activities can aggravate VVD symptoms. *What to do...*

• **Avoid biking and horseback riding,** which rub against the vulva.

• **Don't wear tight pants**—they press on the pudendal nerve.

Better: Wear skirts...skip panty hose or cut out the crotch...don't wear thongs (or any underpants at all if they hurt).

• **If intercourse is painful, stick to sexual activities that do not involve vaginal penetration until the therapies above take effect.** If sex is not painful but itching and/or burning symptoms flare up upon penetration, you may be allergic to your partner's semen—so have him wear a condom.

Vaginal Suppository for Chronic Yeast Infection

Laurie Cullen, ND, naturopathic physician and associate professor of clinical medicine at Bastyr University, Kenmore, Washington, commenting on a recent Italian study quoted in *Prevention.*

In a recent finding, women who placed one probiotic tablet directly in their vaginas nightly for seven nights...then every three nights for three weeks...and then once a week after that had an 87% reduction in yeast infections. The suppository approach may help women for whom conventional therapy has not worked—ask your doctor.

Remedies That Relieve Genital Pain in Women

Joel M. Evans, MD, clinical assistant professor, Albert Einstein College of Medicine, New York City, and founder and director, The Center for Women's Health, Stamford, Connecticut. Dr. Evans is the coauthor of *The Whole Pregnancy Handbook.* CenterForWomensHealth.com

Ladies, have you ever developed an itchy all-over rash that really did go everywhere...or had a sore or an infection (or even a cut from shaving the bikini area) that made your private parts painful or tender?

When discomfort occurs "down there"—especially when there is an open sore or when pain is accompanied by other symptoms that could indicate an infection, such as a fever or vaginal discharge—of course you need to contact your doctor so she can diagnosis the complaint and prescribe treatment. To relieve simple chafing or other minor injuries or irritations, though, there often are steps you can take at home that bring relief.

***Complaint:* A cut or sore in the genital area.**

If you've nicked yourself shaving your bikini area or otherwise injured your genital area, you'll need to give yourself some TLC for a few days to let the problem heal—not easy in an area where everything rubs together. If you've got genital herpes, you'll have already discussed how to handle outbreaks with your doctor, such as by taking oral antiviral medication. But with herpes sores, as with cuts, it's important to keep the area very clean.

To that end, after using the toilet, wipe yourself thoroughly but gently with moistened toilet paper, then pat the area dry with clean toilet paper. Do not use disposable premoistened wipes because these may contain irritating chemicals.

To soothe sores or cuts as they heal apply a topical ointment containing aloe, calendula or shea butter twice daily. If your discomfort is severe or extremely distracting, ask your doctor about using a prescription topical cream that contains a painkilling agent, such as lidocaine, for a few days.

***Complaint:* External itchiness, irritation, inflammation or rash.**

Chafing (for instance, from very tight pants or overzealous cycling) and allergic reactions or sensitivities (to laundry products, personal-care products, clothing fabrics, even toilet paper) are two main reasons why women can end up with a rash in the genital area. Investigate all new products. If you identify a possible suspect, such as a new brand of shower gel or laundry detergent or toilet paper, your course of action is clear—stop using it!

In the meantime, for relief, apply an ice pack to the affected region for 15 minutes or so two or three times daily. You can use an icy gel pack (available at drugstores)...create your own ice pack by placing ice chips in a plastic bag and wrapping it in a towel...or use a bag of frozen peas (peas are small enough to mold comfortably to the shape of your body). Whatever you use, do not apply the ice pack directly to the skin because this could damage the skin—instead, put a thin cloth between you and the ice pack.

It's also helpful to take a cool oatmeal bath once or twice daily—the oatmeal soothes, moisturizes and coats irritated skin. You can buy ready-made oatmeal bath products (such as Aveeno Soothing Bath Treatment Colloidal Oatmeal Skin Protectant or a similar generic brand)...or make your own by running a cup of whole oats through the blender and adding them to the bath water. Soak for 10 to 20 minutes, using only your hands to wash yourself (no soap, washcloth or loofah, which could cause further irritation). Then dry off gently but thoroughly.

Until the area is healed, wear all-cotton underwear (no thongs)...opt for thigh-high or knee-high hose rather than pantyhose...and stick with loose-fitting cotton clothing as much as you can. Avoid panty liners and pads, which can trap moisture, slowing down healing.

***Complaint:* Internal vaginal itching or irritation.**

Though a common culprit here is a recurrent or chronic yeast infection, you don't want to make assumptions. It's best not to use an over-the-counter anti-yeast product on your own because you cannot be sure that you have a yeast infection without going to the doctor. Yeast infections are often confused with bacterial infections, and the treatments are vastly different.

Until you can get to the doctor's office, for temporary relief, try taking frequent baths or sitz baths (using a plastic bowl that sits on top of your toilet seat so you can soak your pelvic area without getting your whole body wet). Use cool water, and soak for about 10 to 20 minutes two or three times daily. Bathing helps soothe the internal irritation and the itching because it dilutes the offending agent.

If it turns out that you are prone to chronic or recurrent yeast infections, for long-lasting relief, you and your doctor will need to work together to determine the underlying cause and find a solution. For example, you might start by trying to identify a trigger, such as latex condoms, and see whether switching to a nonlatex brand helps. Your doctor also may suggest one week of nightly use of a natural douche or vaginal suppositories made with boric acid to help correct the vaginal pH.

Recommended products: Arden's Powder Vaginal Cleansing Douche and Yeast Arrest boric acid suppositories.

Important: If you notice any painless genital symptom—lesion, bump, cyst, discharge—that does not go away within a few days, contact your doctor. Certain sexually transmitted diseases and genital cancers cause no pain at the outset but absolutely must be treated.

Stop Dreading Your Mammogram!

Margarita Zuley, MD, FACR, chief of breast imaging and professor and vice chair of quality and strategic development for the University of Pittsburgh Medical Center department of radiology.

Not looking forward to your next mammogram? You're not alone. Many women experience anxiety in the days leading up to it.

SIMPLE STEPS THAT HELP

There are some simple things you can do to reduce pre-mammogram anxiety and to make the experience itself less unpleasant. *For example...*

- **Limit caffeine intake.** Caffeine can make your breasts more tender. Try decreasing your intake starting a few days before the exam. Don't eliminate caffeine, though, or you'll risk having a caffeine-withdrawal headache.
- **Try Tylenol.** Most women can safely use *acetaminophen* (Tylenol), taken at a standard dose within four hours of the exam, to minimize discomfort.

Bonus: It will reduce any soreness you might experience afterward. Avoid aspirin and other nonsteroidal anti-inflammatory drugs (NSAIDs) such as *ibuprofen* (Motrin, Advil), which can increase the risk for bruising.

- **Exercise before the test.** A recent study conducted by researchers at Barretos Cancer Hospital in São Paulo State, Brazil, found that women who exercised for 20 minutes just prior to their mammograms reported less pain after screening compared with women who didn't exercise—perhaps because the physical activity promoted the release of endorphins, hormones that have a pain-relieving effect. Exercises included warm-ups and stretching... then a series of 10 upper-body moves, such as arm and shoulder circles or interlocking the fingers behind the back and raising the arms.

• **Know what to expect.** Women who feel armed with information about the procedure experience less pain and discomfort from mammograms—likely because they feel less anxiety.

What helps: For first-timers, ask your doctor to walk you through the procedure when he/she prescribes your mammogram. A few days prior to the test, do a dry run to the facility so you know exactly how to get there and, if you're driving, where to find parking.

If possible, bring a friend or family member with you to your appointment for support. The less you have to worry about on the day of your mammogram, the more relaxed—and therefore the less pain—you will feel.

WHAT WORSENS DISCOMFORT

Most women know that mammograms tend to be less uncomfortable during the first two weeks of the menstrual cycle, when the breasts aren't as sensitive. Mammograms are also more accurate when performed on that schedule. This is likely because breast tissue is generally less dense at that time and more easily imaged.

What many women don't know: Certain health conditions can increase pain or discomfort during a mammogram. *What helps women affected by...*

• **Chronic pain.** When scheduling, alert the facility that you have chronic pain. There may be a technologist on staff who is trained in working with chronic pain patients. Continue taking any prescription medications as normal, and be sure to try the general tips above. Never be afraid to speak up if something hurts too much! The compression used for mammograms is based in part on the patient's tolerance.

• **Cold temperatures.** If you have trouble tolerating cold temperatures, ask the technologist for a robe or bring one from home. If your hands get cold, you can ask to wear surgical gloves.

• **Dense breasts.** Roughly 25% of postmenopausal women have dense breasts. This simply means that their breasts have denser, lumpier tissue. Dense breasts tend to be more sensitive to pain and are likely to benefit from a reduction in caffeine intake as described earlier.

• **A lumpectomy.** If you have had this procedure, which involves surgical removal of a suspected cancerous tumor and surrounding tissue, you should return to annual mammogram imaging after surgery. The scar itself may be tender, and the skin may be more sensitive to the touch. Let your mammogram technologist know so that he/she can take any necessary precautions, such as making adjustments in position and compression.

• **Weight issues.** Obese women are nearly twice as likely to cite pain as a mammogram deterrent as nonobese women. Be sure to try the general tips above.

DON'T LET A DISABILITY STOP YOU

Use of a wheelchair or scooter should not prevent you from getting screened for breast cancer.

What helps: When scheduling a mammogram, let the facility where you'll be tested know if you will need assistance undressing... standing...moving your arms...and/or transferring from your wheelchair or scooter. The technologist will work one-on-one with you to make the exam as comfortable as possible.

Help for Cystic Breasts

There are strategies that can help make breasts less cystic and minimize pain. Hormone levels influence fibrocystic breast changes, so to keep these in check, reduce your intake of caffeine and animal fat because they may stimulate estrogen production. Also, ask a nutrition-oriented doctor about supplementing with evening primrose oil (its omega-6 essential fatty acid, called gamma-linolenic acid, may help reduce breast pain)... and with the antioxidant vitamins A, C and E, which have anti-inflammatory effects.

Laurie Cullen, ND, associate professor of clinical education at Bastyr University in Seattle.

Chiropractic Cure for Breast Pain

Mikell Suzanne Parsons, DC, CCN, founder of the Natural Path Health Center in Fresno, California. NaturalPathFresno.com

When the problem is breast pain, a chiropractor may be the last person you'd think to consult. Yet chiropractors are equipped to fix breast pain—though that's rarely the reason why patients go to visit them.

Of course it's wise to alert your primary-care doctor to any breast symptoms you might have. But once serious problems are ruled out, call your chiropractor if discomfort persists. With just a few questions about symptoms and lifestyle, he/she usually can pinpoint the root cause of a woman's breast pain. *Here are three common problems and the treatments that bring relief...*

BREAST PROBLEM #1

Telltale symptoms: Pain is sharp and worsens when you take a deep breath or prod the area...with symptoms arising suddenly (rather than occurring chronically).

Likely cause: Your body is out of alignment in the area where one of the ribs attaches to the sternum, which prevents the lungs from fully expanding as you breathe. What feels like breast pain is actually inflammation of deeper tissues. The misalignment may have occurred when you lifted something heavy, slept in an awkward position or twisted in an unnatural way (for example, by reaching into the backseat while driving).

Solution: The chiropractor usually treats this problem by identifying the specific rib involved and correcting the alignment, either manually or with a handheld, spring-loaded device called an activator that delivers a rapid pulse. In addition, if muscle tissue in the area is affected, she also may do a manual press-and-release treatment called trigger point therapy. Most patients get relief almost immediately.

BREAST PROBLEM #2

Telltale symptoms: Pain is localized primarily on the sides of both breasts...with discomfort that is fairly consistent, occurring more often than not...and often is accompanied by constipation.

Likely cause: The real problem arises some inches south of your breasts, in your intestines—because your body is not detoxifying correctly. When toxins are not eliminated through the digestive system, they get reabsorbed and stored in fatty tissue. Breasts consist primarily of fatty tissue, so toxins can accumulate there and create inflammation.

Solution: Cut caffeine, food additives and processed foods from your diet. Also, consider talking with a nutritionist to determine whether your diet is lacking in any particular detoxifying nutrients, such as the B vitamins. As you reduce your toxic load and resume daily bowel movements, your breast pain should diminish within a matter of days.

BREAST PROBLEM #3

Telltale symptoms: All-over breast achiness occurs nearly all the time...and often is accompanied by dry skin, especially on the hands and shins.

Likely cause: Your diet is too low in healthful fats, perhaps because you try to avoid fats altogether or because the fats you do consume are the unhealthful ones (such as those found in fried foods and baked goods). Healthful fats are needed to build healthy, pliable cell walls. When such good dietary fats are lacking, fatty tissue (including in the breasts) can generate inflammation.

Solution: Boost your intake of foods that provide healthful fats, such as olive oil, avocado and fatty fish...and ask your health-care provider about taking a high-quality fish oil supplement. Breast pain should ease within a few weeks—and as a bonus, your skin will look and feel better, too.

Natural Help for Frequent UTIs

Sergei Frenzel, ND, MD, founder of Integrative Natural Health, a clinic in Milford, Connecticut.

There are several natural ways to treat (and prevent) urinary tract infections. One good approach is to increase your urine flow. You should be drinking about two quarts (eight cups) of water per day when healthy, so try increasing this—up to four quarts per day if you can—when you have a UTI.

Second, you want to adjust your urine's pH (a measure of acidity or alkalinity). The types of bacteria that cause UTIs tend to thrive in a more alkaline environment, so the goal is to make your urine more acidic. Taking 1,000 mg of vitamin C every four to six hours during a UTI helps move urine pH in the right direction.

Third, you can supplement with herbs that have antibacterial qualities, such as echinacea, hydrastis (goldenseal) and/or uva ursi (bearberry). Herbal teas and tinctures are sold in health-food stores...or you can use a combination herbal product, such as Wise Woman Herbals Urinary Tract Formula (WiseWomanHerbals.com).

See your doctor if you are not feeling better within several days or if you experience any worsening of UTI symptoms (such as increased urinary discomfort, fever or back pain).

Natural Help for Painful Periods

Mark A. Stengler, NMD, a naturopathic doctor and founder of the Stengler Center for Integrative Medicine in Encinitas, California. MarkStengler.com

Menstrual cramping, which is characterized by inflammation, is caused by high levels of certain prostaglandins that trigger uterine contractions. Often high prostaglandin levels are accompanied by estrogen dominance, where estrogen levels are too high relative to progesterone. Specific nutrients can balance the ratio between these hormones in patients and greatly relieve cramping.

You can use just one of the remedies below or all of them, depending on what helps you. You need to take most of these remedies all month (as indicated), even though symptoms occur on only a few days, because these remedies work to enhance the release of progesterone...improve circulation...or relax muscles.

- **Vitex.** This herb (also known as chasteberry) improves the production of progesterone and offsets estrogen dominance.

Dose: 160 mg to 240 mg, or 40 drops of tincture daily. Try it for at least three months. If it helps you, you can keep taking it. Don't use vitex if you are taking birth control pills.

- **Pycnogenol.** This pine bark extract contains potent anti-inflammatories and antioxidants. It boosts production of endothelial nitric oxide, which improves circulation and helps to reduce the pain of cramps.

Dose: 100 mg to 150 mg daily.

- **Calcium and magnesium.** These minerals reduce premenstrual syndrome symptoms. Magnesium acts as a muscle relaxant, relieving cramps.

Dose: A daily calcium supplement of 500 mg to 1,000 mg that contains at least half as much magnesium. It may take one to two menstrual cycles to reduce symptoms.

- **Natural progesterone.** For severe menstrual cramps, I recommend bioidentical progesterone cream to reduce estrogen dominance. A typical dose is 20 mg twice daily starting two weeks before menses. Work with a holistic physician who can monitor your hormone levels while you use it.

MAN PAIN

Real Relief for Prostate Pain

H. Ballentine Carter, MD, professor of urology and oncology at Johns Hopkins University School of Medicine, Baltimore. He is coauthor, with Gerald Secor Couzens, of *The Whole Life Prostate Book: Everything That Every Man—at Every Age—Needs to Know About Maintaining Optimal Prostate Health.*

A man who goes to his doctor with prostate-related pain will probably be told that he has prostatitis and that he needs an antibiotic for the infection that is assumed to be causing his discomfort.

In most cases, that diagnosis would be wrong. He probably doesn't have an infection, and antibiotics won't make a bit of difference.

Only 5% to 10% of men with prostate-related symptoms have a bacterial infection. Most have what's known as chronic nonbacterial prostatitis/chronic pelvic pain syndrome (CP/CPPS). It's a complicated condition that typically causes pain in the perineum (the area between the testicles and the anus) and/or in the penis, testicles and pelvic area.

The pain can be so great—and/or long lasting—that it can significantly interfere with a man's quality of life. *Here's how to ease the pain...*

A COMMON PROBLEM

More than one-third of men 50 years old and older suffer from CP/CPPS, according to the National Institutes of Health. In this age group, it's the third- most-common urological diagnosis, after prostate cancer and lower urinary tract conditions.

CP/CPPS isn't a single disease with one specific treatment. The discomfort has different causes and can originate in different areas, including in the prostate gland, the ejaculatory ducts, the bladder or the muscles in the pelvic floor. It can affect one or all of these areas simultaneously.

If you have pelvic pain that has lasted three months or more, you could have CP/CPPS. The pain typically gets worse after ejaculation and tends to come and go. Some men will be pain-free for weeks or months, but the discomfort invariably comes back.

THE UPOINT EXAM

A man with CP/CPPS might not get an accurate diagnosis for a year or more. Many family doctors, internists and even urologists look only for a prostate infection. They don't realize that CP/CPPS can be caused by a constellation of different problems.

You may need to see a urologist who is affiliated with an academic medical center. He/she will be up-to-date on the latest diagnostic procedures and treatments for ongoing pelvic pain.

Recent approach: Researchers recently introduced the UPOINT (urinary, psychosocial, organ specific, infection, neurologic/systemic and tenderness of skeletal muscles) exam. It categorizes the different causes of CP/CPPS and helps doctors choose the best treatments.

Your doctor will perform a physical exam and take a detailed history. He will ask where the pain is, how often you have it and how severe it is. He also will ask if you've had recurrent urinary tract infections, sexually transmitted diseases, persistent muscle pain, etc.

Important: Arrive for your appointment with a full bladder. You might be asked to perform a two-glass urine test. You will urinate once into a container to test for bacteria/cells in the bladder. Then you will urinate a second time (following a prostate "massage") to test for bacteria/cells from the prostate gland.

NEXT STEPS

What your doctor looks for and what he may recommend...

- **Infection.** Even though it affects only a minority of men with pelvic pain, it's the first thing your doctor will check.

Consider yourself lucky if you have an infection: About 75% of men with bacterial prostatitis will improve when they take an antibiotic such as *ciprofloxacin* (Cipro).

The discomfort from an acute infection—pain, fever, chills—usually will disappear within two or three days. You will keep taking antibiotics for several weeks to ensure that all of the bacteria are gone.

In rare cases, an infection will persist and become chronic. Men who experience symptoms after the initial antibiotic therapy will need to be retested. If the infection still is there, they will be retreated with antibiotics.

• **Urinary symptoms.** These include frequent urination, urinary urgency and residual urine that's due to an inability to completely empty the bladder. Your doctor might prescribe an alpha-blocker medication, such as *tamsulosin* (Flomax), to relax muscles in the prostate and make it easier to urinate.

Also helpful: Lifestyle changes such as avoiding caffeine and limiting alcohol...not drinking anything before bedtime...and avoiding decongestants/antihistamines, which can interfere with urination.

• **Pelvic pain.** It is the most common symptom in men with CP/CPPS. It's usually caused by inflammation and/or tightness in the pelvic floor, a group of muscles that separates the pelvic area from the area near the anus and genitals. The pain can be limited to the pelvic area, or it can radiate to the lower back, thighs, hips, rectum or bladder.

Helpful treatments...

• **Kegel exercises to ease muscle tension and pain.** The next time you urinate, try to stop the flow in mid-stream—if you can do it, you're contracting the right muscles. To do a Kegel, squeeze those muscles hard for about five seconds...relax for five seconds...then squeeze again. Repeat the sequence five or 10 times—more often as the muscles get stronger. Do this five times a day.

• **Mind-body approaches,** including yoga and progressive relaxation exercises, can help reduce muscle spasms and pelvic pain.

• **Anti-inflammatory drugs,** such as ibuprofen or aspirin, as directed by your doctor. If you can't take these medications because of stomach upset or other side effects, ask your doctor about trying quercetin or bee pollen supplements. They appear to reduce inflammation in the prostate gland. Follow the dosing instructions on the label.

• **Sitz bath** (sitting in a few inches of warm water) can relieve perianal/genital pain during flare-ups. Soak for 15 to 30 minutes.

Common Symptoms of BPH

- A need to urinate frequently
- Urination that is hard to start or stop
- Weak urination or "dribbling"
- Sensation of an incompletely emptied bladder
- Increased need to urinate at night
- Burning pain accompanying urination
- Recurring bladder infections

Mark Stengler, NMD, a naturopathic doctor and founder of the Stengler Center for Integrative Medicine in Encinitas, California. He is author or coauthor of numerous books, including *The Natural Physician's Healing Therapies* and ***Bottom Line's Prescription for Natural Cures***, and author of the newsletter *Health Revelations*. MarkStengler.com

• **Depression, anxiety or stress.** Therapy and/or stress reduction are an important part of treatment because both approaches can reduce muscle tension. Also, patients who are emotionally healthy tend to experience less pain than those who are highly stressed.

Helpful: Cognitive behavioral therapy, which helps patients identify negative thought patterns and behaviors that increase pain.

I also strongly advise patients to get regular exercise. It's a natural mood-booster that helps reduce stress, anxiety and pain.

Painful Peyronie's Disease

Sheldon Marks, MD, a urologist and microsurgical specialist with a private practice in Tucson, Arizona.

Peyronie's disease is a condition in which scar tissue forms in the penis and causes curvature and sometimes pain during an erection. The condition is usually seen in middle-aged men but can occur at any age.

The exact cause of Peyronie's is not known, but an injury to the penis can cause scar tissue to form. The condition has also been linked to autoimmune disorders, such as scleroderma and lupus. The curvature is usually upward or to one side. In many cases, the curvature is mild and does not progress, but it can become quite severe and painful.

If you think you have Peyronie's, see a urologist as soon as possible. You may need treatment to keep Peyronie's from worsening. Treatment may include oral, topical or injected medication, such as Xiaflex, to soften the scar tissue and reduce pain and curvature. Other therapies to break up scar tissue include high-intensity focused ultrasound or iontophoresis (a painless, low-level electrical application of medication to the area). Mechanical and vacuum devices used to stretch the penis can also help reduce curvature.

If these measures don't produce results, a urologist may recommend surgery to remove scar tissue and replace it with a skin graft. Some men may require a penile implant.

Best Holistic Cures For Men's Urological Problems

Geovanni Espinosa, ND, MS.A.c, director of clinical trials, clinician and co-investigator at the Center for Holistic Urology at Columbia University Medical Center in New York City (HolisticUrology.columbia.edu). He is author of the naturopathic section in *1,000 Cures for 200 Ailments* (Bottom Line Books).

If you've ever had an acute infection of the prostate, you may know that antibiotics often clear up the problem in just a few days.

But as the antibiotics eliminate infection-causing bacteria, these powerful drugs also wipe out "healthy" organisms that aid digestion and help fortify the immune system. You may experience diarrhea, upset stomach or a yeast infection while taking the medication.

What's the answer? Holistic medicine uses alternative therapies, such as dietary supplements, nutritional advice and acupuncture, to complement—or replace—conventional medical treatments, including prescription drugs.

For example, probiotic "good" bacteria supplements help replenish the beneficial intestinal bacteria killed by antibiotics. Ask your doctor about taking 10 billion to 20 billion colony, forming units (CFUs) of probiotics, such as *lactobacillus* or *acidophilus*, two to three hours after each dose of antibiotics.*

Holistic treatments for other urological problems that affect men...**

ENLARGED PROSTATE

Prescription drugs, such as *finasteride* (Proscar) and *doxazosin* (Cardura), can relieve the urgent need to urinate and other symptoms caused by benign prostatic hyperplasia (BPH). But the drugs' side effects often include reduced libido, fatigue and potentially harmful drops in blood pressure. *Holistic approach...*

- **Beta-sitosterol is a plant compound that is found in saw palmetto,** a popular herbal remedy for BPH. Men who do not improve with saw palmetto may want to combine it with beta-sitosterol (125 mg daily).
- ***Pygeum africanum*,** an herb derived from an evergreen tree native to Africa, has anti-inflammatory effects that interfere with the formation of prostaglandins, hormone-like substances that tend to accumulate in the prostate of men with BPH. Take 100 mg two times daily with or without saw palmetto and/or beta-sitosterol.
- **Acupuncture also may help ease BPH symptoms.** It can be used in addition to the remedies described above. The typical regimen is one to two treatments weekly for about four weeks.

Whether you're taking medication or herbs, lifestyle changes—such as drinking less coffee (which acts as a diuretic)...avoiding spicy foods and alcohol (which can irritate the bladder)...and cutting down on fluids—are a key part of managing BPH symptoms.

*To find a doctor near you who offers holistic therapies, consult the Academy of Health & Integrative Medicine, 216-292-6644, AIHM.org. Holistic doctors can help you choose high-quality supplements—these products may contain impurities.

**Because some supplements can interact with prescription drugs, raise blood sugar and cause other adverse effects, check with your doctor before trying any of the therapies mentioned in this article.

CHRONIC PROSTATITIS

Pain and swelling of the prostate (prostatitis) may be caused by inflammation that develops for unknown reasons or by an infection. The prostate enlargement that characterizes BPH, on the other hand, is likely due to hormonal changes that occur as men age. Symptoms of chronic prostatitis, such as pelvic pain and pain when urinating, can linger for months. Conventional medicine has little to offer other than antibiotics. *Holistic approach...*

• **Fish oil and quercetin (a plant-based supplement) are both anti-inflammatories.** The fish oil supplements should contain a daily total of about 1,440 mg of eicosapentaenoic acid (EPA) and 960 mg of docosahexaenoic acid (DHA). Take 500 mg of quercetin twice daily. Fish oil and quercetin can be combined.

Prostatitis: A Natural Treatment Plan

Mark Stengler, NMD, a naturopathic doctor and founder of the Stengler Center for Integrative Medicine in Encinitas, California. He is author or coauthor of numerous books, including *The Natural Physician's Healing Therapies* and *Bottom Line's Prescription for Natural Cures*, and author of the newsletter *Health Revelations*. MarkStengler.com

---

When it comes to men's health, we hear a lot about enlarged prostate and prostate cancer. But there is another prostate ailment that gets much less attention yet affects many men. Prostatitis, a very painful condition, is inflammation of the prostate gland. It can be difficult to diagnose because its symptoms (persistent pain in the pelvis or rectum...discomfort in the abdomen, lower back, penis or testicles...difficult, painful or frequent urination or painful ejaculation) are similar to those of other conditions such as an enlarged prostate or a urinary tract infection.

It is estimated that almost half of all men will be affected by prostatitis at some point in their lives. If the condition lasts for three months or longer, it's considered to be chronic prostatitis.

REASONS BEHIND PROSTATITIS

For a long time, it was thought that prostatitis could be caused only by bacterial infection. That view was dispelled when several studies found that the bacteria in the prostates of both healthy men and men with prostatitis were essentially identical. Still, most mainstream physicians routinely prescribe antibiotics for it—a treatment that is appropriate only if your case is one of a very small number actually caused by bacteria.

Although prostate inflammation is not well understood, the inflammation could be the result of inadequate fluid drainage into the prostatic ducts...an abnormal immune response...or a fungal infection.

PROSTATITIS TREATMENT PLAN

If you experience any of the symptoms of prostatitis mentioned above, see your doctor. Your visit should include a rectal exam to check for swelling or tenderness in the prostate...and a laboratory test of prostatic fluid to check for bacterial infection. (Fluid is released during prostate gland massage.) I also recommend that you have your doctor order a urine culture to test for fungal infection (most medical doctors don't test for this).

In a small number of cases, the lab test does reveal a bacterial infection, and an antibiotic is appropriately prescribed. But if there is no bacterial infection, then I recommend that men with this condition follow an anti-inflammatory, antifungal treatment plan for two months. If symptoms subside but don't disappear, continue for another two months. Even if you don't have a test for fungal infection, I often advise following the antifungal portion of the program (along with the inflammation portion) to see if it helps to relieve symptoms.

FOODS THAT BATTLE PROSTATITIS

• **Anti-inflammatory diet.** If you are thinking, Why is Dr. Stengler telling me again about an anti-inflammatory diet?—I'm telling you because it works. Eating a diet of whole foods and cutting out packaged and processed foods go a long way to reducing inflammation in general and prostate inflammation in particular.

Eat: A variety of plant products to maximize your intake of antioxidants, which are natural anti-inflammatories...coldwater fish such as salmon, trout and sardines, which are high in omega-3 fatty acids...and pumpkin seeds, which are high in zinc, a mineral that helps reduce prostate swelling.

Don't eat: Foods that are high in saturated fat, such as red meat and dairy, which can make inflammation worse. Avoid alcohol, caffeine, refined sugar and trans fats, all of which tend to contribute to inflammation.

- **Antifungal diet.** If you already are following the anti-inflammatory diet above, then you have eliminated refined sugar from your diet. (Fungi thrive on sugar!) Also try eliminating all grains (including whole grains and rice) from your diet. Fungi thrive on these foods.

PROSTATE-PROTECTIVE SUPPLEMENTS

The following supplements have targeted benefits for prostate inflammation. They are safe to take together, and there are no side effects. Many men feel much better within two weeks of taking these supplements.

- **Rye pollen extract.** Studies show that rye pollen extract can relieve the pain of chronic prostatitis. In one study published in *British Journal of Urology*, men with chronic prostatitis took three tablets of rye pollen extract daily. After six months, 36% had no more symptoms and 42% reported symptom improvement. Follow label instructions. The pollen component in rye pollen does not contain gluten, but if you have celiac disease or a severe allergy to gluten, look for a certified gluten-free product.

- **Quercetin.** This powerful flavonoid helps reduce prostate inflammation.

Dose: 1,000 milligrams (mg) twice daily.

- **Fish oil.** In addition to eating anti-inflammatory foods, these supplements are a rich source of inflammation-fighting omega-3 fatty acids.

Dose: 2,000 mg daily of combined EPA and DHA.

ANTIFUNGAL SUPPLEMENTS

Many patients benefit from taking one or more antifungal remedies. Several herbs—such as oregano, pau d'arco, garlic and grapefruit seed extract—have potent antifungal properties. They are available in capsule and liquid form. For doses, follow label instructions. Most patients feel better within two to four weeks of taking antifungal supplements.

Treating Low Testosterone May Relieve Pain

Shehzad Basaria, MD, associate professor of medicine, Harvard Medical School, and medical director, Section of Men's Health, Aging and Metabolism, Brigham & Women's Hospital, both in Boston.

Men feel less pain than women. That's not a judgment call—tests have proven it. For instance, among patients who have chronic pain conditions (such as arthritis or nerve damage) or who undergo identical surgical procedures (such as a knee replacement), women tend to experience more pain than men.

It's not just that men generally are raised to be more stoic or that women are raised to be more sensitive. Rather, a key element in this discrepancy seems to be the hormone testosterone. Though women do produce some testosterone, men naturally produce much more of it.

What does this mean for people whose testosterone levels are abnormally low? They may have increased pain perception. And ironically, opioids—the very drugs that are often used to relieve pain—can significantly reduce testosterone levels, creating a vicious cycle in which patients may require more and more medication to deal with their pain. *Now a fascinating study suggests a possible way to break this cycle...*

TESTING TESTOSTERONE

Men produce testosterone in their testicles, and their normal range of serum testosterone (the total amount in the blood) is between 300 nanograms per deciliter (ng/dL) and 1,000 ng/dL. In women, testosterone is produced in the ovaries, and their normal serum testosterone range is 15 ng/dL to 75 ng/dL. Opioid pain-relieving medications such as *morphine, codeine, fentanyl* and *oxycodone* (OxyContin) are known to reduce testosterone production, sometimes decreasing it to undetectable levels in the blood.

For the new study, researchers enrolled men who were taking opioid medication for chronic pain and whose average testosterone level was 228 ng/dL. Before treatment, all the men underwent various tests to measure their perception of and tolerance for pain. Then they were randomly assigned to one of two groups. In one group, each man used a transdermal (applied to the skin) testosterone gel daily to bring his testosterone level up in the desired range of 500 ng/dL to 1,000 ng/dL. The other group of men used a placebo gel.

After 14 weeks, the tests were repeated to gauge any changes in the men's reactions to...

- **Mechanical pain.** For this test, blunt-edge pins were applied to the forearm. Compared with their scores at the start of the study, the placebo users reported an average increase in perceived pain of eight points on a 100-point scale, while the testosterone users reported a decrease in pain of five points, on average.

- **Cold tolerance.** Here the challenge for each man was to keep his hand immersed in ice-cold water for as long as possible. At the end of the study, the men who had received testosterone were able keep their hands in the water an average of 10 seconds longer than men who had received the placebo.

IF YOU ARE IN PAIN...

This study could hold a clue as to why people often become dependent on opioid medication. It's possible that testosterone replacement therapy could help break this cycle by reducing pain perception and increasing pain tolerance. Additional studies are needed to confirm that theory.

Not all cases of low testosterone are due to opioid use. Other possible causes include obesity, various endocrine disorders, certain inflammatory diseases, excess iron in the blood, and chemotherapy or radiation for cancer treatment. Whether testosterone replacement also might help alleviate pain in these conditions remains to be seen.

Important: The findings from this study do not suggest that patients with normal hormone levels should be given extra testosterone to treat their pain. Excess testosterone can increase the risk for sleep apnea and heart disease and may lead to elevated red blood cell counts.

However, if you have a chronic painful condition or if you experience pain that seems out of proportion to an injury or illness, it is worthwhile to talk with your doctor about having your testosterone level checked and treated if it turns out to be too low.

Hernia or UTI?

Peter N. Schlegel, MD, professor and chairman, department of urology, The Weill Medical College of Cornell University, New York City.

What seems like a hernia in men could be a urinary tract infection (UTI). Typical UTI symptoms include frequent urination, burning on urination and fever—but men can have deep pain within the pelvis or pain radiating to the groin or testicles. These are similar to hernia pains, although pain from a hernia usually occurs during lifting or straining. If pain continues for more than a day or two, see your doctor—and if the pain is constant or accompanied by fever, see the doctor immediately. UTIs are treated with antibiotics.

PART II

Modalities for a Pain-Free Life

CHAPTER 21

Painkiller Dos and Don'ts

Conquer Pain Safely

What's the first thing you do when you're hurting? If you're like most people, you reach for aspirin, *ibuprofen* (Advil, Motrin), *naproxen* (Aleve) or a similar nonsteroidal anti-inflammatory drug (NSAID). Each day, more than 30 million Americans take these popular medications. Another roughly 7 million take a different class of painkiller, *acetaminophen* (Tylenol) each day.

The risks most people don't think about: Even though NSAIDs are as common in most American homes as Band-Aids and multivitamins, few people realize that these medications often cause stomach and intestinal bleeding that leads to up to 20,000 deaths every year in the US. And while previous studies have suggested that these drugs also threaten heart health, an important new meta-analysis found that the risks are more significant than once thought. In fact, ibuprofen and other NSAIDs—taken in doses that many people consider normal—increased the risk for "major vascular events," including heart attacks, by about one-third.

SAFER PAIN RELIEF

The good news is, it's still fine to take an NSAID for arthritis, a headache or other types of short-term pain up to two or three times a week. It is also safe, with your doctor's approval, to take a daily low-dose aspirin—81 milligrams (mg)—to prevent heart attacks and stroke.

What not to do: It is never a good idea to depend on these drugs to relieve chronic pain. *My favorite alternatives to oral NSAIDs (ask your doctor which might work best for your pain)...*

ANALGESIC CREAMS

You've probably seen over-the-counter pain-relieving creams, such as Zostrix and Capzasin. These products contain capsaicin, which

Vijay Vad, MD, a sports medicine physician and researcher specializing in minimally invasive arthritis therapies at the Hospital for Special Surgery in New York City. He is author of *Stop Pain: Inflammation Relief for an Active Life*. VijayVad.com

causes a mild burning sensation and appears to reduce substance P, a neurotransmitter that sends pain signals to the brain. Capsaicin products work well for some people suffering from osteoarthritis or rheumatoid arthritis, back pain, shingles and diabetic nerve pain (neuropathy). *Many people, however, get better results from...*

• **Voltaren Gel.** In the heart study mentioned earlier, oral diclofenac (Voltaren) was one of the riskiest NSAIDs. But a topical version, Voltaren Gel, which is available by prescription, is less likely to cause side effects, even though it's just as effective as the tablets. Voltaren Gel is good for pain in one joint, but if your pain is in several joints, supplements (see below) will offer more relief.

How it's used: Apply the gel (up to four times a day) to the area that's hurting—for example, your knee or wrist.

Helpful: Apply it after a bath or shower, when your skin is soft. More of the active ingredient will pass through the skin and into the painful area. Voltaren Gel should not be combined with an oral NSAID.

PAIN-FIGHTING SUPPLEMENTS

If you need even more pain relief, consider taking one or more of the following supplements. Start with the first one, and if pain has not decreased after eight weeks, add the second, then wait another eight weeks before adding the third, if necessary.

Important: Be sure to check first with your doctor if you take blood thinners or other medications because they could interact.

• **Curcumin.** There's been a lot of research on the anti-inflammatory and painkilling effects of curcumin (the compound that gives the curry spice turmeric its yellow color). One study found that it reduced pain and improved knee function about as well as ibuprofen.

Typical dose: 1,000 mg, twice daily.

• **Fish oil.** A huge amount of data shows that the omega-3 fatty acids in fish oil have analgesic and anti-inflammatory effects.

Scientific evidence: One study found that 60% of patients with neck, back and joint pain who took fish oil improved so much that they were able to stop taking NSAIDs or other medications.

Typical dose: 2,000 mg daily.

HOW TO SAFELY USE TYLENOL FOR PAIN

If you prefer an oral medication over the options mentioned above, ask your doctor about switching from NSAIDs to *acetaminophen* (Tylenol). It's not an anti-inflammatory, but it's an effective pain reliever that doesn't cause stomach upset or bleeding—or trigger an increase in cardiovascular risks. I've found that people who limit the dosage of acetaminophen are unlikely to have side effects.

Caution: Taking too much of this drug can lead to liver damage, particularly if it's used by someone who consumes a lot of alcohol or has underlying liver disease, such as hepatitis. Symptoms include vomiting, sweating and yellowing of the skin, plus eventual pain in the upper right quadrant of the abdomen (the location of the liver). If you experience any of these symptoms after regular use of acetaminophen, seek medical attention immediately.

How to Seek Help for Addiction

No one wants to be labeled an "addict," but fear of that diagnosis shouldn't keep you from seeking expert help. Do not attempt to stop taking your medication cold turkey—this approach may actually be physically dangerous because it will precipitate withdrawal, which can lead to changes in blood pressure, pulse and even cardiac function due to hyperactivity of the nervous system.

Depending on your individual situation, outpatient or inpatient care may be necessary to properly supervise your withdrawal process. A specialist can assess your situation and make a treatment referral—self-diagnosis and selection of treatment are rarely enough. Seek professional help. To find an addiction specialist, consult the American Society of Addiction Medicine at ASAM.org.

Mel Pohl, MD, chief medical officer of Las Vegas Recovery Center in Nevada. Dr. Pohl is coauthor of several books, including *The Pain Antidote and Pain Recovery.* LasVegasRecovery.com

My recommendation: No more than 2,000 mg daily of acetaminophen (this dosage is lower than the limits listed on the label).

Important: In calculating your total daily dose, be sure to factor in all sources of acetaminophen. More than 600 prescription and over-the-counter drugs, including cold and flu medications and allergy drugs, contain the active ingredient acetaminophen.

Example: In a *Journal of General Internal Medicine* overdose study, three drug combinations were most likely to cause an overdose—a pain reliever and a PM pain reliever...a pain reliever and a cough and cold medicine...a sinus medication and a PM pain reliever.

For a partial list of medications that contain acetaminophen, go to KnowYourDose.org/common-medicines.

To be safe: Get a liver function test (usually covered by insurance) every six months if you regularly take acetaminophen.

NSAIDs Can Be Deadly

Lynn R. Webster, MD, vice president of scientific affairs with PRA Health Sciences, a research organization, Salt Lake City. He is author of *The Painful Truth: What Chronic Pain Is Really Like and Why It Matters to Each of Us*. ThePainfulTruthBook.com

Harlan Krumholz, MD, professor of cardiology at Yale School of Medicine, New Haven, Connecticut, and author of *The Expert Guide to Beating Heart Disease: What You Absolutely Must Know*.

The Food and Drug Administration recently strengthened an existing label warning that non-aspirin nonsteroidal anti-inflammatory drugs (NSAIDs) increase the risk for heart attack and stroke. Popular over-the-counter medications including *ibuprofen* (Advil and Motrin) and *naproxen* (Aleve) are among the products affected. Taking these regularly for as little as a few weeks can put people's lives at risk...as could exceeding recommended dosages.

In January 2011, a group of researchers at the University of Bern conducted a meta-analysis of more than 30 randomized trials with a combined total of 116,429 patients taking placebo or NSAIDs. The researchers found abundant evidence of a heightened risk for cardiovascular events and found that taking drugs containing ibuprofen, including brand names such as Motrin and Advil, and those containing naproxen (such as Aleve) raises the likelihood of suffering a stroke.

What to do: If you take an NSAID, keep your dose as low as possible and your duration of use as short as possible. People who have a history of heart disease, kidney disease or stroke should be especially careful to limit NSAID use. Speak with your doctor about options other than NSAIDs.

Flirting With Painkillers: Could You Get Hooked?

Michael Weaver, MD, professor of psychiatry and behavioral sciences, and medical director, Center for Neurobehavioral Research on Addiction, The University of Texas Health Science Center at Houston.

If you've heard about the painkiller-addiction epidemic, you're probably scared of these drugs—even wondering if you could become addicted if you ever needed one.

On the one hand, it is very easy to get hooked on painkillers. On the other hand, if you've been prescribed one of these strong opioids, such as hydrocodone, oxycodone, hydromorphone or fentanyl—which killed the musician Prince in an accidental overdose—and you know exactly how to use it, you don't have to be on a slippery slope to dependency.

What tips the balance? Are you at risk? If you started to get hooked, would you recognize the signs? Would you get help—or even know where to start?

HOW TO KNOW IF YOU'RE AT RISK

Factors that put you in harm's way...

• **Gender.** Women are more likely to become dependent on prescription painkillers than men are, and not only because they are more likely to have chronic pain—women tend to weigh less than men, so when they are prescribed standard doses, they are in effect taking higher amounts, which can jump-start them on the path to dependence. Also, while men are more likely to abuse illegal "hard" drugs such as heroin or cocaine, women are more likely to fall prey to prescription addictions, especially to opioids.

- **A family history of addiction to any substance.** The closer the family member, such as a parent or sibling, the stronger the genetic risk.
- **Symptoms of anxiety and/or depression.** You may knowingly or unknowingly use opioids to numb these symptoms and not just physical pain.
- **A history of abusing another substance**—whether it's nicotine, alcohol, marijuana, stimulants or sedatives.

WARNING SIGNS TO WATCH FOR

Opioid painkillers often are prescribed for chronic pain even though they aren't very effective for chronic pain and should never be the "first line" prescription, according to recent Centers for Disease Control and Prevention guidelines.

Once they are prescribed, often for a hospital procedure, however, some people get used to the drugs' feel-good effects and keep using them...which is to say abusing them. *Here are some signs that that might be happening...*

- **You're using an opioid painkiller for something other than pain**—to improve a bad mood, relieve stress or help you relax or get to sleep.
- **You feel that you have to take a painkiller just to feel normal**—or what you think normal should feel like.
- **You find yourself taking higher doses to have the same effect**—that means you're building up a tolerance.
- **Family members or friends express concern about your painkiller use.**
- **You spend a significant amount of time trying to get your hands on one or more painkillers, using them and recovering from their effects.**
- **You find yourself trying to cut down on your use of painkillers**—to no avail.

WHAT TO DO IF YOU THINK YOU MIGHT BE HOOKED

If any of the above describes you, the first and most important tip is, Don't go it alone. Talk to your doctor about your concerns and your pattern of use, and ask for guidance on the best way to wean yourself from dependence. Dealing with an addiction on your own is always more difficult. It is much easier with help, and there is help available.

Symptoms of opioid withdrawal can feel like a bad case of the flu, without a fever but with nausea, diarrhea, muscle cramps and aches, runny nose and watery eyes. These symptoms often are accompanied by considerable anxiety and powerful cravings to use opioids since that will make the symptoms go away immediately.

To prevent withdrawal symptoms and improve someone's chances of overcoming an opioid addiction, medication-assisted therapy is often recommended. This involves substituting a different opioid such as methadone or buprenorphine, which is much less likely to produce euphoria, for the one that's being abused. It is better to be slowly tapered off over several days or weeks with a longer-acting, less reinforcing opioid with the help of a qualified physician or treatment program. This is what's often referred to as "detox." Naltrexone, which blocks the effects of other opioids if you do use one, may also be prescribed for long-term maintenance.

Over time, with ongoing counseling or other forms of professional help, people can learn skills to help them quit abusing opioids and avoid relapse for the long haul. There are many effective options available, including individual addiction counseling, group therapy, working with a physician who specializes in addiction medicine or participating in an inpatient or outpatient addiction treatment program.

HOW TO AVOID ADDICTION...AND WHEN ADDICTION IS ACTUALLY OK

Of course, if you are at risk for opioid dependence—if you're almost addicted, as it were—the best thing to do is to nip it in the bud before it becomes a full-blown addiction that needs treatment. There are lots of nonopioid pain meds available for many different chronic pain conditions, so talk with your doctor about these.

Finally, it should be noted that continuing use of opioid painkillers can sometimes have a place in medicine. The CDC's new guidelines, for example, make it clear that they don't apply to people who are actively battling cancer pain or who are being given opioids for palliative care at the end of life. For these patients, opioid painkillers can be perfectly appropriate.

What If You Really Do Need an Opioid?

Jane C. Ballantyne, MD, FRCA, professor of anesthesiology and pain medicine, University of Washington, Seattle. Dr. Ballantyne is coeditor of *Expert Decision Making on Opioid Treatments* and president of Physicians for Responsible Opioid Prescribing. Support PROP.org

Every day, more than 115 people in the US die after overdosing on opioids. And the efforts now being made to curtail addiction and stem the shockingly high death and overdose rates are all over the news.

Under-recognized problem: While there's no question that opioid addiction is a serious problem in this country, there are some circumstances where patients need these drugs.

What you need to know...

THE TREATMENT CHALLENGE

Chronic pain (usually defined as lasting three to six months or longer) is widespread, affecting about 100 million American adults.

Yet there's always a balancing act when it comes to treating pain with opioids. About 10% to 20% of the population has risk factors (such as a risk-taking personality) for addiction, even with first use—especially if they have a personal or family history of drug abuse.

And the longer you take these drugs, the more likely you are to become dependent. Drug dependence, which can be a precursor to addiction, compulsive drug use and other harmful behaviors, can occur within 30 days...and even within five days in some patients.

PAIN SPECIALISTS ARE WARY

The majority of doctors, including primary care physicians, receive little training in the best ways to treat pain. Many of these doctors are now nervous about prescribing opioid medications due to increased government oversight (including voluntary opioid-prescribing guidelines issued by the CDC in 2016)...uncertainty, in general, about optimal dosing...and worries about the risk for addiction.

In a survey published in 2017 in *Practical Pain Management* that included more than 3,000 chronic pain patients, nearly 85% reported being in more pain than they were before stricter oversight recommendations were instituted.

Undertreated pain is a real concern when it prevents patients from engaging in normal activities and enjoying a good quality of life. This doesn't mean that doctors should dispense drugs more freely. Many people do better overall when they rely on drug-free methods of pain relief, including things like physical therapy, counseling or support groups. To find such a support group near you, ask your doctor.

SAFER OPIOID USE

Opioids are powerful drugs that need to be monitored. They aren't likely to cause problems when they're taken for a few days for acute pain (after surgery, for example), but long-term use can cause serious side effects, including osteoporosis, digestive problems (such as constipation) and opioid-induced endocrinopathy—decreases in testosterone and other hormones.

I provide long-term opioid prescriptions only for select groups of patients (discussed below). Patients with acute pain—after a back injury, for example—might need opioids, but should take them for as short a time as possible...and only if they can't get adequate pain relief from safer approaches, such as exercise, physical therapy and/or over-the-counter (OTC) *acetaminophen* (Tylenol) or a nonsteroidal anti-inflammatory drug (NSAID), such as *ibuprofen* (Motrin) or *naproxen* (Aleve). Prescription antidepressants or anticonvulsants also can reduce pain regardless of its cause.

With some exceptions, I advise patients never to start treatment with *hydrocodone* and *acetaminophen* (Vicodin), *oxycodone* (OxyContin) or other opioids and to try other pain-relief methods first.

Exceptions: Patients who are terminally ill can have a much higher quality of life when they take high doses of opioids—and not just because of pain relief. Someone with a terminal cancer, for example, might feel more at peace when taking the drugs. Similarly, patients with intractable diseases that impair their ability to function—such as spinal cord injuries, severe multiple sclerosis, etc.—might do better when they take the drugs.

But for those who can do without an opioid, lifestyle approaches, including cognitive behavioral therapy or physical activity, can sometimes relieve pain more than prescription or OTC drugs. Only take an opioid when other approaches don't work...and only take a dose that's high enough to relieve pain but low enough to allow you to function normally. *Also important...*

- **Set limits.** Some doctors continue to write opioid prescriptions too casually.

My advice: Don't take an opioid for short-term pain unless you have a very clear injury—after a car accident, for example. Even then, take the drug for a few days at most. Also: The safest way to take opioid medications—both for acute and chronic pain—is to use them only as needed to control severe or sudden pain...not around-the-clock, unless it's absolutely necessary.

- **Attend a pain clinic.** Patients with complex pain do better when they work with pain specialists at an interdisciplinary clinic (available at most major medical centers), where the medical team typically includes doctors, nurses, psychologists and physical therapists. Opioid medications may be prescribed carefully in these settings, but the emphasis is on other safer, longer-lasting methods of pain relief.

- **Talk to your doctor about dosing.** It's common for patients taking opioids to develop tolerance—they gradually require more medication to get the same relief. This is not the same as addiction. However, the higher doses will increase the risk for side effects, including addiction. Do not change your medication or dose on your own. Get your doctor's advice.

- **Ask about longer-acting drugs.** Patients with acute pain after surgery or an injury often need a fast-acting drug, such as nasal or sublingual (under-the-tongue) fentanyl. But patients with chronic pain usually do better with longer-acting drugs, such as extended-release *oxymorphone* (Opana ER) or a *buprenorphine patch* (Butrans).

Long-acting drugs provide a steady level of medication to stabilize their effectiveness—with fewer "letdowns" that can lead some patients into inappropriate drug-seeking behavior. They're not a perfect solution because patients who take them may be given an additional prescription for a fast-acting drug to control "breakthrough" pain.

Addiction isn't likely to be a problem if you use these powerful medications only when needed and keep in mind the caveats described above.

This Dangerous Moment Leads to Painkiller Addiction

Survey titled "Changes in Substance Abuse Treatment Use Among Individuals With Opioid Use Disorders in the United States, 2004-2013" by researchers in the department of health policy and management and at the Institute for Health and Social Policy, both at Johns Hopkins Bloomberg School of Public Health, Baltimore, published in *Journal of the American Medical Association.*

Study titled "Opioid Prescribing at Hospital Discharge Contributes to Chronic Opioid Use" by researchers at University of Colorado Denver School of Medicine, Aurora, Denver Health Medical Center, University of Colorado School of Medicine, VA Eastern Colorado Health Care System, Denver, Kaiser Permanente Colorado, Denver, published in *Journal of General Internal Medicine.*

Other sources include the Centers for Disease Control & Prevention, the Centers for Medicare & Medicaid Services and *The New York Times.*

For many Americans, the epidemic of painkiller addiction hits close to home—39% of us know someone personally who has been addicted to painkillers, according to the latest Kaiser Family Foundation poll.

Here's what you need to know to protect yourself—and those you love.

THE RISKIEST ADDICTION MOMENT—HOSPITAL DISCHARGE

Here's the scenario: You're not currently taking opioid medications at all. You need to have a procedure at a hospital. When you get discharged, you are given a prescription for an opioid painkiller for the pain. It might be *hydrocodone* (Vicodin, Zohydro), *oxycodone* (Oxycontin, Percocet) or *hydromorphine* (Dilaudid).

Here's why it's risky: Compared with someone given a different kind of painkiller prescription or no prescription at all, you are five times more likely to be a chronic opioid user over the following year. So report researchers at the University of Colorado Anschutz Medical Campus in the *Journal of General Internal Medicine*. One reason, the researchers speculate—the drugs work for pain but also provide euphoria, and it's easy to get addicted even after original post-surgical pain is gone.

BETTER SOLUTIONS FOR CHRONIC PAIN

Chronic pain affects about 100 million Americans, but relying on opioid prescriptions, especially for long-term relief (more than 90 days), greatly increases the risk for adverse side effects—constipation, drowsiness, concentration problems, driving accidents, vision impairment, reduced immunity and, for men, reduced testosterone levels.

Taking opioid medications for chronic pain is a dangerous, and sometimes deadly, slippery slope. To take a different path, work with a knowledgeable practitioner to start by exploring drug-free ways to handle pain.

DO DOCTORS IN YOUR STATE OVER-PRESCRIBE OPIOIDS?

Where you live can be a risk factor, too. The states with the highest prescription opioid addiction rates, according to the Centers for Disease Control and Prevention, are Alabama, Arkansas, Indiana, Kentucky, Louisiana, Michigan, Mississippi, North Carolina, Ohio, Oklahoma, South Carolina, Tennessee and West Virginia. Similar geographical differences also show up in Medicare claims. A map from the Centers for Medicare & Medicaid Services lets you see how your state stacks up against the national average in prescription opioid Medicare claims. Go to CMS.gov and search "Opioid Drug Mapping Tool."

There are many reasons why some states have more opioid prescriptions (and addiction) than others, but one factor may be the prescription patterns of area doctors. So if you live in a high-use state, you may need to be extra-vigilant to avoid falling into a prescription addiction for chronic pain. Ask your doctor if there are better solutions for you.

You May Be Using the Wrong Painkiller

Jianguo Cheng, MD, PhD, professor of anesthesiology and director of the Cleveland Clinic Multidisciplinary Pain Medicine Fellowship Program, and president-elect of the American Academy of Pain Medicine.

Millions of Americans fight their pain and inflammation with an over-the-counter (OTC) nonsteroidal anti-inflammatory drug (NSAID), such as *ibuprofen* (Motrin, Advil) or *naproxen* (Aleve, Naprosyn)—or a prescription anti-inflammatory, such as *celecoxib* (Celebrex). But if you've got heart disease and/or kidney disease, finding a pain reliever that won't worsen your other condition is tricky.

What most people don't realize: Even in healthy people, NSAIDs—especially when taken for longer or at higher doses than directed by a doctor—increase risk for heart attack and stroke and can potentially harm the kidneys. For those who already have heart disease and/or kidney disease, these risks are even greater.

It's widely known that NSAIDs can cause stomach bleeding as a side effect, but the potential risks to the user's heart and kidneys are not nearly as well recognized.

Important: Short-term use of any NSAID (no longer than 10 days) is always preferable to long-term use. In fact, you may not need drugs at all. *Pain relief options if you have...*

HEART DISEASE

Background: NSAIDs raise one's risk for heart attack and stroke by increasing blood clot formation. These medications can also interfere with certain high blood pressure drugs, such as diuretics...angiotensin-converting enzyme (ACE) inhibitors...and beta-blockers, and cause the body to retain fluid—a problem that often plagues people with heart failure.

If you have known risks for heart disease: For people with risk factors such as high blood pressure, diabetes, an enlarged heart or an abnormal EKG reading with no clinical symptoms, NSAIDs may be used, under a doctor's supervision. Celecoxib is generally safer for pain than naproxen or ibuprofen because it is associated with fewer gastrointestinal and/or renal complications.

People treating high blood pressure with an ACE inhibitor drug, such as *captopril* (Capoten) or *benazepril* (Lotensin), should aim for lower doses of celecoxib than typically prescribed (for example, less than 150 mg per day) and use it for no more than 10 days.

If you have known heart disease: NSAIDs increase the risk for new cardiovascular events in people with established heart disease and may lead to heart failure in those with severe heart disease. NSAIDs should be avoided in those with recent heart attack, unstable angina or poorly controlled heart failure. For these individuals, non-NSAID medications, such as *acetaminophen* (Tylenol), may be considered.*

Note: Aspirin is also an NSAID but does not carry the same cardiovascular risks. Low-dose aspirin is widely used for its blood-thinning effects to reduce risk for heart attack or stroke in those who have cardiovascular disease or are at increased risk for it. A doctor should prescribe and monitor such daily aspirin therapy.

KIDNEY DISEASE

Background: NSAIDs can reduce blood flow to the kidneys and/or cause the body to retain fluid, taxing the kidneys.

If kidney disease is mild: It may go unnoticed, except you may have slightly higher blood levels of creatinine (a waste product normally removed by kidneys). Short-term and low-dose NSAIDs, including aspirin, may be used if creatinine levels are not substantially elevated (less than 1.5 mg/dL). Creatinine levels should be monitored if NSAIDs are used in these cases.

If kidney disease is severe: If you have kidney disease and routinely retain extra fluid, it's a severe case. You should avoid all NSAIDs—including daily low-dose aspirin for heart attack prevention. A person with severe kidney disease may use acetaminophen if his/her liver function is normal.

Important: When used as directed, acetaminophen is generally safe but can interfere with liver function when taken in excessive doses (more than 3 g per day) and/or when combined with alcohol.

HEART AND KIDNEY DISEASE

What if you have both heart and kidney problems? If your blood work indicates that your liver function is normal, acetaminophen (see above) can often be used for pain, under a doctor's direction.

NONDRUG PAIN RELIEF

Drugs are not the only option—nor should they even be your first choice—especially if you have heart disease and/or kidney disease. *Nondrug therapies that can reduce or replace your use of pain medication...*

- **Noninvasive.** Physical therapy, aqua therapy, exercise, tai chi and yoga are powerful pain-fighters. Acupuncture and massage have also been shown to help, as have behavioral approaches such as cognitive therapy. Most people see results within days to weeks.
- **Minimally invasive.** Nerve blocks—injected anesthetics or nerve ablations (using heat) that are designed to turn off pain signals—are generally given once every few weeks or months and can produce lasting pain relief without resorting to long-term drug use.

Another option: Neuromodulation, in which a small device (electrodes and a pulse generator about the size of a stopwatch) is surgically implanted to deliver electrical stimulation that disrupts pain signals that travel from

*With some cases of heart disease (and/or kidney disease), a topical NSAID, which is absorbed differently from a pill, may also be an option.

the spinal cord to the brain. This can be used to treat pain in many locations of the body.

- **Surgery.** This is an option if the cause of your pain is identified and can be surgically corrected.

Example: A herniated disk pressing on a nerve may be surgically removed. Of course, nonsurgical methods should be tried first. Surgeries can cause short-term pain and fail to provide the desired level of pain relief and function. Talk to your doctors so that you understand the risks of surgery and have realistic expectations for your outcome.

How Opioid Painkillers Make Pain Worse

A study titled "Morphine paradoxically prolongs neuropathic pain in rats by amplifying spinal NLRP3 inflammasome activation" by Peter M. Grace, PhD, research assistant professor, department of psychology and neuroscience, University of Colorado, Boulder, et al., published in *PNAS Plus*.

In a recent study, animals in pain who received morphine, an opioid, became more sensitive to pain. And that's not even the worst part.

AN INFLAMMATORY JOLT TO THE BRAIN

Whenever nerve cells are damaged, they send distress signals via glial cells in the brain, and you perceive pain. But after morphine, the researchers found, those pain-activated glial cells became more sensitive to the next pain stimuli. As the researchers put it, "Opioids exaggerate pain."

The worst part: It took months for the effect to wear off.

HOW ACUTE OPIOIDS BECOME CHRONIC

The medical community is finally realizing what a big mistake it was to turn so readily to opioids for management of chronic pain—for conditions such as fibromyalgia, for example. Although opioids are still widely prescribed for chronic pain, the latest CDC guidelines state that they should be avoided if possible, with the exception of cancer pain and end-of-life palliative care. Emerging research is also finding new harm from long-term opioid use, including an increased risk for heart disease.

The trickier question is how opioid use for acute pain can turn into long-term dependency. While animal studies such as this one don't tell us exactly how these drugs work in humans, the findings shed some light on how treating acute pain with opioids might lead to the development of chronic pain—by prolonging pain sensitivity.

It's common for doctors to prescribe opioids after an operation, injury or dental procedure. Sometimes they are needed. But if you can use nonopioid medications instead...along with nondrug therapies—you can avoid the risk for this rebound effect.

The Dangers of Combining Painkillers

Joseph Biskupiak, PhD, research associate professor, department of pharmacotherapy, University of Utah, Salt Lake City.

Patients regularly taking an over-the-counter nonsteroidal anti-inflammatory drug (NSAID), such as *ibuprofen* (Advil), and aspirin in the same day had two to three times the risk for ulcers and gastrointestinal (GI) bleeding as those who took either alone.

Theory: Acidity in the GI tract reaches more harmful levels when the painkillers are combined.

If you must take multiple anti-inflammatory drugs: Ask your physician about adding a proton pump inhibitor (PPI) for a limited time, such as *lansoprazole* (Prevacid), to reduce stomach acid.

Pain Pills May Be Dangerous During Pregnancy

Anick Bérard, PhD, professor in the Faculty of Pharmacy at the University of Montreal and director of the Research Unit on Medications and Pregnancy at the Research Center of CHU Sainte-Justine, both in Quebec, Canada.

A recent study suggests that taking NSAIDs during pregnancy can more than double a woman's risk for miscarriage. This is a significant finding in an area that has shown inconsistent research results. So if you are expecting or know someone who is, please take note and spread the word.

Background: In the US, nonprescription NSAIDs include *ibuprofen* (Advil, Motrin) and *naproxen* (Aleve)...in Quebec, Canada (where the new study was done), ibuprofen is the only nonprescription NSAID. In both countries, prescription-strength NSAIDs include ibuprofen, naproxen, *diclofenac* (Voltaren) and *celecoxib* (Celebrex). NSAIDs are among the most commonly used medications during pregnancy, taken by an estimated 17% of expectant mothers. *Here's what researchers found...*

The study involved 4,705 women who miscarried prior to the 20th week of pregnancy, plus a control group of an additional 47,050 women who did not miscarry. Researchers based their analysis of NSAID use on whether each woman had filled a prescription for such a drug immediately prior to or in the first 20 weeks of her pregnancy.

Results: Women who filled one or more prescriptions for NSAIDs were 2.4 times more likely to suffer miscarriages than women who had not received the medication. Though researchers had no way of knowing exactly how much of the medication each woman actually took, miscarriage risk appeared to be elevated no matter what NSAID dosage was prescribed.

Theory: NSAIDs may interfere with hormonelike substances in the uterine lining that affect a woman's ability to maintain a pregnancy. Why might this study be more reliable than previous ones? Because it included a very large number of women...miscarriage diagnoses were confirmed by physicians... and the data on NSAID use were based on actual prescriptions filled and not just on patient recall. Though this study included only NSAIDs purchased by prescription, researchers pointed out that participants could have received prescriptions for nonprescription-strength formulations...and that the purchase of nonprescription NSAIDs would have been equally likely among participants who did miscarry and those who did not miscarry, so this would not have significantly altered the study findings.

Bottom line: Researchers warn that any NSAID use during early pregnancy may increase the risk for miscarriage. Aspirin also should be avoided unless specifically recommended by your doctor because it increases the risk for bleeding.

If you need pain relief during pregnancy: Ask your doctor if it is OK for you to take *acetaminophen* (Tylenol), which is not an NSAID (though it can damage the liver if used improperly).

Harder-to-Abuse Narcotic Available

US Food and Drug Administration, Silver Spring, Maryland.

A new harder-to-abuse narcotic painkiller has been approved. Targiniq ER is a combination of the narcotic oxycodone and naloxone, which blocks the euphoric effects of oxycodone. Naloxone is activated if the pill is crushed, snorted, dissolved or injected, but Targiniq still can be abused by swallowing too many pills. Targiniq is approved for use by patients with chronic pain that has not responded to other medications.

Looking for Pain Relief? Try Prolotherapy

Allan Magaziner, DO, director of Magaziner Center for Wellness in Cherry Hill, New Jersey, and a clinical instructor at University of Medicine and Dentistry of New Jersey in New Brunswick. DrMagaziner.com.

A medical procedure that "tricks" the body into healing itself, prolotherapy treats acute or chronic pain from damaged ligaments, tendons and cartilage. Some studies show significant improvement in patients with injuries or arthritis, especially in the joints, back, neck or jaw. Prolotherapy is used as a first-line therapy or when other treatments fail.

• **How it works.** A physician injects a solution, typically of dextrose (a sugar) and lidocaine (an anesthetic), into the painful area. This provokes minor, temporary inflammation... causing the body to send more blood and nutrients to the spot...which hastens healing.

• **What to expect.** Each session lasts 15 to 30 minutes and includes from one to 20 injections, depending on the areas treated. Patients experience slight discomfort during injection and mild soreness for several days after. Minor pain might need one session...severe pain might require 10 sessions spread over several months.

• **Cautions.** Your doctor may advise you to temporarily reduce or discontinue anti-inflammatory drugs—aspirin, *ibuprofen* (Motrin), *naproxen* (Aleve)—while undergoing prolotherapy. *Acetaminophen* (Tylenol) is okay. If you take blood thinners or other drugs, tell your doctor—extra precautions may be warranted.

• **Finding a practitioner.** Prolotherapy should be administered by a physician trained in the procedure—preferably through the American Association of Orthopaedic Medicine (719-232-4084, AAOMed.org) or Hackett Hemwall Foundation (HHPFoundation.org). Visit these websites for referrals.

Cost: $100 to $400 per session. Because prolotherapy is considered experimental, insurance seldom covers it.

Topical Pain Relievers May Cause Burns

US Food and Drug Administration, Silver Spring, Maryland.

Topical pain relievers may cause burns even after just one application. Over-the-counter creams, lotions, ointments and patches for joint and muscle pain often contain menthol, methyl salicylate and/or capsaicin, all of which can irritate skin. Some users reported a burning sensation, swelling, pain and skin blistering within 24 hours of use. Tightly bandaging or applying heat to areas treated with these products may increase risk.

Drug Overdose Dangers From Pain-Relief Creams

Ellen Marmur, MD, chief of the division of dermatologic and cosmetic surgery, the Mount Sinai Medical Center in New York City.

It's easy not to realize that applying medicines to your skin is not all that different from drinking them in liquid form or swallowing tablets—but it's true. The skin is a permeable membrane and what goes "on" it goes "in" it (this is known as "transdermal" application). And this is why topically applied medications such as pain relief creams or lotions—whether prescription or over-the-counter—can make people very, very sick when used in excess...and in a few recent instances have even proved lethal.

DEATHS FROM SKIN CREAMS

A teenager in New York City, a star on her high-school track team, died after using large quantities of anti-inflammatory products containing methyl salicylate (Bengay is one of several over-the-counter sports creams for muscle aches that contain methyl salicylate). She purportedly used pain-relieving patches and rubbed a large quantity of a sports cream into her sore muscles. Two deaths were linked to other topical painkillers, leading the FDA to issue a warning in 2006 concerning pharmacy-compounded anesthetic creams, which are used before cosmetic procedures such as laser hair removal and skin treatments. The deaths of the two women—in completely separate incidents—occurred after each applied excessive amounts of the creams at home in preparation for laser hair removal.

How can this happen? The active ingredients in the various kinds of numbing creams, ointments and gels (OTC and prescription, depending on the strength) are lidocaine, tetracaine, benzocaine or prilocaine. These are supposed to be applied by trained health-care professionals in doctors' offices, but patients sometimes apply them at home (if directed to do so by their doctor) to save prep time in the office. This appears to be what happened in the deaths of both young women. They applied the creams liberally to their entire legs and, to further absorption, both wrapped their legs in plastic wrap. Since so much cream was applied to large areas of skin, its toxicity was magnified with the result being that the women suffered seizures, went into comas and subsequently died.

Note: If your doctor directs you to apply a painkilling cream at home, have him/her write clear instructions down...and plan to have someone at home with you in case of emergency.

WHAT YOU NEED TO KNOW TO STAY SAFE

These creams are easily obtained, but should be considered serious drugs to be used with the same caution as any other medication. Most importantly, don't use them at home without first reading the dosing instructions carefully and discussing potential dangers with your doctor. Among the early signs of toxicity are feeling fuzzy-headed, blurred vision, dizziness, breathing difficulty and irregular heartbeat. These symptoms should be considered a medical emergency. Go to an ER (don't drive yourself) if you feel this way. Conservative use and medical supervision for any kind of medical cream, including even low-dose prescription and OTC creams, is imperative. We all metabolize differently, so slow and safe is the way to go.

Why You Shouldn't Take Pain Meds Before Exercise

Study by researchers at ORBIS Medical Center, Maastricht, The Netherlands, published in *Medicine & Science in Sports & Exercise.*

Many athletes take ibuprofen—found in Advil and other medicines—or another nonsteroidal anti-inflammatory drug (NSAID) before workouts because they think it will help them exercise more strenuously and prevent muscle soreness afterward.

But: NSAIDs—which can cause damage to the lining of the gastrointestinal (GI) tract—should not be combined with strenuous exercise, which also can cause short-term damage to the GI lining.

Recent finding: Men who took ibuprofen before a workout showed higher intestinal permeability than men who did not—which means that toxins and other bacterial by-products may get into their blood.

Self-defense: If you feel that you need medicine in order to exercise without discomfort, try using acetaminophen, which does not have the GI effects of NSAIDs. Or ask your doctor for a recommendation.

Dangers of Patient-Controlled Pain Medications

Rodney W. Hicks, PhD, RN, FNP-BC, FAANP, UMC Health System Endowed Chair for Patient Safety, and professor, School of Nursing, Texas Tech University Health Sciences Center, Lubbock, Texas.

Patient-controlled pain medications are popular for post-surgical recovery, theoretically enabling people to get what they need when they need it, without having to wait for a nurse...though perhaps that's not so great. A recent study found flaws in the delivery of patient-controlled pain medications that amounted to greater likelihood of medical error. The study examined more than

More Harm from Painkillers...

Heart attack... Older patients taking opioids such as hydrocodone or codeine face a higher risk for heart attack, bone fracture and death, compared with similar patients taking non-narcotic drugs, such as ibuprofen. If an opioid is necessary to control pain, it is best to take the medicine for as short a time as possible in the lowest effective dose.

Daniel H. Solomon, MD, MPH, associate physician, division of pharmaco-epidemiology, Brigham & Women's Hospital, Boston. He led an analysis of painkillers published in *Archives of Internal Medicine*.

Severe liver damage... Several prescription painkillers contain 325 mg of acetaminophen or more. Example: Percocet contains oxycodone and acetaminophen. The most severe liver damage occurred in patients who took more than the prescribed dose or took more than one product containing acetaminophen. OTC products that contain acetaminophen include Excedrin, Nyquil and Sudafed—and Tylenol's only ingredient is acetaminophen.

Jane C. Ballantyne, MD, FRCA, professor of anesthesiology and pain medicine at University of Washington School of Medicine, Seattle.

Hearing loss... In a recent finding, women who regularly took *ibuprofen* (such as Advil or Motrin) or *acetaminophen* (Tylenol) at least twice a week had up to a 24% higher risk for hearing loss than women who used the painkillers infrequently. Other studies have found similar effects in men. These pain relievers may damage the cochlea in the inner ear by reducing blood flow or depleting antioxidants.

Self-defense: Limit painkillers to occasional short-term use—but talk to your doctor before making any changes in your medications.

Study of more than 62,000 women by researchers at Harvard Medical School, Boston, published in *American Journal of Epidemiology*.

Dulled emotions... People who took acetaminophen, the main ingredient in Tylenol and other over-the-counter painkillers, reacted less emotionally to positive and negative photos than participants who took a placebo.

Study of 82 people by researchers at The Ohio State University, Columbus, published in *Psychological Science*.

Infertility... Common pain relievers may undermine fertility. Nonsteroidal anti-inflammatory drugs (NSAIDs), such as *naproxen* (Aleve), may hinder ovulation and reduce levels of the female hormone progesterone. Women who are trying to get pregnant should ask their doctors about alternative pain relievers.

Study by researchers at University of Baghdad, presented at the European League Against Rheumatism Congress in Rome.

9,500 errors that occurred with PCA over a five-year period and found that patients were harmed in 6.5% of those cases—a major difference compared with the 1.5% rate associated with other medication errors.

Perhaps surprisingly, the problems didn't typically result from patients overdosing themselves. Medical errors, including malfunctioning PCA equipment, incorrectly programmed doses (giving 10 mg/mL instead of 1 mg/mL per dose, for example) or incorrect medications, caused the most problems, with human error responsible for about 70% of them.

WHAT CAN PATIENTS DO?

Before your surgery and also for the immediate post-surgical time when you're too foggy to think clearly, have a trusted family member with you to ask for information on the dosing and medications. After you are feeling more alert and aware, take responsibility for this yourself. Know what medication is prescribed and in what dosage and double-check that what you are getting is correct.

Your "trusted person" should be aware of any medication allergies you might have and should remind caregivers of them before medication is administered. "When we start these analgesia pumps on patients, the patients are usually coming out of surgery and that means they're asleep," Dr. Hicks explains. "So if I don't know that the person is allergic to morphine and I start them on a morphine pump...that's trouble." He noted that in this study, the absence of allergy information was an issue. "Part of the problem is where allergies are docu-

Painkillers Can Make Antidepressants Less Effective

Painkillers may make antidepressants less effective. Selective serotonin reuptake inhibitor (SSRI) antidepressants, such as *fluoxetine* (Prozac) and *citalopram* (Celexa), are 25% less effective when the patient also is taking a painkiller, such as *acetaminophen* (Tylenol), *ibuprofen* (Advil) or aspirin. Talk to your doctor about switching to another type of antidepressant, such as *amitriptyline* (Elavil) or *buproprion* (Wellbutrin) if you take painkillers regularly, for example, for arthritis.

Jennifer Warner-Schmidt, PhD, research associate in Dr. Paul Greengard's Laboratory of Molecular and Cellular Neuroscience, The Rockefeller University, New York City, and leader of a study published in Proceedings of the National Academy of Sciences.

mented. Sometimes the nurse uses one sheet, the OR staff another and the MD another."

Also important—the person with you during recovery should be reminded never to push the button delivering the medication for you. Dr. Hicks said there were some instances of "errors related to PCA by proxy." "That means that someone else, likely a family member, pushed the button to administer more pain medication when the patient didn't really need it," he explained. "Let's say you're a patient and you're asleep, and a family member in the room is concerned that you're going to experience pain so he pushes the button for you—that can slow your breathing down so you can't keep your blood oxygen levels up. It's never intentional, but it happens."

The solution: Don't push the button for someone else.

The future will likely bring some changes in how PCA pumps are set up (perhaps with a simpler user interface and a bar-code-scanning system to ensure that the proper drugs are delivered) and how the medications are prescribed in an effort to eliminate those errors. For now, be careful—even when you think you are in charge.

Outside the Opioid Box for Post-Surgery Pain

David Sherer, MD, a board-certified anesthesiologist and president and CEO of Consolidated Medicine, a medical practice and consulting group in Chevy Chase, Maryland. He is coauthor of *Dr. David Sherer's Hospital Survival Guide: 100+ Ways to Make Your Hospital Stay Safe and Comfortable.* His blog on BottomLineInc.com is titled "What Your Doctor Isn't Telling You."

When it comes to postsurgical pain, consider skipping opioids altogether. This won't always be possible because of the severity of some types of pain. It is up to you to decide your own tolerance for pain and how to deal with it.

Consider asking your doctor for the newer injectable forms of the standard anti-inflammatory painkillers. Ibuprofen and naproxen now are available in injectable forms. Another med in this class, injectable ketorolac (see next article on sinus surgery), has been around for decades. These medicines may be appropriate in some cases to give you the pain relief you need.

Also available is a newer form of injectable acetaminophen, better known as Tylenol in pill form. Ofirmev is the brand name of this newer agent and it has shown promise for postsurgical pain relief. Realize, though, that this drug will not have the anti-inflammatory properties of the others mentioned above.

A groundbreaking time-released form of the local anesthetic Exparel has emerged as a novel way to treat surgical pain. This medication, injected by the surgeon or anesthesia provider, can result in longer-lasting pain relief with much fewer side effects as compared to the nonsteroidal anti-inflammatories or narcotic medicines.

Alternative pain relief can be achieved with the use of specific nerve blocks. Ask the anesthesia provider if this is possible. Local anesthetics can be released over time in epidurals and other nerve blocks (for the arm, hand, leg or foot, etc.) with the use of infusion pumps and other devices.

Better Pain Relief After Sinus Surgery

Kevin Welch, MD, assistant professor of otolaryngology, Stritch School of Medicine, Loyola University, Chicago.

Thirty-four patients received either the nonnarcotic drug *ketorolac* (Toradol) or the narcotic fentanyl immediately after undergoing endoscopic sinus surgery.

Result: Ketorolac was just as effective for pain relief as fentanyl but did not have the side effects of a narcotic drug, such as nausea, vomiting and drowsiness.

Self-defense: To avoid the side effects of narcotics, ask your doctor if ketorolac is an option following sinus surgery. It is also used in cardiac and orthopedic surgeries.

Would You Try Medical Marijuana for Pain Relief?

Gregory T. Carter, MD, rehabilitation-medicine specialist and medical director, St. Luke's Rehabilitation Institute, Spokane, Washington.

Would you use cannabis (marijuana) if your doctor recommended it for, say, nerve pain or to help control muscle spasms? Thirty-two states (as of December 2018), plus the District of Columbia, have now legalized it for such medical uses.*

But do the benefits of medical marijuana truly outweigh the risks? Who should consider trying it—and what's the best way to use it safely? *Here, answers to some common questions...*

*Medical marijuana has been legalized in Alaska, Arizona, Arkansas, California, Colorado, Connecticut, Delaware, District of Columbia, Florida, Hawaii, Illinois, Louisiana, Maine, Maryland, Massachusetts, Michigan, Minnesota, Montana, Nevada, New Hampshire, New Jersey, New Mexico, New York, North Dakota, Ohio, Oklahoma, Oregon, Pennsylvania, Rhode Island, Vermont, Washington and West Virginia. Nine states—Alabama, Iowa, Mississippi, Missouri, North Carolina, Tennessee, Texas, Utah and Wisconsin—permit medical marijuana for epilepsy only.

- **Why has marijuana suddenly become so popular as a medical treatment?** There's really nothing new about the medical use of cannabis. It was included in the US Pharmacopeia (the official authority for prescription and over-the-counter drugs) until the early 1940s, when, due largely to political opposition, it was removed. For this reason, it has been difficult to study cannabis for medical purposes.

The US government still classifies cannabis as a Schedule 1 drug—that is, a substance with no medical benefits and a high potential for abuse. Although federal law prohibits the use of medical marijuana, doctors now prescribe it instates where it has been legalized by the state legislatures.

- **What conditions is marijuana most likely to help?** Several—but because research has been impeded by political considerations, the level of evidence varies for each condition.

Beginning nearly 30 years ago, the prescription drug *dronabinol* (Marinol) was approved by the FDA for treating appetite loss in AIDS patients. It's a synthetic version of one of the active compounds in cannabis.

Since then, cannabis has been shown to relieve nausea in cancer patients. Unlike the synthetic version, it's not a single agent. It contains 80 to 100 different medicinally active compounds known as cannabinoids.

Recent lab and animal studies suggest that cannabis can be an effective treatment for cancer itself. The active compounds have been shown to limit tumor invasiveness and the activation of chemical signals that stimulate growth in some types of cancers.

Patients who have nerve pain often get more relief with cannabis than with other prescription medications, such as *gabapentin* (Neurontin). Cannabis also has been used successfully to treat muscle spasms, seizures and other neurological conditions such as multiple sclerosis. And it seems to be effective at controlling the tics and behavior problems caused by diseases such as Tourette's syndrome. Some people also use it for fibromyalgia, glaucoma and post-traumatic stress disorder, but studies are mixed.

- **If my doctor prescribes cannabis, what type should I buy?** Cannabis dispensaries (in states where medical uses are permitted) typically sell many different strains, which affect users in different ways. The best medical strains have a high concentration of cannabidiol (CBD) and cannabinol (CBN), with relatively small amounts of tetrahydrocannabinol (THC), the compound responsible for most of the intoxicating effects.

Bear in mind that even in states that have legalized it, insurance does not cover the cost of medical marijuana, which ranges from $200 to $500 an ounce.

• **Is it better to smoke medical marijuana or eat it?** Neither. It's unlikely that the small amount of smoke from medical doses increases the risk for emphysema or other lung diseases, but the smoke does contain carcinogens. Why take chances? Edible forms of cannabis—such as baked goods, shakes and candies—are effective, but it's difficult to control your intake. The absorption rate will depend on what's already in your stomach, and it can take up to two hours to feel the effects. Plus, a recent study found that cannabinoid concentrations in edibles often are mislabeled (about one-quarter of the products tested were stronger than their labels indicated).

The best way is to use a vaporizer. The medicinal compounds vaporize at a much lower temperature than is required for combustion (smoking). The inhaled vapor gives the same rapid onset as smoking—you'll feel the effects within a few minutes. Vaporized cannabis is safer than inhaled smoke. Vaporizers are sold online and at dispensaries for around $100 to as much as $400.

You can also buy sublingual tinctures at dispensaries. You put a few drops under your tongue. You'll feel the effects almost as quickly as from smoking. This form of medical marijuana can be just as effective as other forms, but concentrations are not standardized, so it can be a bit harder to provide the correct dose.

• **What is the right dose?** Everyone reacts differently to cannabis, and some strains are more potent than others. If your doctor prescribes cannabis, don't leave the office without detailed instructions—how much to use...how often...and what to expect.

Marijuana also interacts with certain medications you may be taking, such as sedatives, including the tranquilizer *lorazepam* (Ativan) and the sleep drug *zolpidem* (Ambien), so be sure to also discuss all medications you take.

• **What are the risks?** Your motor skills and reaction times will be diminished, particularly within the first few hours. You don't want to engage in other tasks that require serious concentration while the drug is active in your body, which varies widely depending on the person and the strain of cannabis but is typically four to six hours.

• **What about addiction?** Few people who use cannabis for medical purposes will become dependent, develop cravings or go on to abuse other drugs. But the potential for addiction is obviously a concern, just as it is with alcohol and some types of medication. If you have a history of alcoholism or other forms of addiction, talk to your doctor about this before using cannabis.

Finally, if you're not getting it legally, you should still tell your doctor that you're using marijuana so he/she can advise you of the risks. Because marijuana can raise your heart rate (even doubling it), there's a concern for people who are already at risk for heart attack or stroke. It's also dangerous (and illegal) to drive while you're under the influence of marijuana.

CBD: The "No High" Marijuana Extract

Hyla Cass, MD, an integrative physician in private practice in Los Angeles. She is author of several books, including *Natural Highs, 8 Weeks to Vibrant Health, Supplement Your Prescription* as well as *Your Amazing Itty Bitty Guide to Cannabis* and an upcoming, more in-depth book, *The Miracle of CBD.* CassMD.com

If you follow the headlines, you know that many states have legalized the medical use of cannabis, the plant more commonly known as marijuana or hemp.

Recent development: An increasing body of scientific evidence shows comparable medical benefits from an extract of the marijuana/

hemp plant that does not contain the psychoactive compound tetrahydrocannabinol (THC), which causes that signature high.

Known as cannabidiol, or CBD, it most often is taken in a formula that combines other related plant compounds (cannabinoids and terpenes) for much greater efficacy. CBD has been the focus of more than 8,000 published studies showing that it can help with a variety of common health problems.

HOW DOES CBD WORK?

CBD's therapeutic effects are tied to the body's endocannabinoid system (ECS), a complex "communication system" that was discovered by Israeli scientist Raphael Mechoulam, PhD. The ECS is comprised of cannabinoid receptors found throughout the body to balance vital functions, including the central nervous system and the cardiovascular, hormonal and immune systems.

When there's an imbalance in the ECS, conditions such as anxiety and pain develop. CBD helps rebalance this messenger system. *Here's how CBD can help with...*

ANXIETY

Widely used antianxiety medications, such as *alprazolam* (Xanax), *lorazepam* (Ativan) and *clonazepam* (Klonopin), to mention a few, are highly addictive and commonly cause side effects, including drowsiness, dizziness, fatigue, headaches and blurred vision. CBD, on the other hand, is equally effective, much safer and rarely produces side effects (see the next column).

Scientific evidence: A review article published in *Neurotherapeutics* looked at a variety of experimental and clinical data and concluded that the evidence "strongly supports CBD as a treatment for generalized anxiety disorder, panic disorder, social anxiety disorder, obsessive-compulsive disorder and post-traumatic stress disorder."

PAIN RELIEF

Staggering numbers of people who suffer from chronic pain become addicted to opioid pain medications or, worse, die of an overdose. But CBD can often relieve chronic pain—without the risk for addiction.

Scientific evidence: In both human and animal studies, CBD is increasingly being studied for a variety of pain-relieving effects. For example, a study published in *British Journal of Pharmacology* found that CBD was "safe and effective" in the prevention and reduction of neuropathic pain due to the chemotherapy drug paclitaxel.

SEIZURES AND MORE

CBD can prevent seizures in patients with epilepsy. It also has been miraculous for children with Dravet's syndrome, a condition that can cause hundreds of seizures a day and has not been effectively treated with medication. I often advise patients in my integrative medical practice, where I treat various conditions, to try CBD for painful health problems such as fibromyalgia, Crohn's disease, irritable bowel syndrome and migraine.

SHOULD YOU CONSIDER CBD?

Based on my clinical experience, CBD can be used effectively and safely for the conditions described earlier. Side effects are rare—generally sleepiness, diarrhea and weight gain (or weight loss).

Important: Even though CBD has a good safety profile, you should check with your doctor before trying it if you are taking medication. Certain medications, including chemotherapy agents, anti-epilepsy drugs and the

Ointments vs. Oral Drugs for Pain

Painkilling ointments are as effective as oral drugs for certain types of pain.

Recent finding: Topical NSAIDs treated pain associated with osteoarthritis in the knee and hand and musculoskeletal injuries, such as tendinitis, as effectively as oral NSAIDs. Topical NSAIDs are absorbed through the skin, so there is little risk for gastrointestinal bleeding. Currently, only three are available, all by prescription—Voltaren Gel, the Flector Patch and liquid Pennsaid.

Roger Chou, MD, professor of medicine, division of general medicine and geriatrics, School of Medicine, Oregon Health & Science University, Portland.

blood thinner *warfarin* (Coumadin), may be affected. For a list of potential drugs that may interact with CBD, go to MedLinePlus.gov and search "cannabidiol."

HOW TO USE CBD

Even though hemp-derived CBD oil is legal in many states, the federal Drug Enforcement Agency still classifies CBD as an illegal narcotic due to its association with the marijuana plant. To avoid any issues related to the federal regulations, which are being sorted out in the courts, CBD products often are labeled "hemp oil."

When using this type of CBD product, follow label instructions for dosing, starting low and gradually increasing the dose until you get the desired result. Response to CBD is very individualized. If you have questions, you can consult a health-care professional who has experience prescribing CBD. CBD is available for oral use in tincture and capsules. There also are lotions, creams and other topicals that are useful for arthritis, migraines and other painful conditions and skin ailments such as acne and psoriasis.

To ensure purity and quality: Look for a non-GMO hemp oil product that has a certificate of analysis (check the company's website), stating the amount of the various cannabinoids and terpenes, and that it does not contain chemical solvents, pesticides, mold or bacteria.

Most important, look for a reputable manufacturer, some of which are listed here: CV Sciences (CVSciences.com)...Charlotte's Web (CWHemp.com)...and Elixinol (Elixinol.com). You also can purchase the CBD that I prescribe to my patients at CassMD.com/hempoil.

The Legal Fight Over CBD

James Anthony, Esq., an attorney in Oakland, California, specializing in cannabis-related law.

You can buy CBD—cannabidiol, the therapeutic yet noneuphoria-inducing marijuana component—online and in some health-food stores even if your state doesn't allow it. But is it legal to do so?

That's now being battled out in federal courts. While a US law makes it legal to sell marijuana-plant products such as hemp and hemp oil that have only trace amounts of THC (the compound in marijuana that makes people high), the Federal Drug Enforcement Agency still classifies CBD (the marijuana compound that doesn't make people high) as an illegal narcotic—like heroin.

As a consumer, though, you're almost certainly safe—it's highly unlikely that you'd get into legal trouble for buying or using a CBD product. The real target of the federal prohibition seems to be sellers, not buyers.

If your state allows the sale of medical marijuana—you can find out by going to Governing.com and searching for "marijuana map"—go to a state-licensed dispensary. If your state doesn't allow medical marijuana and you want to try using CBD, you still might be able to find it for sale...if not, you always have the option of ordering online.

CHAPTER 22

Drug-Free Protocols for Pain Relief

Live Pain-Free Without Drugs

Chronic pain from an injury, arthritis or nerve damage can be so uncomfortable that the sufferer will do almost anything to relieve it—including regularly using over-the-counter (OTC) painkillers that can cause stomach upset, internal bleeding and even death...and/or prescription narcotics that can lead to addiction and cognitive impairment.

But chronic pain sufferers often do not need these drugs...or can take them far less often. *Newest thinking on when—and when not—to take drugs for pain...*

SAFER WAYS TO MANAGE PAIN

More and more scientific evidence now shows that various nondrug approaches can be highly effective in fighting chronic pain.

It's well-known that people who are overweight can help curb their pain by losing weight and reducing the mechanical stress placed on the body. But recent research has uncovered another key factor—fatty tissue actually secretes inflammatory compounds that increase pain and pain-sensitivity. *Other nondrug approaches to relieve chronic pain...**

1. Exercise the right amount. Some chronic pain sufferers avoid exercise, while others overdo it. But exercise can help.

A recent study found that the majority of back patients who performed stretching and strengthening exercises for 15 minutes, three days a week—with a day off in between to allow muscles to recover—had a 50% reduction in pain. The patients were allowed to use the painkiller hydrocodone with acetaminophen, but only as needed. In those who used medi-

*The nondrug approaches described in this article can be used at the same time, but it is helpful to initially use them one at a time for one to two weeks each so you can determine which approach works best for you.

Vijay Vad, MD, a sports medicine physician and researcher specializing in minimally invasive arthritis therapies at the Hospital for Special Surgery in New York City. Dr. Vad is the author of *Stop Pain: Inflammation Relief for an Active Life*. VijayVad.com

cation but didn't exercise, pain was reduced by only 33%.

Why does exercise help? For one thing, it increases blood flow to injured tissues. This promotes a flow of nutrients that accelerates healing and reduces pain. Exercise also increases the body's production of endorphins, neurotransmitters that have effects that are similar to morphine and other narcotic painkillers.

Important: Exercise must be tailored to each individual to help strengthen specific parts of the body and avoid additional injury. Walking and swimming are good choices for most patients because they put little stress on muscles and joints. If you're not sure what type of exercise and/or how much would be best for your chronic pain, consult your doctor or a physical therapist.

2. Supplement with vitamin D. Low vitamin D levels have been linked to chronic pain—in part because the vitamin curbs inflammation. You can potentially get enough vitamin D from sun exposure, but up to one-third of Americans are deficient. Most people can get adequate vitamin D by spending 10 to 15 minutes in the sun without sunscreen twice a week. Sunscreen should be used at other times.

In people who suffer more pain in the winter, it may have less to do with cold temperatures than with the lack of sunshine and vitamin D production. Because food generally does not provide significant levels of the vitamin, I suggest taking a vitamin D supplement.

Typical dose: 1,000 IU to 2,500 IU daily. To determine the best dose for you, get an annual blood test to check your vitamin D level.

3. Take ginger or turmeric daily. Both are potent anti-inflammatories that reduce pain as effectively as ibuprofen and other NSAIDs. They do this by blocking the enzyme COX-2, which causes inflammation. Unlike NSAIDs, ginger and turmeric do not block the COX-1 enzyme—a lack of COX-1 is what leads to gastric bleeding.

Scientific evidence: A yearlong study published in the journal *Osteoarthritis and Cartilage* found that participants with osteoarthritis of the knee who took ginger supplements had significant relief from knee pain. Other studies have found that turmeric also can reduce pain from knee osteoarthritis.

Typical dose: Follow label instructions. Ginger and turmeric supplements are available at most health-food stores.

Caution: Ginger and turmeric have mild blood-thinning effects. If you take *warfarin* (Coumadin) or another blood-thinning medication, or medications to lower blood sugar or blood pressure, check with your doctor before using ginger or turmeric supplements.

4. Use fish oil. It's well established that omega-3 fatty acids in fish can help reduce cardiovascular disease, arthritis and other conditions. That's because omega-3s are among the most potent anti-inflammatory agents found in nature.

Scientific evidence: A study at the University of Pittsburgh School of Medicine found that 59% of patients with neck or back pain who were given omega-3s experienced enough pain reduction that they were able to stop using NSAIDs.

Typical dose: 2,000 mg daily.

Caution: Fish oil can have a mild blood-thinning effect, so consult your doctor before taking it.

5. Take care of your mental health. Patients with chronic pain tend to experience higher-than-normal levels of stress, fatigue and depression—all of which, in turn, increase pain in most patients.

If you're depressed—symptoms include changes in sleep habits, difficulty concentrating, unexplained changes in appetite and/or a loss of interest in things that you used to enjoy—see a therapist. About 20% to 25% of patients with both chronic pain and depression will experience a significant reduction in pain just from treating the depression.

6. Increase REM sleep. Patients who don't get enough rapid eye movement (REM) sleep tend to be more sensitive to pain. Researchers speculate that decreased amounts of this deep sleep boost levels of amino acids, such as glutamate, which increase pain signal transmission.

You can't directly target REM when increasing sleep. However, those who get a good night's sleep naturally get more REM.

My advice: To promote restful sleep, spend a few minutes doing deep-breathing exercises just before you go to bed. Breathing slowly and deeply stimulates the lower lobes of the lungs and activates the part of the nervous system that reduces stress as well as pain.

FOR ACUTE PAIN...

Acute pain should be promptly treated with lifestyle measures as well as prescription or OTC painkillers. Pain that is reduced or eliminated within six to eight weeks is less likely to become a lifelong problem than pain that isn't treated quickly.

Important: If you're suffering from acute or chronic pain but don't know the cause, see your doctor.

The Natural Pain Cures You Need to Try

Heather Tick, MD, clinical associate professor in both the departments of family medicine, and anesthesiology and pain medicine. She is the author of *Holistic Pain Relief.*

If you're among the estimated 25% of adults in the US who live with moderate-to-severe chronic pain, from conditions such as arthritis, headaches and fibromyalgia, you may be so desperate for relief that you decide to try a powerful opioid—and take your chances with side effects.

Sadly, these drugs don't stop the root cause of the pain—they simply block the intensity of pain signals that a patient feels. While opioids can be appropriate for acute conditions (including broken bones and postsurgical pain), they rarely are the best choice for chronic pain.

What's more, a recent study published in *JAMA: The Journal of the American Medical Association* found that long-acting opioids, such as OxyContin or *fentanyl* (Duragesic), increase one's risk for death by 65%—due to heart attack and other cardiovascular events.

THE PAIN MEDICINE PARADOX

It's an unfortunate paradox that pain medicine can actually worsen pain. In fact, researchers are now finding that patients who are weaned off opioids, using such nondrug therapies as physical therapy and relaxation exercises instead, actually can experience less pain than they did while on opioids, and they have a greater sense of well-being and function better.

Here's what happens: It's relatively easy to develop a tolerance to an opioid, which requires increasingly higher doses for the drug to work. Even when properly prescribed, chronic high doses of these medications can trigger a condition called hyperalgesia, which results in new pain sensitivity either in the primary area of pain or in a new area. For example, a patient who takes an opioid for low-back pain may begin to develop neck pain and headaches.

The good news: Nonopioid therapies that stimulate the parasympathetic nervous system—the branch of the nervous system that helps us feel calm and relaxed—can be highly effective for pain relief. *Here are ways to trigger the parasympathetic system's pain-fighting mechanism...**

• **Autogenic training.** Autogenic training (AT) is a relaxation technique based on a set of affirmations (self-directed statements) that are designed to reverse the physical effects of stress. You can buy AT recordings online, in which a person with a soothing voice says the affirmations...or you can repeat them to yourself or make your own recording, using a script like the one below.

What to do: Sit or lie in a comfortable, quiet room. Repeat each of the following statements three times, then dwell on each statement for about 30 seconds afterward. Try to truly feel each sensation in the script. Do this daily.

I am completely calm.

*Consult your doctor before trying these methods or the supplement described here—especially if you take blood thinners or have a chronic medical condition such as hypertension.

My arms feel heavy and warm.
My legs feel heavy and warm.
My heartbeat is calm and regular.
My abdomen is warm and comfortable.
My forehead is pleasantly cool.
My shoulders are heavy and warm.

• **Ujjayi breathing.** Stress causes us to breathe shallowly from the chest instead of deeply from the belly. This leaves stale air trapped in the bottom of the lungs and hinders delivery of healing oxygen to muscles. Any deep-breathing technique can stimulate the parasympathetic system, but Ujjayi (pronounced oo-ja-EE) breathing is particularly effective.

What to do: To get the hang of this technique, inhale deeply through your nose and exhale through your open mouth, gently constricting the muscles at the back of your throat and making a HAAAH sound, as if you were trying to fog up a mirror. Then try to make the same sound on the inhale.

Once you've achieved the correct sound, close your mouth and breathe in and out through your nose, making the HAAAH sound on both the inhale and exhale. Spend equal time (at a pace that's comfortable for you) inhaling and exhaling several times a day. When you first start this technique, try to do it for six minutes at a time. You can work up to 15 to 20 minutes at a time.

Important: If you have a favorite deep-breathing technique of your own, feel free to use that—just be sure that you keep the flow of air constant, and you don't hold your breath for longer than a beat. Otherwise, you will stimulate the sympathetic nervous system, triggering the pain response.

ANOTHER NONDRUG SOLUTION

In addition to the approaches described above, the following supplement can help ease pain by reducing inflammation...

• **Turmeric.** This mildly bitter spice is a powerful analgesic with impressive anti-inflammatory powers. A 2014 study suggested it may be as effective as ibuprofen in reducing the pain of knee osteoarthritis.

Capsules are one option to try. But if you like the taste, try making "Golden Milk."

What to do: Combine one-quarter cup of turmeric with one-half cup of water in a pot, and blend to create a thick paste. Heat gently, adding a pinch of ground black pepper and drizzling in water as needed to maintain a thick but stirrable consistency.

Refrigerate the mixture in a glass container, and add one heaping teaspoon to an eight-ounce glass of warm water mixed with a little almond milk every day. You can add some honey to cut the bitterness. Or use warm broth instead of water and a dash of ginger and/or garlic for a tasty soup.

To Fight Chronic Pain, Wear This Under Your Clothes

Gary Kaye, founder and chief content officer, Tech50+, Oxford, Connecticut.

Study titled "Transcutaneous electrical nerve stimulation: review of effectiveness" by researchers at Leeds Metropolitan University, UK, published in *Nursing Standard.*

Chronic pain can be insidious. But what if you could relieve chronic pain almost anywhere in your body just by wearing a discreet band on your leg?

There is a new product on the market that makes that claim—and believe it or not, it has received FDA approval.

It's called Quell, and it's a band that you strap around your lower leg to stop pain you're feeling in your neck, back, shoulder and elsewhere on your body (although it doesn't work for headaches). The device, designed by researchers from MIT and Harvard, has been approved by the Food and Drug Administration as a medical device that can be sold to the public without a prescription for relief of chronic pain. It can be used while you're awake and/or while you're sleeping.

AN ESTABLISHED TREATMENT

The basic technology underlying the Quell device has been around for decades—transcutaneous electrical nerve stimulation (TENS). If you've had physical therapy, you may have had TENS—tiny electrodes attached to your body and hooked up to a battery pack deliver a tingling sensation. These neural pulses are believed to release natural brain chemicals that block pain signals. With Quell, the technology has been adapted and miniaturized so you can wear it.

While TENS doesn't work for every patient, studies show that it can relieve pain in many people with conditions such as chronic low-back pain, neuropathy (nerve pain) and fibromyalgia. A recent meta-analysis of randomized clinical studies found strong evidence that TENS is more effective than placebo for chronic musculoskeletal pain and moderate evidence that it is effective for neuropathy. "In addition," the report said, "the general consensus from clinical experience is that TENS helps patients to manage their pain."

SHOULD YOU TRY IT?

Because the FDA approved Quell based on the efficacy of the underlying TENS technology, the company didn't need to submit independent studies showing that the Quell device itself is effective. But an earlier version called Sensus was tested with physicians who used it on their chronic-pain patients, and more than 50% of the patients were still using it six months later, a sign that they were getting relief. According to the company, two-thirds of Quell users take less pain medication and 81% report an improvement in chronic pain. The company also offers a 60-day money-back guarantee in case Quell doesn't work for you. That said, it would be preferable if there were published, peer-reviewed studies of the new device.

If you decide to give it your own personal trial, let your doctor know—especially if you are being treated for a chronic pain condition. That way, you can monitor your progress together and work out any issues as you attempt to reduce your use of pain medications. While this nerve stimulation is generally safe and without significant side effects—one reason the FDA has approved it for use without prescription—it should not be used if you have a cardiac pacemaker, implanted defibrillator or any other implanted metallic or electronic device...if you are prone to seizures...or if you are pregnant. (Nor does it work for every kind of pain, such as migraine pain, although there's another wearable device for that, Cefaly.)

The cost, which at present is not covered by insurance, is about $299 for the device—plus about $30 a month for replacement electrodes. You can learn more at QuellRelief.com.

Acupuncture: The Go-To Pain Fighter

Roger Batchelor, DAOM, LAc, doctor of acupuncture and Oriental medicine and associate professor of acupuncture at the National University of Natural Medicine in Portland, Oregon.

Got a backache? If you're like most people, you probably reach for a bottle of *ibuprofen* (Motrin). If the pain is more severe—say, a broken bone or a piercing ache after surgery—you, like millions of Americans, may be prescribed a highly addictive opioid, such as *oxycodone* (OxyContin) or *hydrocodone* (Vicodin).

Now: Acupuncture, an ancient form of healing that has been practiced and refined for centuries, is increasingly being used in the US as the go-to treatment for pain relief. About three million American adults receive acupuncture each year, with chronic pain being the number-one reason—whether it's back, neck or shoulder pain, chronic headache or osteoarthritis.

HOW ACUPUNCTURE EASES PAIN

If the thought of being stuck with needles sounds more pain-inducing than pain-relieving, there are a few details you need to know. It's true that acupuncture involves "needling"—or the insertion of needles through your skin. But it's worth noting that the typical acupuncture needle is sterile and no wider than a strand of hair.

When these needles are inserted by a skilled acupuncturist, it doesn't hurt. The most that some people feel is a mild tingling or pinprick sensation at the outset. During a typical session for a pain-related condition, the acupuncturist might use 10 to 20 needles, often placed in such areas as the limbs, back and scalp.

The needles are inserted into specific "acupoints" throughout the body, based on the ancient Chinese philosophy that our health is governed by the uninterrupted flow of qi (pronounced "chee"), or bioenergy, through the body. According to the principles of traditional Chinese medicine, when one's bioenergy becomes blocked, it builds up like water behind a dam, leading to pain and/or dysfunction. Needling a combination of acupoints—there are thousands of them—can relieve qi blockages and elicit the body's natural healing response.

Needling also signals the brain and spinal cord to produce chemicals and hormones, such as endorphins, that function as the body's own pain relievers, as well as natural anti-inflammatory compounds.

The result: Less need for pain medication. Many patients also feel less stress and sleep better following acupuncture—benefits that also help them cope with pain.

So what happens when you go for acupuncture? You'll be asked to lie on an exam table for the treatment. You can usually remain clothed, though you may need to remove a shirt or your socks, for example, if they are covering an area that will be needled. In some cases, you may prefer to change into a gown provided by the practitioner. You can expect to see your acupuncturist once or twice weekly for five to 10 sessions that last about one hour each. Not all insurance (including Medicare) covers acupuncture. Check with your insurer.

ACUPUNCTURE FOR OPIOID WITHDRAWAL

On the heels of a shocking report that more than 64,000 Americans died from drug overdoses in 2016, the US Department of Health & Human Services recently declared the abuse of pain-relieving opioids a public health emergency.

Not only does acupuncture lessen the need for opioids, it can help opioid-addicted individuals through the painful withdrawal process. When a person addicted to opioids first quits, he/she will experience unpleasant withdrawal symptoms, including insomnia, pain, leg cramps, irritability, nausea and constipation.

Medications such as *methadone* (Dolophine or Methadose) and *buprenorphine* (Subutex) are prescribed to ease withdrawal but tend to backfire. Methadone must be taken daily, with each dose providing pain relief for about four to eight hours. However, methadone is highly addictive, and misuse of this drug can be fatal. Buprenorphine can cause side effects such as muscle aches, nausea, constipation, sleep problems, irritability and more.

Acupuncture, on the other hand, has no side effects...may help prevent relapse...quells cravings...and does not require the patient to take yet another drug.

It's all about the ears: When treating people addicted to opioids, many acupuncturists follow an auricular, or ear-focused, acupuncture protocol endorsed by the US National Acupuncture Detoxification Association (NADA). Auricular acupuncture is based on the belief that points on the ears correspond to different areas of the brain and body. The NADA-approved protocol, also called acudetox or 5-Needle or 5NP ear acupuncture protocol, involves inserting three to five needles into each ear at specific points.

For opioids such as OxyContin, one to three months of daily acupuncture are needed to get through the worst of the detox process.

To get more information on the NADA-approved protocol, visit AcuDetox.com. For general pain relief, you can find an acupuncturist with multiple years of training and certification at NCCAOM.org.

A NEWER APPROACH

With electroacupuncture (EA), a newer form of acupuncture that was developed in the 1950s, the needles may be connected to a small unit that provides painless mild electrical stimulation. The electricity mimics the act of a practitioner physically maneuvering the needle, sending a stronger signal to the body. Even though you may feel a mild electric tingle with electroacupuncture, it is not uncomfortable and should feel relaxing.

Numerous studies show that different types of naturally occurring pain-relieving hormones are released at different EA frequencies. Needles are typically left in for 20 to 40 minutes.

Important finding: In a study in the journal *Pain*, women who received EA prior to abdominal surgery needed 60% less morphine in the 24 hours following the operation. Besides reducing the need for addictive pain medications, acupuncture also counters the most common side effects of opioids—including nausea, dizziness, urinary retention, constipation and lethargy.

Note: People with pacemakers should avoid EA to prevent unnecessary interference with the device.

WHAT ABOUT ACUPRESSURE

For certain conditions, acupressure—applying pressure or massaging acupoints—can be as effective as acupuncture.

How it works: Massaging one point on the body can relieve symptoms in other parts of the body via pathways called meridians.

You can try acupressure for 30 to 60 seconds once or more daily on yourself or another person for…

Frontal headache: Massage the fleshy spot between the thumb and pointer finger with firm pressure. This point is known as Large Intestine 4.

Neck pain: Massage the spot located below the base of the skull, in the space between the two vertical neck muscles. This point is known as Gallbladder 20.

Note: During opioid withdrawal or after surgery, traditional acupuncture is more appropriate than acupressure.

Do Magnets Work for Pain?

Michael Weintraub, MD, clinical professor of neurology at New York Medical College in Valhalla, and Mt. Sinai School of Medicine in New York City.

Hard floors and old shoes may leave you with foot, leg and back pain. Do the "as-seen-on-TV" magnets you step on work to relieve body aches?

Not really, says Michael Weintraub, MD, clinical professor of neurology at New York Medical College in Valhalla, and Mt. Sinai School of Medicine in New York City. Most "therapeutic" magnets sold in malls and on television don't work—but that doesn't mean magnet therapy is bunk.

In a landmark study of 375 people published in 2003 in *Archives of Physical Medicine and Rehabilitation*, Dr. Weintraub showed that wearing magnetic insoles constantly for four months provided significant relief for many people with diabetic foot pain and numbness.

Medical magnets also help some individuals with finger, wrist, neck or back pain. According to a Mt. Sinai/University of Tennessee study, magnets worn on the abdomen can lessen disability from chronic pelvic pain in women. Magnets come in many different forms, including knee braces, wrist wraps and bracelets.

No one knows why magnets often are effective in relieving pain.

One popular theory: Magnets increase blood flow, boosting the delivery of oxygen and nutrients to the affected tissues. The stronger the magnet (measured in a unit called a gauss), the better the relief. A typical refrigerator magnet measures 10 gauss and has no effect on pain. Effective therapeutic magnets seem to range in strength from 450 gauss to more than 10,000 gauss. However, Dr. Weintraub points out that manufacturers usually do not list the strength of magnets and, when they do, the numbers often are wrong. Two reputable brands—Nikken (888-669-8859, Nikken.com) and Bioflex Medical Magnets, Inc. (864-310-6370, BaermannMagnetics.com).

Use magnets throughout the day for several weeks to see whether they work for you.

Helpful: Keep a pain journal to gauge their effect over time.

Although therapeutic magnets have no known side effects, consult your doctor before treating pain with magnets. They usually are not recommended for pregnant women or people with internal defibrillators, pacemakers or insulin pumps. Nor should they be placed over drug-delivery patches or open wounds.

Homeopathy Help for Pain and More

Edward Shalts, MD, DHt, a homeopathic doctor with a private practice in New York City. He is author of two books—*The American Institute of Homeopathy Handbook for Parents* and *Easy Homeopathy*. HomeopathyNewYork.com

Homeopathy is a type of treatment that can be used for a wide range of ailments. It uses minute doses of natural substances to stimulate the body's self-healing response. The right homeopathic remedy can shorten the duration of symptoms, with relief often beginning in as little as 15 minutes. It also can help prevent relatively benign conditions from evolving into more dangerous ones. It can reduce the dosage of conventional medication required to manage some chronic diseases or eliminate the need for medication altogether. Unlike conventional drugs, which have the potential to produce unpleasant side effects, homeopathic remedies are exceedingly safe.

Important dosage information: For the following remedies, a dose is three pills (pellets) of 30C concentration unless otherwise noted. Allow the pills to dissolve under your tongue. Also, unless otherwise noted, follow these instructions for pain relief…

If you don't notice any change in symptoms after 30 minutes, don't repeat the dose. Try another homeopathic remedy or conventional medicine.

If you feel somewhat better after 30 minutes but not completely better, repeat the dose.

If your symptoms have improved dramatically, don't take another dose unless the problem comes back.

The rule of thumb is to take no more than three doses at 30-minute intervals over two hours—if that doesn't work, talk to your doctor. Also, talk to your doctor before taking any medication or supplement.

All remedies mentioned here are available at most health-food stores and many pharmacies.

HEADACHE

• ***Iris versicolor.*** Frequently indicated for classic migraine headaches that begin with visual aura and end with vomiting. It also is for blurry vision, and sometimes even blindness during headache. Take every 15 minutes, a maximum of three times. Stop if there is a significant improvement earlier.

HERPES ZOSTER (SHINGLES)

Take one of these remedies twice a day for three days. If there is no effect or you feel worse, discontinue.

• **Apis mellifica.** For shingles lesions on the face.

• **Arsenicum album.** For burning pain.

• **Ranunculus bulbosus.** The remedy of choice for shingles on the left side of the chest.

INDIGESTION

Take either of the following three times a day for one day. Stop if the condition improves earlier. Also, discontinue if there is no effect after three doses.

• **Nux vomica.** For indigestion from overeating in general, along with irritability and cramping pains.

INSECT BITES AND STINGS

Take either remedy below every 15 minutes for a total of three times.

• **Apis mellifica.** For stings and bites from bees and other small insects, such as spiders.

What Is Rolfing?

Structural Integration (SI) is a bodywork technique that focuses on the fascia, the protective connective tissue that surrounds the muscles. Founded by Ida P. Rolf, the technique also is sometimes known as "rolfing." SI therapists use pressure and stretching to lengthen and manipulate fascia to enhance body alignment and balance. SI is based on the theory that through the force of gravity and injury, the body's structure becomes misaligned…and fascia shortens, resulting in pain and stiffness. I find that SI is helpful for those with muscle or spine pain. You can find out about practitioners near you from the Rolf Institute of Structural Integration, Rolf.org, 303-449-5903.

Mark A. Stengler, NMD, a naturopathic doctor and founder of the Stengler Center for Integrative Medicine in Encinitas, California. He is author or coauthor of numerous books, including *The Natural Physician's Healing Therapies* and *Bottom Line's Prescription for Natural Cures*, and author of the newsletter *Health Revelations*. MarkStengler.com

The site of the bite is typically hot to the touch, red and swollen.

• **Ledum palustre.** For stings and bites by large insects (wasps, for example). The site of the bite is cold to the touch and has a bluish tinge.

SPRAINS AND STRAINS

Take any of the remedies listed below three times a day for two to three days. Discontinue after three days.

• **Arnica montana.** For a sore, bruised feeling. Often indicated for people who have over-exercised after a long break.

• **Bryonia alba.** For ankle sprains and strains.

• **Rhus toxicodendron.** The most frequently recommended remedy for these conditions. You also can apply Rhus tox ointment twice a day.

WRIST CONDITIONS

• **Ruta graveolens.** A specific remedy for wrist problems. Take three times a day for three days. For long-standing wrist strain, take three 12C pellets once a day every day for a month.

STRESS

• **Nux vomica.** For overworked, stressed-out, career-oriented people. Also for anger in people who work many hours in a row and are on edge and whose nerves feel raw. Take the dose. Repeat after 15 minutes, then again after another 15 minutes.

Craniosacral Therapy Helps Chronic Pain

Thomas A. Kruzel, ND, practices CST at the Rockwood Natural Medicine Clinic in Scottsdale, Arizona. He is the former vice president of clinical affairs and chief medical officer at the Southwest College of Naturopathic Medicine in Phoenix.

Can a gentle scalp massage really cure illnesses and injuries as diverse as carpal tunnel syndrome and Bell's palsy—not to mention healing long-ago trauma and emotional distress? As a matter of fact, it can—if you put yourself in the hands of a trained and skilled craniosacral therapist. Of the many alternative therapies, craniosacral therapy (CST) is surely one of the most unusual. CST is a variation of osteopathic and chiropractic medicine, where a therapist gently places his/her hands atop your skull and feels for the oscillation frequency—the small degree of movement that the skull bones naturally retain throughout life. This is a subtle motion of the membrane encasing the cerebrospinal fluid in the brain and spinal cord down to the sacrum, the bone at the bottom of the spine. The therapist gently manipulates the bones to bring them back into proper alignment. It feels like a very gentle massage, but CST is a potent healing therapy for a wide variety of disorders, including chronic pain, headaches, carpal tunnel syndrome, fibromyalgia, learning disabilities, depression, post-traumatic stress disorder, vertigo, whiplash injury, TMJ, herniated disc pain and musculoskeletal problems. While surprising and somewhat inexplicable, even many skeptics acknowledge that "sometimes it just works."

HOW CST WORKS

CST is based on research from the early part of the last century by osteopathic doctor William Garner Sutherland, DO. His work centered on the theory that the skull bones have a rhythm that he called the "breath of life" and others call "the vital force." The theory now associated with CST, besides one of treating illness, is that physical or emotional trauma, even from birth, can cause a disturbance in this oscillation that can last for years. Cerebrospinal fluid affects nerves that control all tissues in the body, so any disruption can contribute to a wide range of problems. It's believed that restoring its natural flow enables the body to begin healing itself.

Here in the US, thousands of osteopathic doctors, naturopathic doctors, chiropractors and massage therapists are also CST practitioners. But you probably won't be surprised to learn that the medical world considers CST just this side of loony. Skeptics say its very basis is impossible because the skull bones fuse completely in childhood. CST practitioners respond that this is not so—the skull bones have motion throughout life. They say that even the elderly continue to respond well to CST.

The concept of opening up cerebrospinal fluid flow is connected to underlying chiropractic principles in which "communication channels" are realigned throughout the body. CST does not itself heal problems—it releases inertia and congestion, thereby returning homeostasis and enhancing the body's ability to heal and regulate itself.

According to Thomas Kruzel, ND, a CST practitioner, the hardest part of his CST training was learning to discern the motion in the skull, which he describes as something like an undulation. When a patient comes to see him, he places his hands on his/her head to get an exact sense of this person's motion. This gives him information he uses in clearing restrictions in the pumping of the fluid through the brain, into the spinal column and the emanating nerve roots. Sometimes he may also gently manipulate the lower part of the spine in an osteopathic fashion to restore tandem movement in the sacrum and the spine.

WHAT WILL YOU FEEL?

Patients don't always feel the change as it is occurring, he says, but they often experience a kind of gastrointestinal release such as a gurgling in the bowels when the fluid is freed up.

Injury victims can benefit from this procedure. One of Dr. Kruzel's patients had been severely injured in a car accident. She had many broken bones and went through a year of physical rehab, but even after her physical injuries had healed she struggled with depression and pain. When she came to Dr. Kruzel, he found that she had almost no cranial motion because the flow of the fluid had been truncated when her pelvis broke. He treated her regularly for a time and today she is doing very well physically and mentally.

Patients remain fully clothed for CST treatment. Sessions usually last 30 minutes to one hour. Patients may come only one or two times, or several times a week for a number of months. Elderly patients tend to check in for a session once every few months. Costs vary by area of the country and many insurance plans cover the cost when treatment is from an osteopathic or naturopathic doctor.

The technique may seem simplistic, even magical—but craniosacral therapy is actually a precise skill a good therapist has trained long and hard to learn. You can find a CST practitioner near you by going to the site of osteopathic doctor John Upledger, DO, OMM, Upledger.com. Another resource is the Biodynamic Craniosacral Therapy Association of North America (CraniosacralTherapy.org), which provides CST standards. Since quality may vary widely in the absence of national standards, it's helpful to get a recommendation from someone you trust who has personal experience with a particular therapist.

Pet Therapy for Pain

Julia Havey, RN, senior systems analyst, department of medical center information systems, Loyola University Health System, Maywood, Illinois.

Pets can reduce the need for pain medicine. In a recent finding, patients who received pet therapy after joint-replacement surgery needed 50% less pain medicine than those who did not. Animal-assisted therapy—typically done during five- to 15-minute sessions during which the patient may talk to the animal or perhaps take the dog for a walk—improves patients' emotional and physical health.

Get More Sleep to Feel Less Pain

Timothy Roehrs, PhD, director of research, Sleep Disorders and Research Center, Henry Ford Hospital, and adjunct professor of psychiatry, department of psychiatry and behavioral neuroscience, Wayne State University, both in Detroit.

Are you suffering from chronic pain or anticipating a painful procedure such as surgery? There's a simple way to reduce your sensitivity to pain. All you need to do is get a little more sleep, a small but encouraging new study suggests.

Participants were all healthy, pain-free and mildly sleep-deprived (as confirmed by tests that measure daytime sleepiness). They habitually slept for an average of seven hours and 42 minutes per night.

Half of the participants (the control group) were instructed to maintain their usual sleep pattern for the four consecutive nights of the study, while the other half were told to spend 10 hours in bed per night. The sleep-encouraged participants ended up sleeping an average of 1.8 hours longer per night than the control group did.

Now here's the pain part. At the start and end of the four-day study period, each participant underwent pain testing using what is called a radiant heat stimulus. Volunteers were told to move their fingers away as soon as they felt any pain from the heat source. The maximum heat generated was 101.6°F—not particularly hot, but painful if a sensitive fingertip is steadily exposed to it.

Researchers measured how many seconds each participant kept his or her finger on the hole.

What they found: Volunteers who had gotten the extra sleep kept their fingers on the heat source for 10 seconds, on average—versus just eight seconds for those who had continued to short-change their slumber.

Keep in mind: The test measures the point at which people first feel pain, not their ability to tolerate pain—so the extra sleep didn't just help people "tough it out," but rather actually diminished their perception of pain.

Though this study focused only on acute pain, additional sleep probably helps reduce sensitivity to virtually any type of physical pain, whether chronic or temporary.

DRUG-FREE PAINKILLING PRESCRIPTION: ZZZZZZ

Granted, time spent in lying in bed isn't exactly equal to time spent actually sleeping. However, if you stay in bed longer than usual—nine to 10 hours is a good goal—you're bound to sleep more than usual, too.

If you know that pain lies ahead: You can plan ahead to reduce pain sensitivity before a potentially painful medical procedure (such as a root canal, elective surgery or tough physical therapy session) or grueling physical challenge (running a marathon, competing in a tennis tournament). Simply spend nine to 10 hours in bed per night for at least four nights before that pain-inducing event. While pain sensitivity may be reduced somewhat after only two or three nights of extra sleep, four or more nights generally are needed for any meaningful reduction.

If you're already in pain: The pain from an existing injury (a sore back, a broken bone) or a chronic ailment (such as arthritis) can make it tough to get even a normal amount of sleep, much less any extra rest. If that's your situation, consider talking with a naturopathic doctor about dietary changes and supplements that can help you sleep.

If these natural approaches aren't enough to completely solve your sleep problems, your doctor may suggest a short course of prescription sleep-inducing medication or a consultation at a sleep center, a specialized clinic where insomnia and other sleep problems are diagnosed and treated. To find a sleep center near you, visit the website of the American Academy of Sleep Medicine.

Change Your Sleep Position To Relieve Pain

Mary Ann Wilmarth, PT, DPT, chief of physical therapy at Harvard University in Cambridge, Massachusetts. She is also the founder and CEO of Back2Back Physical Therapy, a private practice based in Andover, Massachusetts. Back2BackPT.com

---

Sleep positions can sometimes be tricky. Certain positions can help—or worsen—common health problems.

The best—and worst—sleep positions for seven common ailments...

SHOULDER PAIN

Sleeping on your back is often a good option if you have shoulder pain. To avoid compressing shoulder nerves, tendons and/or joints, make sure that your head, neck and shoulders are in a neutral position. Put a small pillow under your head (with a rolled-up towel under your neck, if needed). You may even want to put a small towel roll or pillow under your shoulder to give it more support, if needed.

Should you sleep on your side when your shoulder hurts? And if so, which side? It depends on the cause of your shoulder pain.

For sprains and rotator cuff injuries: When opting for side-sleeping, most people with this type of shoulder pain are most comfortable hugging a pillow with the painful shoulder up.

Some people, however, are more comfortable—and hurt less in the morning—if they sleep with the painful side down. The joint will be supported by the mattress, and your weight will keep the affected shoulder from moving. Just be sure to place a pillow in front of your chest and under the painful shoulder for support.

For arthritis: The irritation and inflammation can worsen if you sleep on the painful shoulder. Keep pressure off the affected joint by lying on your back or on the other side with the arm supported by hugging a pillow.

KNEE PAIN

Do not lie on your stomach if you have knee pain—whether it's from arthritis, an injury or a surgical procedure. The pressure on the kneecap can be painful. Also, people who sleep on their stomachs often stretch out the back of the knee joint. This can cause an overextension of the hamstring and the knee joint, leading to pain in the knee or hamstring.

Better: Sleep on your side with a pillow between your knees. The pillow should be thick enough so that the top leg remains in alignment with the hip. This prevents the top hip from dropping down, which can stress the leg and the spine. The pillow reduces friction and pressure on the knees and keeps the legs in proper alignment.

Another choice: Sleep on your back. You may want to sometimes use a small pillow or towel roll under your knees.

Caution: If you have arthritis or any acute injury and use a pillow in this way often, it can increase swelling in your knees and limit the knees' range of motion. For this reason, you might need to alternate between side-lying and sleeping on your back throughout the night or on different nights.

BACK PAIN

Back-sleeping is a good position for people with back pain. However, if you're lying flat on your back, you may feel more comfortable with a pillow under your knees. This will eliminate an excessive arch between your lower back and the mattress.

Self-test: If you can easily slip your hand into an open space between your lower back and the mattress, raise your knees a little more. Your lower back should be flat against your hand.

For back pain, you may also find it comfortable to sleep on your side with a pillow between your legs.

NECK PAIN

If your neck is tight and/or painful, do not sleep on your stomach.

Reason: Unless you sleep with your face pressed into the mattress, you'll need to turn your head to the side. This puts a lot of stress on the neck joints as well as the muscles and soft tissues in the neck and upper back.

Better: Sleep on your side with a pillow under your neck. The pillow should fill the distance between your neck and shoulder. You can use a special pillow for side-sleeping with more support for your neck and a cutout for your head (available online or from home-goods stores). Alternately, you can use a rolled-up towel to give your neck more support. You also can sleep on your back as long as you don't prop up your head too high, which will strain your neck. (Usually one pillow is enough.)

FOOT PAIN

If you have extreme pain on the sole of your foot, you may have plantar fasciitis. This condition causes painful inflammation of the tissues on the bottom of the foot. If you have plantar fasciitis, it will likely worsen if you sleep on your stomach.

Reason: You generally point your feet when you're on your stomach. This shortens the muscles of the calf and soles of the feet and can cause painful cramps.

You will do better if you sleep on your back or side using a pillow between the legs. If you must sleep on your stomach, at least hang your feet over the end of the bed so that your feet and ankles are in a more neutral position.

ACID REFLUX

If a burning sensation from reflux keeps you up at night, you'll feel better if you elevate the upper half of your body with a wedge pillow, often made of foam. There are also special pillows that slip between the box spring and mattress (or under the mattress on a platform bed) to elevate the head of the bed. Risers for the head of the bed also can be used.

If you have heartburn: Sleeping on your left side often is advised. In this position, the esophagus is higher than the stomach to help prevent the backwash of stomach acid.

HOW TO CHANGE HOW YOU SLEEP

Suppose that you are a side-sleeper, but you know that you should be sleeping on your back. Before you go to sleep, think about the position that you want to maintain and start in that position. Remind yourself of this whenever you happen to wake up and return to the desired position.

It may take a few weeks (or even months), but the mental reminders and time in the desired position will eventually change the way that you sleep most of the time.

IS IT TIME TO REPLACE YOUR MATTRESS?

If you can't remember when you bought your mattress, you're probably due for a new one. Mattresses start to sag and lose their support after about eight or 10 years.

Choose a mattress that's on the firm side or firm but with some cushioning on top, such as a plush-top mattress. About every three months, rotate the mattress. Flip it over if it has two sleep sides.

Also: Invest in more pillows. You can use them in different ways when you need more support or padding—for example, between your legs, for hugging and under your knees. Depending on the size of the pillows, two to four will generally be enough to provide added support for your body.

Myotherapy: Drug-Free Help for Back, Shoulder, And Hip Pain

The late Bonnie Prudden helped create the President's Council on Youth Fitness in 1956 and was a leading authority on exercise therapy. In 2007, she received the Lifetime Achievement Award from the President's Council on Physical Fitness and Sports. She authored 18 books, including *Pain Erasure.*

Bonnie Prudden was a longtime physical fitness advocate who lived until she was 97. She was able to move pain-free despite having arthritis that led to two hip replacements by using a form of myotherapy ("myo" is Greek for muscle) that she developed more than 30 years ago.

Now: Tens of thousands of patients have successfully used this special form of myotherapy, which is designed to relieve "trigger points" (highly irritable spots in muscles) that develop throughout life due to a number of causes, such as falls, strains or disease.

By applying pressure to these sensitive areas and then slowly releasing it, it's possible to relax muscles that have gone into painful spasms, often in response to physical and/or emotional stress.

A simple process: Ask a partner (a spouse or friend, for example) to locate painful trigger points by applying his/her fingertips to parts of your body experiencing discomfort—or consult a practitioner trained in myotherapy.*

*To find a practitioner of Bonnie Prudden's myotherapy techniques, go to BonniePrudden.com. If you are unable to find a practitioner near you, call local massage therapists and ask whether they are familiar with the techniques.

If you're working with a partner, let him know when a particular spot for each body area described in this article is tender.

Pressure should be applied for seven seconds (the optimal time determined by Prudden's research to release muscle tension) each time that your partner locates such a spot.

On a scale of one to 10, the pressure should be kept in the five- to seven-point range—uncomfortable but not intolerable.

The relaxed muscles are then gently stretched to help prevent new spasms.

If you prefer to treat yourself: Use a "bodo," a wooden dowel attached to a handle, and a lightweight, metal "shepherd's crook" to locate trigger points and apply pressure. Both tools are available at 520-529-3979, BonniePrudden.com, for $10 and $39.95.

For areas that are easy to reach, use the bodo to locate trigger points and then apply pressure to erase them. For spots that are difficult to reach, use the shepherd's crook to find and apply pressure to trigger points.

As an alternative to the specially designed tools, you can use your fingers, knuckles or elbows on areas of the body that can be reached easily. Common types of pain that can be relieved by this method...*

SHOULDER PAIN

Finding the trigger point: Lie facedown while your partner uses his elbow to gently apply pressure to trigger points that can hide along the top of the shoulders and in the upper back. If you are very small or slender, your partner can use his fingers instead of his elbow.

Place one of your arms across your back at the waist while your partner slides his fingers under your shoulder blade to search for and apply pressure to additional trigger points. Repeat the process on the opposite side.

While still lying facedown, bend your elbows and rest your forehead on the backs of your hands. With his hands overlapped, your partner can gently move all 10 of his fingers along the top of the shoulder to locate additional trigger points.

Pain-erasing stretch: The "shrug" is a sequence of shoulder exercises performed four times after myotherapy and whenever shoulder tension builds.

From a standing or sitting position, round your back by dropping your head forward while bringing the backs of your arms together as close as possible in front of your body. Extend both arms back (with your thumbs leading) behind your body while tipping your head back and looking toward the ceiling.

Next, with both arms at your sides, raise your shoulders up to your earlobes, then press your shoulders down hard.

LOW-BACK PAIN

Finding the trigger point: Lie facedown while your partner stands to your right and reaches across your body to place his elbow on your buttocks in the area where the left back pocket would appear on a pair of pants. For seven seconds, your partner should slowly apply pressure to each trigger point—not straight down but angled back toward himself.

Repeat on the other side. If the pressure causes slight discomfort, your partner has found the right spot! If not, your partner should move his elbow slightly and try the steps again. Two to three trigger points can typically be found on each buttock.

Pain-erasing stretch: Lie on your left side on a flat surface (such as a bed, table or the floor). Bend your right knee and pull it as close to your chest as possible.

Next, extend your right leg, keeping it aligned with the left leg and about eight inches above it.

Finally, lower the raised leg onto the resting one and relax for three seconds. Perform these steps four times on each leg.

HIP PAIN

Finding the trigger point: The trigger points for hip pain are often found in the gluteus medius, the muscle that runs along either side of the pelvis.

Lie on your side with your knees slightly bent. Using one elbow, your partner should scan for trigger points along the gluteus medi-

*Check with your doctor before trying this therapy if you have a chronic medical condition or have suffered a recent injury.

us (in the hip area, roughly between the waist and the bottom seam of your underpants) and apply pressure straight down at each sensitive spot for seven seconds.

The same process should be repeated on the opposite side of your body.

Pain-erasing stretch: Lie on your left side on a table with your right leg hanging off the side and positioned forward. Your partner should place one hand on top of your waist and the other hand on the knee of the dangling right leg.

This knee should be gently pressed down eight times. The stretch should be repeated on the opposite side.

Spa Indulgences with Proven Health Benefits

Michael Tompkins, RN, LMT, a registered nurse and a licensed massage therapist, is CEO and general manager of Hilton Head Health, a weight loss and wellness resort in South Carolina.

Spa patrons today are very selective with their services, trending toward therapies with demonstrable results...and prime examples include the following four treatments. Each generally is safe, though it is important to check with your doctor first if you are pregnant or have a medical condition. *Consider trying...*

- **Mud therapy.** Certain types of mud contain magnesium and other beneficial minerals that moisturize and nourish the skin and help draw toxins out of pores—which is why mud therapy may ease dermatologic conditions such as acne, eczema and psoriasis.

Therapeutic mud also may help relieve arthritis pain, as several recent studies show.

What to expect: At some spas, you can take an actual mud bath, immersed up to your neck in warm mud. More typically, warm mud is applied directly to body areas that are painful (such as joints) or to areas that you want to draw toxins from, such as the face. The treated area is wrapped in gauze for 20 minutes or so...then the wrapping is removed and the mud rinsed away.

Note: Therapeutic mud usually has a strong sulfur smell, which some people may find unpleasant.

- **Mineral water bath.** The special water used for this treatment is rich in minerals such as magnesium, potassium, calcium, sodium and sulfur, which are thought to have anti-inflammatory, antibacterial and/or moisturizing properties. In addition to research demonstrating benefits for improving the skin condition psoriasis, several recent European studies showed encouraging results from treating osteoarthritis with mineral water baths.

How it is done: You soak some or all of your body (up to the neck) in a tub full of warm mineral water for 15 to 30 minutes.

- **Massage.** A massage not only feels fantastic and leaves you blissfully relaxed, it also loosens tight muscles and releases waste products (such as lactic acid) that can lead to muscle stiffness and soreness. Numerous studies show additional benefits—for instance, massage can help alleviate pain, including chronic low-back pain...reduce blood pressure...boost the immune response and promote healing in patients suffering from burns or cancer...reduce aggression...ease depression...and improve sleep.

There are many types of massage.* While some people like intense hands-on pressure, massage does not have to be painful to be therapeutic. *Options...*

- Swedish massage, the most popular, combines kneading and long muscle strokes using light to medium pressure.
- Hot stone massage uses the warmth of basalt stones to penetrate muscles, loosening them prior to gentle, relaxing tissue manipulation.
- Shiatsu massage aims to restore the natural flow of energy to your meridian points through gentle finger and palm pressure.
- Thai massage combines rhythmic holds and stretches that promote energy flow while reducing tension.

*To seek out massage therapists trained in healing therapy, visit Associated Bodywork & Massage Professionals at MassageTherapy.com, for a therapist in your area.

- Deep tissue massage is intense, using maximum pressure to release chronic muscle tension.
- Athlete's massage involves intense, constant pressure with targeted stretching.

- **Reflexology.** This therapy is based on the concept that certain areas of the foot correspond to various parts of the body. For instance, the toes are associated with the head and neck...the arch of the foot corresponds to the internal organs...and the ball of the foot corresponds to the chest and lungs. By applying manual pressure to certain zones on the foot, reflexologists aim to remove energy blockages and bring the body into ideal balance. From a Western perspective, studies show that stimulating and massaging the foot can reduce fatigue and stress, promote circulation and strengthen immunity.

Evidence: In a Korean study, middle-aged women were trained to do reflexology on themselves daily for six weeks. By the end of the study, participants showed significant improvement in measures of stress, depression and immune system response, plus reduced systolic blood pressure.

Recommended: If you want a genuine reflexology experience (rather than a simple foot massage), confirm that the spa's reflexologist is certified by the American Reflexology Certification Board or a state certification program.

Gua Sha: Hands-On Therapy For Muscle and Joint Pain

Arya Nielsen, PhD, licensed acupuncturist and gua sha researcher, department of integrative medicine, The Center for Health and Healing, Beth Israel Medical Center, New York City. Dr. Nielsen, considered the Western authority on gua sha, is author of *Gua Sha: A Traditional Technique for Modern Practice.* GuaSha.com

You may never have heard of gua sha—but if you experience recurrent muscle or joint pain, particularly in the back, neck or shoulder, this drug-free hands-on therapy is certainly worth learning about.

An East Asian healing technique, gua sha (pronounced gwah sah) is typically performed by an acupuncturist, but no needles are used. Instead, the practitioner uses a round-edged, handheld instrument on a particular area of the body to repeatedly "press-stroke" (stroke while applying gentle pressure) without breaking the skin.

The purpose is to alleviate what in Chinese medicine is called "blood stagnation." The press-stroking motion forces red blood cells out of the tiny capillaries and into the surrounding tissues. The capillaries are not broken and there is no external bleeding. However, numerous tiny reddish spots of blood called petechiaedo appear just beneath the skin's surface, giving the area a rashlike appearance. (This is not the same as bruising—a bruise represents traumatic damage to the tissue and can take a week or more to heal, but with gua sha the tissue is not damaged.) The red blood cells immediately begin to be reabsorbed. This stimulates the immune system, promoting healing over a period of days.

IF YOU WANT TO GIVE GUA SHA A TRY...

Gua sha often is done on the back, neck, shoulders and hips, though it can be used on other parts of the body. Sometimes the area treated is the painful spot itself, but other times it is an area that corresponds with a certain organ or body channel (meridian), according to the traditions of Eastern medicine.

A gua sha session usually lasts about 10 minutes.

To the patient, gua sha feels invigorating. It does not hurt if done correctly. Even babies and children can be treated without a problem. The red marks raised on the skin immediately begin to change and fade and are completely gone within a few days. After a session, it is best to drink water and moderate your activity.

The number of sessions needed varies based on patients' conditions. The cost of treatment depends on the training of the practitioner and your location, as with most medical treatments. Check your insurance—it may pay for the treatment if it covers care by an acupuncturist.

Gua sha often can be safely used even on people who have a condition such as diabetes, who are pregnant or who use anticoagulant medication, but for safety's sake, it is essential to be treated by a qualified licensed practitioner who is trained in gua sha. Acupuncturists often have such training, as do some physical therapists and massage therapists. To find a practitioner, contact licensed acupuncturists in your area and ask about their level of experience with the technique. You can find nearby acupuncturists and verify their licensure through your state's department of public health, office of consumer affairs, office of professional regulators or similar agency.

Lasers That Relieve Pain, Lasers That Heal

Mark A. Stengler, NMD, naturopathic doctor and founder of the Stengler Center for Integrative Medicine in Encinitas, California. He is author or coauthor of numerous books, including *The Natural Physician's Healing Therapies* and *Bottom Line's Prescription for Natural Cures*, and author of the newsletter *Health Revelations*. MarkStengler.com

Cold laser therapy, so called because it is unlike older types of lasers that use very hot, high-energy beams of light, also is known as low-level laser treatment (LLLT). I use LLLT in my clinic to relieve many types of musculoskeletal pain, including arthritis and strained or inflamed muscles, joints, tendons and ligaments.

HOW IT WORKS

LLLT uses different wavelengths to penetrate to varying depths—from just below the skin's surface to four to five inches deep. Depending on the area being treated, the therapy may employ one or more wavelengths during a treatment session. The laser in my clinic, like many others now in use, enables me to vary the frequency of wavelengths.

Once these photons reach their target depth, they produce a variety of effects that help reduce pain and accelerate healing by...

- **Improving blood vessel dilation,** which increases blood flow to the treated area.
- **Inhibiting the pain-signaling activity of nerve cells.**
- **Increasing production of serotonin,** the neurotransmitter associated with well-being.
- **Enhancing immune activity in the area being treated.**

Numerous studies have demonstrated LLLT's effectiveness. One 2009 study published in *The Lancet* was an analysis of 16 randomized controlled studies of LLLT for neck pain. The researchers concluded that patients were about 70% more likely to experience reduced pain following LLLT, compared with those given a placebo treatment. Similarly, a 2008 study published in *American Journal of Sports Medicine* found that recreational athletes with chronic Achilles tendinopathy who received LLLT combined with therapeutic exercises had faster recovery times. The laser group recovered after four weeks of treatment, compared with 12 weeks for the control group, which received no laser therapy.

When I use LLLT, I usually pass the laser over the affected area for five to 10 minutes per treatment. I often administer one to two treatments per week until symptoms resolve. Many people notice at least some improvement in pain, soreness and stiffness after just one treatment, and 90% of my patients notice a significant reduction in pain within two to three treatments. Benefits can last from weeks to months depending on the individual and the problem being treated. If desired, LLLT also can be used in conjunction with other therapies, such as physical therapy, anti-inflammatory medications and acupuncture. Laser treatments for conditions such as sinusitis and tinnitus work similarly.

Here's an example: Joe, 40 years old, had had acute sinusitis for two days. He was very uncomfortable because of the pressure-like pain in his head. In addition to treating him with nutritional supplements for sinusitis, I also performed a laser treatment. His symptoms cleared up immediately. For the next four hours, mucus drained from his nostrils, relieving his symptoms completely.

LLLT typically costs $50 to $75 per session. Some health insurance companies cover it. Many naturopathic doctors, physiotherapists, chiropractors and acupuncturists, as well as some holistic medical doctors, are trained in LLLT. When choosing a practitioner, ask whether he/she has attended formal seminars in this type of therapy.

People with cancerous tumors should not have this treatment because it may aggravate their condition. Lasers have not been tested on pregnant women.

Ginger Compress for Pain Relief

Study by researchers at Edith Cowan University, Perth, Western Australia, published in *Journal of Holistic Nursing.*

When placed on the lower backs of people with osteoarthritis for 30 minutes daily, a warm ginger compress reduced overall pain and fatigue by half after just one week. The ginger compress was a cotton cloth soaked in a hot ginger infusion (two teaspoons of ground ginger to one-half cup of very hot water), squeezed well so that it was just moist.

Theory: Topical ginger seems to warm and relax the musculoskeletal system, increasing mobility. The compress likely will work on pulled muscles and achy joints, too.

Roll Away Your Pain

Mary Ann Wilmarth, DPT, OCS, chief of physical therapy at Harvard University Health Services in Cambridge, Massachusetts, and former director of the Doctor of Physical Therapy (DPT) Program at Northeastern University in Boston. She is also the founder and CEO of Back2Back Physical Therapy in Andover, Massachusetts.

Studies show that a foam roller helps ease age-related muscle tightness, reduce exercise-induced muscle soreness and prevent injuries by warming up muscles before workouts and improving range of motion.

Foam-rolling is also helpful for a variety of common conditions, especially any kind of tendinitis (such as patellar tendinitis affecting the knee or Achilles tendinitis affecting the foot and ankle)...and muscle imbalances due to overuse (such as tennis elbow or golfer's elbow). Rolling out the tighter side of the muscle helps bring both sides into balance.

Why does rolling help so much? Moving your body back and forth across a foam roller increases restorative blood flow that helps promote muscle healing. A foam roller can also help reduce muscle soreness by physically dispersing lactic acid—a substance that accumulates in your muscles during intense exercise. To target specific parts of the body, do each of the following exercises for 15 to 60 seconds daily. *Common problem areas and some of the best new foam rollers...*

• **Hamstrings.** Tight hamstrings (the back of your thighs) are a common problem for people who sit for long hours (at a desk or behind the wheel of a car), run or bike. Tight hamstrings often lead to low-back pain. Because the hamstrings tend to be less sensitive than other muscles in your body, the increased stimulation provided by a textured roller (as opposed to a smooth roller) often works well.

One example of a good-quality textured roller is the Stott Pilates Two-in-One Massage Point Foam Roller ($69.99, Target.com). Its spikes target trigger points and deeply massage muscle tissue.

What to do: While sitting on the floor with your legs extended in front of you, with knees slightly bent, place the textured roller directly underneath your hamstrings, perpendicular to the muscles. While using your arms to support your weight, slowly roll your hamstrings up and down the roller, from buttocks to knees and back, adding pressure to the roller.

When you reach a trigger point (an area of tightness or increased soft tissue tension), either move back and forth on it or hold steady for 30 seconds (or until the knot "releases"). You'll feel the tissue soften and tightness melt away. This process may be a bit painful, but the discomfort should dissipate when you move off the roller.

• **Quads and hip flexors.** Walkers and runners and people with knee tendinitis often have tight hip flexors, the muscles that extend from the pelvis to the knee. Anyone who sits a lot needs to stretch and roll the quadriceps muscles on the front of the thighs and the hip flexors.

Baton-shaped foam rollers have handles on either side and are ideal for rolling out the quadriceps muscle or anytime you want to better control the pressure and intensity of the rolling (as opposed to lying atop a roller and applying your body weight). For this reason, baton rollers are especially helpful for people who are sensitive to pain. They also allow other people, such as a physical therapist or spouse, to roll your muscles for you.

What to do: Begin by sitting down on the floor with your legs extended in front of you. (For stability, place a rolled-up towel beneath your "sit bones"—at the base of your buttocks.) Bend your right leg slightly, with your knee falling out to the side, and position the baton at the top of your left leg, perpendicular to your thigh. Roll down and away to just above the left knee, as if you're rolling out dough with a rolling pin, then lift up, return to the top of the leg and repeat. Do the same steps on the other leg.

Good products: The GRID STK Foam Roller ($34.99, TPTherapy.com) has a three-dimensional surface...the TheraBand Roller Massager ($18.49, Amazon.com) is ridged. The texture you choose is a matter of personal preference.

• **Back and shoulder blades.** Ball-shaped massagers work well for hard-to-reach knots such as those in your upper or lower back, between the shoulder blades or in the piriformis muscle in the upper buttocks. A good choice for back and shoulder blade pain is the Tiger Ball Massage-on-a-Rope ($27.95, TigerTailUSA.com). If you're looking for deeper penetration, try a textured ball such as the RumbleRoller Beastie ($24.95, OPTP.com, RambleRoller.com).

What to do: For a tight or painful upper back, stand with your back to a wall, placing the ball in the space between your shoulder blades. Bend your knees slightly and push your body weight into the ball, making small circles with the ball. Avoid letting the ball directly press on your spine, which could be painful.

Minifoam rollers are another option that allows you to pinpoint trigger points on your back and shoulder blades. A product such as the GRID Mini Foam Roller ($24.99, TP Therapy.com) easily fits in a desk, gym bag or suitcase.

Virtual Reality Relieves Pain

Brennan Spiegel, MD, professor of medicine, director of Health Services Research and director of the master's degree program in health delivery science, all at Cedars-Sinai Health System in Los Angeles.

Imagine this: You are lying in a hospital bed after surgery when you begin to feel a stabbing pain. Desperate for relief, you look for your daily dose of pain medication. Not so fast. Soon, you may reach instead for a set of virtual-reality goggles.

Using virtual reality (VR) for pain is not some sci-fi snake oil. This high-tech therapy, which immerses you in a three-dimensional, multisensory world of cinematic grandeur, is on the cutting-edge of pain relief approaches.

Scientific evidence: New research shows that VR significantly reduces many types of pain and may lessen (or, in some cases, replace) the need for pain medication—a well-timed breakthrough given the addiction epidemic that's being fueled by pain medicine such as opioids.

What you need to know about this exciting new advance...

VIRTUAL REALITY IN ACTION

So what's it like to experience VR? Once you slip on the somewhat clunky-looking headset or even a simpler pair of special goggles, you'll be ready to watch three-dimensional, 360-degree streaming video complete with sound that depicts a wide variety of vibrantly colored realistic scenes—either photographed or animated. You'll hear the sounds associated with

> **Reflexology Works for Pain**
>
> Reflexology can reduce pain by 40% and may be as effective as drugs, a recent study claims. Reflexology involves applying pressure to specific points on the hands, feet or ears—that is believed to stimulate the body's production of pain-relieving endorphins in the brain and spinal cord. (See chapters 11 and 17 for specific exercises.)
>
> Study of reflexology by researchers at University of Portsmouth, England, published in *Complementary Therapies in Clinical Practice.*

that scene and even experience vibrations or other sensations for a completely immersive experience.

Depending on the purpose of the VR therapy—whether you need to focus your mind to distract yourself from pain, for example, or you need relief from anxiety—you may view scenes that give you the feeling of swimming with dolphins in the ocean...lobbing snowballs while hurtling through an animated snowscape...or relishing the splendor of a gushing waterfall.

VR therapy has been used successfully by scientists for years to help treat the symptoms of conditions such as stroke, post-traumatic stress disorder, social phobia and burns. In hospitals, VR therapy is used as needed with children to distract them from painful or scary procedures, such as getting blood drawn.

Until recently, however, VR therapy was too expensive and not widely available. That's now changing.

REDUCING PAIN MEDICATION

Many people who use VR continue to have pain reduction even after discontinuing the therapy. Scientists theorize that VR may somehow reset the brain, making some people less susceptible to peripheral pain signals for a period of time.

Scientists are also investigating whether VR can reduce the use of painkillers after an acute injury, such as a broken leg, or postoperatively—for example, after hip- or knee-replacement surgery.

VR EQUIPMENT

Cedars-Sinai and other medical centers use a VR kit provided by the company AppliedVR (go to AppliedVR.io). This kit consists of a Samsung headset and Galaxy phone at a cost of $800. A subscription to access the library of visualizations is extra.

But do not let that cost overwhelm you. You can use your own smartphone to access VR therapy by buying a headset (available on Amazon.com for about $20 to $100) and then streaming VR content by buying an app or going to YouTube.com. Look online for lists of highly rated VR apps.

Important: The VR therapy used in hospitals is prescribed for specific conditions. When using VR therapy on your own, try it on a trial-and-error basis. For example, if you are looking to relax or alleviate anxiety, you can search "VR and beach" or "VR and relax," and try out different scenes. There may be minor side effects, such as dizziness. People with dementia, epilepsy, nausea and certain other conditions should not use VR therapy without checking with their doctors.

HOW TO ACCESS VR THERAPY

Several hospitals across the country are conducting clinical trials on the use of VR therapy for pain management (including neuropathic pain and phantom limb pain) and other conditions such as attention deficit hyperactivity disorder (ADHD), traumatic brain injury, fear of heights and more.

To find a VR trial near you: Go to Clinical Trials.gov, type in "virtual reality" and choose your state or a nearby state.

The Healing Power of Biofeedback

Aubrey Ewing, PhD, past president of the Association for Applied Psychophysiology and Biofeedback. He maintains a private psychological services and biofeedback practice in Boynton Beach, Florida. DrEwing Online.com

---

Biofeedback helps us gain control of our bodies with the aid of technology. It uses electrical sensors, attached to different parts of the body, to monitor physiological activity, such as skin temperature, sweat gland activity, muscle tension and/or heart rate.

Readings of these measurements are displayed or "fed back" to patients on a monitor (in the form of cues such as beeps or flashing lights). This process enables patients to become aware of their bodies' physiological activity, especially involuntary activity that they are not usually aware of, including feeling certain muscles or heart rate. They can then learn how to use thoughts to control the body.

What's new: Advances in technology have made biofeedback more precise, improving treatments for conditions ranging from arthritis to anxiety and insomnia. *Examples of painful conditions biofeedback can help…*

- **Arthritis.** In an analysis of 25 studies in *Arthritis Rheumatology*, biofeedback was shown to reduce arthritic pain and disability. Exactly how biofeedback helps isn't clear. But by increasing blood flow to the joints, biofeedback may reduce or muffle the perception of pain intensity.

- **Temporomandibular joint (TMJ) disorder.** The headache, facial pain and/or ear pain of TMJ can be severe and hard to treat. Studies have shown that biofeedback can help TMJ by reducing tension in the muscles around the jaw joints and by promoting general relaxation.

BIOFEEDBACK BASICS

Depending on the individual, about eight to 12 biofeedback sessions are needed for medical problems such as arthritis. Biofeedback for such conditions as anxiety and insomnia sometimes requires 30 to 50 sessions. There are no side effects with biofeedback, and it generally is safe for everyone.

FINDING A PRACTITIONER

If you are interested in biofeedback, ask your doctor whether it might help you. One-hour biofeedback sessions cost $60 to $150. Some insurance companies pay for biofeedback therapy.

To find a qualified practitioner, contact the Association for Applied Psychophysiology and Biofeedback, Inc. (800-477-8892, AAPB.org and click on "Find a Provider") or the Biofeedback Certification International Alliance (720-502-5829, BCIA.org).

Try DMSO for Quick Pain Relief

Mark A. Stengler, NMD, a naturopathic doctor and founder of the Stengler Center for Integrative Medicine in Encinitas, California. He is author or coauthor of numerous books, including *The Natural Physician's Healing Therapies* and *Bottom Line's Prescription for Natural Cures*, and author of the newsletter *Health Revelations*. MarkStengler.com

For immediate pain relief for burns, sprains, back pain or arthritis I often offer my patients a little-known favorite remedy called dimethyl sulfoxide (DMSO), a remarkable topical alternative medication for pain that has its own remarkable history. *Find out how it can help you…*

CONTROVERSIAL DMSO

The fascinating story of DMSO began in the 1960s, when Stanley Jacob, MD, head of the organ transplant program at Oregon Health Sciences University in Portland, was investigating compounds that might help preserve organs for transplant. DMSO, which had been used as an industrial solvent, attracted his attention because of the way it penetrates skin without damaging it. He experimented with DMSO and found that it could relieve pain. From the start, DMSO was highly controversial—and some were worried that this "miracle" drug had harmful side effects, although nothing specific was found.

THE POWER OF DMSO

DMSO works in several ways. First, as a topical compound, it has analgesic properties and reduces pain quickly—which is why it is great for rubbing on sore muscles and joints. Second, DMSO is rich in sulfur—and sulfur is found in every cell and is essential for life. Third, DMSO dissolves and transports other substances through the skin, which makes it a great carrier and helper in getting other substances into sore or damaged tissues.

Where to get DMSO: You can buy DMSO for basic pain relief at health-food stores and online at HerbalRemedies.com and Jacob Lab, the website of Dr. Stanley Jacob (JacobLab.com). It generally comes in two concentrations, with either 70% or 90% DMSO. Most people find pain relief with the 70% solution. At Jacob Lab, the 70% gel costs $28 for four ounces. This may seem expensive compared with many conventional pain relievers such as NSAIDs, but it works so effectively, has no side effects and is often needed only short-term, so my patients don't mind spending the extra money.

How to use DMSO: Make sure your hands are clean before applying DMSO, especially since it is efficient at transferring substances through the skin. For acute injuries, apply up to four times daily. For chronic conditions, apply twice daily. It can be used for a few days, a few weeks or indefinitely, depending on the condition. Apply a small amount to the painful area and rub it in. Wash your hands after applying DMSO so that the excess is not absorbed by your skin.

Within minutes of applying DMSO, many people experience a taste of sulfur or garlic in their mouths that can last for several hours. In general, this is not a big problem. People who are allergic to sulfites can use DMSO. (There is no such thing as an allergy to sulfur.)

Turn On the Water for Pain Relief!

Mark A. Stengler, NMD, a naturopathic doctor and founder of the Stengler Center for Integrative Medicine in Encinitas, California. He is author or coauthor of numerous books, including *The Natural Physician's Healing Therapies* and *Bottom Line's Prescription for Natural Cures*, and author of the newsletter *Health Revelations*. MarkStengler.com

If you think about it, you probably already use water to heal—ice packs for injuries…steam inhalation for congestion…and a soak in a hot tub to ease sore muscles.

But you might not know that constitutional hydrotherapy, a treatment that involves applying hot- and cold-water-soaked towels to the body, is an incredibly effective and easy-to-do treatment that can also relieve pain.

HOW CONSTITUTIONAL HYDROTHERAPY WORKS

The contrast between the application of hot and cold towels—and the body's response to these changes in temperature—is what makes constitutional hydrotherapy so effective. Heat dilates the blood vessels, cold contracts them. The alternating dilation and contraction creates a pumping action that improves circulation through the blood vessels to the skin and internal organs. With improved circulation comes a reduction in congestion and inflammation. I have even used this treatment for patients with pneumonia as one component of an overall treatment program.

HOW TO DO IT

You can do hydrotherapy at home by yourself, although it is easier (and less messy!) with the help of someone who can place the hot and cold towels on various parts of your body. Note that this method works for all conditions mentioned. *Here's how…*

- **Lie on your back in bed or on the floor if it is comfortable for you.** (If you are worried about getting the bed wet, use a water-resistant covering on top of the bed.)
- **Have the helper cover your bare chest and abdomen with one thick (bath) towel that has been soaked in hot water and wrung out (as hot as is tolerable).** The towel should be moist. Be careful not to burn your skin.
- **Cover the hot wet towel with a dry towel.**
- **Place a blanket on top of the dry towel.** Remain bundled up in these layers for five minutes.
- **Next, replace the hot towel with thin towels that have been soaked in cold water (as cold as you can tolerate) and wrung out—the towels should still be moist.**
- **Cover the cold towels with a dry towel and the blanket.** This phase of the treatment should take about 10 minutes, the time it takes for the towels to reach body temperature.
- **Turn over onto your stomach and repeat the process, this time with the towels placed on your back.** Again, five minutes of hot-towel treatment should be followed by 10 minutes covered with thin, cold towels.

• **After the treatment, drink at least eight ounces of water and rest for at least 15 minutes.** The water helps flush out any toxins that have been released during the treatment. Rest allows you to readjust to room temperature before standing up.

If you have an acute condition such as bronchitis, do constitutional hydrotherapy once or twice daily. For a chronic condition such as arthritis or for detoxification, use constitutional hydrotherapy five times weekly. Constitutional hydrotherapy can be used safely by patients of all ages. However, consult with a holistic physician when using hydrotherapy with an infant, when pregnant or if you have cardiovascular disease, diabetes or asthma.

No More Chronic Pain

The Calmare pain therapy treatment relieves chronic neuropathic pain from diabetes, shingles, herniated disks, chemotherapy, reflex sympathetic dystrophy (RSD) and other causes. The FDA-approved device uses electrodes applied to the skin to transmit "no-pain" messages to the brain. Patients usually undergo 10 to 12 daily treatments, each lasting less than one hour. For a list of centers that offer Calmare therapy, go to Calmarett.com and click on Facilities.

C. Evers Whyte, MS, DC, pain expert and founder and director of the New England Center for Chronic Pain, Stamford, Connecticut. NECCP.com

You Can Get Relief From Pain, Nausea, Depression and More

Diane E. Meier, MD, director of the Center to Advance Palliative Care (CAPC), a national organization devoted to increasing the number and quality of palliative care programs in the US.

Until recently, palliative care—a type of medical care that focuses on making a person who is seriously ill as comfortable and pain-free as possible—was used only when death was imminent.

Now: Palliative care is being extended to people suffering from any stage of serious illness.

This approach has many benefits. The patient has a better quality of life...families and caregivers get more support...and medical costs are reduced. In fact, a recent study published in *Archives of Internal Medicine* found that palliative care saved hospitals up to $374 per patient per day (in pharmacy, laboratory and intensive-care costs).

To learn more about this new vision of palliative care—and how more people can take advantage of it—we spoke with Diane E. Meier, MD, one of the world's leading experts on this type of medical care and a recent winner of the prestigious MacArthur "Genius" Fellowship.

How does palliative care differ from other types of medical care?

Palliative care, which primarily is offered in hospitals (usually on an inpatient basis, but sometimes to outpatients), focuses on easing suffering by putting an emphasis on relief of a patient's pain and other symptoms, as well as overall improvement in his/her quality of life. For example, it complements ongoing care by helping patients control pain, reduce nausea, improve appetite, relieve fatigue and/or depression—and live a meaningful life despite the limitations of illness.

Palliative care can help a Parkinson's disease patient, for example, carry on with daily life by relieving such symptoms as joint pain and shortness of breath.

Are there any other advantages of palliative care?

There are several. For one, most physicians cannot always spend a great deal of time discussing treatment goals and options. A palliative care team, however, is able to give patients as much time as they need to get the information and guidance that is necessary to make the best medical decisions.

With palliative care, patients also get a team of specialists. Depending on an individual's needs, the palliative care team may include doctors, nurses, social workers, psychologists, massage therapists, chaplains, pharmacists and nutritionists.

Who is eligible for palliative care?

Doctors can administer palliative care to anyone who has been diagnosed with a serious, life-threatening or progressive illness that causes debilitating symptoms.

Diseases treated with palliative care include cancer, chronic obstructive pulmonary disease (COPD), congestive heart failure, kidney or liver failure, Parkinson's disease, dementia and autoimmune disorders, including multiple sclerosis and lupus erythematosus.

Palliative care may be particularly helpful for people with a serious or chronic illness who have been admitted to the hospital three or more times in the past year...if they visit an emergency room once a month or more...if their illness stops responding to ongoing treatment...and/or if basic life functions—such as breathing or eating—are affected. But people can take advantage of palliative care at any time—even immediately after diagnosis or during the early stages of disease.

Palliative care generally is covered by insurance.

Is palliative care the same as hospice?

Definitely not. If a doctor suggests palliative care, it does not necessarily mean that you are close to dying. It simply means that you could benefit from more extensive care to give you a better quality of life.

How does palliative care help support the patient's family?

Palliative care provides emotional support for family members, helps them navigate the health-care system and provides guidance to assist them and their loved ones in making difficult treatment choices.

What's the best way to seek out palliative care?

The first step is to approach your doctor. Sadly, most practicing physicians were not trained in palliative care, and your doctor may not know much about it. If you feel you need help describing palliative care, give your doctor a copy of this article.

Take this opportunity to clarify your understanding of your diagnosis, disease progression or treatment. And tell your doctor whether—and how much—your disease is limiting your life due to pain, depression or other factors.

What if the hospital my doctor is affiliated with doesn't offer palliative care?

At some point, all hospitals will offer palliative care. However, if your doctor is not affiliated with a hospital that provides this type of care, you may have to be proactive and seek out a hospital that does.

You can check the website of the Center to Advance Palliative Care, GetPalliativeCare.org, to see which hospitals in your area offer palliative care. Click on "Access the Provider Directory," and search your hometown as well as surrounding cities.

About 1,300 US hospitals now offer palliative care. Once you find a nearby hospital on the list, ask your doctor for a referral to the hospital's palliative care team.

CHAPTER 23

Foods, Supplements and Herbs for Overall Pain Relief

How to Eat to Relieve Chronic Pain

Most people don't realize that dietary changes—eating certain foods and avoiding others—can have a big effect on chronic pain, such as joint pain, back and neck pain, headaches and abdominal pain.

HEAL YOUR DIGESTIVE TRACT

Pain anywhere in the body is almost always accompanied, and made worse, by inflammation. The inflammatory response, which includes the release of pain-causing chemicals, can persist in the body for decades, even when you don't have redness or other visible signs.

Common cause: A damaged mucosa in the innermost lining of the intestines. The damage can be caused by food sensitivities...a poor diet with too much sugar or processed foods...or a bacterial imbalance, among many other factors. A weakened mucosal lining can allow toxic molecules to enter the body, where they then trigger persistent inflammation.

If you suffer from chronic pain—particularly pain that's accompanied by intermittent bouts of constipation and/or diarrhea—your first step should be to heal the damaged intestinal tissue. *To do this...*

- **Eat a variety of fermented foods.** They are rich in probiotics, which will help the mucosa heal. Most people know that live-culture yogurt is a good source of probiotics...but yogurt alone doesn't supply enough. You can and should get more probiotics by eating one

Mel Pohl, MD, a physician who specializes in treating addiction and chronic pain. He is the medical director of the Las Vegas Recovery Center and author, with Katherine Ketcham, of *The Pain Antidote: The Proven Program to Help You Stop Suffering from Chronic Pain, Avoid Addiction to Painkillers—and Reclaim Your Life.*

Heather Tick, MD, the Gunn-Loke Endowed professor for integrative pain medicine at the University of Washington, Seattle, where she is a clinical associate professor in the department of family medicine and the department of anesthesiology and pain medicine. She is the author of *Holistic Pain Relief: Dr. Tick's Breakthrough Strategies to Manage and Eliminate Pain.*

or more daily servings of fermented foods such as sauerkraut or kimchi (Asian pickled cabbage).

Because most highly processed fermented foods—such as canned sauerkraut—will not give you the live probiotics you need, select a product that requires refrigeration even in the grocery store. You also can take a probiotic supplement, which is especially important for people who take antibiotics or who don't eat many fermented foods.

• **Eat more cherries and berries.** All fruits contain healthy amounts of antioxidants, which are important for reducing inflammation and pain. Inflammation is associated with tissue swelling, pressure on nerves and decreased circulation, which contribute to pain. Cherries (along with blueberries, cranberries and blackberries) are particularly helpful because they're rich in anthocyanins, chemicals that relieve pain even more effectively than aspirin. Cherries do have a fairly short season, but frozen cherries and 100% cherry juice offer some of the same benefits, though nothing takes the place of fresh organic produce.

In a study, researchers at University of California–Davis found that men and women who ate a little more than a half pound of cherries a day had a 25% reduction in C-reactive protein (CRP), a clinical marker for inflammation.

Bonus: The vitamin C in cherries and other berries has additional benefits. It's used by the body to build and repair joint cartilage, important for people with joint pain caused by osteoarthritis. Like anthocyanins, vitamin C also is a potent antioxidant that can reduce CRP.

• **Give up sugar.** By now, many of the hazards of sugar, including weight gain and cardiovascular damage, are well known—but most people don't know that consuming sugar increases pain.

What's the link with chronic pain? A high-sugar diet causes the body to produce advanced glycation end products (AGEs), which trigger massive amounts of inflammation.

And it isn't only sugar per se that does the damage. The American College of Clinical Nutrition has reported that foods with a high glycemic index—these include white bread, white rice and other "simple" carbohydrates that are quickly converted to glucose during digestion—increase inflammation even in healthy young adults. For those with arthritis or other ongoing painful conditions, even a slight increase in inflammation can greatly increase discomfort.

Try to eliminate added sugar and processed carbohydrates from your diet. Give up candy, soda, baked goods and highly refined grains. If you really enjoy a bit of sugar in your morning coffee, go for it. Treat yourself to the occasional sweet dessert. But in my experience, people with chronic pain usually do better when they give up sugar altogether.

Exception: It's good to avoid sweets, but make an exception for an ounce or two of dark chocolate daily. Chocolate that contains at least 70% cocoa is very high in antioxidants. It reduces inflammation, improves brain circulation and lowers blood pressure, according to research. And because it's a sweet treat, it will make it easier for you to say no to the nasty stuff like cake, cookies and ice cream.

LESS MEAT AND ALCOHOL

• **Limit red meat.** Red meat, especially the organic, grass-fed kind, does have valuable nutrients and can be part of a healthy diet. But eaten in excess (more than three ounces daily), red meat increases inflammation. If you eat more than the amount above, cut back. At least half of each meal should be foods grown in the ground—such as vegetables, nuts and seeds. One-quarter should be whole grains, and the rest should be protein, which doesn't always mean animal protein. Other good proteins include lentils, beans and tempeh.

• **Cook "cooler."** You might struggle with pain control if grilling is one of your favorite rituals. Meats and other foods exposed to prolonged, high-heat cooking—on the grill, in the broiler, pan-frying and deep-fat frying—generate high levels of AGEs. Increased pain is just one of the risks—some research has linked AGEs to heart disease, diabetes and possibly even Alzheimer's disease.

You'll do better with cooler cooking methods, such as simmering and sautéing and moderate-heat (around 350°F) roasting. Slow-cookers are another good choice. I don't advise patients with chronic pain to give up grilling, broiling or pan-frying altogether. Just remind yourself to use these methods less often—say, once a week. Let your pain be your guide. If it's getting worse, make bigger changes.

• **Cut back on alcohol.** Actually, no alcohol is the best choice for people with chronic pain. Alcohol irritates intestinal tissue and allows bacteria to pass into the blood more readily. The presence of bacteria will increase inflammation even if you don't develop obvious symptoms of infection.

Listen to your body. Some people can have an occasional beer or a glass of wine without noticing any change in their pain levels. If you're one of them, go ahead and imbibe on occasion.

• **Switch to olive oil.** The heart-healthy benefits aren't the only reasons to use extra-virgin olive oil in place of polyunsaturated vegetable oils (such as canola). Olive oil contains a substance called oleocanthol, which interferes with the inflammatory COX-1 and COX-2 enzymes. People who consume olive oil have lower levels of prostaglandins, the same pain-causing neurotransmitters that are blocked by aspirin.

Use olive oil just as you would other cooking oils—by drizzling some on pasta or salads, for example, or using it when you sauté vegetables or fish.

• **Eat more vegetables.** If you are expecting an exotic recommendation here, sorry—because what you really need to eat to reduce inflammation in your body is lots and lots of vegetables—raw, steamed, sautéed, baked or roasted. Vegetables contain cellulose, a type of fiber that binds to fats and some inflammatory substances and carries them out of the body in the stools. The antioxidants in vegetables, such as the lycopene in tomatoes and the indole-3-carbinol in crucifers such as broccoli, cabbage and Brussels sprouts, further reduce inflammation.

This part of your pain-reduction strategy is pretty simple, really: There is not a vegetable on the planet that will worsen your pain... and most of them, if not all, will help reduce your pain. For easy, general dietary guidelines, just follow the well-known, traditional Mediterranean-style diet, which includes lots of vegetables, fish (fish oil is anti-inflammatory), small amounts of red meat and olive oil.

• **Eat seafood twice a week.** The omega-3 fatty acids in cold-water fish (such as salmon, sardines and trout) are among the most potent anti-inflammatory agents. Studies have shown that people who suffer from morning stiffness and joint tenderness do better when they consume more omega-3s. You can get by with fish-oil supplements, but they're unnecessary if you eat fatty fish at least twice a week.

• **Don't forget spices.** Turmeric and ginger are great spices for pain relief and can replace salty and sugary flavor enhancers. Ginger tea is a delicious pain fighter. Also, garlic and onions are high in sulphur, which helps in healing.

• **Drink plenty of water—between eight and 10 glasses a day.** It helps the kidneys and liver filter toxins (such as pesticide residues) from the body. Even though the liver breaks down about 95% of the toxins you ingest, the by-products can linger in the blood and other tissues. Water dilutes the concentration and reduces the inflammatory effects.

Also helpful: Green tea. It provides extra water along with catechins, antioxidants that reduce inflammation and pain.

Plant-Based Diet for a Pain-Free Life

Harris H. McIlwain, MD, rheumatologist and pain specialist with Florida's largest rheumatology practice, and adjunct professor at University of South Florida College of Public Health, both in Tampa. He is coauthor, with Debra Fulghum Bruce, PhD, of *Diet for a Pain-Free Life*.

Being overweight and having a poor diet are crucial factors that cause chronic pain. Fatty tissue is an endocrine (hormone-producing) organ, just like other organs in the body. Studies show that patients who are overweight produce high levels of cytokines, C-reactive protein and other proinflammatory chemicals—substances that promote joint and tissue damage and increase pain.

Good news: Losing as little as 10 pounds can significantly reduce inflammation, pain and stiffness—regardless of the underlying cause of the discomfort. People who combine weight loss with a diet that includes anti-inflammatory foods (and excludes proinflammatory ones) can reduce pain by up to 90%. The effect rivals that of ibuprofen and similar painkillers—without gastrointestinal upset or other side effects.

PAIN-FREE DIET

The saturated fat in beef, pork, lamb and other meats is among the main causes of painful inflammation. People who eat a lot of meat (including poultry) consume arachidonic acid, an essential fatty acid that is converted into inflammatory chemicals in the body.

Although a vegetarian diet is ideal for reducing inflammation and promoting weight loss (no more than 6% of vegetarians are obese), few Americans are willing to give up meat altogether.

Recommended: A plant-based diet that includes little (or no) meat and poultry…at least two to four weekly servings of fish…and plenty of fiber and anti-inflammatory foods. Patients who follow this diet and limit daily calories to about 1,400 can lose 10 to 25 excess pounds within three months.

Helpful: It takes at least two to three weeks to establish new dietary habits. People who give up meat entirely usually find that they don't miss it after a few weeks—while those who continue to eat some meat may find the cravings harder to resist.

My favorite cookbooks: *Vegan with a Vengeance* by Isa Chandra Moskowitz and *Pike Place Public Market Seafood Cookbook* by Braiden Rex-Johnson.

Here are the best painkilling foods and beverages. *Include as many of these in your diet as possible…*

RED WINE

Red wine contains resveratrol, a chemical compound that blocks the activation of the COX-2 enzyme, one of the main substances responsible for pain and inflammation. Resveratrol may be more effective than aspirin at relieving pain from osteoarthritis and other inflammatory conditions.

Other beverages made from grapes, such as white wine and grape juice, contain some resveratrol, but not as much as red wine.

Servings: No more than two glasses daily for men, and no more than one glass for women.

Alternative source of antioxidants for nondrinkers: Two or more cups of tea daily. Both green and black teas contain epigallocatechin-3 gallate (EGCG), a chemical that blocks the COX-2 enzyme.

BERRIES AND PINEAPPLE

Virtually all fruits contain significant amounts of antioxidants, which prevent free radical molecules from damaging cell membranes and causing inflammation. Berries—particularly blueberries, cranberries and blackberries—are among the most powerful analgesic fruits because they're high in anthocyanins, some of the most effective antioxidants. One-half cup of blueberries, for example, has more antioxidant power than five servings of green peas or broccoli.

Fresh pineapple contains the enzyme bromelain, which is in the stem and fruit of the pineapple and inhibits the release of inflammatory chemicals. It has been shown in some studies to reduce arthritic pain. I advise patients with sports injuries to eat pineapple because of its healing powers.

Servings: At least two half-cup servings weekly, more if you're suffering from injuries or an arthritis flare-up. Bromelain also can be taken in supplement form—200 milligrams (mg) to 300 mg, three times daily before meals.

FISH

I advise patients to substitute oily fish (such as salmon, tuna and sardines) for meat. Fish has little saturated fat (the main proinflammatory nutrient in the American diet) and is high in omega-3 fatty acids. Omega-3s increase the body's production of inhibitory prostaglandins, substances that lower levels of inflammatory chemicals and can reduce arthritis pain.

Servings: Two to four three-ounce servings of fish weekly or 1,000 to 2,000 mg of fish oil (available in capsule form) daily. If you don't like fish or want to maintain a vegetarian diet, omega-3s also are found in flaxseed, walnuts and soy foods.

WHOLE GRAINS AND BEANS

These are among the best sources of B vitamins—especially important for people who eat a lot of processed foods, which are usually deficient in these nutrients. Studies suggest that vitamins B-1 (thiamin), B-6 (pyridoxine) and B-12 (cyanocobalamin) may reduce inflammation.

Other B vitamins, such as B-3 (niacin), also reduce inflammation and may increase natural steroid levels and reduce the risk of osteoarthritis.

Servings: At least one-half cup of whole grains and/or beans daily.

Good choices: Brown rice, lentils, chickpeas, black beans and kidney beans.

Bonus: Grains and beans are high in fiber. High-fiber foods promote weight loss by increasing a sense of fullness and maintaining optimal blood sugar levels.

Spicy Spice Relieves Pain, Helps with Weight Loss

Joshua Levitt, ND, a naturopathic physician and medical director at Whole Health Natural Family Medicine in Hamden, Connecticut. He is author of *The Honey Phenomenon* and numerous other books and articles. WholeHealthCT.com

You know cayenne as a spicy, flavorful powder made from dried, red chili peppers. But the natural intensity of cayenne and its active ingredient capsaicin affect more than your taste buds.

It's the only natural compound that—when applied topically—can degrade substance P, a neurotransmitter that tells the brain to transmit pain signals. With less substance P, there's less pain—which is why capsaicin is a common ingredient in many creams, ointments and salves for pain problems such as arthritis, nerve pain, foot pain and back pain.

Little-known benefit: Cayenne can also help you lose weight. Capsaicin and other compounds in cayenne work because they have several effects that help you shed pounds—they suppress appetite...increase calorie-burning ("basal metabolic rate")...and burn up ("oxidize") body fat.

In a recent meta-analysis of nine studies on capsaicin and weight loss, published in *Critical Reviews in Food Science and Nutrition*, researchers concluded that the spice "could be a new therapeutic approach in obesity."

How to get more: For patients who want to lose weight, I usually recommend adding cayenne to the diet or using low-dose (2 mg) capsaicin supplements daily. (High-dose supplements can irritate the gastrointestinal tract.)

As a weight-loss aid, I recommend drinking one or more cups a day of warm water with a pinch of cayenne, juice from half a lemon, a teaspoon of honey and ground ginger (using a chunk of fresh ginger the size of half your thumb, from knuckle to tip). Cayenne is also excellent in marinades for fish and poultry and sprinkled on eggs. Plus, it adds a kick to salad dressings.

Ginger and Turmeric for Pain

Holly Phaneuf, PhD, expert in medicinal chemistry and author of *Herbs Demystified*. She is a member of the American Chemical Society and is conducting research on exercise and herb use.

You've probably heard that turmeric is a brain booster and that ginger helps ease nausea. But credible scientific evidence shows that many herbs that are well known for treating a particular ailment also work for pain.* *For example...*

*If you use prescription drugs and/or have a chronic medical condition, such as diabetes, cancer or heart disease, speak to your doctor before trying herbal remedies. In some cases, herbs may interfere with medication or cause an undesired effect on a chronic medical problem. Women who are pregnant or breast-feeding also should consult a doctor before taking herbs.

GINGER

Ginger is widely used to treat nausea, including that due to motion sickness (one-quarter to one-half teaspoon of ginger powder)...and chemotherapy (one to two teaspoons daily of ginger powder). Ginger is believed to quell queasiness by stopping intense stomach motions that can interfere with digestion.

What else ginger can do: Relieve arthritis pain. With its aspirin-like effects, ginger inhibits both COX-1 and COX-2 enzymes, two substances that are involved in the production of inflammatory hormones known as prostaglandins.

Typical dose: One-quarter to one-half teaspoon daily of ginger powder.

TURMERIC

In India, turmeric is a popular remedy for indigestion. It contains curcumin, an oily, yellow pigment that appears to prevent gut muscles from contracting and cramping.

What else turmeric can do: Relieve arthritis, morning stiffness and minor sprains. Turmeric reduces levels of an inflammatory, hormone-like substance known as PGE2. In lab studies, researchers also are finding that turmeric helps prevent colorectal and skin cancers, but its cancer-fighting mechanism has not yet been identified.

In addition, turmeric is being studied for its possible role in decreasing risk for Alzheimer's disease. Test tube and animal studies suggest that turmeric interferes with the formation of amyloid plaque, a hallmark of this neurodegenerative disease.

Recommended: Consume turmeric powder regularly by adding it to food, such as Asian dishes.

Caution: Because turmeric can cause gallbladder contractions, people with gallbladder problems should avoid the herb.

What Relief! Natural Ways To Curb Your Pain

Mark A. Stengler, NMD, a naturopathic doctor and founder of the Stengler Center for Integrative Medicine in Encinitas, California. He is author or coauthor of numerous books, including *The Natural Physician's Healing Therapies* and *Bottom Line's Prescription for Natural Cures*, and author of the newsletter *Health Revelations*. MarkStengler.com

In light of the dangers from prescription and OTC drugs, what safe alternatives are available to you? There are many natural supplements that I recommend.

NATURE'S PAIN RELIEVERS

If you take prescription or OTC pain medication, work with a naturopathic physician, holistic medical doctor or chiropractor who will incorporate natural pain fighters into your treatment regimen. With his/her help, you may be able to reduce your dosage of pain medication (natural pain relievers can be used safely with prescription or OTC painkillers)—or even eliminate the drugs altogether.

Natural pain-fighting supplements are even more effective when combined with physical therapies, such as acupuncture, chiropractic, magnet therapy or osteopathic manipulation (a technique in which an osteopathic physician uses his hands to move a patient's muscles and joints with stretching, gentle pressure and resistance). Physiotherapy (treatment that uses physical agents, such as exercise and massage, to develop, maintain and restore movement and functional ability) also is helpful.

Coffee Relieves Pain

The caffeine in coffee raises the body's level of dopamine, which causes pleasurable sensations that counteract pain. Caffeine also narrows swollen blood vessels in the brain that are associated with certain types of headaches, such as migraines. If you usually drink one cup of coffee a day, a second one may make you feel better when you get a headache.

Robert Kaniecki, MD, director, The Headache Center, University of Pittsburgh School of Medicine.

Here are—in no special order—the best natural pain relievers, which can be taken alone or in combination…

• **Methylsulfonylmethane (MSM)** is a popular nutritional supplement that relieves muscle and joint pain. According to Stanley Jacob, MD, a professor at Oregon Health & Science University who has conducted much of the original research on MSM, this supplement reduces inflammation by improving blood flow. Your cells have receptors that send out pain signals when they're deprived of blood. That's why increased blood flow diminishes pain.

MSM, a natural compound found in green vegetables, fruits and grains, reduces muscle spasms and softens painful scar tissue from previous injuries. A double-blind study of 50 people with osteoarthritis of the knee found that MSM helps relieve arthritis pain.

Start with a daily dose of 3,000 mg to 5,000 mg of MSM. If your pain and/or inflammation doesn't improve within five days, increase the dose up to 8,000 mg daily, taken in several doses throughout the day. If you develop digestive upset or loose stools, reduce the dosage. If you prefer, you can apply MSM cream (per the label instructions) to your skin at the painful area. This product is available at health-food stores and works well for localized pain. MSM has a mild blood-thinning effect, so check with your doctor if you take a blood thinner.

• **S-adenosylmethionine (SAMe)** is a natural compound found in the body. The supplement is an effective treatment for people who have osteoarthritis accompanied by cartilage degeneration. SAMe's ability to reduce pain, stiffness and swelling is similar to that of NSAIDs such as ibuprofen and naproxen, and the anti-inflammatory medication Celebrex. There's also evidence that SAMe stimulates cartilage repair, which helps prevent bones from rubbing against one another. A 16-week study conducted at the University of California, Irvine, compared two groups of people who were being treated for knee pain caused by osteoarthritis. Some took 1,200 mg of SAMe daily, while others took 200 mg of Celebrex. It took longer for people to get relief from SAMe, but by the second month, SAMe proved to be just as effective as Celebrex.

Most patients with osteoarthritis and fibromyalgia (a disorder characterized by widespread pain in muscles, tendons and ligaments) who take SAMe notice improvement within four to eight weeks. Many studies use 1,200 mg of SAMe daily in divided doses. In my experience, taking 400 mg twice daily works well. It's a good idea to take a multivitamin or 50-mg B-complex supplement daily while you're taking SAMe. The vitamin B-12 and folic acid contained in either supplement help your body metabolize SAMe, which means that the remedy goes to work faster.

• **Kaprex** is effective for mild pain caused by injury or osteoarthritis. It is a blend of hops, rosemary extract and oleanic acid, which is derived from olive leaf extract. Rather than blocking the body's pain-causing enzymes, these natural substances inhibit pain-causing chemicals called prostaglandins.

In a study sponsored by the Institute for Functional Medicine, the research arm of the supplement manufacturer Metagenics, taking Kaprex for six weeks reduced minor pain by as much as 72%. I recommend taking one 440-mg tablet three times daily. Kaprex is manufactured by Metagenics (800-692-9400, Metagenics.com), the institute's product branch. The product is sold only in doctors' offices. To find a practitioner in your area who sells Kaprex, call the toll-free number. Kaprex has no known side effects and does not interact with other medications.

• **Proteolytic enzymes,** including bromelain, trypsin, chymotrypsin, pancreatin, papain and a range of protein-digesting enzymes derived from the fermentation of fungus, reduce pain and inflammation by improving blood flow. You can find these natural pain fighters at health-food stores in products labeled "proteolytic enzymes." Take as directed on the label. Bromelain, a favorite of athletes, is available on its own. Extracted from pineapple stems, bromelain reduces swelling by breaking down blood clots that can form as a result of trauma and impede circulation. It works well for bruises, sprains and surgical recovery. If you use bromelain, take 500 mg three times daily between meals. (See page 480 for more on digestive enzymes.)

Repair is a high-potency formula of proteolytic enzymes that I often recommend. It is manufactured by Enzymedica (to find a retailer, call 888-918-1118 or go to Enzymedica.com). Take two capsules two to three times daily between meals. Don't take Repair or any proteolytic enzyme formula if you have an active ulcer or gastritis. Any enzyme product can have a mild blood-thinning effect, so check with your doctor if you take a blood thinner.

• **PainMed** is homeopathic gel that provides quick relief. It is remarkably effective for relieving the pain of arthritis, muscle soreness and spasms, sprains, strains, stiffness, headaches (especially due to tension) as well as injuries, including bruises.

A 60-year-old woman came to my office suffering from severe arthritis pain in both hands. I gave her a bean-sized dab of PainMed that she applied directly to the skin on her hands. After a few applications in the span of 30 minutes, her pain was reduced by 90%. She did not need to apply the gel again for two weeks. I witnessed a similar result with a retired National Football League player. He had severe chronic hip pain from past injuries. With one application of the gel, his pain was relieved by 70% for two full days.

PainMed is a combination of nine highly diluted plant and flower materials, including arnica, bryonia, hypericum and ledum. Like other homeopathic remedies, it promotes the body's ability to heal itself. A bean-sized dab works well for anyone who has pain. It should be spread on the skin around the affected area. Following an injury, use it every 15 minutes, for a total of up to four applications. As the pain starts to diminish, apply less often. Do not reapply the gel once the pain is gone. PainMed does not sting, burn or irritate the skin. It is clear, has no odor, does not stain and dries quickly. Because it has so many uses and works so rapidly, PainMed is a good first-aid remedy to have on hand. To order, contact the manufacturer, GM International, Inc., at 800-228-9850.

Four Natural Painkillers… And How to Use Them

Mark A. Stengler, NMD, a naturopathic medical doctor and leading authority on the practice of alternative and integrated medicine. Dr. Stengler is author of the *Health Revelations* newsletter, author of *The Natural Physician's Healing Therapies* (Bottom Line Books), founder and medical director of the Stengler Center for Integrative Medicine in Encinitas, California. MarkStengler.com

The four herbs described below can help with a variety of ailments, from headaches to arthritis pain.

How the remedies can help you…

For the conditions listed below, take the first natural painkiller on the list for four weeks. If you notice an improvement, stay with it. If not, try the next one. They are all available at health-food stores or online.

Caution: Women who are pregnant or breast-feeding should not take these remedies, because they have not been studied in these populations.

• **For headache (tension or migraine),** take white willow bark.

• **For inflammatory bowel disease,** take Boswellia, curcumin.

• **For low-back pain,** take devil's claw, white willow bark, curcumin.

• **For muscle aches and pains,** take white willow bark, curcumin.

• **For menstrual pain,** take white willow bark.

• **For osteoarthritis,** take Boswellia, white willow bark, devil's claw.

• **For rheumatoid arthritis,** take Boswellia, curcumin, devil's claw.

• **For tendonitis,** take devil's claw, curcumin, white willow bark.

The remedies…

BOSWELLIA

What it is: Part of India's Ayurvedic healing tradition, Boswellia (*Boswellia serrata*) comes from a tree found in India, Northern Africa and the Middle East. The tree yields a milky resin containing boswellic acids, substances that inhibit the body's synthesis of inflammatory leukotrienes. A study of patients with knee arthritis found that Boswellia extract relieved pain and stiffness as well as daily doses of the prescription drug *valdecoxib* (Bextra). And Boswellia's benefits persisted for one month longer than those of Bextra.

Dose: Take 750 mg of a standardized extract containing 60% to 65% boswellic acid two to three times daily for as long as symptoms last.

Recommended brand: Solgar Boswellia Resin Extract (877-765-4274, Solgar.com).

Side effects: While generally safe, Boswellia has been known to cause occasional mild digestive upset.

CURCUMIN

What it is: Curcumin (*diferuloylmethane*), a constituent of turmeric, is the pigment compound that gives the spice its distinctive yellow coloring. In one study of rheumatoid arthritis patients, 1,200 mg daily of curcumin extract improved morning stiffness and joint swelling.

Dose: Take 500 mg of standardized turmeric extract (containing 90% to 95% curcumin) three times daily.

Recommended brands: New Chapter Turmericforce (888-874-4461, NewChapter.com) and Life Extension Super Curcumin (855-990-1945, LifeExtensionVitamins.com).

Caution: It has blood-thinning properties, so do not take curcumin if you take blood-thinning medication, such as *warfarin*, unless monitored by a physician. Do not take curcumin if you have gallstones since it can cause gallstones to block bile ducts.

DEVIL'S CLAW

What it is: Devil's claw (*Harpagophytum procumbens*), a shrub found in southern Africa, works similarly to many pharmaceutical pain relievers—by blocking the action of pain-promoting compounds in the body—but without damaging the digestive tract. In studies involving people with chronic low-back pain, devil's claw extract proved as effective as prescription pain relievers.

Dose: Devil's claw extract is available in capsules. Look for 1.5% to 2% harpagoside, one of the active ingredients. Take 1,000 mg three times daily of a standardized extract.

Recommended brand: Nature's Way Standardized Devil's Claw Extract (800-962-8873, NaturesWay.com).

Side effect: The only significant potential side effect is diarrhea.

WHITE WILLOW BARK

What it is: White willow bark is a pain reliever that has anti-inflammatory and blood-thinning benefits similar to those of aspirin, but unlike aspirin, it doesn't appear to damage the stomach lining. For centuries, the bark of the white willow (*Salix alba*), a tree found in Europe and Asia, was noted for its pain-relieving qualities. Its active ingredient is salicin, which the body converts to salicylic acid, a close cousin to aspirin (acetylsalicylic acid). One study conducted in Haifa, Israel, involved 191 patients with chronic low-back pain who took one of two doses of willow bark extract or a placebo daily for four weeks. Researchers found that 39% of patients taking the higher dose of willow bark extract had complete pain relief, compared with only 6% of those taking a placebo. The participants who benefited the most took willow bark extract that contained 240 mg of the compound salicin, the active-constituent in this herbal remedy.

Dose: Take 120 mg daily of white willow bark extract capsules. If this amount does not reduce pain, try 240 mg.

Recommended brand: Solaray White Willow Bark (Solarayproducts.com).

Caution: Don't take this if you have an aspirin allergy and for one week before undergoing surgery. White willow bark is a blood thinner, so take it only while being monitored by a physician if you take blood-thinning medication.

Magnesium for Pain

Magnesium supplements, in the form of magnesium malate, can relieve pain. This natural muscle relaxant doesn't provide the powerful pain relief of a pharmaceutical agent, but it certainly has fewer side effects.

Thomas H. Reece, DO, ND, former medical director of the Southwest Naturopathic Medical Center in Scottsdale, Arizona, Dr. Reece now practices at the Preventive Medical Center of Marin in California.

Digestive Enzymes May Be Your Answer to Pain Relief

Leo Galland, MD, director of the Foundation for Integrated Medicine in New York City. He is the author of *Power Healing*. MDHeal.org

Digestive enzymes not only help relieve digestive problems (such as flatulence, heartburn and abdominal pain), they can also have powerful healing effects for other ailments, such as arthritis and sinusitis, that have nothing to do with the digestive system.

WHAT ARE DIGESTIVE ENZYMES?

Digestive enzymes are present in saliva, the stomach and the small intestine. Their job is to break down the food you eat into smaller components.

After about age 50, the pancreas produces only about half the amount of digestive enzymes that it did when you were younger. Some individuals find that they have less gas, bloating or fullness when they take an enzyme supplement during or after meals.

When to consider taking a digestive enzyme for pain (you can find these supplements at health-food stores or online)...

- **Arthritis.** A study published in *Clinical Rheumatology* found that a European product known as Phlogenzym, a blend of the enzymes bromelain and trypsin and rutosid (a flavonoid), was as effective at treating osteoarthritis of the knee as a commonly prescribed anti-inflammatory drug. Researchers believe that this particular mix of enzymes may help with all forms of osteoarthritis.

What to try: Consider buying Phlogenzym online from a European pharmacy. Take two capsules three times daily, on an empty stomach. Phlogenzym's major ingredients—bromelain, trypsin and rutosid—also can be found in US health-food stores. Follow dosage instructions on the products.

Caution: If you take these enzymes for arthritis relief, be sure to do so only under the supervision of a physician. In some individuals, the protein-digesting components can damage the lining of the stomach.

- **Sinusitis.** Bacterial sinusitis usually responds to antibiotics, but some people can have chronic sinusitis that lasts 12 weeks or more—even when they are taking medication.

What to try: Bromelain or other protease enzymes (with protease or trypsin on the label). They are not a replacement for antibiotics if you have a stubborn bacterial infection, but they can help to reduce inflammation and discomfort while the infection is active and even while you are taking an antibiotic.

How to take it: Follow the directions on the product label. The dosing directions will depend on the specific enzymes, concentrations, etc.

Neprinol Stops Pain

Andrew L. Rubman, ND, director, Southbury Clinic for Traditional Medicines, Southbury, Connecticut, Naturopath.org.

You may not have heard of this painkiller. Neprinol, it's called, and it addresses a number of problems that involve chronic pain, inflammation and conditions associated with both, including—and these are just a few on a long list—arthritis, chronic sinusitis, coronary vascular disease and multiple sclerosis. Neprinol's primary ingredients are the vegetable-derived enzymes nattokinase and serrapeptase, but it also contains Co-Q10 and several other ingredients.

Neprinol breaks down and removes excess fibrin, which is a protein essential to clotting, used by the body to repair what it perceives as injury. However, excess fibrin is also produced by the body due to inadequate management of stressors, thus leading to a growing list of inflammation-based conditions. Neprinol works by clearing the way for restoration of healthy tissue and then supporting that process.

MANY DON'T REALIZE THEY NEED NEPRINOL

Excess fibrin is a problem that many adults have, but few are aware of. As mentioned above, fibrin is the structural scaffolding with which the body responds to injury and inflammation to help stabilize tissue and initiate repairs as part of the healing response. In fact, that scar tissue is actually made of bundles of fibrin. This becomes problematic when a chronic inflammatory condition, such as arthritis, is present. Fibrin is supposed to be produced responsively, then taper off and eventually dissolve, but when production becomes chronic, the stage is set for trouble. For example, fibrin laid down on the artery lining, in response to inflammation, may cause LDL cholesterol to contribute to plaque formation, since it disturbs normal blood flow and forms a sticky surface to cling to.

ENTER NEPRINOL

Neprinol's ability to break down excess fibrin helps to slow the degenerative processes of aging and many diseases. It's a powerful supplement, best used under medical supervision tailored to each patient's health issues and treatment regimen. For example, a person on long-term corticosteroid or anticoagulant therapy would require close initial physician monitoring to determine effective dose levels.

There is a downside, however. Neprinol is expensive—about $90 for a 150-capsule bottle, which will last a month or two, depending on your dosage. But it's worth the cost. I've seen patients have a dramatic decrease in abdominal, pelvic and breast pain and tenderness associated with PID (pelvic inflammatory disease), IBS, GERD, mastitis, fibromyalgia and other conditions, within days of starting the supplement. Many patients do well with an occasional capsule, though individuals with serious inflammatory conditions may be prescribed many capsules a day—as many as six or eight, depending on what the health practitioner thinks is best.

Make sure to tell your doctor about Neprinol and why you believe it should be considered in your treatment protocol.

The one precaution for its use: Suspend taking it for several days before surgery since the supplement affects blood clotting and blood viscosity and wounds need fibrin to initially heal.

The Neprinol product that I recommend is made by Arthur Andrew Medical. You can obtain more information about Neprinol at Nepri nol.net. You can also purchase at Amazon.com.

Top Herbal Inflammation Fighters

Mark Blumenthal, founder and executive director of the American Botanical Council (ABC), Herbal Gram.org. He is the editor and publisher of the ABC's journal, *HerbalGram*, and the senior editor of several books, including *The ABC Clinical Guide to Herbs.*

In addition to making appropriate lifestyle changes, consider taking one or more herbal remedies that have shown significant anti-inflammatory properties in clinical trials. These herbs have been used for centuries as natural remedies.

ZYFLAMEND HERBAL COMBINATION

Zyflamend is a popular herbal anti-inflammatory product that contains extracts of turmeric, ginger and rosemary (which has antioxidant and anti-inflammatory properties). Among the other herbs found in Zyflamend are holy basil (used in India's traditional Ayurvedic medicine for its immune-boosting and anti-inflammatory properties) and the Chinese herb *Polygonum cuspidatum* (a rich source of resveratrol, the powerful antioxidant that also is found in grapes).

Anti-inflammatory benefits: Zyflamend lowers the body's general inflammatory response.

Cancer-fighting benefits: Zyflamend has been studied as a therapy for a type of prostate inflammation called high-grade prostatic intra-epithelial neoplasia (HGPIN), which is associated with precancerous changes in prostate cells. Zyflamend may be able to return these precancerous cells back to their normal state. Zyflamend may inhibit the proliferation of human prostate cancer cells, as well.

To purchase Zyflamend: Go to the website of the manufacturer, New Chapter, Inc. (New Chapter.com), or call 888-874-4461.

ROSE HIP

An extract of a certain type of rose hip called *Rosa canina* is especially high in the anti-inflammatory chemical glycoside of mono- and diglycerol.

Anti-inflammatory benefits: Clinical trials have shown rose hip extract to benefit osteoarthritis of the knee, hip, wrist and neck. Another trial of rheumatoid arthritis sufferers showed significant improvement in their pain, movement and quality of life after six months of treatment with rose hip extract.

Recommended product: Swanson Ultra Danish Rose Hips i-flex (dried powder of a special type of rose hip), available from Swanson Health Products (800-824-4491, SwansonVitamins.com).

Chronic Pain Linked to Low Vitamin D

Chronic pain is the leading cause of disability in the US. In a recent study, it was found that patients with low vitamin D levels required twice as much narcotic pain medication to manage symptoms as those with adequate levels.

Theory: Vitamin D deficiency leads to low bone density, which can create achy pain throughout the body.

Best: Ask your doctor about testing your blood level of vitamin D and supplementing if it is below 20 nanograms per milliliter.

Thomas H. Reece, DO, ND, former medical director of the Southwest Naturopathic Medical Center in Scottsdale, Arizona, Dr. Reece now practices at the Preventive Medical Center of Marin in California.

The Right Probiotic Can Help Your Pain

Gary B. Huffnagle, PhD, professor of internal medicine at the University of Michigan Medical School in Ann Arbor and coauthor of *The Probiotics Revolution: The Definitive Guide to Safe, Natural Health Solutions Using Probiotic and Prebiotic Foods and Supplements.*

Until recently, probiotics were mostly known for their ability to help prevent or alleviate various digestive problems.

Now: Research has uncovered several other health benefits—for example, these beneficial intestinal microorganisms also boost immunity and reduce the severity of certain autoimmune conditions, such as rheumatoid arthritis and asthma.

What you need to know…

THE RIGHT PROBIOTIC

Consuming probiotics is one of the smartest things you can do for your health.

What you may not know: Some probiotics—available as over-the-counter (OTC) supplements and in certain fermented food products, such as many brands of yogurt and buttermilk—have been found to be more effective than others for treating certain conditions.

What's more, because everyone's intestinal microflora—the term for the many billions of different bacteria and fungi that populate your gut—is unique in its exact makeup, a probiotic that's effective for someone else might not work for you, and vice versa.

Best approach: Try one probiotic product (such as those described in this article) for two weeks and see if you feel better. Probiotics are extremely safe. While some people may experience slight gastrointestinal disturbance, such as intestinal gas or bloating, from a given probiotic, this can be alleviated by reducing the dosage.

If you don't see clear benefits after two weeks, try a different probiotic from the same category (listed on the next page).

Even though most research has focused on the benefits of single types (strains) of microorganisms, many people benefit from combining two or more probiotics, and a number of probiotic products also contain multiple strains.

Once you find a probiotic you respond well to, I recommend taking it daily even in the absence of any specific health complaint—just like a daily multivitamin and mineral supplement.

Choose products from well-known manufacturers, such as Sustenex, Culturelle and Align, that include information on the label about the type of micro-organisms and number of viable bacteria, or colony-forming units (CFUs), they contain. Follow the label recommendation on dosage. Studies indicate that probiotics are equally effective when taken with or without food.

FOR DIGESTIVE PROBLEMS

In addition to promoting the growth of beneficial bacteria in the gut, probiotics aid digestion by inhibiting the proliferation of harmful bacteria and other micro-organisms in the intestines.

If you suffer from digestive problems, including diarrhea, constipation, bloating, gastroesophageal reflux disease or irritable bowel syndrome (IBS), try one of the following OTC probiotics...

- **Bifidobacterium.** This group, one of the major types of intestinal bacteria, includes *Bifidobacterium infantis* (found in Align, sold in capsule form)...*Bifidobacterium bifidus* (a common ingredient of many pro-biotic supplements, such as those by Source Naturals and Nature's Way)...and *Bifidobacterium animalis* (contained in Activia yogurt).

Important scientific evidence: In a 2006 randomized study of 362 women with IBS, those who took B. infantis in a daily dose of 10 million CFUs showed significant improvement after four weeks, compared with a placebo group.

- ***Bacillus coagulans.*** This species of bacteria (found in Sustenex Probiotic products, sold in capsule and chewable forms, and Digestive Advantage capsules) can survive for an extended time in the digestive tract, which is believed to increase the probiotic's effectiveness. In a 2009 study of 44 people with IBS, those receiving a daily dose of B. coagulans reported significant improvement.

FOR ALLERGIES, ASTHMA, ARTHRITIS, ECZEMA AND MORE

As a first-line probiotic for allergies, asthma, eczema or other autoimmune-related disorders, I recommend trying either B. coagulans—shown in a 2010 study to significantly reduce rheumatoid arthritis pain compared with a placebo—or one of the following...

- **Lactobacillus.** Another major category of probiotics, this genus includes the widely used *Lactobacillus acidophilus*, contained in many probiotic supplements and yogurt products (including Brown Cow, Stonyfield Farm and some Dannon yogurts)...*Lactobacillus GG* (the active ingredient in Culturelle capsules and powder)...and *Lactobacillus casei* (contained in the yogurt drink DanActive).

- ***Saccharomyces boulardii.*** This probiotic is actually a strain of yeast. Although most people think of yeast as something to be avoided—as in a yeast infection, for example—S. boulardii helps fight disease-causing organisms. S. boulardii is available in capsule form in Florastor and in products by Jarrow Formulas, Nutricology, Swanson, NOW Foods, Douglas Labs and others.

PROBIOTIC-BOOSTING DIET

Certain foods, known as "prebiotics," stay in the digestive tract for an extended period of time, where they stimulate the growth of many types of beneficial bacteria.

Try to include as many of the following prebiotic foods in your diet as possible each day. For example...

- **Foods rich in natural antioxidants**—especially those found in colorful fruits and vegetables, such as berries, citrus fruits, peppers, tomatoes, broccoli, spinach, asparagus and okra...dark beans and nuts...and green tea.

- **Foods high in soluble fiber**—including legumes, such as peas, lentils and pinto beans... oat bran...carrots and Brussels sprouts...apples, pears and prunes...and root vegetables, such as onions and unprocessed potatoes.

To further boost soluble fiber consumption: Talk to your doctor about taking a daily psyllium supplement, such as Carlson Psyllium Fiber Supplement or Metamucil. Follow label instructions.

At the same time, minimize your intake of processed foods containing sugar, white flour and other refined carbohydrates—all of which promote the growth of harmful bacteria in the digestive tract.

Chinese Herbal Remedies You Can Make Yourself

Daisy Dong, LAc, OMD, a licensed herbalist and professor at Southwest Acupuncture College in Boulder and a senior acupuncturist at The Center for Integrative Medicine at University of Colorado Hospital in Aurora.

Modern Western medicine can achieve some true miracles—like transplanting a heart or removing a brain tumor. But when it comes to easing the discomfort of minor injuries and aches, conventional over-the-counter ointments may not help as much as you would like. So, why not consider some herbal remedies that have provided healing help for thousands of years? Traditional Chinese Medicine (TCM) offers natural topical remedies that can soothe joint pain, sprains and minor burns and promote healing.

Some TCM herbal remedies are simple enough for you to make and use at home (though for any serious injury or significant ongoing pain, you should see a health-care professional first). The recipes below were provided by Daisy Dong, LAc, OMD, a licensed herbalist and professor at Southwest Acupuncture College.

Ingredients for these remedies are available at many herbal stores and Asian markets as well as online (Dr. Dong recommended Spring Wind Dispensary). Ask for the herbs by their Chinese names and/or their Latin or common names. Herbs often are measured in grams, so you may want to invest in a small kitchen scale... or, in most cases, you can use the familiar teaspoon, tablespoon and cup measurements that also are provided.

Important: These are topical remedies, meant to be applied directly to the affected area. Do not ingest them! Used as directed, they have no side effects.

FOR ACHY JOINTS: HONG HUA LINIMENT

This remedy invigorates blood flow to reduce blood stasis (stagnation) in the joint... lessens swelling...and eases aching pain.

Note: The preparation must soak for a week before it is ready to use, so make a batch to keep it on hand, ready for when you need it. *Ingredients...*

50 g (10 tsp.) dried, raw hong hua (also called carthamus)
300 ml (1¼ cups) of 70% isopropyl rubbing alcohol

To prepare: Place the hong hua into a container that has a tight-fitting lid and pour the alcohol over the herb. Cover and refrigerate for one week. Strain the liquid through cheesecloth, removing and discarding all solid remnants of the herb. Store the liquid liniment, tightly covered, in the refrigerator for up to three months.

To use: Up to four times per day as needed, soak a cotton ball or gauze pad in the liniment, then rub on the aching joint. Avoid getting the liniment on your clothing as it may stain.

FOR SPRAINS: HUANG LIAN SALVE

This remedy reduces blood stasis...combats inflammation...and alleviates pain. All herbs for this salve should be purchased in powdered (granule) form. For maximum effect, the salve should be prepared fresh each day, Dr. Dong recommended, but the dry ingredients can be combined ahead of time and stored for easy future use. *Ingredients...*

30 g (6 tsp.) huang lian (coptis root)
12 g (2½ tsp.) yan hu suo (corydalis rhizome)
12 g (2½ tsp.) hong teng (sargentodoxa vine)
10 g (2 tsp.) bai zhu (atractylodes rhizome)
10 g (2 tsp.) qiang huo (notopterygium root)
10 g (2 tsp.) du huo (pubescent angelica root)
10 g (2 tsp.) mu xiang (saussurea)
3 g (⅔ tsp.) xue jie (dragon's blood)
Fresh egg whites

To prepare: In a container, combine all herbs (not the egg whites) and mix together thoroughly. Cover and store this powdered mixture in a dry place until ready to use. When the remedy is needed, combine 6 g (1¼ tsp) of the mixed powder with one fresh egg white and stir to form a pasty salve.

To use: Rub the salve on the affected area, cover with gauze and leave on for one to two hours. Apply once daily until pain is gone. Avoid applying to skin that is broken or cut.

FOR MINOR BURNS: DANG GUI SALVE

Applied to small burns that are reddened or blistered, this salve helps eliminate toxins... invigorates blood flow...and moistens skin to promote tissue healing and regrowth. *Ingredients...*

30 g raw, sliced dang gui (Chinese angelica root)
120 g (8 Tbsp.) sesame oil
30 g (2 Tbsp.) beeswax

To prepare: In a frying pan, fry the raw, sliced dang gui with the sesame oil for several minutes until the herb turns blackish and the oil changes color. Remove from heat. With a slotted spoon, remove and discard the dang gui. Add the beeswax to the hot oil and stir quickly until completely mixed. Pour the mixture into an oven-safe container and place in a 200°F oven for about one hour, stirring mixture two or three times as it bakes. Toward the end of the baking time, check the consistency by placing a small amount of the mixture on a metal spoon and putting it in the freezer for one minute—ideally, it should be soft and pasty (no longer watery but not yet hard) when mixture is the proper consistency. Remove the mixture from the oven and stir again to mix well. Let cool, then transfer to a glass or metal container. Cover and store in the refrigerator for up to nine months.

To use: Spread 1 Tbsp. of salve on a gauze pad and apply to the burned area, changing the dressing once or twice daily, Dr. Dong recommended. Repeat applications until the burned tissue heals.

The Wonders of Aloe

Mark A. Stengler, NMD, a naturopathic doctor and founder of the Stengler Center for Integrative Medicine in Encinitas, California. He is author or coauthor of numerous books, including *The Natural Physician's Healing Therapies* and *Bottom Line's Prescription for Natural Cures*, and author of the newsletter *Health Revelations*. MarkStengler.com

Aloe can be used topically or internally (juice or capsule form). All forms are available at health-food stores. *How aloe can help you...*

- **Digestive disorders.** Aloe juice has been found to ease stomach ulcers...inflammatory bowel disease...Crohn's disease...and ulcerative colitis. Aloe also can help constipation. But people with these digestive disorders should be cautious when using aloe products that contain aloe latex (from the milky part of the plant) since this component of aloe can be a powerful laxative.
- **Skin conditions.** Aloe cream expedites the healing of cold sores. Because of its anti-inflammatory and emollient properties, it also can ease psoriasis, eczema and hemorrhoids. Apply an aloe vera cream three times daily.
- **Arthritis.** Taking aloe (either orally or topically) can help joint pain.

How to use aloe: When buying a topical gel, look for a product that contains at least 80% aloe. When drinking aloe juice, start with one teaspoon daily. Add a teaspoon daily to see how well you tolerate it until you reach six teaspoons daily, either on its own or mixed in water or some other juice. Pregnant women and children under age 13 should not use any aloe products orally. Since aloe may lower blood sugar, people with diabetes should speak to their doctors before taking aloe orally.

Comfrey Ointment Is Back to Relieve Your Pain

Mark Blumenthal, founder and executive director, American Botanical Council, Austin, Texas.

Can modern science turn an ancient healing herb with potentially dangerous toxicity into a safe salve? That was the goal of a German company that has created a product from an herb—comfrey—used traditionally to heal wounds and ease pain. Taking comfrey as a tea or capsule can harm your liver, and in fact, the US Food and Drug Administration (FDA) has advised the herb industry to not use comfrey as an ingredient in supplements. But now the herb is on the market again and may make a big comeback here as a topical ointment for treating back pain, arthritis, sprains and wounds. If you have pain, it sounds wonderful…but is it safe, and should you try it?

A HEALING HERB THAT…HARMS

You might wonder why a toxic herb has a long tradition as a healing remedy.

Here's why: It is "very effectual…for outward wounds and sores in the fleshy or sinewy part of the body," wrote the great 17th-century British physician-herbalist Nicholas Culpepper in his *Complete Herbal* (originally published in 1653), adding that comfrey "give[s] ease to pained joints." It's been used internally for purposes as diverse as treating gout and aiding bone healing (hence the nickname knitbone) and, as recently as the 1970s and 1980s, it was all the rage in teas and capsules as well as in topical preparations.

That all changed in a flash when scientists discovered that comfrey can contain significant amounts of pyrrolizidine alkaloids (PAs), which can be very toxic to the liver. Sales dropped…comfrey disappeared from the shelves…the FDA issued a safety warning about oral comfrey products. Comfrey teas and capsules? Gone.

Topical comfrey preparations such as creams, ointments and salves remained on the market. The problem is that dangerous PAs can penetrate the skin, too, and build up in the bloodstream to levels that are dangerous to the liver. When used carefully—no more than 10 days at a time…no more than four to six weeks total in a year…never on open wounds (sorry, Culpepper!)…not in children or pregnant or nursing women…not in people with liver disease—topical comfrey may be used in relative safety.

However, relative safety may not be what you are looking for! That's why there's a new product that promises to make it really safe—PA-free comfrey. To learn more, we spoke with Mark Blumenthal, executive director of the nonprofit American Botanical Council in Austin, Texas.

MODERN SCIENCE RENEWS AN ANCIENT SALVE

According to Blumenthal, a few herbal product companies, all outside the US, now cultivate varieties of comfrey with very low levels of PA, and then they test the product to make sure it is PA-free.

In the US, only one PA-free comfrey product is currently available—Traumaplant Comfrey Cream. It's manufactured in Germany and became available in the US in 2013. The cream is made from the flowers, stems and leaves of a special variety of comfrey that has been developed to be very low in PAs and then is run through a PA-removing extraction process—with the result that there are no detectable PAs in the product.

The new PA-free cream can be used not only for pain but also for cuts and abrasions, since there is no concern that PAs would get into the bloodstream. With PA-free comfrey, the beneficial compounds that promote tissue regeneration are able to work without danger of liver problems.

WHAT COMFREY HELPS

Although much of the research has been supported by manufacturers with an interest in selling comfrey, it has been published in peer-reviewed journals, finding effectiveness for…

- **Sprains.** A randomized study compared seven days of topical comfrey to seven days of topical diclofenac (a prescription nonsteroidal anti-inflammatory sold as Voltaren Gel). It was "observer blind," meaning that the health professionals didn't know which ointment each patient was getting.

Results: Comfrey led to a bigger reduction in pain at rest (92%) than the prescription product (85%), pain during motion decreased 83% with comfrey and 72% with diclofenac, and swelling decreased 81% with comfrey and 69% with diclofenac.

- **Back pain.** A randomized, double-blind study compared comfrey cream with a placebo cream for 120 participants with back pain. After five days, those who rubbed on the comfrey cream reported 95% reduction in pain intensity during movement, compared with just 38% reduction for placebo users.

- **Osteoarthritis.** A randomized, double-blind study showed that after a three-week treatment with comfrey cream (three times daily), participants with osteoarthritis of the knee reported 55% less pain at rest and during movement. Participants using a placebo cream reported 11% improvement. Comfrey users also reported higher quality of life and more mobility.

• **Wound healing.** A randomized, double-blind study compared the use of two comfrey creams, one with the same amount found in the Traumaplant preparation (10%), and the other with just 1%, in people with fresh abrasions. After two to three days, wounds were 49% smaller in participants treated with the full-strength comfrey, compared with 29% smaller in those treated with 1% cream.

THE FUTURE OF COMFREY

So now that comfrey cream without PAs is available, will an oral formulation soon be on the market? Probably not. Comfrey has been shown to be effective in clinical trials for contusions, bruises, osteoarthritis, back pain and other indications that are best treated with topical comfrey extracts, not oral formulas. So there would be no benefit. It's not recommended that people sip comfrey tea.

But if you experience joint or muscle pain and you don't want to reach for a pharmaceutical painkiller or anti-inflammatory medications (with their risks and side effects), this modern new version of an ancient healing salve with established safety is good news. Traumaplant is available online and in several department stores.

Natural Topical Treatments For Acute Pain

Jill Stansbury, ND, assistant professor and chair of the department of botanical medicine at the National College of Natural Medicine in Portland, Oregon. She is the coauthor of *Herbs for Health & Healing*. JillStansbury.net

Oils, ointments and soaks provide quick relief from the pain of muscle strains and arthritis flare-ups. For mild discomfort, try any one of the remedies below...for severe pain, use two or more. Do not use on broken skin or take internally. If skin irritation develops, discontinue use.

• **Arnica, from a daisylike plant, improves blood flow and reduces inflammation.**

To use: For stiff, aching pain, rub a palmful onto the sore area two to three times daily.

Recommended brand: Gaia Herbs Arnica Oil (800-831-7780, GaiaHerbs.com), $10.99 for one ounce.

• **Castor oil comes from the castor bean plant.** Used topically, it helps blood cells function properly...combats autoimmune diseases...and relieves pain and inflammation.

To use: Just rub a palmful onto skin of the affected area (it can be messy, so you might want to do it at bedtime).

Recommended brand: Frontier Natural Products Co-op Castor Oil (844-550-6200, FrontierCoop.com), $16.09 for 32 ounces.

• **Epsom salts contain magnesium sulfate, which fights infection and inflammation and relaxes muscles.**

To use: Fill a basin or bathtub with comfortably hot water, and mix in the desired amount of Epsom salts. The stronger you make the mixture, the more effective it is—try two to three cups of salts per tub of water. Soak the affected area for 15 to 20 minutes once or twice daily, then rinse if desired.

Recommended brand: TheraSoak from SaltWorks (800-353-7258, SaltWorks.us), $9.99 for a five-pound bag.

• **Heat rub.** Topical pain relievers (Bengay, Icy Hot) contain organic compounds, such as camphor, menthol and/or methyl salicylate. They work by creating a feeling of heat that overrides the nerves' transmission of pain.

To use: Products are available as ointments, creams or skin patches. Follow the manufacturer's instructions for the best amount and frequency of use.

Warning: Methyl salicylate is toxic if used in excess. Do not exceed recommended dosages. Never use multiple heat rubs at once. Do not use with a heating pad or while taking medication from the salicylate family, such as aspirin or antacids.

Recommended brand: Tiger Balm Red (TigerBalm.com), about $10 for four ounces, available at select drugstores and health-food stores.

Chamomile for Pain Relief

Jamison Starbuck, ND, a naturopathic physician in family practice and a guest lecturer at the University of Montana, both in Missoula. DrJamisonStarbuck.com

While many people think of drinking a cup of chamomile tea to help them relax or sleep (which it does), this herb also has several lesser-known benefits. For example, as an antispasmodic, chamomile helps control muscle spasms, as may occur with irritable bowel syndrome or diverticulitis pain. The herb also has antiseptic (germ-fighting), carminative (digestion-supporting and gas-reducing qualities) and analgesic (pain-fighting) properties. For example, dried chamomile flowers can be used to make a topical compress that relieves the pain, irritation and/or infection of sties, pinkeye, bug bites, acne, eczema, burns and hemorrhoids.

What to do: In a pot, pour three ounces of boiling water over one tablespoon of dried chamomile flowers. Cover and let sit for 10 minutes, then put the moist flowers and remaining liquid in gauze and place it directly over the skin condition you want to treat. Cover with a dry towel, and leave in place for 15 minutes. Repeat this hourly as needed. You can also use chamomile tea bags to make a compress.

How: Put as many tea bags as you need to cover the affected area in a pot, and moisten thoroughly with boiling water. Let cool slightly, then apply over the area and cover with a dry towel. Let sit for 15 minutes.

Caution: People who are allergic to ragweed may also be allergic to chamomile.

CHAPTER 24

Exercises, Stretches and Alignment for Pain Relief

How to Exercise Despite Pain

Exercise is the magic elixir. It protects the heart, strengthens bones, lifts mood, increases energy, improves memory, boosts metabolism and prevents disease. But how can you get these benefits if your body hurts?

That is the problem for millions of Americans with chronic pain, especially knee pain or back pain. You want to exercise, but getting over that "pain hump" while you exercise is just too tough.

The irony is that pain not only makes regular exercise tougher—it also makes it more important. Why? It's a path toward less pain and a greater ability to do everyday tasks.

To learn how to get exercise when jogging or even walking is painful, we spoke with physical therapist Marilyn Moffat, PT, DPT, PhD. She homed in on two of the biggest obstacles that keep most people away from pain-relieving exercise—knee pain and back pain. *Her recommendations...*

FINDING YOUR OWN PATH

I'll provide exercises below that almost everyone can do. But no single exercise is perfect for everybody, and your unique limitations and physical condition will dictate your ideal activity. Many people with chronic joint or back pain benefit from a detailed individual plan developed with a physical therapist. Ask your health-care provider for a recommendation or go to the website of the American Physical Therapy Association (MoveForwardPT.com), and click on "Find a PT" at the top of the page. It's always a good idea to check with your doctor before beginning a new exercise program.

When trying these exercises, start slowly, be cautious and pay attention to doing them correctly.

Marilyn Moffat, PT, DPT, PhD, a practicing physical therapist and professor of physical therapy at New York University, New York City. She is author of two books for the lay audience and four professional books in the field. Steinhardt.nyu.edu/faculty/Marilyn_Moffat

Important: Many people may need to build up to the "hold" times. For example, if an exercise calls for you to hold a pose for 30 seconds and that's too hard, try doing it for 10 seconds. If even that's too hard, just hold it as long as you can. You'll get stronger over time.

Stop immediately if any particular movement causes sharp pain, especially in a joint area. On the other hand, muscle fatigue (even burn) should be expected, especially with strengthening exercises. It's a good thing!

Let's get moving...

IF YOU HAVE KNEE PAIN

The best way to reduce knee pain is to increase the strength and flexibility in the muscles that support your knee. The key is to find exercises that permit pain-free range of motion. That means taking the load off the joint as much as possible. Walking in waist-deep water is a great way to do this—but not everyone has regular access to a pool. *Alternatives...*

• **Seated straight-leg raises** build up the quadriceps, which help support the knees.

What to do: Sit on the floor with your back against a wall. With one knee bent and the other leg straight out in front of you, wrap your hands around your bent leg, then slowly raise the straight leg up, keeping the knee as straight as possible—hold for 30 seconds. Then slowly lower the straight leg back to the floor. Do the exercise two or three times on each side.

• **Bridges** strengthen the hamstrings and quadriceps (key knee muscles), as well as the glutes and both the front and back of your body's core.

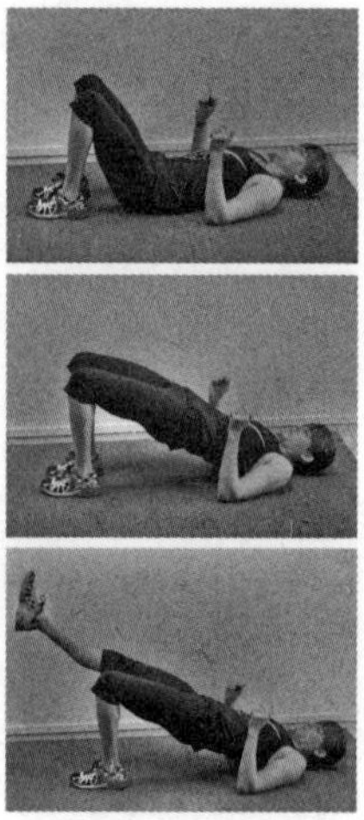

What to do: Lie on your back with your knees bent, and your feet and upper arms on the floor. Bend your elbows to a 90-degree angle, with your fingers pointing to the ceiling. Lift your glutes (butt muscles) off the floor, then straighten one leg out in the air at the level of the opposite knee and hold for 30 seconds. Bend the knee down, put your foot back on the floor and lower your butt. Alternate legs. Do this exercise two or three times per leg.

IF YOU HAVE BACK PAIN

People with spinal stenosis (narrowing of the spaces within the spine) or other degenerative changes in the low back have a hard time with many exercises. Even walking can be difficult with spinal stenosis because each step slightly extends the spine, which narrows the spinal canal, exacerbating the pain.

What helps: Increasing flexibility and core strength. Yoga planks with the spine straight or slightly rounded are especially beneficial—they strengthen the core muscles that support the back as well as the arm and leg muscles. Pay attention to good form.

• **Basic front plank.** Start on your hands and knees with your hands directly under your shoulders and your knees directly under your hips. Straighten one leg all the way back, then the other leg, and you should be in perfect position. (If weight bearing on straight arms is too difficult, do a plank on your forearms.) Tuck your chin in so that your neck is straight and you are looking at the floor. Your spine should be in a straight line and not arched. Maintain as straight a line as is comfortable from your head through to your ankles. Hold for 30 seconds. Do two or three times.

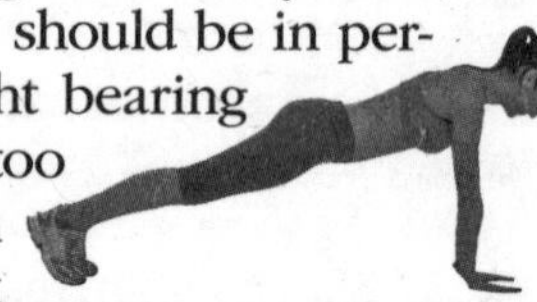

• **Side plank** also strengthens the core muscles and the arms and legs. Start by lying on your right side and with your right hand directly under your right shoulder. Ideally your feet should be stacked one on top of the other, but it's fine to start with the bottom knee bent. Lift your hips off the floor, and keep a straight line from your head through your shoulder, hips and feet. As you lift your hips, push your right hand into the floor. (Again, if weight bearing on a straight arm is too difficult, do the side plank on your forearm.) Hold for 30 seconds. Alternate sides. Do two or three times on each side.

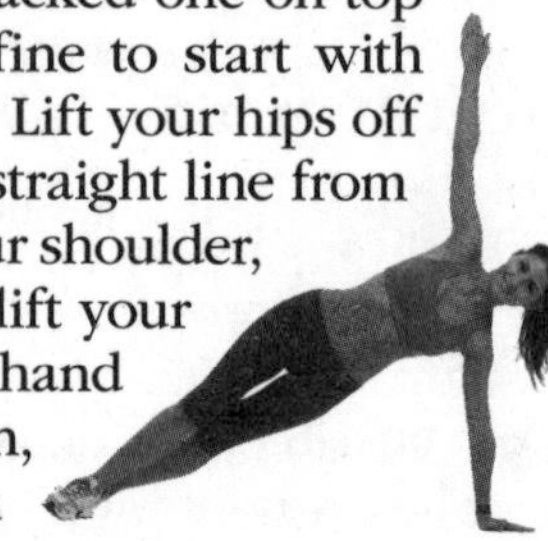

AEROBIC FITNESS FOR ANYONE WITH PAIN

Whether you have pain in your knees or back (or hips or somewhere else), getting aerobic activity to improve your circulation and protect your heart can be challenging. But it's vital! *Here are ways to do it...*

Recumbent exercise bikes (the kind where you are seated against a backrest) and seated stepper machines allow you to build your aerobic capacity. Being seated while doing aerobic exercise usually is easier for your back and reduces the forces on your knees that would occur if you were using a treadmill. The seated stepper, which resembles a recumbent elliptical machine, engages your arms as well as your legs. Many gyms have these machines.

What about walking? It's great if you can do it comfortably.

Tip: To absorb impact, wear sneakers that have good cushioned bottoms, add gel inserts into the sneakers and wear padded socks.

When walking on a treadmill, use the handrails for support and to off-load some of the force of the body weight on your back and knees.

When walking outside, choose school tracks or nature paths if possible—and consider walking poles (available online). They help to absorb some impact, engage your upper body, help intensify your workout and improve stability. Be sure to use two poles for the best balance and posture.

Photo of bridge exercise series: Courtesy of Dr. Marilyn Moffat; photos of plank exercises: Gettyimages/blanaru.

RX for Pain—A Simple Exercise Can Do the Trick

Joel Harper, personal trainer in New York City who designs workouts for Olympic athletes, celebrities, musicians and business executives. JoelHarperFitness.com He is creator of the best-selling DVDs *Firming After 50* and *Slim & Fit*. He is also author of *Mind Your Body* and writes the "Your Personal Mind-Body Coach" blog at BottomLineInc.com. Photo courtesy Joel Harper.

Before you turn to surgery or drugs for back or neck pain or carpal tunnel syndrome, try a simple exercise instead. Many of the most common injuries and disorders affecting joints, muscles, tendons, ligaments and/or nerves can be prevented, and often relieved, with targeted exercises and stretches. These work as massage for your muscles. (If the exercise or stretch starts to hurt, ease up.)

CARPAL TUNNEL PAIN

Carpal tunnel syndrome is caused by pressure on the median nerve that passes through a narrow "tunnel" in the wrist. Even a small amount of swelling or inflammation in this area can cause numbness, tingling and weakness. People who perform repetitive motions of the hand and wrist—such as assembly-line workers and those who often use computers—have a high risk of getting it. *Exercises that help...*

- **Wrist twists.** Get down on your hands and knees. Rotate your hands so that your middle fingers on each hand are facing directly toward the same knee, thumbs on the outside. Keep your elbows soft and your head down. Maintain this position for about five deep inhales. It helps to gently relax into the position. Gradually walk your knees away from your fingers to increase your stretch.

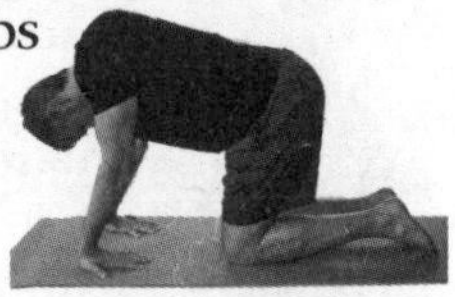

- **Wrist circles.** This movement "opens up" the wrist and reduces tightness. With your elbows bent, hold both hands in front of your torso, with the palms facing up. Rotate your hands/wrists in a complete circle five times. Then do five more circles in the opposite direction.

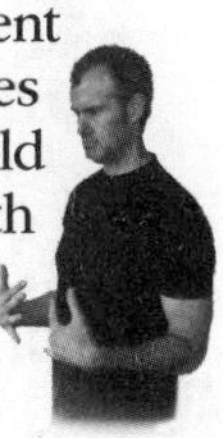

Important: It's normal for one wrist to be tighter than the other. Rotating both wrists simultaneously a few times a day will help keep the muscles balanced.

NECK PAIN

This is another malady of the computer age. People who work on computers often spend hours in the same hunched-over position without taking breaks to stretch.

Fact: Neck pain usually is caused by shoulder tension. Exercises that target the neck aren't the most effective, because they don't address shoulder tightness. *Exercises that help...*

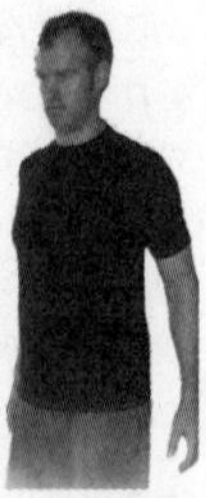

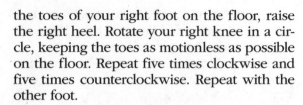

• **Shoulder rolls.** Stand straight, with your arms relaxed at your sides. Roll your shoulders in a backward circle slowly five times. Then roll them forward five times.

• **Chicken wing.** Place the back of your right hand on your right hip, with your palm facing out. Your elbow should jut out like a chicken wing. With your left hand on your right elbow, gently pull the right elbow toward your belly button. Keep your left and right shoulders at the same height. Hold the stretch for five deep inhales with your chest lifted, then repeat on the other side.

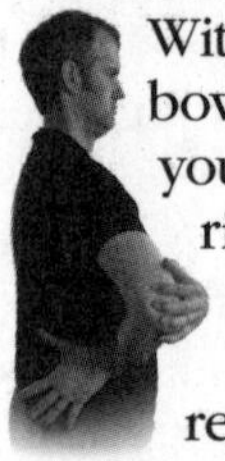

LOW-BACK PAIN

The back stretches recommended by most trainers temporarily will relieve tightness and pain, but they don't affect muscles in the hips. Tightness in the hips pulls the spine out of alignment, which can cause painful contractions in muscles in the lower back. *Exercises that help...*

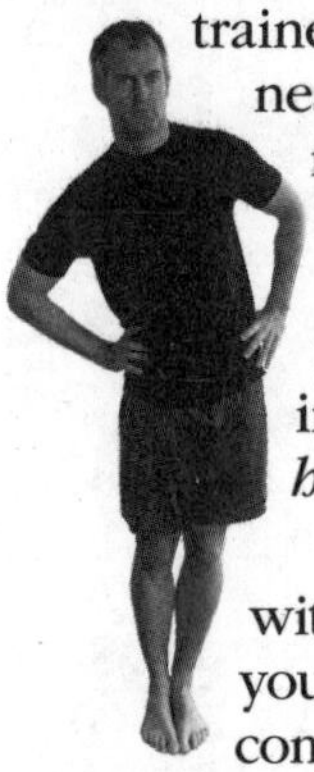

• **Hip rolls.** Stand up straight with your hands on your hips and your feet perfectly together. Make a complete circle with your hips, rotating to the right. Do this five times. Repeat in the other direction.

• **Wall hammock.** Sit on the floor with your back against a wall, your left foot flat on the floor and your left knee bent. Cross your right ankle over your left knee. From this position, slide your tailbone toward the base of the wall to cause a stretch. Hold the position for about 20 seconds, then relax. Switch legs, and do the stretch again.

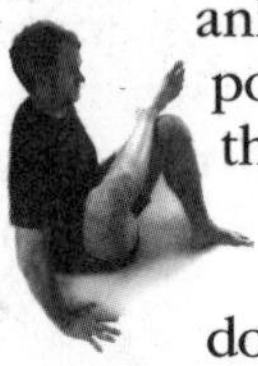

PLANTAR FASCIITIS

This is a painful inflammation of the plantar fascia, the band of connective tissue that runs from the heel bone along the bottom of the foot toward the toes. *Exercise that helps...*

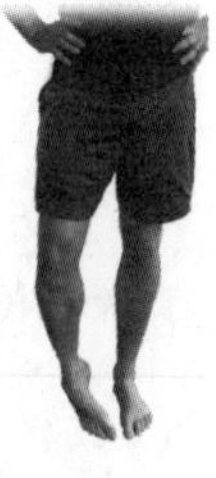

• **Toe rolls.** Stand up straight with your hands on your waist. Keeping the toes of your right foot on the floor, raise the right heel. Rotate your right knee in a circle, keeping the toes as motionless as possible on the floor. Repeat five times clockwise and five times counterclockwise. Repeat with the other foot.

SHOULDER PAIN

Shoulders often hurt because of inflammation or a small tear in the ligaments that make up the rotator cuff, the four major muscles and tendons in the shoulder.

Start by doing shoulder rolls, described at the top of the x-ray page. *Another exercise that helps...*

• **Shoulder squeezer.** Lie on the floor on your right side, with your knees slightly bent. Prop your right arm up on your triceps, with the back of the upper part of your arm flat on the floor and the fingers of your hand pointing up. Place your left hand on the back of your right wrist, and very gently press until your right palm is going toward the floor. Hold for three deep inhales, relax and then repeat once. Then switch sides.

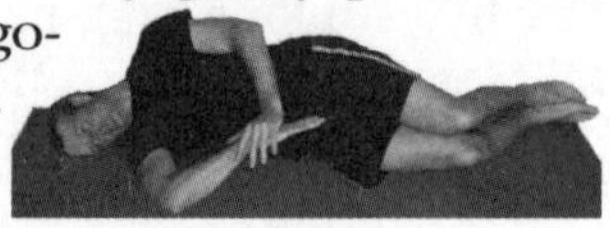

SHIN SPLINTS

They're common in runners and those who engage in stop-and-start sports, such as tennis, soccer and basketball. Repetitive and excessive force on the muscle on top of the shinbone (the same muscle that lifts the toes) can cause inflammation and/or "micro-tears" in the muscle fibers. *Exercise that helps...*

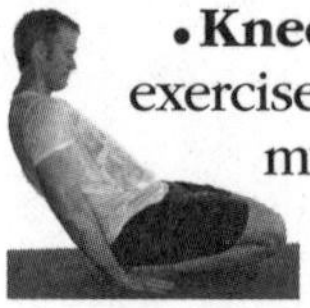

• **Knee lifts.** This is among the best exercises for reducing tightness in the muscle and, in some cases, helping shin splints heal more quickly. Do this exercise very slowly and only if you don't have knee problems. (If you have knee problems, talk with your doctor or physical therapist.)

Kneel on the floor so that you're sitting on your heels, with your shins flat on the floor. Lean back slightly, and put your palms on the floor next to each heel and your thumbs on the arches of the bottoms of your feet. Using your hands for support, press down with your arms to raise your shins slightly off the floor.

At this point, you will be balancing on your hands and toes. Hold the stretch for five to 10 deep inhales, then repeat five times.

Simple Stretches That Really Do Relieve Pain

Ben Benjamin, PhD, a sports medicine and muscular therapy practitioner, founder of The Benjamin Institute in Cambridge, Massachusetts. He is the author of several books, including *Listen to Your Pain: The Active Person's Guide to Understanding, Identifying, and Treating Pain and Injury*. BenBenjamin.com

If you suffer from pain or stiffness due to an injury, arthritis or even a neurological disorder, such as Parkinson's disease or multiple sclerosis, a type of bodywork known as Active Isolated Stretching (AIS) may give you more relief than you ever thought possible.

What makes AIS different: While most other stretching techniques recommend doing each stretch for 30 seconds or longer, AIS uses brief, two-second stretches that are done eight to 10 times each.

What's the advantage of quick, repeated stretches? This approach gives the muscle a full stretch without triggering its stretch reflex—an automatic defense mechanism that causes the muscle to contract and ultimately undo many of the stretch's benefits. The result is that muscles stretch more efficiently and avoid the buildup of waste products that lead to muscle soreness.

Developed by American kinesiologist Aaron Mattes about 35 years ago, AIS also stretches each muscle group at a variety of different angles, thus stretching all muscle fibers equally.

A MINI REGIMEN

To get a sense of AIS, try the stretches in this article. While doing each one, slowly count to yourself "one-one thousand, two-one thousand"—never any longer than two seconds. Always exhale while performing the stretch and inhale as you return to the starting position.

The first repetition of each stretch should be gentle...the second should go up to the point where you begin to feel resistance. Subsequent repetitions should push just beyond this point (with the help of your hands, a rope or other aid, if necessary) to go a few degrees further each time, thus providing a maximum stretch. If you feel discomfort during a stretch, stop the stretch at that point. If a stretch feels painful from the start, then skip it.

Daily AIS exercises that help relieve common types of pain...*

SHOULDER STRETCHES

Purpose: To help prevent muscle strain and joint sprain by increasing flexibility.

1. With your right elbow bent, position your right arm at a 90-degree angle in front of your body. Place your right palm on the back of your right shoulder. Exhale and extend your flexed arm upward as far as possible. Gently assist the stretch with your left hand. Repeat eight to 10 times on each side.

2. With your right elbow bent and your right arm positioned at a 90-degree angle in front of your body, place your right palm on the back of your right shoulder. Drop a two- to three-foot rope over your right shoulder and grasp the bottom of it with your left hand. Gently pull the rope to move your right arm upward behind your neck at a 45-degree angle for a maximum stretch. Return to the starting position after each repetition. Repeat eight to 10 times on each side.

NECK STRETCHES

Purpose: To help prevent neck injuries, relieve stiffness and improve range of motion.

1. Tuck your chin as close to your neck as possible. Put both your hands on the back of your head and, while keeping your back straight, gently bend your neck forward, bringing your chin as close to your chest as you can. Return to starting position. Repeat 10 times.

2. Gently bend your head to the right side, moving your right ear as close as possible to the top of your right shoulder. Exhale and place your right hand on the left side of your head to gently extend the stretch. Keep your left shoulder down. Focus your eyes on a point directly in front of your body to keep

*Check with your doctor before performing these movements.

your head in an aligned position. Repeat 10 times on both sides.

GETTING STARTED

For people who are new to AIS, I advise working with an AIS practitioner for hands-on instruction. If the movements are done incorrectly, you will get no benefits and could even hurt yourself. To find a practitioner near you, go to StretchingUSA.com and click on the "Practitioner Directory" link. Sessions are not typically covered by insurance and usually range from $50 to $150 per session. The website also offers books, including *Specific Stretching for Everyone*, and DVDs if you prefer to learn a complete AIS regimen on your own.

Better Movement = Less Pain

Patricia A. Buchanan, PhD, movement-improvement expert focusing on the Feldenkrais Method in Toledo, Ohio. She previously was an associate professor in the physical therapy program at Des Moines University. DrPatBuchanan.com

Many people have never heard of the Feldenkrais Method, but there are plenty of reasons why it should be on your radar. It can be used to resolve chronic musculoskeletal pain, speed recovery from injuries and/or surgery and provide relief from chronic conditions such as fibromyalgia. So what exactly is it…and how can it help you?

IT'S HOW YOU MOVE

The Feldenkrais Method (developed by Moshe Feldenkrais, DSc, an Israeli physicist, mechanical engineer and martial arts expert, after he suffered a serious knee injury) helps people become aware of the habitual movements that could be causing pain or discomfort and teaches them to replace these motions with movements that are less stressful to the body. With practice, the new movements become ingrained and automatic, and discomfort or pain is greatly minimized—pain meds can often be reduced or even stopped.

Example: If you have hip pain, you might unconsciously contract the large muscles that surround the hip joint in an effort to protect the painful area from more injury or pain. You might start to keep these muscles tight all the time—whether you're standing, sitting, walking or sleeping. This forces other muscles to overcompensate…causes imbalance in the body…and eventually increases pain and stiffness.

Research on this treatment's effectiveness for pain relief continues to mount. In a small study published in *Journal of Occupational Rehabilitation*, industrial workers who had Feldenkrais therapy showed significant reduction in neck and shoulder complaints compared with the physical therapy group. And research at California State University, Northridge, found that Feldenkrais was effective in reducing pain and decreasing disability in men and women (average age 52) with chronic low-back pain.

Important: The Feldenkrais Method is not a substitute for medical care but is often used to complement conventional medical treatment. If you have acute or severe pain, see your doctor for an evaluation before starting this treatment.

LEARNING THE METHOD

Certified Feldenkrais practitioners often have a background in physical therapy or massage, but all undergo a three-and-a-half-year accreditation program. They conduct both individual lessons (known as Functional Integration) and group sessions (Awareness Through Movement).

During individual lessons (sessions last 30 to 60 minutes), the practitioner will first ask what the client hopes to achieve—typically it will be relief from back, neck, hip or shoulder pain or recovery of mobility/function after an injury or surgery.

The practitioner will observe the client's movements/posture and use hands-on touch to discover where he/she is tight and how his movements are painful or inefficient. During a session, the client will be guided through a variety of movements, which could include everyday actions such as bending, walking or getting up from a chair.

The practitioner will then develop a lesson plan that's tailored to specific goals—for instance, how to climb stairs or raise arms with less pain or how to sit at a computer with less muscle tension.

During group sessions, the practitioner will lead a class through a series of slow movements. As in the one-on-one sessions, clients discover which movements can be done without pain and movement options for various functions such as reaching, getting up from a chair, etc. A movement that feels right for you might not work for the person next to you. These sessions last about an hour.

Some people get relief in one session while others need more. Some have lessons every week, like going to a regular yoga or Pilates class.

Feldenkrais sessions are not usually covered by insurance, but check with your provider. Individual sessions can run $100 or more, but group sessions typically cost $15 to $25. There are about 1,200 Feldenkrais practitioners in the US. To find a practitioner in your area, consult the Feldenkrais Guild of North America, Feldenkrais.com.

It is best to work with a practitioner who can give you customized instruction, but CDs, DVDs and MP3 downloads (available at FeldenkraisResources.com) can give you an overview of the process.

Not just for pain: As mentioned earlier, people often try the Feldenkrais Method because they suffer from chronic pain, but it's also popular among athletes, musicians and other physically healthy people who want to learn how to move with more efficiency and less tension. It can benefit people with multiple sclerosis as well.

This Special Form of Physical Therapy Can Heal Your Pain

Ming Chew, PT, a physical therapist with a private practice in New York City. He is author of *The Permanent Pain Cure.* MingMethod.net

Most conventional doctors' approach to orthopedic pain and injuries is "medicate or cut." But there are alternatives.

Before resorting to powerful drugs or surgery, people who suffer from aching knees, backs, shoulders, hips or necks owe it to themselves to first try physical therapy.

Secret to permanent pain relief: A specialized form of physical therapy that focuses on fascia (the tough sheet of connective tissue found in all parts of your body) is one of the most effective—yet underused—cures for joint pain.

WHY DOES IT WORK?

Over time, the fascia (pronounced fash-ee-uh) throughout your body can become less flexible from lack of exercise. Repetitive movements, such as typing, knitting, golfing or tennis playing...bad posture...or trauma, including bruising or surgery, also affect the fascia. When the fascia tightens, your muscles no longer contract properly. This results in muscle weakness that can lead to aches and pains in other parts of the body.

Important: If the fascia is injured, it won't show up on a magnetic resonance imaging (MRI) scan, which doctors routinely use to diagnose orthopedic problems. But unhealthy fascia often is the underlying cause of joint and muscle pain.

THE KEY TO HEALTHY FASCIA

To check the resilience of your fascia, place your palm flat on a table and spread your fingers as wide as possible. Using the thumb and index finger of your other hand, pinch a fold of skin on the back of your flattened hand. Pull it up and hold it for five seconds. Then let go. If the skin snaps back and becomes completely flat instantaneously, your fascia is highly elastic and healthy. If it takes longer than two seconds, your fascia has lost some elasticity.

For the health of your fascia...

- **Stay hydrated.** The fascia in your body is 70% water. For proper hydration, drink at least 64 ounces of filtered water or purified bottled water per day if you're male or 48 ounces daily if you're female.
- **Eat an anti-inflammatory diet by limiting sugar consumption** (including fruit juices and sweets), trans fats ("partially hydrogenated oils" found in many packaged and fast foods) and fried foods.

• **Take supplements to further reduce inflammation.** For example, ask your doctor about taking 1.5 g to 2.5 g of fish oil per day (taken with meals)...and a daily joint-support supplement that combines glucosamine and chondroitin (components of joint tissue and cartilage, respectively)—consult a naturopathic or integrative medicine physician for advice on specific dosages and any precautions that should be taken when using these supplements.

STRETCHING TIGHT FASCIA

The following three fascial stretches address some especially common problem areas.

Important: Always warm up with two minutes of continuous movement, such as jogging in place or performing arm circles, before stretching.*

• **Hip flexor stretch.** This stretch affects the psoas, a muscle that runs down either side of the pelvis, connecting the base of the spine to the hip bones. Tight psoas muscles are a major—and under-recognized—cause of low-back pain as well as hip and knee pain.

What to do: Place a chair on each side of your body. Kneel on your right knee and place your left leg in front of you with your left foot flat on the ground and your left knee bent 90 degrees. Place the palm of each hand on the seat of each chair.

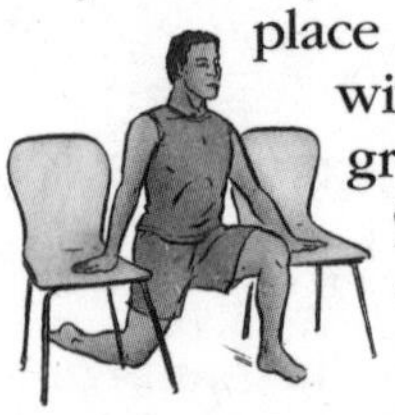

Next, tilt your entire torso to the left. While maintaining this tilt, rotate your torso to the right.

Lift your chest and tuck your chin to your chest. Clench your buttocks to press your right hip forward. To avoid arching your back, contract your abdominal muscles.

Finally, while pressing your right foot downward, imagine that you're dragging your right knee forward and contract the muscles you would use to do this. You should feel a deep stretch in the front of your right hip. Hold for 20 seconds, keeping your buttocks firmly contracted. Relax for 10 seconds, then hold for 30 seconds more. Switch legs and repeat on the other side.

*These stretches should not be performed by pregnant women or people with bone cancer, acute pain or recent muscle tears or strains.

• **Shrug muscle stretch.** This stretch affects the trapezius muscle, which runs from the lower back to the outer shoulder and base of the skull. The stretch can help relieve neck stiffness, which is often due to a tight trapezius.

What to do: While seated or standing, hold your right arm five inches out from your hip, elbow straight. Bend your wrist slightly behind your body and drop your chin to your chest. Rotate your chin to the right about 30 degrees, and hold it there while you tilt the upper part of your head to the left. Press your right shoulder down hard, away from your ear and hold for 20 seconds. You should feel a stretch from the back of your head to the outer edge of your right shoulder. Rest for 10 seconds, then hold for 30 seconds more. Repeat on the left side.

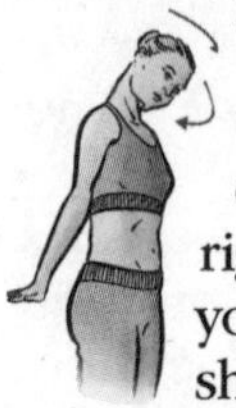

• **Biceps stretch.** This stretch helps with a range of problems, including shoulder pain, tennis elbow and golfer's elbow. It also strengthens muscles in the mid-back, which helps improve posture. For this stretch, you'll need a chair and a low table.

What to do: Place the chair back against the table and sit with your feet flat on the floor. Put both arms on the table behind you with the backs of your hands facing down. Pull both shoulders backward and lift your chest. Next, walk both feet slightly leftward so your torso is rotated to the left. Straighten your right elbow and bend your right wrist up, touching the fingers and thumb of your right hand together in a point (your left hand should remain flat on the table).

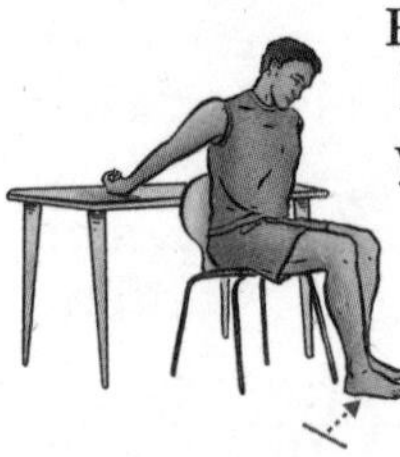

Next, tilt your head to the left, and rotate it to the left so that the right side of your neck feels a stretch. Then drop your chin to your left collarbone. It should feel like a strap is being pulled from the top front of your shoulder to your elbow. Hold for 20 seconds. Rest for 10 seconds, then hold for 30 seconds more. Switch sides and repeat.

Illustrations by Shawn Banner.

Age-Defying Moves

Marilyn Moffat, PT, DPT, PhD, professor of physical therapy at New York University in New York City and coauthor of *Age-Defying Fitness*.

Physical therapy exercises you can do at home help your body retain youthful vigor. How? By improving posture, balance, flexibility and strength. The anti-aging moves below are quick and simple and require no equipment. For seated exercises, sit in a straight-backed chair, feet flat on floor and hip-width apart.

All exercises: To do a "set," repeat each move three times, breathing slowly and deeply...relax momentarily between each repetition. Aim for two or three sets daily.*

- **Improved Posture.** Poor posture makes your spine curve and jaw jut forward (as shown at right), causing back and neck pain and compressing the lungs. These moves correct head alignment and strengthen mid-back muscles.

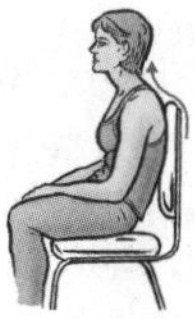

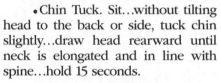

- Chin Tuck. Sit...without tilting head to the back or side, tuck chin slightly...draw head rearward until neck is elongated and in line with spine...hold 15 seconds.

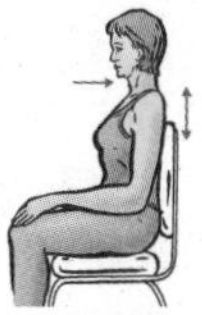

- Isometric Elbow Press. Sit...bend elbows to a 90-degree angle so hands are in front of you, held in relaxed fists. Keeping your back against the chair back, press elbows backward against the chair back, using the pressure to help straighten spine...hold 15 seconds.

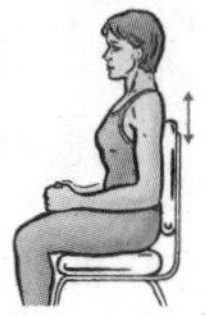

- **Better Balance.** Avoiding falls requires keeping your balance while moving.

- Tandem Walk. Stand straight, abdominal muscles ("abs") tight, head aligned with spine. Stepping forward, place right foot directly in front of left foot, so right heel touches left toes (as if on a tightrope). Walk this way for 15 feet. Start slowly...increase your pace gradually as balance improves.

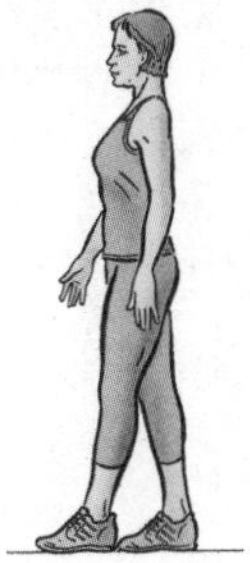

*It's always best to check with your doctor before starting a new exercise routine, especially if you have joint pain or any other physical challenges.

- **Greater Flexibility.** Being flexible helps prevent muscle and joint injuries. For these moves, sit with hips six to 10 inches from the chair back.

- Behind-the-Back Shoulder Stretch. Reach left hand over left shoulder, palm facing your back...bring right hand up behind your back, palm facing away from you. Gently move left hand down and right hand up for 30 seconds, trying to get tips of third fingers of each hand to touch. Switch hand positions and repeat.

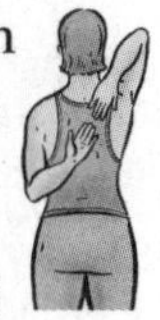

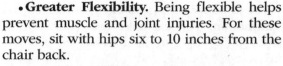

- Sit-and-Reach. Straighten right knee and place right heel on floor, toes pointed toward ceiling. With one hand on top of the other, lean forward, trying to touch toes of right foot...hold 30 seconds. Switch to left leg. (If you have low bone density or a history of spine fractures, skip this exercise.)

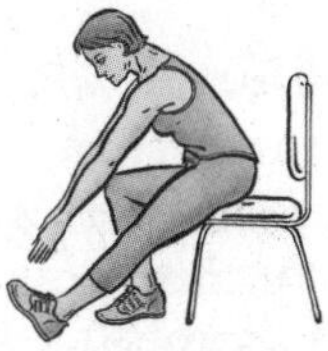

- **Increased Strength.** The stronger you are, the easier it is to do just about anything.

- Plank Position. Get down on all fours, hands flat on floor and directly below shoulders. Tightening abs and keeping head aligned with spine, extend one leg and then the other until toes are curled under and on the floor in "push-up" position. Hold position, with body perfectly straight, for 15 to 30 seconds (do not lower yourself into a push-up)...return to hands and knees.

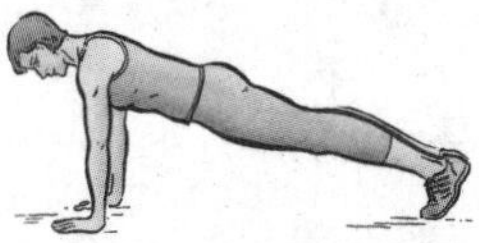

Illustrations by Shawn Banner.

Yoga Fights Pain

Chronic pain sufferers should hit the yoga mat. Chronic pain can cause loss of gray matter in the brain, which can lead to memory loss, cognitive impairment, emotional problems and reduced pain tolerance.

New finding: Practicing yoga can actually increase gray matter in the brain, including in the area related to pain tolerance.

M. Catherine Bushnell, PhD, scientific director, National Center for Complementary and Integrative Health, Bethesda, Maryland.

Resistance Bands: A Fun and Easy Way To Get Much Stronger

Karl Knopf, EdD, the author of *Injury Rehab with Resistance Bands* and coauthor of the *International Sports Sciences Association's Senior Fitness Certification Course.* He also sits on the board of directors for PBS's *Sit and Be Fit*. Dr. Knopf is the retired coordinator for the Adaptive Fitness Therapy Program and Life Long Learning Institute at Foothill College in Los Altos, California.

If you've ever been in physical therapy, you've likely used a stretchy latex tube or flat strip called a resistance band. It is incredibly effective at building strength and endurance…easing lower back pain and arthritic discomfort…and improving balance.

What you may not know: Resistance bands are a safe way to build strength on your own if you have a bad back, joint pain or other problems that can make weight-lifting off-limits. Once your health-care provider gives you the green light, first try whatever moves below are right for your condition without a band—to make sure you can do the motion without pain or discomfort before adding resistance. (If there is discomfort, check in again with your doctor for advice.) Ideally, these exercises should be done three to four times a week.

If you have low-back pain: It is often due to weak abdominal muscles…tight hamstrings and quadriceps…and/or tight hip flexors (the muscles that connect the legs to the torso). Your goal is to strengthen the abdominals, the lower back muscles and the glutes while reducing hip flexor tension. *What helps…*

- **Pelvic lifts.** While lying on your back, place a band across your hips and grab each end, placing your fists on the floor. Slowly lift your hips to a comfortable height (a 45-degree angle from hips to shoulders is ideal), engaging your glutes (the muscles in your buttocks). Count to one, then return to start position. Repeat 15 times.

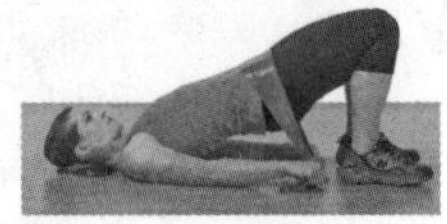

If you have hip pain or hip arthritis: Years of overuse or being overweight can turn good hips bad. The moves below help promote the stability and mobility that healthy hips need. *Note*: If you've had a hip replacement or have severe hip issues, consult your doctor for specific exercises.

- **Seated leg press.** This works the quadriceps (the stronger the leg muscles are, the less stress is placed on painful joints). Sit in a chair, both hands gripping either end of a band so that you can loop the band around your right foot. Keeping your left foot on the floor, lift the right leg up, gently resting the right foot in the middle of the band. Extend your right leg out in front nearly all the way, then crisscross the band once to keep your foot from slipping off. Pull elbows back to the waist. Slowly bring the right knee in toward your chest, stopping when knees reach a 90-degree angle, and press back out, without locking your knee. Switch sides. Start with just a few reps and gradually build up.

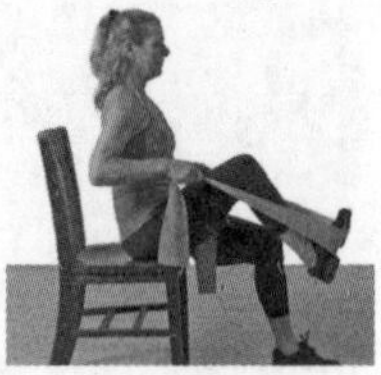

- **Hip extension.** Attach a flat band or tubular band* (see photo) to a door using a door anchor strap (available online or in sporting goods stores). Facing the door, attach the other end of the band to your right ankle. Move far enough away from the door to place some tension on the band. Keeping a slight bend in the left leg, slowly extend your right leg backward, engaging the glutes. You can grasp a chair for balance. Hold for one to two seconds before returning to the start position. Repeat 10 to 15 times. Switch sides.

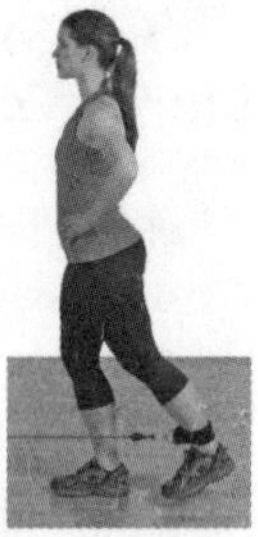

If you have a knee injury: Knees are meant to straighten and bend. Any other movement, such as twisting and pivoting, places them at risk. Healthy knees demand strong quadriceps, which provide stability and support. *What to do…*

- **Forward lunge.** Stand with your left foot in the middle of your band and grab the ends with each hand at a location that provides ad-

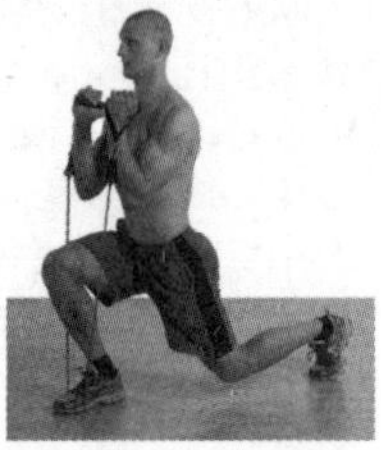

*People who have had pain or arthritis often like to use a tubular band. It is less likely to tear or snap—and comes with easy-to-grip handles.

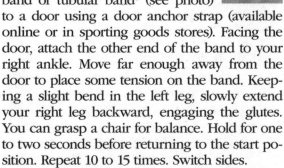

equate resistance. Typically, your elbows will be waist-high, arms bent. Slide your right foot backward, attempting to lower your right knee as low as you comfortably can—to the floor if possible. Now transfer your weight back to your left leg as you push up through your left quad and glutes until standing. You should feel an increase in resistance in your left leg as you rise up. Repeat three to five times. Switch sides.

WHAT TO LOOK FOR...

Resistance bands are available online or in sporting goods stores for about $20 or less. They come in a rainbow of colors, each representing a different intensity. They also come in different lengths—the longer the length, the less resistance. For most beginners, I advise starting with a three- to six-foot flat band. To increase the intensity, you can "choke up" on the band before moving up to a band with a higher level of resistance.

Stretch Away Your Pain

Joseph Tieri, DO, an osteopathic physician who is an adjunct professor at Touro College of Osteopathic Medicine in Middletown, New York, and co-owner of Stone Ridge Healing Arts in Stone Ridge, New York. Dr. Tieri is also the author of *End Everyday Pain for 50+: A 10-Minute-a-Day Program of Stretching, Strengthening and Movement to Break the Grip of Pain*. EndEverydayPain.com

Those everyday aches and pains that we all experience are commonly chalked up to arthritis. But that condition is the true cause far less often than most people realize.

While your doctor may order an MRI, discover arthritis or a bulging disk, and blame your musculoskeletal pain on that, studies reveal that arthritis and other degenerative conditions often can be detected on the films of pain-free middle-aged and older people. Age-related musculoskeletal aches and pains that result from tension and misalignment are far more common than arthritis but don't show up on film. As a result, many patients resort to medicine or even surgery for arthritis or herniated disks when that's not the real source of their pain.

Instead, it's poor posture combined with the inactivity of everyday living and underused joints that leads to stiffness and pain, whether it's shoulder pain, hip pain, back pain, etc.

Good news: Doing strategic stretching, strengthening and range of motion exercises for just a few minutes a day is enough to keep your muscles supple, your joints lubricated and everyday aches and pains at bay. Incorporate each of these moves into your daily routine to prevent various types of pain and to help relieve it.

Note: Hold each stretch for 30 seconds if you're younger than age 65...and for 60 seconds if you're 65 or older.

Most of the benefit comes from the first stretch, so one repetition is sufficient. *However, you can repeat these stretches throughout the day whenever your back, neck, hips and/or shoulders feel tight or stiff...*

• **Shoulder and chest stretch.** This is one of the most important—and simplest—moves you can do to reverse the rounded-shoulder posture that affects so many people.

What to do: Lie on the floor (on an exercise mat, if you like), face up, arms straight out to the sides in a "T" position with palms up. That's it! Believe it or not, this very simple stretch helps loosen the tight, shortened muscles in the front of your neck, shoulders and chest.

• **Neck stretch.** This stretch reverses the tension caused when one's head juts forward—common when driving or typing. It also elongates and aligns the neck, creating space for disks between the vertebrae, which lessens the odds of a bulging or herniated disk.

What to do: Begin by lying flat on your back on a bed or a mat on the floor (a wedge mat as shown in the photo below may be more comfortable for older individuals). Allow your head to relax for a few seconds. Then reach up and place

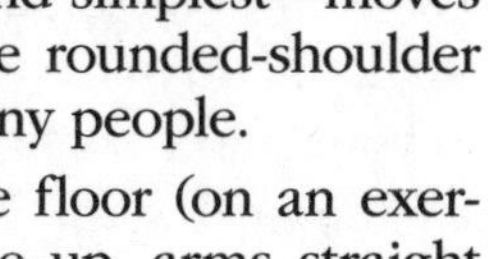

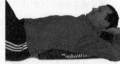

the fingers of both hands in the space beneath your neck. With fingertips touching, move them to the bottom of your head. Now move your fingers up, pushing or sliding the back of your head upwards, feeling the back of your neck elongating. Then hold.

Note: This movement may tilt your head down a bit, but the back of your head should stay in contact with the bed or mat at all times.

• **Psoas stretch.** The psoas (pronounced "SO-az") is the most important muscle you've never heard of—it's the main muscle connecting the spine to the legs, and it works with other muscles to stabilize the lower spine and promote proper body alignment. The psoas often weakens with age and inactivity, leading to lower back and hip pain and poor posture.

What to do: Start by lying flat on your belly (on an exercise mat, if you wish) with your forehead resting on the backs of your crossed hands. Allow your stomach to relax and notice the natural curve of your lower back. For many older patients, this provides enough of a stretch—if so, continue doing this daily for a week or two until you no longer feel the stretch in your lower back, which means you're ready for the next step—slowly press up onto your forearms (Sphinx) or your palms (Cobra). Remember, keeping your belly relaxed as your lower back gently stretches is more important than trying to lift higher.

• **Piriformis stretch.** The piriformis is a small muscle that runs diagonally from the bottom part of the spine to the upper thighbone on each side of the body. Asymmetry can develop after years of driving with your right foot on the gas pedal, crossing your legs the same way or sleeping in the same position, which can cause pain in the hips and lower back.

What to do: Sit in a chair with both feet on the floor. Rest your right ankle on top of your left thigh, just above the knee. Keeping your back straight, gently bend forward at the waist until you feel a stretch in your right thigh and glute. Then repeat on the other side.

Feel-Great Posture Secrets

Kathleen Porter, author of *Ageless Spine, Lasting Health* and director, Natural Posture Solutions, LLC, Portland, Oregon. NaturalPostureSolutions.com

Standing the wrong way can worsen such conditions as osteoporosis, arthritis, lower back pain and neck and shoulder pain. Conversely, when you hold your body correctly it extends your spine—not only does this do wonders for back pain, it also gives ample support and space to the internal organs and nerves and enhances circulation. Just reading those words feels good, doesn't it?

THREE RULES TO UNLEARN

There are three common postural rules we should all work to unlearn. Correcting these particular behaviors will go far toward making many of us feel a whole lot better.

Posture myth #1: **Tuck your butt.** A common instruction when standing up straight is to "tuck your butt" (or your tailbone) under.

Problems it causes: Tucking your butt takes your legbones out from under you. Your legs should be like vertical posts to properly support your weight. Otherwise, the muscles in your back, shoulders and/or neck must work harder.

Posture myth #2: **Hold your chest high.** Many people think the proper stance is to squeeze back the shoulder blades, angling the breastbone (sternum) slightly up and toward the sky. It's the way that soldiers and athletes typically stand—and don't they look like great role models for good posture?

Better Posture Eases Pain

People feel more powerful, in control and able to tolerate pain when they stand tall. Better posture may increase levels of testosterone, which improves pain tolerance and decreases stress hormones.

Vanessa Bohns, PhD, assistant professor, department of management sciences, University of Waterloo, Ontario, Canada, and Scott Wiltermuth, PhD, assistant professor of management and organization, USC Marshall School of Business, Los Angeles.

How this hurts: Lifting the chest displaces the ribcage, tightens neck muscles, compresses the spine and works many muscles—when the goal is to keep them tension-free. You'll often hear people say that they love to stretch, but that's really an indication of stored-up tension caused by unnatural posture. A body in correct alignment has no tight muscles that need relief!

***Posture myth #3:* Suck in your belly.** Give it a try—hold those stomach muscles tight. Are you breathing? Are you more relaxed?

Why it's wrong: Tensing the belly tightens the diaphragm, putting pressure on the lungs and making it harder to breathe fully—plus it triggers the motion of tilting and tucking the pelvis toward the back, flattening your bottom. This tilted pelvis shifts the pelvic floor muscles out of place, making it harder for them to support the organs in the lower abdomen and putting excessive tension in the lower back. Also, a tight belly interferes with the work of certain muscle groups—the oblique and transversus abdominis. These are the deepest abdominal muscles—they wrap around the torso, running from the ribs to the pelvis, and are crucial to proper alignment and supporting the core of the body.

THE RIGHT WAY TO STAND

Start by looking down at your feet, with your shoulders back (keeping the plumb line in mind). Hold your sternum perpendicular to the floor and lift your ribs by pulling up from the lower ribs in the back.

Helpful mental image: Picture yourself as a marionette with strings attached to the back of your lower ribs and just inside the back of each of your armpits. Now imagine the strings being gently drawn up behind you. Roll each shoulder in a circular motion forward, around, up and back—letting the shoulder come to rest right on top of the rib cage. Lift your face just enough to see comfortably in front of you as you imagine that a string at the base of your skull pulls just a bit of length into the back of your neck. Relax your belly muscles as well. Take a minute and breathe.

Returning to proper alignment is not a quick fix, and it almost always feels awkward at first. As many times a day as you can remember, visualize yourself as a skeleton. This will help you focus on what is happening with your bones, muscles and joints as well as on the corrections you need to make.

The Right Way to Stand and Walk for More Energy and Less Pain

Mitchell Yass, DPT, a Florida–based physical therapist and creator of the Yass Method for treating chronic pain. He is also the author of *The Pain Cure Rx: The Yass Method for Diagnosing and Resolving Chronic Pain* and the PBS special *The Pain Prescription.* MitchellYass.com

When you are standing or walking, do you ever think about where you are placing your feet? Of course not! We are not designed to have to think about these things. Posture and movement are subconscious, and they are supposed to take care of themselves. Right?

Well...not exactly. Over time, any aspect of the body can (and does) go off track. When it comes to standing or walking, your feet may gradually move closer together until your heels touch or, worse, your feet begin to cross. The dangerous effect of this phenomenon is that you stop using your skeleton to support you and instead begin to depend almost exclusively on muscle.

The result: The muscles responsible for supporting the body when you stand or walk take on a much bigger load than they were designed for, becoming overused and strained. This will lead to the sense that you have weights around your ankles, making standing or walking very hard. You may begin to feel that even the smallest walk, let's say from one side of a room to another, feels like you've walked miles. When you are out, you may begin to feel that you need to sit down to rest every block or two because you are so tired—yes, even from this little level of activity.

My great concern here is that you will seek medical attention regarding this "fatigue" factor. Once the medical system gets involved, you will have batteries of tests for your heart, lungs, your metabolic status (such as checking for diabetes). You may even be checked for depression—all because you feel very tired doing what is seemingly very little activity.

Let's break down the actual mechanics of what's going on here so you don't end up being misdiagnosed and sent down a path of medication and erroneous treatment.

Think about the force of gravity that is always pushing down on you. Gravity pushes down in a vertical line directly perpendicular to the ground. If the skeleton is properly aligned to be perpendicular to the ground, then your skeleton can support this load. The bones require no energy to achieve this support. They are simply building blocks placed in alignment with the force (gravity) so they absorb that force.

The proper alignment of the leg bones from the pelvis to the foot is when the foot is directly under the hip joint. This means that you should keep about five to six inches between your feet whenever you stand or walk.

Let's try this simple experiment...

Stand in front of a full-length mirror with your feet directly under your hips. Notice that in this stance, your legs are perpendicular to the ground.

Place your feet next to one another, aligned with the midline of the body. Try to hold this stance for one minute. See how hard you are working to support yourself?

Next, place your feet directly under your hips and stand for one minute. Notice how you are exerting dramatically less energy this time? That is because your skeleton is now taking a large portion of the force of gravity rather than your muscles.

Now that you understand that the most efficient and proper positioning of your feet is directly under your hips, how do maintain it? *You need to do two things...*

- **Correct your faulty movement pattern.** It takes 21 days for a new movement pattern to be ingrained in the brain and considered to be the correct pattern. So for 21 days you need to keep consciously correcting yourself whenever your feet are not being maintained at hip-width distance while standing or walking. After 21 days of conscious effort and strengthening your gluteus medius (see below), your feet will remain under your hips subconsciously.

- **Strengthen the muscles that sit at the side of the pelvis—the gluteus medius muscles.** They are responsible for keeping your feet hip-width apart. The exercise to be performed is *hip abduction.* This exercise is surely sounding familiar to you by now. I've also advised it for helping to resolve low-back pain, knee pain, plantar fasciitis and preventing recurring sprained ankles. The stronger your gluteus medius muscles, the easier it will be to keep the feet hip-width apart.

This exercise can be performed either lying on your side or standing. To do it correctly, make sure you do not go too far when moving your leg outward. People falsely believe that more range of motion is better, but in this case too much range of motion means you are using the lower back muscle to create the motion, not the gluteus medius (hip muscle). The gluteus medius muscle can only move the leg out to the point where it is parallel with the hip joint. Any outward motion beyond that is created by the lower back muscle.

HIP ABDUCTION

To do the exercise lying down, lie on your side with the knee of the bottom leg bent and the top leg straight. The top leg should run in a continuous line from the torso—if the leg is angled in front of the torso, you would use the wrong muscle. Start to raise the top leg off the supporting leg until your top leg is parallel with the floor. As you lift, try to turn the leg in slightly so the heel is the first part of the foot that is moving. This puts the gluteus medius in the optimal position to raise the leg. Once your leg reaches parallel to the floor, begin to

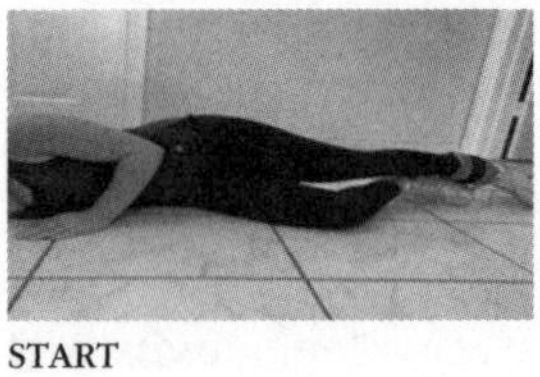

START

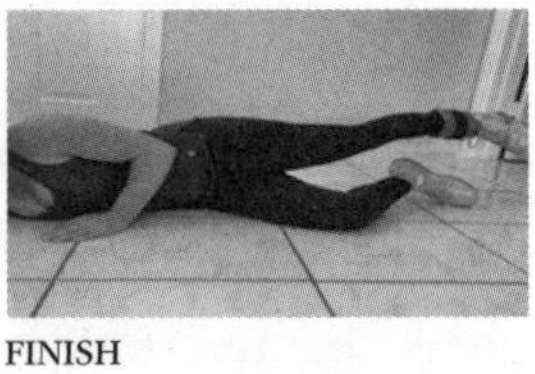

FINISH

lower it back onto the supporting leg.

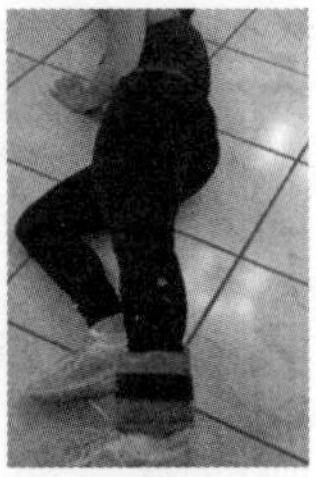

SIDE VIEW

If you prefer to stand, the outward movement is similar to when lying down—lead with the heel, and don't move your leg too far to keep the exercise focused on the gluteus medius. Holding on to a sturdy table or chair while you perform the exercise will make it easier to use proper form.

Perform this exercise three times a week. At each session, performed three sets of 10 repetitions with a one-minute break between sets. Gradually increase the resistance used until the muscles involved are strong enough to perform your functional activities without straining and emitting symptoms.

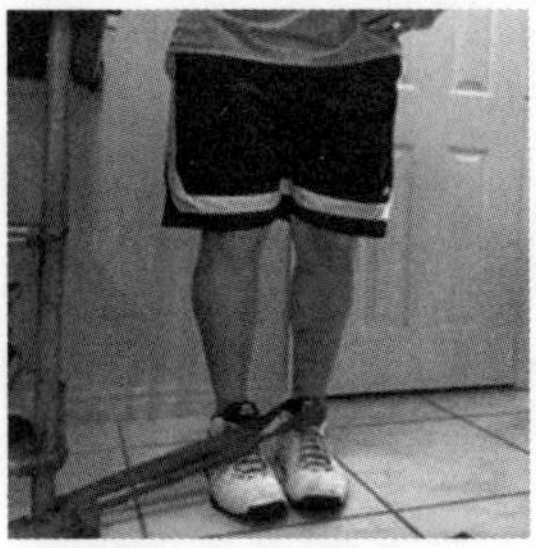

START

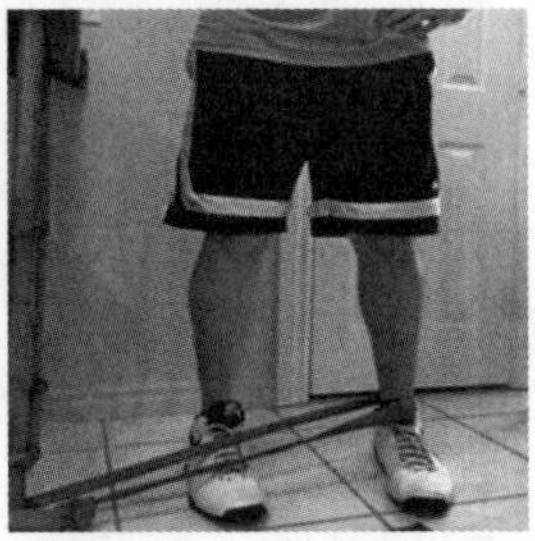

FINISH

Will it be a tough three weeks? Sure. But it's worth the effort! You will find it easier to perform all weight-bearing activities, and you will be able to do them for longer periods of time. You will also decrease the chances of straining other muscles that work in conjunction with these muscles. So you can prevent back pain, hip-region pain, groin pain, knee pain and even ankle pain by strengthening the gluteus medius muscles and relearning to place your feet under your hips. For the ladies out there, this may seem a bit manly, but I assure you—your quality of life will increase so substantially that a little change in how you move will be well worth it.

CHAPTER 25

Mind-Over-Body Pain Relief

The Mind-Body Cure For Chronic Pain Helps Headaches, Back Pain And More

From backaches and headaches to wrist pain caused by carpal tunnel syndrome, chronic pain continues to be an enormous problem in this country. Why is that? Because the average doctor persists in the mistaken belief that pain is a structural disorder only.

It's now quite clear that most chronic pain is the result of an emotionally induced physical condition—which, in turn, is the result of hidden conflict between our conscious and unconscious minds.

This mind-body cycle of pain is known as tension myositis syndrome (TMS).

THREE-STEP SEQUENCE

Chronic pain typically occurs as a result of a three-step sequence...

1. You're under pressure. It might be psychological stress caused by perfectionism or another self-induced pressure...or an external pressure, such as a demanding boss.

2. Growing pressure gives rise to rage and frustration. These feelings lie within the unconscious mind only. That's because they're simply too frightening to be acceptable to your conscious mind. You're not even aware of their existence—despite the fact that they can be very intense.

3. To keep angry feelings from spilling over into consciousness, your subconscious mind directs your attention to your body. It

John E. Sarno, MD, who died in 2017, was professor of clinical rehabilitation medicine at New York University School of Medicine and an attending physician at The Rusk Institute of Rehabilitation Medicine, both in New York City. He was author of several best-selling books, including *Healing Back Pain: The Mind-Body Connection* and *The Divided Mind: The Epidemic of Mindbody Disorders.*

does so by activating your autonomic nervous system, which controls digestion, respiration, circulation and other involuntary functions. Upon activation, the autonomic nervous system reduces blood flow to a particular muscle, tendon or nerve. Exactly which part of the body is affected varies. The decrease in circulation deprives the tissues of oxygen. That causes pain.

STOPPING CHRONIC PAIN

To stop pain caused by TMS, you don't need painkilling medication...or surgery...or physical therapy. What you need is an understanding of the three-step sequence. Once you acknowledge that pain stems from the subconscious mind's efforts to protect your conscious mind from troubling emotions, you can get on with the cure...

Have a doctor rule out physical causes. You must be absolutely certain that there is no serious disease causing your pain—cancer, for example.

Important: Despite what many doctors believe, spinal disc abnormalities are rarely the cause of back pain. In a 1984 study, back-pain sufferers proved to be no more likely to have spinal disc degeneration or bone spurs than people who did not have back pain. In a similar study, researchers detected disc abnormalities in 64 people—none of whom had back pain.

- **"Talk" to your brain.** This sounds silly, but it works. If you feel a twinge of pain, silently tell your brain that you know what it is doing—you can even tell it to increase the blood flow to the painful area. Put your brain on notice that you're no longer going to let yourself be affected by its efforts to shield you from negative emotions.

Accept that pain is caused by repressed emotions. It can be very hard to admit that emotions are causing your pain—especially if a doctor has told you that the culprit is a slipped disc or another structural problem...or physical stress, such as that caused by typing for hours a day. Of course, your conscious mind is desperately trying to deny that emotions are the cause. It doesn't want to experience those emotions—or even admit they exist.

- **Make a written list of the possible sources of your psychological stress.** In making the list, remember that most distress is internally generated. Two common examples...

Example #1: **Perfectionism.** Because you're so eager to excel at everything you do, you're highly critical of yourself—and overly sensitive to criticism from others.

Example #2: **The need to be liked.** You try to be good and nice to everyone—because you want everyone's love, admiration and respect. "Goodism" is just as stressful as perfectionism—and just as likely to cause frustration and rage.

External causes of distress might include a mean boss, an argumentative spouse, a meddlesome relative or another person with whom you have a difficult relationship.

It could also be serious financial trouble or simply a sense of having too little time to get things done.

Even happy experiences—marriage, job promotion, a new baby—create pressure. And pressure creates unconscious rage.

By reading and rereading your list—and reminding yourself of the true cause of your pain—you'll "cure" the pain. Most people who use this technique become pain-free within eight weeks.

- **Review your list on a daily basis.** Spend at least 30 minutes a day thinking about each item on your list and how it could be causing pressure in your life. Resolve to take action to defuse the pressures you can change...and to accept the pressures you cannot change.

- **Visualize your rage.** Imagine yourself in a blind fury. That is the experience your unconscious mind is having to cope with on a continuing basis. Now consider what might happen if you gave free rein to your rage. You could ruin your marriage, lose your job—even wind up in jail. Your conscious mind is as frightened of these experiences as you are. That's why it chooses to hide your rage from you.

- **Resume physical activity.** Once your pain has largely subsided, go back to exercising, lifting heavy objects, using a computer keyboard, etc. Start slowly, and build up over a period of weeks.

If you're afraid to resume normal activity, it means that your unconscious mind is still in charge. You've got more mind-body work to do.

• **Understand "location substitution."** Say you've just gotten over a bad case of back pain—and now your elbow has started to hurt. Chances are that the brain has simply picked a new spot in your body to cause pain to distract you from your rage. Realize the same pain process is happening once again—only in another part of your body. Once again, the pain should disappear.

STAY PAIN-FREE FOREVER

To keep pain at bay, you must continually remind yourself that pressure causes unconscious, frightening rage...and your brain distracts your attention from that rage by creating pain. Tell yourself this again and again, and you should stay pain-free for the rest of your life.

Mind-Touch Combo To Relieve Pain

Beth Darnall, PhD, assistant professor, department of anesthesiology and perioperative medicine, Oregon Health & Science University, Portland.

We generally assume that when something hurts, the pain is caused by a real biological event—a wound, an infection, a sprain. But this isn't always the case. For instance, consider the dramatic example of phantom limb pain, in which people experience sensations—most often pain—in an arm or leg that has been amputated. It's puzzling...and oddly fascinating...all the more so now that neuroscientists have discovered that they can use mirrors (in a complicated arrangement) to trick the brain into "seeing" the missing limb as present—and that doing so causes the pain to stop! There's more research where UK scientists have started to develop simpler tricks that people with any kind of pain can do themselves—no mirrors needed (no drugs either)—to "fool" their brains into perceiving less pain. It involves simply touching your own body in a certain way. It sounds so appealing—does it really work?

THE BRAIN'S POINT OF VIEW

The technique involves a process that scientists call "brain signaling." An ample body of research has shown that often the brain does not distinguish between what is real (that you can see and touch) and what it just believes to be true based on experience. Furthermore, research shows that just thinking negatively about pain can create biochemical changes that show up in MRI brain scans when areas associated with pain light up. In other words, people can literally grow their pain through their thoughts—so it also makes sense that people can use their brains to banish it.

MIND OVER PAIN

So what can we do with this intriguing research finding? *Here's advice on how to put it to use right now...*

The first step is to become aware of the extent to which chronic pain triggers anxiety and catastrophic thinking (chronic thoughts and feelings of helplessness and doom). This increases stress and worsens pain, so it is crucial to establish ways to calm and center your body and mind—otherwise you'll be at the mercy of anything in the environment, including your own body. Cognitive behavior therapy can be a good way to learn how to eliminate anxiety and catastrophic thinking, noting that studies show that such therapy actually can change—physically change—the neural networks of the brain and make them healthier.

As far as the self-touch method for pain relief, the technique is called "bilateral tactile stimulation." You can learn to use it on yourself for pain relief—though it's important to start with a practitioner in order to experience how it is properly done.

Note: Psychotherapists trained in either Eye Movement Desensitization Reprocessing (EMDR) or Emotional Freedom Technique (EFT) are the ones most likely to be familiar with this technique.

How it works: Sitting in front of the client, the therapist leads him/her through a guided visualization or deep-relaxation exercise while lightly and rapidly tapping one side and then the other of (for example) the back of the knees or hands—a place that is easy to reach and comfortable but not the painful spot. This is done for one to three minutes. *This works to reduce pain in the following ways...*

Tapping while also doing a guided visualization seems to help patients encode positive images, feelings and thoughts more quickly.

In turn, this helps put a stop to the cycle of pain, stress and the body's inflammatory response by keeping the brain from focusing on helplessness and how much it hurts.

Lastly, this technique can help deepen the relaxation response, thereby releasing the muscle tension that pain causes and, with it, the pain itself. In other words, the tapping helps to encode and anchor information in the brain, including the information that the patient is fully relaxed and pain-free.

THE AT-HOME VERSION

Once you are familiar with the process and feel ready to try it on yourself, here is an at-home process to follow...

Sit or lie down in a comfortable position. Because it is crucial to feel calm before using this technique, listen to a relaxation-response CD (many are available online and at health-food stores), meditate or do some diaphragmatic breathing to first get centered.

Once you are relaxed and calm, focus on envisioning positive images. Create an image of yourself hurting less and functioning better. Concentrate on how good it feels to move without pain...to experience joy...or to accomplish goals you set for yourself.

Now, alternating one side of the body and the other, tap your knees, legs or upper arms—whatever location you have chosen where you can easily reach and you have sensation (no numbness). Using the opposite hand (e.g., left hand on right knee, right hand on left knee), tap at a rate of two or three taps per second, all the while continuing your positive imagery, as described above. Start with sessions of about three minutes, and gradually add more time in later sessions if you wish.

As you become more practiced at this simple pain-relief technique, try to expand your vision of yourself, creating new visualizations where you picture yourself moving more easily around your life, pain-free, exercising and engaging in other activities you enjoy. Keep tapping as you do this...consider it a source of positive energy that you can "tap" at any time you wish!

Hypnosis: Painful Problems It's Been Proven to Help

Marc I. Oster, PsyD, a psychologist and professor of clinical psychology at the Illinois School of Professional Psychology at Argosy University in Schaumburg, Illinois. He is a fellow and past president of the American Society of Clinical Hypnosis and the recipient of the Milton H. Erickson Award for Scientific Excellence in Writing on Clinical Hypnosis.

Don't confuse medical hypnosis with the flamboyant stage shows that feature a swinging watch, a performer in a glittery jacket and volunteers from the audience, all quacking like ducks.

Hypnosis-enhanced therapy is a legitimate treatment for various medical problems—and unlike many treatments, it is noninvasive and totally safe.

Here are specific painful conditions hypnosis can help...

IRRITABLE BOWEL SYNDROME

IBS is a mysterious, often debilitating condition that causes cramps and intermittent episodes of diarrhea, pain and constipation. Medications to treat it often aren't very effective.

Several well-designed studies of hypnotherapy for IBS have shown that IBS patients who were treated with hypnosis had "substantial, long-term improvement" of gastrointestinal symptoms, along with less anxiety and depression. It's possible that hypnosis alters how the central nervous system responds to intestinal signals. It also diverts people's attention from their intestinal sensations and causes them to perceive less discomfort.

PAIN RELIEF

Hypnosis doesn't necessarily reduce pain, but it does alter how people react to it. Studies have shown, for example, that hypnotized dental patients have a higher pain threshold. They also have less anxiety, which reduces sensitivity to pain.

One study, which looked at patients with burn injuries, used virtual-reality technology to induce hypnosis. Patients wore a fiber-optic helmet that immersed them in a make-believe environment. As they descended into a snowy, three-dimensional canyon, an audiotape with a clinician's voice prepared them for what they would experience during the treatment of the burn.

Result: They had a decrease in both pain and anxiety—and their need for potent painkillers was reduced by half.

LESS SURGICAL PAIN

Another study of cancer patients found that those who had a single, 15-minute hypnosis session prior to their surgery required less sedation and experienced less nausea, pain and fatigue than those in a nonhypnosis group.

Mount Sinai researchers analyzed 20 studies on hypnosis and surgery, and they found that in 89% of cases, hypnotized surgical patients had less pain, used less pain medication and recovered faster.

HOW YOU CAN TRY HYPNOSIS

Because of its long association with parlor tricks, hypnosis still is a subject of confusion.

A few facts: You don't go into a trance during hypnosis...you are more in control of yourself than usual, not less...and you won't do anything that you don't want to do.

A specially trained therapist will use guided imagery to focus and direct your imagination. It is the same technique sometimes used during meditation.

Example: While you relax, the therapist will encourage you to breathe slowly and deeply...to imagine a soothing scene (such as walking in the woods)...and to keep your mind focused on just that one thing. This is known as the induction phase. Your brain activity slows, but you still are focused and alert.

At this point, medical hypnosis diverges from traditional meditation. While you are in a relaxed state, the therapist will guide your thinking toward particular issues.

Suppose that you have arthritis and that your arm always hurts. The therapist might describe a scene in which you're walking to a lake... submerging yourself in icy water...and feeling your arm go pleasantly numb. The positive effects can last for minutes to hours to forever.

Research has shown that people who are mentally and physically relaxed are more receptive to taking in new ideas and feeling in new ways.

To find a hypnotist who can help you, look for a licensed health-care professional who offers hypnosis as only one part of his/her practice. Someone who only does hypnosis may not have the understanding of health-care issues to properly diagnose and treat you. The webites for the American Society of Clinical Hypnosis and the Society for Clinical & Experimental Hypnosis have referral pages that can help you find an expert in your area.

Expect to complete between four and 10 sessions. The cost per session is about the same as you would pay for other types of counseling.

Example: Depending on where you live, you might pay about $150 for a session with a psychologist. You will pay less if you see a social worker, nurse or mental-health counselor.

Most insurance companies do not cover hypnosis per se, but they may cover therapy that includes hypnosis. Medicare covers "hypnotherapy" for certain conditions.

Visualize Your Way To Healing the Pain

David E. Bresler, PhD, president and cofounder of the Academy for Guided Imagery and a pioneer in the field of guided imagery techniques. He is the author of numerous books, including *Free Yourself from Pain.*

People often are surprised to find out that they can use their imaginations to heal. Visualization, a form of guided imagery in which you use your imagination to gain a greater understanding of yourself, has been proven to help relieve pain and other symptoms of disease. *So sit down and get comfort-*

able—and experience the positive effects of this safe and pleasurable mind-body therapy…

• **We don't know exactly why guided imagery works,** but studies have shown that it can help patients ease the symptoms of many chronic conditions (such as arthritis and fibromyalgia) and psychological problems (such as depression and anxiety).

Best: Practice visualization for five to 20 minutes once or twice a day. There is no harm in doing it as frequently as you like. *Follow these steps…*

1. Quiet your breathing. Sitting comfortably in a quiet place, begin to slow down your breathing. Let it become more regular…deeper…quieter. Quieting yourself will enable you to focus your mind's power on any symptoms you are experiencing.

2. Release tension. Imagine a ball of energy that starts in your lower abdomen and rises to your forehead as you inhale. As you exhale, the imaginary ball goes down your spine and your legs and then into the ground. As this "energy sponge" travels around your body, it absorbs and drains away any tension, tightness, pain or discomfort as you breathe.

3. Bring to mind any symptom that is present. Allow an image to form in your mind's eye that represents or symbolizes a symptom (pain, palpitations) or condition (diabetes, cancer, arthritis). Someone with allergies might imagine them as pollen, red or yellow lights, creatures, energy fields, smells or tastes. Examine the image and notice what part seems to be most uncomfortable.

4. Imagine that your body can heal the symptom. Create an inner healing movie in your mind's eye by imagining that your body is using all of its resources to heal what is most uncomfortable.

Example: A woman with peripheral neuropathy viewed the pain as "fire ants chewing on the nerve." With the help of guided imagery, she learned to focus on her breathing and to imagine that, with each breath, the nerve could release its own natural "insecticide," causing the ants to become smaller and fewer in number. This helped to significantly reduce the intensity of her pain.

5. Create an inner adviser. You can base this image on a mentor or teacher who, in the past, provided you with wise advice, encouragement and guidance. You might ask the adviser, "What can I do to speed up healing?" or, "Am I doing anything that is getting in the way of healing?" You might discover that your body needs more sleep or a change in diet, for example. And with your adviser's help and support, you will be more likely to try it—and succeed.

WORK WITH A PRACTITIONER

Many patients benefit from following instructions on guided imagery CDs or audiotapes, which can be purchased online. You also can work with a certified guided imagery professional. To find one in your area, visit the Academy for Guided Imagery website, AcadGI.com.

Immerse Yourself to Relieve Pain

David H. Bradshaw, PhD, research assistant professor, department of anesthesiology, Pain Research Center, University of Utah, Salt Lake City.

If you suffer from some type of chronic pain and tend to get anxious about it (or if you tend to be an anxious person in general), you've probably been told umpteen times by well-meaning friends, "Just try to not think about the pain"…and of course, that's easier said than done!

Scientists at the Pain Research Center at the University of Utah in Salt Lake City have discovered a way that people can stop thinking about their pain…interestingly, this strategy works best for people who tend to be anxious or nervous!

PAIN, PAIN GO AWAY

For this study, researchers gathered 143 men and women, ages 18 to 55, who were healthy and free of chronic pain. Participants were given questionnaires that assessed how much general anxiety they had. Then they went through three phases of the experiment. During one phase, they sat still while, at random times, they were given fingertip shocks to produce pain. Researchers chose to shock the participants rather than study people with chronic pain, because it made the data easier to measure and control. During another phase, participants got the random shocks while individually performing an "easy" task. The easy task was listening to a familiar melody (for instance, "Twinkle, Twinkle, Little Star") and shouting "bad" when they heard a wrong note. During a third phase, they got the random shocks while individually performing a "hard" task. The hard task was similar to the easy task—but the researchers made the wrong notes more subtle and therefore more difficult to detect. How much each participant was "aroused" (or bothered) by the painful shocks was assessed by measuring changes in pupil dilation, palm sweatiness and electrical activity in the brain. *Here's what the researchers found...*

***Finding #1:* This first discovery was not incredibly surprising.** As you would expect, the more difficult the task that the participants were engaged in, the less they felt the pain.

***Finding #2:* The second discovery was much more interesting.** Participants who had shown themselves to be anxious types on the general anxiety questionnaire and who performed the tasks well (signaling greater engagement) experienced the least amount of pain during the experiment—less pain, even, than participants who tended to have relaxed, worry-free personalities and performed the task well.

That's the opposite of what was expected. And that's why this study is so remarkable—it suggests that by becoming fully engaged in a task, some of the people who need pain relief the most can finally get it.

RULES OF ENGAGEMENT

Of course, the type of task that the study participants performed isn't something that you can easily replicate at home, but there are other, similar ways that you can intensely engage your mind to relieve your pain. For example, if you want to make it less likely that your sore neck or bad back is going to bother you, forget passive activities such as watching TV. Even reading a book, while it isn't passive mentally, is usually not very challenging—so most books aren't likely to provide the kind of immersion that will really beat your pain.

More likely to help are virtual-reality video games (the kind where you take on the role of a character onscreen, navigate your way through different virtual environments and make decisions along the way). In fact, research has shown that even burn patients have less pain when they play such games. Or if you're listening to music, you can engage with it by singing or tapping along with your foot—because it forces you to pay closer attention to the rhythm, melody and lyrics. Another strategy you could try anywhere—even at work, where you can't exactly sing along to music or play video games—is to breathe deeply. Inhale for 10 seconds, exhale for 10 seconds, and repeat this for at least a few minutes, focusing your mind on your breath and nothing else.

It is interesting to realize that the mind has so much power over our pain. Any pain reduction due to distraction is likely to be only temporary...but even brief relief is better than no relief. So when you are in pain, before you pop a pill, see if getting immersed in something doesn't take the edge off—and if you are a worrywart, try this technique with confidence!

Photos for Pain Relief?

Naomi Eisenberger, PhD, assistant professor of psychology, director of the Social and Affective Neuroscience Laboratory, Director of the Social and Affective Neuroscience Laboratory as well as codirector of the Social Cognitive Neurosciences Laboratory, University of California at Los Angeles.

We all take comfort from the presence of a loved one during tough times—and here is a way to tap into those feelings even if that person isn't able to be physically present. Researchers have found that bringing a picture of a loved one to a medical procedure can help make it less painful—literally.

Naomi Eisenberger, PhD, assistant professor of psychology at University of California, Los Angeles, led a team exploring how social support can help people cope with physical pain. Twenty-five female undergraduate students were recruited to participate in a study that they were told would "explore how people respond to comforting and uncomfortable stimuli." The study required participants to bring a loved one to the one-hour session.

To produce the "uncomfortable stimuli," researchers placed a probe onto each participant's forearm. It could be heated to a temperature high enough to cause pain but not high enough to create a burn. As the probe heated up, each subject was asked to rate the level of pain on a scale of 0 to 20.

There were six different scenarios tested for each participant: holding the hand of her loved one...holding a stranger's hand...holding a "stress ball" to squeeze to release tension... gazing at a computer screen on which was displayed a photo of the loved one...a photo of a stranger...or a photo of a chair.

Predictably enough, participants felt less pain while holding the hands of their loved ones compared with when they held either a stranger's hand or the stress ball. But it also turned out that simply looking at a loved one's photo greatly reduced pain—in fact, more effectively even than holding the loved one's hand.

So this is easy advice you can put to use right away—carry a photo of your partner, family or a friend (or all of them!) with you to look at when something hurts. You can do this for others, too—if you can't be with someone you love who is sick or having a medical procedure, send a photo and explain why you think it will help—chances are, it will.

Curse to Reduce Pain, But Don't Overdo It!

Swearing is a common response to an injury—and a recent study suggests why. Volunteers were asked to keep their hands in ice water for as long as possible while repeating either a neutral word or the swear word of their choice.

Results: Swearers tolerated the discomfort longer, perhaps because cursing triggers a fight-or-flight response that reduces pain perception.

But: Don't make it a habit—swearing more often may make it less effective at relieving pain.

Richard Stephens, PhD, lecturer, school of psychology, Keele University, Staffordshire, UK, and leader of a study of 64 people.

Pain Recovery Affected by Spouse's Behavior

Laura Leong, PhD candidate, Wayne State University, Detroit.

Researchers observed communication patterns between 78 adults with chronic pain and their spouses.

Result: The male patients' pain, marital satisfaction and depression were more affected by their spouse's negative and/or unsupportive behavior than were the female patients'.

Theory: Pain may be disruptive to the husband's traditional role as provider, making men vulnerable to a spouse's negative responses.

If you or your spouse suffers from chronic pain: See a psychologist or social worker who can counsel the couple, not just the pain patient.

Paint Away Your Pain

Allan I. Basbaum, PhD, chair of the department of anatomy at the University of California, San Francisco, and editor-in-chief of *Pain*.

Measuring and characterizing pain so that it can be understood and treated is a real challenge in the medical world, with even the most sophisticated facilities and physicians resorting to simplistic scales using numbers and happy/sad faces to quantify the intensity of a particular patient's experience. Adding insult to injury is the matter of how isolated people with chronic pain often feel —they not only must cope with the physical suffering, but also with the emotional toll of being set apart from the rest of the world, cut off from physical activities and feeling like a burden, a whiner, a nag. If only others could see chronic pain, the way you can look at an injury and imagine how bad it must hurt or watch the numbers rise on a thermometer and identify with how sick someone must be to have such a high fever. Just being understood often can make people feel a little better and also help the doctor provide better treatment. One way this is being done today is through art.

HEALING ARTS

Many hospitals in this country now offer some form of art therapy as a way to help patients express what they are feeling, emotionally as well as physically. Of course, the experience of pain has long been portrayed on canvas.

Some of the immediate benefits patients derive from the exercise of demonstrating what pain feels like through artwork…

- **It gives people a nonverbal way to express their problem without being judged or having others get fed up,** figuratively rolling their eyes as if to say "there he/she goes again." Family and other loved ones are much more responsive to the person's suffering when they see it on paper.

- **Doctors and other health care providers, who are often confounded on how to appropriately treat a patient with chronic pain, have more information to work with.** Being able to express the level of pain through imagery can help a patient who may be under-medicated to make clear what he/she is feeling.

- **Art helps express the emotional content in the perception of pain, which can have a healing effect.** Along with showing the physical aspect of pain, art allows people to express the powerful psychological aspects of the pain experience. Because constant pain becomes part of a person's sense of self, making pain visible to the world helps them take ownership of it, often bringing some feeling of control.

THE ARTIST WITHIN

If you have no ability or training in art, you may believe that attempting to draw physical and/or emotional pain is off-limits for you. But lack of artistic ability or training doesn't matter in the least. For instance, children who have limited ability to express in words what they are going through can demonstrate clearly what is happening to them just using stick figures. In one therapeutic session, several children suffering from migraine headaches drew simple but insightful sketches of their pain—one made a circle to represent his head and slashed a black X across it…another drew a similar circle head but added arrows piercing it. Artistically speaking, some drawings of pain are good and some are not, but all of them are expressive. And that, of course, is the goal.

If you find the concept interesting, but aren't sure how to get started, here are some ideas to experiment with…

- **Create a self portrait, using any materials (or pictures of items) you'd like.** One suggestion from a website called the Art Therapy blog (ArtTherapyBlog.com) is to use a brown paper bag as the starting point and draw, paint and decorate with bits of fabric and whatever else you find evocative of your experience.

- **Make a collage,** using materials (or pictures of items) that have relevance to your pain (for instance, a prescription label, string tied in knots, a photo of a sharp knife) to express the intensity, frequency or any other aspect of pain that you find particularly overwhelming.

- **Keep a "sketchbook diary" of drawings describing your experience with pain,** including times you are immobilized and/or times you can function more normally. Don't limit yourself to literal images—try playing with patterns, scribbles, words and letters, or anything else that comes to mind. (For more ideas, visit VeryWellMind.com and search Art Activities for Stress Relief.)

There are no painful side effects to using art to express away your pain.

Brain Wave Therapy for Pain, Parkinson's and More

Celeste De Bease, PhD, medical psychologist and bioneurofeedback therapist, based in Bala Cynwyd, Pennsylvania.

People with epilepsy, Parkinson's disease, attention deficit disorder (ADD) or addictions may be able to learn how to "think themselves better" by altering their brain waves to improve their symptoms. A new form of treatment called neurotherapy (also known as neurofeedback) is similar to biofeedback but has a unique focus on controlling brain wave activity rather than skin temperature, heart rate, breathing and muscle tension.

Neurotherapy is now used with a wide scope of health issues, including not only those listed above but also autism, chronic pain, post-traumatic stress disorder, depression and anxiety. Medical psychologist and bioneurofeedback therapist Celeste De Bease, PhD, explains how.

HIGH-TECH MIND-BODY MEDICINE

According to Dr. De Bease, many neurological problems involve disordered brain waves. Neurofeedback helps patients learn to set them right.

The brain produces brain waves at varying electrical frequencies measured in hertz (cycles per second). (Just to compare, the current used for household electricity is 60 Hz here in the US.) *Brain wave electrical frequencies include…*

- **Delta**—1 to 3 Hz and the slowest of all, is mostly seen during sleep.
- **Theta**—4 to 7 Hz, a state of deep relaxation that can bring bursts of creative insight. It occurs during daydreaming and advanced meditation.
- **Alpha**—8 to 13 Hz, a pleasurable, relaxed state associated with being calm and lucid. it occurs in some forms of meditation and sometimes with dream sleep.
- **Beta**—14 to 30 Hz, is the frequency produced during normal waking activities, when you are processing information for daily living, problem solving and the like.
- **High Beta**—any Beta over 21 Hz, these waves show that the brain is in its racing mode associated with anxiety and tension.

Many patients with neurological problems tend toward either under- or over-arousal of the brain. Neurofeedback teaches methods to gain control by using video display (like a video game) images that correspond to different brain waves. Working with the therapist, people can learn ways to produce faster or slower waves. Even children can do this.

MIND CONTROL?

Dr. De Bease explained that people with ADD or depression, or who suffer from mental fog and lethargic thinking in general, benefit from learning how to speed up their brain waves—those who need to slow them down to calm over-arousal include people with compulsions, autism, post-traumatic stress disorder, chronic-pain disorders, epilepsy and insomnia. Parkinson's disease patients can benefit from slower brain waves that relax their nervous systems and contribute to better motor functioning.

Neurofeedback technology is continuing to evolve. Where there used to be just a few approaches, therapists now have many well-researched training protocols to work with, and their techniques become more customized as the science and training are refined. For instance, placement of electrodes varies depending on the issue being addressed—for people with ADD, Dr. De Bease places electrodes on the scalp directly above the frontal cortex, which controls the function of paying attention.

PRACTICAL ADVICE

The goal of neurotherapy is to recognize how it feels to operate in the desired brain wave activity range and to then learn how to get there at will. Effective training typically takes 10 or more sessions, depending on the problem. Prices vary by area and may range from $50 to more than $100/session. Some health insurance plans cover neurofeedback for some conditions, but usually only after you get a diagnosis and prescription from your doctor.

Dr. De Bease calls neurotherapy "a powerful technique," but cautions that it is crucial to find a Biofeedback Certified Professional (BCP) who is well-trained specifically in this technique, especially in light of the fact that many who call themselves qualified have completed just a weekend training program. Look for a practitioner who is certified by the Biofeedback Certification Institute of America (BCIA.org). This means that, among other credentials, the practitioner has had 25 hours of practice mentored by a BCIA-approved practitioner and 100 patient/client sessions reviewed and approved by BCIA. (For more on biofeedback, see chapter 22, "Drug-Free Protocols for Pain Relief.")

Neurofeedback can benefit healthy people, too. Dr. De Bease said she works primarily with medical conditions but knows many therapists who focus on performance enhancement, which includes training athletes, business professionals and even members of the military in the use of neurofeedback. Certainly this is a therapy worth looking into—it's noninvasive and drug-free, not terribly expensive, and may help with many conditions.

How Compassion Relieves Chronic Pain

Emma Seppälä, PhD, science director, Center for Compassion and Altruism Research and Education, Stanford University, California, and author of *The Happiness Track: How to Apply the Science of Happiness to Accelerate Your Success.*

If you suffer from chronic pain, and perhaps the angry emotions that hurting all the time can lead to, there's a drug-free treatment that takes only 15 minutes a day and can bring real relief.

It's called compassion meditation. It's not like "regular" meditation. Rather than letting your mind wander, you actively direct your thoughts—toward kindness and altruism. Don't believe this could relieve your pain? Rigorous scientific studies have found that it can—and it even may help you live longer.

THE SCIENCE OF KINDNESS

At the Center for Compassion and Altruism Research and Education at Stanford University School of Medicine, we study compassion and altruistic behavior and their health effects. *Here's what recent research at our center and other institutions has found...*

- **Chronic pain—and anger.** Among people with chronic pain, a nine-week compassion meditation program at Stanford University led to significantly reduced pain severity and greater pain acceptance by the end of the program, according to a study published in *Journal of Compassionate Health Care.* One way it helped was that it reduced levels of anger, based on self-evaluations of the patients. Anger has been shown to be an important predictor of chronic pain symptoms, and cultivating compassion has been shown to positively influence how we process emotions, reducing the tendency toward negativity, including anger.

- **Post-traumatic stress disorder (PTSD) symptoms.** In a study at the Veterans Administration's Puget Sound Health Care System in Seattle, published in *Journal of Traumatic Stress,* researchers found that when veterans with post-traumatic stress disorder (PTSD) practiced loving-kindness meditation (a form of compassion meditation) for 12 weeks, they experienced a reduction in PTSD symptoms and depression. The benefits were still evident three months later.

- **Migraines.** A study from University of Massachusetts Medical School in Worcester, published in *Pain Management Nursing,* found that migraine sufferers who learned loving-kindness meditation in a single session experienced a 33% decrease in pain and a 43% reduction in emotional tension.

- **Longevity.** While there's certainly no conclusive evidence that learning to be compassionate to yourself and to others will help you live longer, there are intriguing clues that it might.

The connection: Telomeres, which are "caps" on the tips of each strand of DNA on your chromosomes. A study from Massachusetts General Hospital and Harvard Medical School, published in *Brain, Behavior, and Im-*

munity, found that people experienced in practicing loving-kindness meditation have longer telomeres, which are associated with greater longevity.

HOW TO PRACTICE COMPASSION MEDITATION

With roots in Buddhist philosophy, compassion meditation aims to strengthen feelings of compassion and empathy toward yourself and other people—to generate feelings of kindness toward yourself and others. It's different from the well-known "mindfulness" meditation, which is mostly focused on calming the mind and increasing awareness. In compassion meditation, rather than letting your thoughts come and go without judgment, you focus your attention in specific ways as you silently repeat benevolent phrases or visualize kind wishes.

The goal is to express your intention to move from judgment or dislike to caring, compassion, acceptance and understanding. Compassion meditation involves bringing to mind people you know and love, feeling their love and spreading caring feelings toward strangers or even people you find challenging.

It isn't hard to do. To do it, sit quietly, close your eyes, breathe gently and silently repeat a phrase designed to evoke a feeling of goodwill toward yourself, such as "May I be happy, healthy and strong." Then, extend the good wishes to someone you feel thankful for, then to someone you're indifferent to, then to someone you find challenging and finally to the world at large.

Practicing loving-kindness or compassion meditation is a way to stretch the "muscles" of kindness, caring and empathy toward everyone and to remember our common humanity. The key is to give your "compassion muscles" a regular workout by practicing regularly, just as you might any other skill. Doing so will help you cultivate more loving relationships, greater happiness and better health…and could noticeably reduce your chronic pain.

An Easier Way to Meditate Your Pain Away

Fadel Zeidan, PhD, assistant professor of neurobiology and anatomy, Wake Forest School of Medicine, Winston-Salem, North Carolina.

Research shows that training in mind-fulness-based stress reduction (MBSR) can help you manage pain. The training includes learning "mindfulness meditation," in which you sit quietly and focus on your breath, while acknowledging but not judging thoughts and feelings.

Problem: The mindfulness program is eight weeks long, includes daily homework assignments and a full day of silent retreat and requires a trained professional to teach you the technique. In other words, it takes a lot of time, and you can't do it on your own.

Solution: Three, 20-minute sessions of mindfulness meditation may accomplish the same result, says a new study.

MORE MINDFULNESS, LESS PAIN

Led by Fadel Zeidan, PhD, researchers at the University of North Carolina, Charlotte, conducted three experiments on 22 people.

First—since everyone's perception of pain is different—they figured out pain levels for each participant by administering an electric shock to the forearm at several levels of intensity and asking each participant to rate the pain on a scale, with 2 being "low pain" and 4 being "high pain."

Then, they divided the students into two groups.

One group was taught a simple form of mindfulness meditation in three 20-minute training sessions, each of which included a period of meditation.

Next, they again administered the electric shocks to both groups.

The nonmeditators had the same level of pain perception—a 2 was still a 2 and a 4 was still a 4. But the meditators now required a much higher level of electric shock to create the same pain perception of 2 and 4.

"The short course of meditation was very effective on pain perception," says Dr. Zeidan, an assistant professor of neurobiology and anatomy at Wake Forest University School of Medicine, in North Carolina. "In fact, it was kind of freaky. I was ramping up the shocks to what was previously perceived as a high level of pain, and their arms would be jolting back and forth because the current was stimulating a motor nerve, yet they would still be asking, 'Is that a 2?' It was very surprising."

The researchers then tested whether or not the distraction of doing a difficult math problem or practicing a relaxation technique could match the decreased pain perception from mindfulness meditation.

Again, the meditators had a lower perception of pain—both at the low and high levels—than those doing the math problem or relaxing. And those who were the most mindful (as measured by a questionnaire called the Freiburg Mindfulness Inventory) perceived the least pain. The meditators also had significantly less anxiety.

"These data suggest that a decrease in anxiety and the ability to sustain focus on the present moment can attenuate the feeling of pain," wrote Dr. Zeidan and his colleagues, in *The Journal of Pain*.

But not only did the meditators have a lower perception of pain while meditating.

The researchers found the meditators continued to have a lowered awareness of pain, outside of meditation. In short, they had lessened pain's ability to distract and disturb.

"This was totally surprising," says Dr. Zeidan. "We did not expect to find a change in general sensitivity to pain."

"This is the first study to demonstrate the efficacy of such a brief intervention on the perception of pain," he continues. "We already knew that meditation has significant effects on pain perception in long-term practitioners whose brains seem to have been completely changed—but we didn't know you could do this in just three days."

Why it works: "It's attention," says Dr. Zeidan. "Mindfulness training lessens the awareness of and sensitivity to pain because it trains a person's brain to pay attention to sensations in the present, rather than anticipating future pain or dwelling on emotions caused by pain. It teaches you that distractions, thoughts and feelings are momentary and don't require a label or judgment, because the moment is already over. With the meditation training, you can acknowledge the pain, realize what it is, but just let it go and bring your attention back to the present, without anxiety."

A SIMPLE WAY TO MEDITATE

This study shows that meditation is a much easier way to manage pain than previously thought, says Dr. Zeidan. In fact, even self-taught mindfulness might work to reduce the perception and burden of pain, he says.

Here are instructions to practice a simple mindfulness meditation...

- **Sit comfortably.**
- **Close your eyes.**
- **Focus on the feeling of the breath as it flows in and out of the nostrils.**
- **Nonjudgmentally become aware of your thoughts,** sensations and feelings, while maintaining focus on the breath in the nostrils.

If you are distracted by thoughts, sensations or feelings, simply acknowledge and release the distraction, and bring attention back to the breath.

Practice for 15 or 20 minutes, once a day.

Resources: On the second day of the study, the meditators had a guided mindfulness

Meditation Beats Morphine

Mindfulness meditation, a technique that focuses on awareness and acceptance of daily thoughts and feelings, activates areas of the brain that reduce pain intensity, recent research finds.

Details: Adults who meditated for 20 minutes a day for four days before being touched with a hot probe reported feeling up to 44% less pain than those who did not meditate—which was twice the benefit provided by opioid drugs such as morphine.

Fadel Zeidan, PhD, assistant professor of neurobiology and anatomy, Wake Forest School of Medicine, Winston-Salem, North Carolina.

meditation, listening to a 20-minute tape by Jon Kabat-Zinn, PhD, author of *Full Catastrophe Living* (Delta), the classic text on mindfulness-based stress reduction.

You can find mindfulness meditation training on the Internet, says Dr. Zeidan. Youtube.com has several videos that explain mindfulness and/or that guide you through a session of meditation.

Bottom line: "Use mindfulness to change your perception of pain—and that should help alleviate the feeling of that pain," says Dr. Zeidan.

Index

B

C

I

N

Don't miss these other titles from Bottom Line books and newsletters

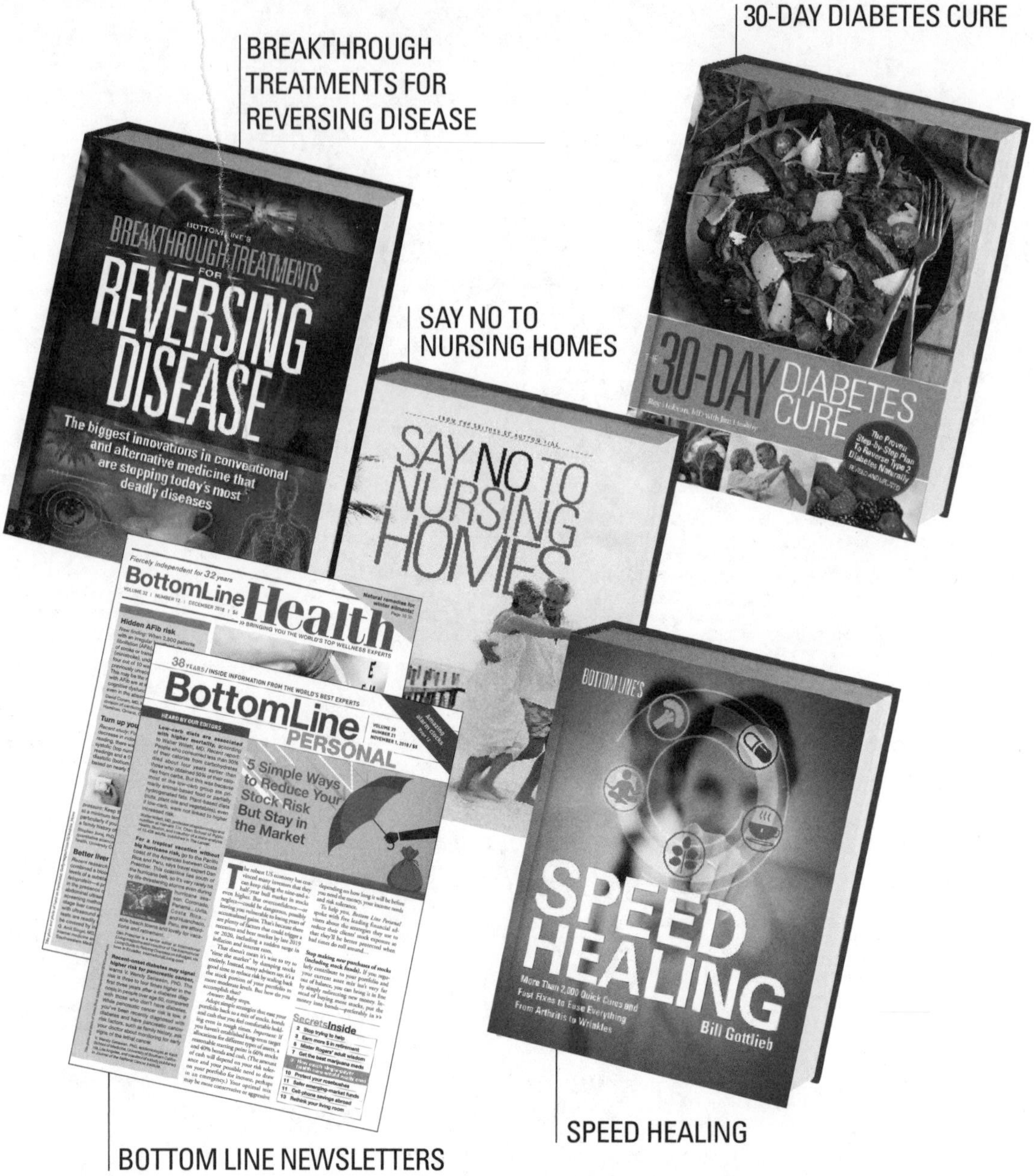

SHOP NOW FOR THE LATEST BREAKTHROUGHS

BOTTOMLINESTORE.COM